T0337867

**Ethics in Veterinary Practice**

# Ethics in Veterinary Practice

Balancing Conflicting Interests

*Edited by*

**Barry Kipperman, DVM, DACVIM, MSc, DACAW**
*Instructor, Veterinary Ethics*
*University of California at Davis*
*School of Veterinary Medicine*
*Davis, CA, USA;*
*Adjunct Associate Professor*
*Department of Veterinary Medicine and Surgery*
*University of Missouri*
*College of Veterinary Medicine*
*Columbia, MO, USA*

**Bernard E. Rollin, PhD**
*University Distinguished Professor Emeritus*
*Professor of Philosophy*
*Professor of Animal Sciences*
*Professor of Biomedical Sciences*
*University Bioethicist*
*Colorado State University*
*Fort Collins, CO, USA*

**WILEY** Blackwell

*Registered Office*
John Wiley & Sons, Inc., 111 River Street, Hoboken, NJ 07030, USA

*Editorial Office*
111 River Street, Hoboken, NJ 07030, USA

For details of our global editorial offices, customer services, and more information about Wiley products visit us at www.wiley.com.

Wiley also publishes its books in a variety of electronic formats and by print-on-demand. Some content that appears in standard print versions of this book may not be available in other formats.

*Library of Congress Cataloging-in-Publication Data*
Names: Kipperman, Barry, 1958- author. | Rollin, Bernard E., author.
Title: Ethics in veterinary practice : balancing conflicting interests / edited by Barry Kipperman, DVM, DACVIM, MSc, DACAW, Instructor, Veterinary Ethics, University of California at Davis, School of Veterinary Medicine, Davis, CA, USA, Adjunct Associate Professor, Department of Veterinary Medicine and Surgery, University of Missouri, College of Veterinary Medicine, Columbia, MO, USA, Bernard Rollin, PhD, University Distinguished Professor Emeritus, Professor of Philosophy, Professor of Animal Sciences, Professor of Biomedical Sciences, University Bioethicist, Colorado State University, Fort Collins, CO, USA
Description: Hoboken : John Wiley & Sons, 2022. | Includes bibliographical references and index.
Identifiers: LCCN 2021053307 | ISBN 9781119791195 (hardback) | ISBN 9781119791218 (pdf) | ISBN 9781119791225 (epub) | ISBN 9781119791256 (ebook)
Subjects: LCSH: Veterinary medicine--Moral and ethical aspects. | Veterinarians--Professional ethics.
Classification: LCC SF756.39 .K57 2022 | DDC 179/.3--dc23/eng/20211206
LC record available at https://lccn.loc.gov/2021053307

Cover Images: (left) © Digital Zoo/Getty Images; (center) Courtesy of Penney Adams; (right) © Shanelle Hulse/EyeEm/Getty Images
Cover design by Wiley

Set in 9.5/12.5pt STIXTwoText by Integra Software Services Pvt. Ltd, Pondicherry, India

SKY10035140_071822

# In Memoriam—Dr. Bernard E. Rollin (1943–2021)

In 2002 I was suffering from conditions inherent to the veterinary profession and referral practice that regularly limited my capacity to help my patients. Having received no training in ethics in veterinary school, I wasn't prepared for this. I knew something was wrong, but I couldn't articulate it. As one would call a rabbi, priest, or therapist for help, I called Bernie. He commiserated with my circumstance, taught me about the concept of moral stress, and a friendship was born. I asked if he would be willing to participate in roundtable discussions on ethics at national veterinary meetings. It was Bernie's star power that opened the door to get ethics discussions on the map. These efforts changed my perspective from being a victim to feeling empowered.

Bernie inspired my interest in veterinary ethics, especially by his landmark books *An Introduction to Veterinary Medical Ethics* (2006) and *Animal Rights and Human Morality* (2006). He presented what I perceived as "doing the right thing for animals" in erudite, yet understandable and compelling language. Bernie supported my decision to pursue a Master's degree in animal welfare and ethics, writing a letter of reference, and being my faculty advisor for my dissertation. When I was appointed to teach ethics at UC Davis, my first call to share my elation was to Bernie. We collaborated on two research projects published in 2018 and 2020. In the fall of 2020, we decided to work together on a new ethics text. In addition to writing two chapters and editing, Bernie was instrumental in suggesting ideas for chapter topics and suitable expert authors.

Bernie became ill while this book was in the final editing stages, and he passed away yesterday, prior to its publication. Even though I understood that he was very ill, I cried when his wife Linda called me with the terrible news.

We were at a meeting in Las Vegas many years ago after an ethics session, when a student of his approached us to tell him what an influence he had on her life. I'll never forget that moment, as those of us entrusted with teaching can only dream about having such a profound impact on our students.

Bernie's life undoubtedly similarly touched many of this book's authors and readers. He was an iconic figure, a force in the animal rights movement, and a hero to many. His views validated those who questioned the status quo regarding how animals are treated. The animals have lost a brilliant, fearless, and persuasive advocate, and I have lost a mentor, colleague, and friend. For Bernie, ethics was an instrument to improve the lives of animals. He taught me that advocacy and ethics are complementary. I hope that this book honors and perpetuates his legacy.

Barry Kipperman
November 20, 2021

# Contents

# List of Contributors

**Melissa Bain, DVM, DACVB, MS, DACAW**
Professor, Clinical Animal Behavior
Department of Veterinary Medicine and
Epidemiology
University of California at Davis
School of Veterinary Medicine
Davis, CA, USA

**Michael J. Blackwell, DVM, MPH**
Assistant Surgeon General, USPHS (Ret.);
Director, Program for Pet Health Equity
Center for Behavioral Health Research
University of Tennessee, Knoxville
Knoxville, TN, USA

**Timothy E. Blackwell, DVM, MSc, PhD**
Belwood, Ontario
Canada

**Gary Block, DVM, MS, DACVIM**
Ocean State Veterinary Specialists
East Greenwich, RI, USA

**Larry Carbone, DVM, PhD, DACLAM, DACAW**
Director of Institutional Animal Care
and Use Program (retired)
University of California, San Francisco
San Francisco, CA, USA

**Sathya K. Chinnadurai, DVM, MS, DACZM,
DACVAA, DACAW**
Senior Vice President of Animal Health
and Welfare
Chicago Zoological Society
Brookfield, IL, USA

**Jim Clark, DVM, MBA**
Instructor, Professional Skills
University of California at Davis
School of Veterinary Medicine
Davis, CA, USA

**Barbara de Mori, PhD**
Professor
Department of Comparative
Biomedicine and Food Science
Ethics Laboratory for Veterinary
Medicine, Conservation, and Animal
Welfare
University of Padua
Legnaro, Italy

**Julie D. Dinnage, DVM**
Executive Director (retired)
Association of Shelter Veterinarians
Apex, NC, USA

**Christian Dürnberger, PhD**
Unit of Ethics and Human-Animal
Studies
Messerli Research Institute
University of Veterinary Medicine
Vienna Medical University, Vienna,
University Vienna
Vienna, Austria

**Michael Dutton, DVM, MS, DABVP (Canine
& Feline Practice, Avian Practice, Exotic
Companion Mammal Practice, Reptile &
Amphibian Practice), CVPP, CertAqV**
Managing Veterinarian

Weare Animal Hospital
Weare, NH, USA;
Hopkinton Animal Hospital
Hopkinton, NH, USA

**Thomas Edling, DVM, MSpVM, MPH**
Chief Veterinary Officer
American Humane
Washington, DC, USA

**David Favre, JD**
Professor of Law
Michigan State University
East Lansing, MI, USA

**Brian Forsgren, DVM**
Gateway Animal Clinic (retired)
Cleveland, OH, USA;
Consultant
The Stanton Foundation

**Jackie Gai, DVM**
Director of Veterinary Services
Performing Animal Welfare Society
(PAWS)
San Andreas, CA, USA

**Carol Gray, BVMS, MA, PhD, MRCVS**
Principal Lecturer in Veterinary Nursing
Hartpury University
Gloucester, UK;
Honorary Research Associate
University of Liverpool
School of Law and Social Justice
Liverpool, UK

**Herwig Grimm, PhD**
Unit of Ethics and Human-Animal
Studies
Messerli Research Institute
University of Veterinary Medicine
Vienna Medical University Vienna,
University Vienna
Vienna, Austria

**Carrie Jurney, DVM, DACVIM**
Not One More Vet
San Francisco, CA, USA;

Jurney Veterinary Neurology
Redwood City, CA, USA

**Barry Kipperman, DVM, DACVIM, MSc,
DACAW**
Instructor, Veterinary Ethics
University of California at Davis
School of Veterinary Medicine
Davis, CA, USA;
Adjunct Associate Professor
University of Missouri
College of Veterinary Medicine
Columbia, MO, USA

**Andrew Knight, BSc (Vet. Biol.), BVMS, PhD,
MANZCVS (Animal Welfare), Dip ECAWBM
(AWSEL), Dip ACAW, FRCVS, PFHEA**
Professor of Animal Welfare and Ethics
& Founding Director
Centre for Animal Welfare
University of Winchester, UK;
Adjunct Professor
Griffith University
School of Environment and Science
Queensland, Australia

**Joy Mench, PhD**
Professor Emeritus
Department of Animal Science and
Center for Animal Welfare
University of California at Davis
Davis, CA, USA

**Bea Monteiro, DVM, PhD, PgDip**
Research Advisor
Université de Montréal
Faculty of Veterinary Medicine
Saint-Hyacinthe, QC, Canada

**Liz H. Mossop, BVM&S, MMedSci (Clin Ed),
PhD, FRCVS**
Deputy Vice Chancellor
University of Lincoln
Brayford Pool
Lincoln, UK

**Shaw Perrin, DVM**
Large Animal Services

College of Veterinary Medicine
The Ohio State University
Columbus, OH, USA

**Anne Quain, BA (Hons), BScVet (Hons),
BVSc (Hons), MVetStud, GradCertEdStud
(HigherEd), MANZCVS (Animal Welfare),
Dip ECAWBM (AWSEL)**
Senior Lecturer
Sydney School of Veterinary Science
University of Sydney, Sydney, Australia

**David W. Ramey, DVM**
Ramey Equine
Chatsworth, CA, USA

**Sheilah Robertson, BVMS (Hons), PhD,
DACVAA, DECVAA, DACAW, DECAWBM
(AWSEL), MRCVS**
Senior Medical Director
Lap of Love Veterinary Hospice Inc.
Lutz, FL, USA;
Courtesy Professor
Department of Small Animal Clinical
Sciences
University of Florida
College of Veterinary Medicine
Gainesville, FL, USA

**Narda G. Robinson, DO, DVM, MS, FAAMA**
President, CEO
CuraCore MED and CuraCore VET
Fort Collins, CO, USA

**Bernard E. Rollin, PhD**
University Bioethicist
University Distinguished Professor
Professor of Philosophy
Professor of Animal Sciences
Professor of Biomedical Sciences
Colorado State University
Fort Collins, CO, USA

**Andrew Rowan, BS, MA (oxon), DPhil**
President, WellBeing International
Potomac, MD, USA;
Adjunct Professor
Tufts Cummings School of Veterinary
Medicine

N. Grafton, MA, USA

**Martha Smith-Blackmore, DVM**
Visiting Fellow
Brooks McCormick Jr. Animal Law &
Policy Program
Harvard Law School
Cambridge, MA, USA;
President
Forensic Veterinary Investigations,
LLC
Boston, MA, USA

**Svenja Springer, Dr.med.vet, PhD**
Unit of Ethics and Human-Animal
Studies
Messerli Research Institute
University of Veterinary Medicine
Vienna Medical University Vienna,
University Vienna
Vienna, Austria

**Bernard Unti, PhD**
Senior Principal Strategist,
Communications
Humane Society of the United States
Washington, DC, USA

**Jennifer Walker, MSc, DVM, PhD,
DACVPM**
Director Quality and Care
Danone North America
White Plains, NY, USA

**James W. Yeates, BVSc, BSc, PhD, MBA,
DWEL, FRCVS**
Chief Executive Officer
World Federation for Animals
Boston, MA, USA

**Miriam A. Zemanova, PhD**
Research Fellow
University of Fribourg
Environmental Sciences and Humanities
Institute
Fribourg, Switzerland;
Scientific Associate
Animalfree Research
Bern, Switzerland

# Foreword

Ethical discussions among veterinary students or veterinarians sometimes center on our obligations to animals, animal owners, or on the societal responsibilities facing veterinarians. In these conversations, one frequently discovers that some practices are deemed essentially good and need to be perpetuated, while others are inherently bad and should be avoided. Until these discussions become more informed, veterinarians struggle with this dualist vision where it may be a challenge to find common ground on which to agree.

As we learn and think about these complicated issues, we are reminded of the wise words of Oscar Wilde: "The truth is rarely pure and never simple." It is soon clear that things are hardly ever black and white, and a broad range of colors permeates these discussions. When this first happens, we struggle to refine our answers, and finding a defensible position becomes a greater challenge. An understanding of veterinary ethics becomes fundamental in shaping these opinions.

Veterinarians deal with conflicting situations daily. We may be expected to conduct procedures we find objectionable because our hospital offers them. We deal with clients who make requests with which we disagree. We witness practices unacceptable in one species being done in others. We can improve the condition of a patient but may be prevented from taking care of them. Our responses to many of these circumstances have an ethical foundation. Unfortunately, traditional veterinary education models emphasize the mechanics of how to do certain things rather than how to decide whether it is a good idea to do them, and both questions are equally relevant.

It is in this context that *Ethics in Veterinary Practice* becomes an important academic resource for our profession. It offers critical background to pertinent issues that veterinarians frequently encounter, provides a framework for evaluating ambiguity, and discusses the implications of these relevant and critical decisions.

The introductory chapters focus on the relevance of ethics to decisions about animal welfare and the parallel that exists between ethics and the laws that regulate our interactions with animals. In the clinical ethics section, economic issues and medical errors are discussed; the authors also reflect upon the relevance of the social contract that veterinarians enter and how this impacts our professional behavior. This book includes chapters focusing on the main categories of veterinary practice so those interested in a particular species or niche can proceed to a deeper level in their reflection. Finally, the concluding chapters include an overview of current ethical issues, like animal pain and our responsibility in alleviating it, and our duty in defending animals from mistreatment. Included sections additionally explore issues associated with the use of animals in education and the impact that cognitive dissonance and decisions conflicting with our personal values have on veterinarians' mental health.

Veterinarians have a commitment, dictated by our professional oaths, to ensure that the health and welfare of animals under our care are protected. Veterinarians must do this with integrity while juggling the interests of the client, the needs of their veterinary practice, and the concerns of society. It is easy to agree that, in doing so, veterinarians are involved in ethical decisions. *Ethics in Veterinary Practice* provides a necessary structure to help veterinarians navigate some of these difficult considerations. It is a must-read for veterinary professionals whom society entrusts with the care of our animals.

*Jose M. Peralta, DVM, PhD*
*Diplomate of the American College of Animal Welfare*
*European Veterinary Specialist in Animal Welfare Science, Ethics and Law*
*Professor of Animal Welfare*
*College of Veterinary Medicine*
*Western University of Health Sciences*

# Preface

It has been more than 15 years since Dr. Bernie Rollin published the last textbook on veterinary ethics in North America. Since then, the field of veterinary ethics has expanded internationally, resulting in a steady increase in papers addressing ethical concerns. This book incorporates this literature for those interested in veterinary ethics regarding longstanding concerns such as medically unnecessary surgery and what the profession should do to mitigate the consequences of economic limitations on veterinary care, and emerging issues such as the use of animals in veterinary education and ethics consultation services. Bernie and I are fortunate to have assembled an impressive array of global scholars and practitioners who have contributed to this effort. This book comprises four sections: fundamental principles and concepts that inform the remainder of the chapters; clinical ethical concerns relevant to all veterinary clinicians; ethical implications in the veterinary profession by practice type, so the practitioner can focus on issues relevant to their niche in the profession and so students can prepare for what they may encounter in practice; and the last section addresses emerging concerns in veterinary ethics. Dr. Rollin taught and wrote about veterinary ethics for over 40 years, and I have been fortunate enough to stand on his shoulders for the past 20 years. I hope this book encourages you to think about these issues, reminds you of your beliefs about the moral status of animals, and inspires you toward creating a more ethical veterinary profession.

*Barry Kipperman*

# Introduction

When I prepared to write the first edition of my book *Animal Rights and Human Morality* in the late 1970s, it seemed clear to me that social concern about animal treatment, relatively embryonic then, would inevitably proliferate and become a major social issue. Since the publication of my book *An Introduction to Veterinary Medical Ethics* in 2006, much has occurred that is relevant to veterinary ethics. Public concern regarding farm animal welfare and confinement and the use of animals for research, testing, and education has increased dramatically, and with that public expectation of veterinary involvement in addressing these issues. A social movement for increasing the economic value of companion animals has steadily gained momentum, as have the demands for augmented legal status of these animals. Veterinary specialization continues to grow (including a specialty in animal welfare) as has veterinarian utilization of complementary and alternative medicine and hospice and palliative care. Concern with animal pain and distress and their control has proliferated beyond what I ever dared hope for, evidenced by the recent acknowledgment of veterinary professionals to prevent and alleviate fear, anxiety, and stress. Studies are documenting what common sense would suggest: that animals are stressed when visiting or staying in veterinary hospitals. All of these, of course, pose major ethical challenges for the veterinary profession.

This new textbook reflects these concerns, and contains new material on professionalism, ethical dilemmas, futile intervention, economic issues, medical errors, access to veterinary care, the welfare concerns of brachycephalic dogs, animals in zoos, aquaria, and free-ranging wildlife, corporate veterinary medicine, animal use in veterinary education, animal pain, animal maltreatment, death, moral stress, and the future of veterinary ethics. I hope this will help the veterinary community engage these issues.

I am often asked, "When will you retire?" My reply is when they carry me out. As long as I'm physically and mentally healthy, I will continue my battle for what Gandhi called the "most disenfranchised members of society." I have been blessed to have the opportunity to work in this area and would not have chosen any other path. I have seen many hideous and evil things, and I have seen enough good to balance it out. While much has improved, too much remains the same for billions of animals. Individuals can effect meaningful change and I hope this book inspires others to do so. There is no better legacy than diminishing the suffering one confronts.

Bernard E. Rollin

# Acknowledgments

I'm thankful to my mother for fostering a reverence for animals, and to all my interns, associates, technicians, clients, and students for challenging me and asking tough questions during my career as an internist and instructor. To my friends and colleagues Dr. Larry Gilman for supporting me throughout my career and who texted me, "You've found your niche!", after attending one of my first lectures as an instructor, and Dr. Rene Gandolfi, a veterinarian by day and closet philosopher, who gave me the book *A Philosophical Basis of Medical Practice* 25 years ago, and who had the vision to initiate ethics discussions at local veterinary association meetings. I'd like to recognize Dr. Jose Peralta and Dr. Jim Reynolds for encouraging me to pursue specialization in animal welfare, and Dr. Fritha Langford at the University of Edinburgh for accepting me into the Master's program which inspired my transition from clinical practice to academia. I'm appreciative of the time, expertise, and knowledge of our contributing authors and to the editors at Wiley for seeing the book to its fruition. I wish to acknowledge Jerry Tannenbaum for his *Veterinary Ethics* textbook, which acted as my sole resource for many years when faced with ethical questions and who provided me with an opportunity to teach ethics as a guest speaker in his class at UC Davis. This book is dedicated to Dr. Bernard Rollin, one of the pioneers in the field of veterinary ethics.

Barry Kipperman

*Linda Rollin on behalf of Bernard Rollin:*
*Because of the passing of Bernard Rollin while this book was in its final stages, he did not have the opportunity to write a section acknowledging those responsible for producing this book. Instead, as his wife of 57 years, who knew well to whom Bernie was grateful for their contributions to his work, I try here to express what I know were his feelings.*

Bernie was grateful for the contributions to his work, this book, and those that preceded it, to many:

To every student he ever taught, including those in his classes and those in the gym who would listen to his ideas and provide some of their own.

To the graduate students who carried the torch to future generations of students and others.

To the academics from all over the world who came to Colorado to work with him, and who provided a global perspective to his ideas while giving him the opportunity to share his thinking worldwide, as well as those who translated his writings into many other languages, thereby broadening the influence of his ideas.

To every co-author or contributor to the books he authored, without whose work the books would have been diminished, and to those who crafted the clever ethical questions that provided a platform for him to teach by answering them.

To every layperson, mechanic, barber, or waitstaff who had no doubts that animals are sentient (unlike academics who would quibble over it), and who, upon learning what he did, agreed with his views, applauded him, and regaled him with their own stories.

To the farmers and ranchers who inspired his understanding of husbandry, and to those who took his ideas and ran with them, improving the lives of the creatures they raised.

To the editors who made his books better, even as they enraged him with their demands for footnotes.

To the innumerable veterinarians who offered their perspectives and insights, and who inspired his work to provide an ethical foundation for what they do.

To the representatives of the many organizations that invited him to talk to them, and who offered hospitality, whether near to home or in faraway places that he might otherwise never have visited.

To all those who cannot easily be categorized, who influenced and inspired, by happenstantial meeting, or by decades-long friendship.

**Section 1**

**A Fundamental Basis for Veterinary Ethics**

# 1

## Why Do Animals Matter? The Moral Status of Animals

*Bernard E. Rollin*

## Philosophers and Moral Status

Ever since human beings began to think in a systematic, ordered fashion, they have been fascinated by moral questions. Is moral concern something owed by human beings only to human beings? Twenty-five hundred years of moral philosophy have tended to suggest that this is the case, not by systematic argument, but simply by taking it for granted. An entity has moral status "If ... its interests morally matter ... for the entity's own sake" (Stanford Encyclopedia of Philosophy 2021). In other words, moral status relates to our duties, responsibilities, and obligations to others. Few thinkers have come to grips with the question of what makes a thing a moral object, and one wonders why. Surely the question of whether animals are direct objects of moral concern is a legitimate subject for inquiry. Yet, while examining the history of philosophy, there is very little discussion of the moral status of animals. What has prompted our ignoring of this question? Perhaps a cultural bias that sees animals as tools. Or, perhaps, a sense of guilt mixed with fear of where the argument may lead. For if it turns out that reason requires that other animals are as much within the scope of moral concern as are humans, we must view our entire history as well as all aspects of our daily lives from a new perspective.

Immanuel Kant (1724–1804) argued that only rational beings can count as moral agents and that the scope of moral concern therefore extends only to rational beings. He believed that only humans could entertain, understand, and formulate statements that are universal in scope, therefore only humans are rational. In contrast, animals were believed to be subject to stimulus and response reactions. Kant concluded that only rational beings are "ends in themselves": that is, beings that are not to be used as means to achieve some immediate or long-term goal. Animals had only instrumental value: any worth they had related to their usefulness to humans. The position linking rationality, language, and moral status may briefly be outlined as follows:

1) Only humans are rational.
2) Only humans possess language.
3) Only humans are objects of moral concern.

But if only rational and linguistic beings fall within the scope of moral concern, it is difficult to see how infants, children, the mentally disabled, the senile, or the comatose can be considered legitimate objects of moral concern. This shows that rationality and language do not represent a necessary condition for moral concern.

*Ethics in Veterinary Practice: Balancing Conflicting Interests*, First Edition. Edited by Barry Kipperman and Bernard E. Rollin.

In a tradition most frequently associated with St. Thomas Aquinas (1225–1274) and Kant and incorporated into the legal systems of most civilized societies beginning in the late eighteenth century, cruelty to animals (see Chapter 20) was vigorously proscribed, though animals themselves were denied moral status. Most legal definitions of cruelty involve three criteria: (i) expert evidence of physical or mental suffering beyond a reasonable doubt; (ii) the suffering was unnecessary, unjustified, or illegitimate; and (iii) an intention to cause harm. Aquinas and Kant argued that allowing cruelty to animals would have a pernicious psychological effect upon humans; that is, if people are allowed to be cruel to animals, they will eventually abuse people, which is socially undesirable. Therefore, humans had only indirect duties to animals.

Why can we not broaden the anti-cruelty ethic to cover other animal treatment? It is because only a tiny percentage of animal suffering is the result of deliberate, malevolent acts. Cruelty would not cover animal suffering that results from industrial agriculture, safety testing of toxic substances on animals, and all forms of animal research. People who raise animals for food in an industrial setting, or who do biomedical research on animals, are not driven by desires to hurt these creatures. Rather, they believe they are doing social good, providing cheap and plentiful food, or medical advances, and they are in fact traditionally so perceived socially.

This left utilitarianism (see Chapter 4) as the source of the only clearly articulated basis for a robust animal ethic in the history of philosophy before the 20th century. Profound and intellectually bold utilitarian thinkers included Jeremy Bentham (1748–1832) and John Stuart Mill (1806–1873), who based candidacy for moral status on sentience, the ability to experience emotions and feel pleasure and pain. Bentham famously affirmed that: "The question is not, Can they reason? nor Can they talk? but, Can they suffer? Why should the law refuse its protection to any sensitive being? The time will come when humanity will extend its mantle over everything which breathes" (Bentham 1996). Since animals can feel pain and pleasure, according to Bentham, they belong within the scope of moral concern.

This approach was appropriated by Peter Singer (1946–) in his revolutionary book *Animal Liberation* (Singer 1975), the first contemporary attempt to ground full moral status for animals. Singer argues that species membership alone should not determine moral status, and is speciesism, a form of discrimination no different than racism or sexism (Singer 2009). Singer has argued, for utilitarian reasons, that the only way to ameliorate the suffering of farm animals raised in industrial animal factories is to stop eating meat and adopt a vegetarian, if not vegan, diet. A moment's reflection reveals the implausibility of this suggestion. People will not give up meat even when counseled to do so by their physicians to improve their own health or even to save their own lives, so the chances that they will do so in the face of a philosophical argument are exceedingly small. In other words, not only must a successful animal ethic be logically consistent and persuasive, but it must also suggest real solutions that people can both advocate and adhere to.

The fundamental question for anyone attempting to extend all or part of our socio-ethical concerns to other creatures is this: are there any morally relevant differences between people and animals that compel us to withhold the full range of our moral machinery from animals? Answering this question occupied most of the thinkers who were trying to raise the moral status of animals. While most philosophers working on this question did not affirm that there is no moral difference between the lives of animals and the lives of humans, there was a consensus among them that *the treatment of animals by humans needs to be weighed and measured by the same moral standards by which we judge the moral treatment of humans.*

On the other hand, there are a considerable number of thinkers who have tried to deny a continuum of moral relevance across humans and animals and have presented arguments and criteria that support the concept of moral cleavage between the two. Many of these claims are theologically based. Most famous, perhaps, is the omnipresent Catholic view that humans have immortal souls and animals do not. Such claims include the ideas that humans are more powerful than animals, are superior to animals, are higher on the evolutionary scale than animals, have dominion over animals, are capable of reason and language while animals are not, even that humans feel pain while animals do not. These arguments draw a hard and fast line between humans, who have thoughts and feelings, and animals, who do not. The superior position of humans does not serve as adequate grounds for excluding animals from moral concern. One can argue that humans are obligated to behave morally toward other creatures precisely *because* of their superior power. Just as we expect fair and benevolent treatment at the hands of those capable of imposing their wills upon us, so ought we extend similar treatment to those vulnerable to us.

Of all the philosophical arguments to exclude animals from the moral arena, the most damaging are those going back to Rene Descartes (1596–1650) that deny thought, feeling, and emotion to animals. This view perpetrated the notion that animals were nothing more than machines, devoid of souls. This paradigm justified live vivisection of animals without anesthesia or pain management. It is common sense that we cannot have obligations to entities unless what we do to them, or allow to happen to them, *matters* to them. Therefore, we cannot have direct moral obligations to cars. If I destroy your friend's car, I have not behaved in an immoral way toward the car but only toward its owner, to whom the condition of the car matters. For this reason, anyone advocating for higher moral status for animals cannot let claims about lack of sentience in animals go unchallenged and unrefuted.

In my experience, most people will acknowledge a continuum from animals through humans, as Charles Darwin (1809–1882) did. Most people will affirm that animals have thoughts, feelings, emotions, intentions, pain, sadness, joy, fear, and curiosity. Even more important to the inclusion of animals within the scope of moral concern is the point that most people share empathetic identification with animals, particularly regarding their pain and suffering. All forms of mattering to an animal are determined by what Aristotle referred to as its *telos*, or unique nature. Every living thing is constituted of a set of activities making it a living thing. How each living being actualizes these functions and fulfills these needs determines its *telos*. If we are to adopt *telos* as the basis for ethical obligations to animals, as our societal ethic has done for people, we can considerably broaden what is included in the scope of moral concern. For this reason, to enjoy moral status, an animal must have the kind of *telos* whose violation creates some *negative mode of awareness*. My contention is that animals have needs and desires flowing from their *telos*, which when thwarted, frustrated, or simply unmet, result in negative feelings and poor welfare. Consequently, entrance into the moral arena is determined by someone's being alive and having interests and needs that can be helped or harmed by a being who can act morally.

## Evidence of Social Change for Animals

The past 60 years have witnessed a dazzling array of social ethical revolutions in Western society. Such moral movements as feminism, civil rights, environmentalism, affirmative action, consumer advocacy, pro- and anti-abortion activism, homosexual rights, children's rights, the student movement, and anti-war activism have forever changed the way governments and public institutions comport themselves. This is equally true for private enterprise: to be successful, businesses must be seen as operating solidly in harmony with changing and emerging social ethics. It is arguable that morally-based boycotting of South African business was instrumental in bringing about the end of apartheid, and similar boycotting of some farm products in the United States led to significant improvements in the treatment of farm workers. It is *de rigueur* for major corporations to have reasonable numbers of minorities visibly peopling their ranks, and for liquor companies to advertise on behalf of moderation in alcohol consumption. Cigarette companies now press upon the public a message that cigarettes kill and extol their involvement in protecting battered women; and forestry and oil companies spend millions (even billions) to persuade the public of their environmental commitments. Socially and environmentally responsible investment funds are ubiquitous, and reports of child labor or sweatshop working conditions can literally destroy product markets overnight.

Of importance to the veterinary profession, legal mandates that a veterinarian must be a member of Institutional Animal Care and Use Committees that provide oversight for animal research, the proliferation of veterinary specialists (including those in animal welfare and behavior), and the public's acknowledgment of companion animals as members of the family are testaments to the evolution of the moral status of animals.

Not only is success tied to accord with social ethics but, even more fundamentally, freedom and autonomy are as well. Every profession – be it medicine, law, or agriculture – is given freedom by the social ethic to pursue its aims. In return, society basically says to professions it does not understand well enough to regulate, "You regulate yourselves the way we would regulate you if we understood what you do, which we don't. But we will know if you don't self-regulate properly and then we will regulate you, despite our lack of understanding." For example, Congress became concerned about excessive use of antibiotics in animal feeds to promote growth and prevent disease and concluded that veterinarians were a major source of the problem. In 2016, Food and Drug Administration officials removed all over-the-counter access to antimicrobials that are both used in human medicine and given to livestock in feed or water. Those drugs now can be given only with veterinarian approval for disease-related reasons (Burns 2019).

One major social ethical concern is an emphasis on the treatment of animals used by society for various purposes. It is easy to demonstrate the degree to which these concerns have seized the public imagination. Legislators acknowledge receiving more letters, phone calls, e-mails, and personal contacts on animal-related issues than on any other topic.

Whereas 40 years ago one would have found no bills pending in the US Congress relating to animal welfare, recent years have witnessed dozens of such bills annually, with even more proliferating at the state level. Federal bills have ranged from attempts to prevent duplication in animal research, to saving marine mammals from becoming victims of tuna fishermen, to preventing importation of ivory, to curtailing the parrot trade. State laws passed in large numbers have increasingly prevented the use of live or dead shelter animals for biomedical research and training, have abolished cage confinement of animals raised for food, and have focused on myriad other areas of animal welfare. Eight states have abolished the steel-jawed leghold trap, as have some 85 countries. When Colorado's politically appointed Wildlife Commission failed to act on a recommendation from the Division of Wildlife to abolish the spring bear hunt (because hunters were liable to shoot lactating mothers, leaving their orphaned cubs to die of starvation), the public ended the hunt through a referendum (Willoughby 2013). Now, most people in western states oppose spring bear hunting (NSSF 2019).

Interest in the welfare of horses has led to US federal laws that includes measures to stop the widespread doping of racehorses and increase track safety, keep horse slaughter plants shuttered, and boost funding to stop the cruel soring of Tennessee walking horses (Block and Amundson 2020). Municipalities have passed ordinances ranging from the abolition of rodeos and circuses to the protection of prairie dogs.

Even more dramatic, perhaps, is the worldwide proliferation of laws to protect laboratory animals. In the United States, two major pieces of legislation, which I helped draft and defend before Congress, regulating and constraining the use and treatment of animals in research were passed by the US Congress in 1985, despite vigorous opposition from the powerful biomedical research and medical lobbies. This opposition included well-financed, highly visible advertisements and media promotions indicating that human health and medical progress would be harmed by implementation of such legislation. There was even a less than subtle film titled *Will I Be All Right, Doctor?* – the query coming from a sick child, the response coming from a pediatrician who affirmed, in essence, "You will be if 'they' leave us alone to do as we wish with animals." With social concern for laboratory animals unmitigated by such threats, research animal protection laws moved easily through Congress and have been implemented at considerable cost to taxpayers. When I testified before Congress on behalf of this law in 1982, a literature search in the Library of Congress turned up no papers in the scientific literature on laboratory animal analgesia and only two on animal analgesia, one of which said, "there ought to be papers." A Google Scholar search now finds over three million papers and book chapters on animal pain (see Chapter 19).

In 1986, the UK superseded its pioneering Cruelty to Animals Act of 1876 (the first national legislation to regulate animal experimentation) with new laws aimed at strengthening public confidence in the welfare of experimental animals (HMSO 1986). Many other countries have moved or are moving in a similar direction, even though some 90% of laboratory animals are rats and mice, not the most cuddly and lovable of animals. Research on great apes has been truncated across the world. In 2021, the European Parliament voted overwhelmingly in favor of a resolution to phase out animal experiments (Block and Amundson 2021).

Many animal uses seen as frivolous by the public have been abolished without legislation. Toxicological testing of cosmetics on animals has been curtailed; companies such as The Body Shop have been wildly successful internationally by totally disavowing such testing; Orca performance exhibits at SeaWorld ended in 2016 in response to a documentary *Blackfish*, which highlighted their miserable conditions and confinement; and greyhound racing in the United States has declined, in part for animal welfare reasons. In 2017, Ringling Bros. ended circuses founded on exotic animal acts after 146 years, and zoos that were little more than prisons for animals (the state of the art during my youth) have all but disappeared, and the very existence of zoos is being increasingly challenged (Pierce and Bekoff 2018) despite the public's unabashed love of seeing animals. And, as Gaskell and his associates' work has revealed (1997), genetic engineering has been rejected in Europe not, as commonly believed, for reasons of risk but for reasons of ethics: in part for reasons of animal ethics. Similar reasons (i.e. fear of harming cattle) have, in part, driven European rejection of bovine somatotropin (BST).

## Animals in Agriculture and Research

Inevitably, agriculture has felt the force of social concern with animal treatment – indeed, it is arguable that contemporary concern in society with the treatment of farm animals in modern production systems blazed the trail leading to a new ethic for animals. As early as 1965, British society took notice of what the public saw as an alarming tendency to industrialize animal agriculture by chartering a group of scientists under the leadership of Sir Rogers Brambell, the Brambell Commission, which affirmed that any agricultural system failing to meet the needs and natures of animals was morally unacceptable (Brambell 1965). Though the Brambell Commission recommendations enjoyed no regulatory status, they served as a moral lighthouse for European social thought. In 1988, the Swedish Parliament passed, virtually unopposed, what the *New York Times* called a "Bill of Rights" for farm animals, abolishing, in a series of timed steps, the confinement systems currently dominating North American agriculture (Lohr 1988). The European Union has moved in a similar direction, banning sow stalls (gestation crates) for pigs and battery cages for egg-laying hens in 2013, and the European Parliament recently voted to ban the use of cages in animal agriculture by 2027 (Kelly 2021).

Although the United States has been a latecomer to progress on agricultural issues, things have moved rapidly. My own work attests to this tendency. In 2007, over two days of dialogue, I convinced Smithfield Farms, the world's largest pork producer, to phase out gestation crates. Most dramatically, I was able to broker an agreement between the Humane Society of the United States (HSUS) and the Colorado Livestock Association passing a jointly sponsored farm animal welfare law in Colorado in 2008, abolishing sow stalls and veal crates. In 2008, the Pew Commission, on which I served as the advocate for farm animal welfare, called for the end of high-confinement animal agriculture within 10 years, for reasons of animal welfare, environmental despoliation, human and animal health, and social justice. Citizen ballot initiatives pressed by the HSUS abolishing sow stalls, battery cages, and veal crates have passed in 12 states. Cage-free egg production is now proliferating across the United States.

Evolving societal values are the basis of this progress for animals. While 58% of US adults believe that "most farmed animals are treated well" (Anthis 2017), 77% of consumers noted they are concerned about the welfare of animals raised for food (ASPCA 2016). The agriculture community in the United States has been far behind societal concerns. There is one monumental conceptual error that is omnipresent in the agriculture industry's discussions of animal welfare – an error of such magnitude that it trivializes the industry's responses to ever-increasing societal concerns about the treatment of agricultural animals. When one discusses farm animal welfare with industry groups or with the American Veterinary Medical Association (AVMA), one finds the same response – animal welfare is solely a matter of "sound science."

Those of us serving on the Pew Commission (2008) (better known as the National Commission on Industrial Farm Animal Production), which studied intensive animal agriculture in the United States, encountered this response regularly during our communications with industry representatives. For example, one representative of the Pork Producers, testifying before the Commission, answered that while people in her industry were quite "nervous" about the Commission, their anxiety would be allayed were we to base all of our conclusions and recommendations on "sound science." Hoping to rectify the error in that comment, as well as educate the numerous industry representatives present, I responded to her as follows: "Madam, if we on the Commission were asking the question of how to raise swine in confinement, science could certainly answer that question for us. But that is not the question the Commission, or society, is asking. What we are asking is, ought we to raise swine in confinement? And to this question, science is not relevant."

Questions of animal welfare are at least partly "ought" questions: questions of ethical obligation. The concept of animal welfare (see Chapter 2) is an ethical concept to which, once understood, science brings relevant data. When we ask about an animal's welfare, we are asking about what we owe the animal, and to what extent. A document called the CAST Report, first published by US agricultural scientists in the 1980s, affirmed that the necessary and sufficient conditions for attributing positive welfare to an animal were represented by the animals' productivity (Council for Agricultural Science and Technology 1981). A productive animal enjoyed positive welfare; a nonproductive animal had poor welfare.

This notion was fraught with many difficulties. First, productivity is an economic notion predicated of a whole operation: welfare is predicated of individual animals. An operation such as caged laying hens may be quite profitable if the cages are severely overcrowded, yet the individual hens do not enjoy good welfare. Second, equating productivity and welfare is, to some significant extent, legitimate under husbandry conditions, where the producer does well if and only if the animals do well, and square pegs, as it were, are fitted into square holes with as little friction as possible (as when pigs live outside). Under industrial conditions, however, animals do not naturally fit in the niche or environment in which they are kept and are subjected to "technological sanders" that allow producers to force square pegs into round holes – antibiotics, feed additives, hormones, air-handling systems – so the animals do not die and produce more and more kilograms of meat or milk. Without these technologies, the animals could not be productive. We will return to the contrast between husbandry and industrial approaches to animal agriculture.

The key point here is that even if the CAST Report definition of animal welfare did not suffer from the difficulties outlined, it is still an ethical concept. It essentially says, "What we owe animals and to what extent is simply what it takes to get them to create profit." This in turn would imply that the animals are well off if they have only food, water, and shelter, something the industry has sometimes asserted. Even in the 1980s, however, there were animal advocates and others who took a very different ethical stance on what we owe farm animals. Indeed, the famous Five Freedoms articulated in the UK by the Farm Animal Welfare Council (FAWC) during the 1960s represents quite a different ethical view of what we owe animals, when it affirms that:

> The welfare of an animal includes its physical and mental state, and we consider that good animal welfare implies both fitness and a sense of well-being. Any animal kept by man, must at least, be protected from unnecessary suffering. We believe that an animal's welfare, whether on farm, in transit, at market or at a place of slaughter should be considered in terms of "five freedoms" (Animal Welfare Committee n.d.):

1) **Freedom from Hunger and Thirst** – by ready access to fresh water and a diet to maintain full health and vigor.
2) **Freedom from Discomfort** – by providing an appropriate environment including shelter and a comfortable resting area.
3) **Freedom from Pain, Injury or Disease** – by prevention or rapid diagnosis and treatment.
4) **Freedom to Express Normal Behavior** – by providing sufficient space, proper facilities and company of the animal's own kind.
5) **Freedom from Fear and Distress** – by ensuring conditions and treatment which avoid mental suffering.

Clearly, the two definitions contain very different notions of our moral obligation to animals. Which is correct, of course, cannot be decided by gathering facts or doing experiments – indeed which ethical framework one adopts will in fact determine the shape of science studying animal welfare. To clarify: suppose you hold the view that an animal is well off when it is productive, as per the CAST Report. The role of welfare science in this case will be to study what feed, bedding, temperature, etc. are most efficient at producing the most meat, milk, or eggs for the least money – much what animal and veterinary science does today. On the other hand, if you take the FAWC view of welfare, your efficiency will be constrained by the need to acknowledge the animal's natural behavior and mental state, and to assure that there is minimal pain, fear, distress, and discomfort – not factors in the CAST view of welfare unless they have a negative impact on economic productivity. Thus, in a real sense, sound science does not determine your concept of welfare: rather, your concept of welfare determines what counts as sound science!

The failure to recognize the inescapable ethical component in the concept of animal welfare leads inexorably to those holding different ethical views talking past each other. Thus, producers ignore questions of animal pain, fear, distress, confinement, truncated mobility, bad air quality, social isolation, and impoverished environment unless any of these factors impact negatively on the "bottom line." Animal advocates, on the other hand, give such factors primacy, and are totally unimpressed with how efficient or productive the system may be.

A major question obviously arises here. If the notion of animal welfare is inseparable from ethical components, and people's ethical stances on obligations to farm animals differ markedly across a highly diverse spectrum, whose ethic is to predominate and define, in law or regulation, what counts as "animal welfare"? It is to this issue we now turn.

What is the nature of the emerging new ethical thinking that underlies and informs the dramatic social changes I've discussed? Although society has always had an articulated ethic regarding animal treatment, that ethic has been very minimalistic, leaving most animal conduct to people's personal ethic, rather than to the social ethic. Since biblical times, that limited social ethic has forbidden deliberate, willful, sadistic, deviant, purposeless, unnecessary infliction of pain and suffering on animals, or outrageous neglect, such as not feeding or watering. Beginning in the early nineteenth century, this set of prohibitions was articulated in the anti-cruelty statutes of the laws in all civilized societies (Leavitt 1978). But even in biblical and medieval times, the social ethic inveighed against cruelty. The Old Testament injunctions against yoking an ox and an ass together to a plow, or muzzling the ox when it is being used to mill grain or seething a calf in its mother's milk, all reflect concern with and abhorrence for what the Rabbinical tradition called *tsaar baalei chaiim* – the suffering of living things. In the Middle Ages, St. Thomas Aquinas (Aquinas 1956), while affirming that, lacking a soul, animals enjoyed no moral status, nonetheless, strictly forbade cruelty, on the grounds that permitting such behavior toward animals would encourage its spreading to human beings. Numerous serial killers have evidenced early abusive behavior toward animals.

For most human history, until some six decades ago, the anti-cruelty ethic served as the only socially articulated moral principle for animal treatment. Except for a few sporadic voices following in the wake of Darwin's articulation of human–animal continuity, no one spoke of animals' rights: nor did society have moral concepts for animal treatment that went "beyond cruelty." The obvious question that presents itself is this: what has occurred during the past 60 years that led to social disaffection with the venerable ethic of anti-cruelty and to strengthening of the anti-cruelty laws, which now make cruelty a felony in all 50 states?

In a study commissioned by the US Department of Agriculture (USDA) to answer this question, I distinguished a variety of social and conceptual reasons (Rollin 1995):

1) *Changing demographics and consequent changes in the paradigm for animals.*
    At the start of the twentieth century, more than half the population was engaged in producing food for the rest; today only some 1.5% of the US public is engaged in production agriculture (USDA). One hundred years ago, if one were to ask a person in the street, urban or rural, to state the words that come into their mind when one says "animal," the answer would doubtless have been "horse," "cow," "food," "work," etc. Today, however, for most of the population, the answer is "dog," "cat," "pet." Repeated studies show that most of the pet-owning population views their animals as members of the family (Ballard 2019) and virtually no one views them as an income source.

2) *We have lived through a long period of ethical soul-searching.*
    For almost 60 years, society has turned its "ethical searchlight" on humans traditionally ignored or even oppressed by the consensus ethic – blacks, women, the handicapped, and other minorities. The same ethical imperative has focused attention on our treatment of the non-human world – the environment and animals. Many leaders of the activist animal movement in fact have roots in earlier movements – civil rights, feminism, homosexual rights, children's rights, and labor.

3) *The media has discovered that "animals get clicks."*
    One cannot surf across the television or internet without being bombarded with animal stories, real and fictional (a *New York Times* reporter once told me that more time on cable TV in New York City is devoted to animals than to any other subject).

Animal books related to "the inner or secret lives of animals" or "what animals are thinking" arouse incredible interest and are commonly assured to be best sellers. Animals have their own Facebook and Twitter pages!

4) *Strong and visible arguments have been advanced in favor of raising the moral status of animals by philosophers and activists* (Singer 1975; Regan 1983; Francione 2000; Scully 2002; Sunstein and Nussbaum 2004; Rollin 2006; Pacelle 2011; Cochrane 2012).

5) *Changes in animal use demanded new moral categories.*

In my view, while all the reasons listed here are relevant, they are nowhere nearly as important as the precipitous and dramatic changes in animal use that occurred after World War II. These changes were, first, huge conceptual changes in agriculture and, second, the rise of significant amounts of animal research and testing.

For virtually all human history, animal agriculture was based foursquare in animal husbandry. Husbandry, derived from the old Norse word "hus/band," bonded to the household, meant taking great pains to put one's animals into the best possible environment one could find to meet their physical and psychological natures or *telos*, and then augmenting their ability to survive and thrive by providing them with food during famine, protection from predation, water during drought, medical attention, help in birthing, and so on. Thus, traditional agriculture was roughly a fair contract between humans and animals, with both sides being better off by virtue of the relationship. Husbandry agriculture was about putting square pegs into square holes, round pegs into round holes, and creating as little friction as possible doing so. So powerful is the notion of husbandry, in fact, that when the Psalmist seeks a metaphor for God's ideal relationship to humans, he seizes upon the shepherd in the 23rd Psalm: "The Lord is my shepherd; I shall not want; He maketh me to lie down in green pastures; He leadeth me beside still waters; He restoreth my soul." We wish no more from God than what the husbandman provides for his sheep. In husbandry, a producer did well if and only if the animals did well, so productivity was tied to welfare. No social ethic was thus needed to ensure proper animal treatment: only the anti-cruelty laws designed to deal with sadists and psychopaths were needed to augment husbandry. Self-interest virtually assured good treatment.

After World War II, this beautiful contract was broken by humans. Symbolically, at universities, departments of animal husbandry became departments of animal science, defined not as care, but as "the application of industrial methods to the production of animals" to increase efficiency and productivity. With "technological sanders" – hormones, vaccines, antibiotics, air-handling systems, mechanization – we could force square pegs into round holes, and place animals into environments where they suffered in ways irrelevant to productivity. If a nineteenth-century agriculturalist had tried to put 100,000 egg-laying hens in cages in a building, they all would have died of disease in a month: today such systems dominate.

The new approach to animal agriculture was not the result of cruelty, bad character, or even insensitivity. It developed rather out of perfectly decent, *prima facie* plausible motives that were a product of dramatic, significant historical and social upheavals that occurred after World War II. At that point in time, agricultural scientists and government officials became extremely concerned about supplying the public with cheap and plentiful food for a variety of reasons. First, after the Dust Bowl and the Great Depression, many people in the United States had soured on farming. Second, reasonable predictions of urban and suburban encroachment on agricultural land were being made, with a resultant diminution of land for food production. Third, many farm people had been sent to both foreign and domestic urban centers during the war, thereby creating a reluctance to return to rural areas. Fourth, having experienced literal starvation during the Great Depression, the American consumer was, for the first time in history, fearful of an insufficient food supply. Finally, projection of major population increases further fueled concern.

When the above considerations of loss of land and diminution of agricultural labor are coupled with the rapid development of a variety of technological modalities relevant to agriculture during and after World War II and with the burgeoning belief in technologically-based economies of scale, it was inevitable that animal agriculture would become subject to industrialization. This was a major departure from traditional agriculture and a fundamental change in agricultural core values – industrial values of efficiency and productivity replaced and eclipsed the traditional values of "way of life" and husbandry.

There is thus no question that industrialized agriculture, including animal agriculture, is responsible for greatly increased productivity. Milk yield from cows has more than doubled in the past 40 years, hens now lay 300 eggs per year instead of 115, and chickens raised for meat now mature in 42 days when it used to take 80 days to reach market weight. It is equally clear that the husbandry associated with traditional agriculture has changed significantly because of industrialization. One of my colleagues, a cow-calf cattle specialist, said that the worst thing that ever happened to his department was betokened by the name change from animal husbandry to animal science. No husbandry person would ever dream of feeding sheep meal, poultry waste, or cement dust to cattle, but such "innovations" are entailed by an industrial/efficiency mindset.

Animal producers are also responsible for new types of animal suffering on at least four fronts:

1) Production diseases from the new methods the animals are subjected to. Lameness and pain are accepted as commonplace in dairy cattle, pigs, chickens raised for meat, and laying hens as a consequence of their environment and immobility. Mastitis in dairy cattle is associated with increased milk production. "Shipping fever" refers to the frequent onset of infectious disease due to immunosuppression from the stress of transport. Animal welfare scientist Dr. Temple Grandin has referred to this as "the new normal." The ideas of a method of production creating diseases that were "acceptable" would be anathema to a husbandry agriculturalist.

2) Most farm animals endure routine husbandry procedures including tail docking, castration, disbudding/dehorning, debeaking, and branding without the use of analgesics to address pain (Kleinhenz et al. 2021).

3) Another new source of suffering in industrialized animal agriculture results from physical and psychological deprivation: lack of space, lack of companionship for social animals, premature separation of dairy calves from their mothers, inability to move freely, boredom, austerity of environments, and so on. Since the animals evolved for adaptation to extensive environments but are now placed in truncated environments, such deprivation is inevitable. This was not a problem in traditional, extensive agriculture.

4) The huge scale of industrialized agricultural operations and the small profit margin per animal militate against the sort of individual attention that typified much of traditional agriculture. In traditional dairies 60 years ago, one could make a living with a herd of 50 cows. Today, one needs literally thousands. In the United States, dairies may have 10,000 cows. The USDA notes that large-scale farms generating one million dollars or more in income make up about 3% of farms but 44% of all revenues (USDA 2022). In these confinement systems, caretakers may not be "animal smart": the "intelligence," such as it is, is in the mechanized system. Instead of husbandmen, workers in animal factories are minimum wage, often animal-ignorant labor. So, there is often no empathy with, or concern for, the animals.

These sources of suffering are not captured by the vocabulary of cruelty: nor are they proscribed or even acknowledged by the laws based on the anti-cruelty ethic. Furthermore, they typically do not arise under traditional agriculture and its ethic of husbandry.

Many years ago, I experienced some sharply contrasting incidents that dramatically highlight the moral difference between intensive and extensive agriculture. That particular year, Colorado cattle ranchers, paradigmatic exemplars of husbandry, were afflicted by a significant diarrhea problem in their herds. Over two months, I talked to a half-dozen rancher friends of mine. Every single one had experienced trouble, and every one had spent more on treating the disease than was economically justified by the calves' monetary value. When I asked these men why they were being what an economist would term "economically irrational," they were quite adamant in their response: "It's part of my bargain with the animal; part of caring for them," one of them said. It is, of course, the same ethical outlook that leads ranch wives to sit up all night with sick calves, sometimes for days in a row. If the issues were strictly economic, these people would hardly be valuing their time at 50 cents per hour – including their sleep time!

Now in contrast to these uplifting moral attitudes, consider the following: one of my animal scientist colleagues related to me that his son-in-law was an employee in a large, total confinement swine operation. As a young man he had raised and shown pigs, keeping them semi-extensively. One day he detected a disease among the feeder pigs in the confinement facility where he worked, which necessitated killing them with a blow to the head, since this operation did not treat individual animals, their profit margin being allegedly too low. Out of his long-established husbandry ethic, he came in on his own time with his own medicine to treat the animals. He cured them! Management's response was to fire him for violating company policy! He kept his job and escaped with a reprimand only when he proved that he had expended his own – not the company's – resources. He continued to work for them but felt that his mental health had suffered in virtue of what I have called the *moral stress* (see Chapter 22) he experienced every day: the stress growing out of the conflict between what he was told to do and how he morally believed he should be treating the animals. Eventually, he left agriculture altogether. The above-detailed contrasting incidents, better than anything else I know, eloquently illustrate the large gap between the ethics of husbandry and industry.

In addition, in the mid twentieth century there arose large-scale use of animals in research and testing for toxicity. This too was an unprecedented use of animals, lacking the fairness of husbandry agriculture. A moment's reflection on the development of animal research and high-technology agriculture elucidates why these innovations have led to the demand for a new ethic for animals in society. In a nutshell, these new developments represent a radically different playing field of animal use from the one that characterized most of human history; in the modern world of agriculture and animal research, the traditional anti-cruelty ethic grows increasingly less applicable as only a small percentage of suffering is a result of intentional cruelty of the sort condemned by the anti-cruelty ethic and laws. Few people have ever witnessed overt, intentional cruelty, which is thankfully rare.

On the other hand, people realize that biomedical and other scientific research, toxicological safety and vaccine potency testing, uses of animals in teaching, pharmaceutical product extraction from animals, and so on all produce far more suffering than does overt cruelty. This suffering comes from creating disease, burns, trauma, fractures, and the like in animals to study them; producing pain, fear, learned helplessness, aggression, and other states for research; poisoning animals to study toxicity; and performing surgery on animals to develop new operative procedures. In addition, suffering is engendered by the housing of research animals. The discomfort and suffering animals used in research experience by virtue of being housed under conditions that are convenient for us, but inimical to their biological natures – for example, keeping rodents, who are social, nocturnal, burrowing creatures, isolated in polycarbonate crates under artificial, full-time light – far exceed the suffering produced by invasive research protocols. Even the utilization of carbon dioxide as the most common method to end the lives of these animals primarily reflects human expediency, despite this being known to be aversive, causing fear and air hunger before death (Makowska et al. 2009).

Now it is clear that researchers and farmers are not intentionally cruel – they are motivated by plausible and decent intentions: to cure disease, advance knowledge, ensure product safety, and provide cheap and plentiful food. Furthermore, the traditional ethic of anti-cruelty and the laws expressing it had no vocabulary for labeling such suffering, since researchers were not maliciously intending to hurt the animals. Indeed, this is eloquently marked by the fact that the cruelty laws exempt animal use in science and standard agricultural practices from their purview. Therefore, a new set of concepts beyond cruelty and kindness was needed to discuss the issues associated with burgeoning research animal use and industrial agriculture.

## The Way Forward for Animals

Given that the old anti-cruelty ethic did not apply to animal research or confinement agriculture, society needed new ethical concepts to express its concern about these new uses. Plato taught us a very valuable lesson about effecting ethical change. If one wishes to change another person's – or society's – ethical beliefs, it is much better to remind than to teach, or, in my martial arts metaphor, to use judo rather than sumo. In other words, if you and I disagree ethically on some matter, it is far better for me to show you that what I am trying to convince you of is already implicit – albeit unnoticed – in what you already believe. Similarly, we cannot force others to believe as we do (sumo): we can, however, show them that their own assumptions, if thought through, lead to a conclusion different from what they currently entertain (judo). These points are well exemplified in twentieth century US history. Prohibition was sumo, not judo – an attempt to forcefully impose a new ethic about drinking on the majority by the minority. As such, it was doomed to fail, and in fact people drank more during Prohibition. Contrast this with civil rights legislation in the 1960s. As a Southerner, then President Lyndon Johnson realized that even Southerners would acquiesce to the following proposition:

> All humans should be treated equally, and black people were human – they just had never bothered to draw the relevant conclusion.

If Johnson had been wrong about this point, if "writing this large" in the law had not "reminded" people, civil rights would have been as ineffective as Prohibition!

Society is faced with the need for new moral categories and laws to deal with animal use in science and agriculture and to limit the animal suffering with which it is increasingly concerned. At the same time, recall that Western society has inexorably extended its moral categories for humans to people who were morally ignored or invisible – women, minorities, the handicapped, children, citizens of the developing world. But new and viable ethics do not emerge *ex nihilo*. So, a plausible and obvious move is for society to continue in its tendency and attempt to extend the moral machinery it has developed for dealing with people, appropriately modified, for animals. And this is precisely what has occurred. Society has taken elements of the moral categories it uses for assessing the treatment of people and is in the process of modifying these concepts to make them appropriate for dealing with new issues in the treatment of animals, especially their use in science and confinement agriculture.

What aspect of our ethic for people is being so extended? One that is in fact quite applicable to animal use is the fundamental problem of weighing the interests of the individual against those of the general welfare. Different societies have provided different answers to this problem. Totalitarian societies opt to devote little concern to the individual, favoring instead the state, or whatever their version of the general welfare may be. At the other extreme, anarchical groups such as communes give primacy to the individual and very little concern to the group – hence they tend to enjoy only transient existence. In our society, however, a balance is struck. Although most of our decisions are made to the benefit of the general welfare, fences are built around individuals to protect their fundamental interests from being sacrificed to the majority. Thus, we protect individuals from being silenced even if the majority disapproves of what they say; we protect individuals from having their property seized without recompense even if such seizure benefits the general welfare; and we protect individuals from torture even if they have planted a bomb in an elementary school and refuse to divulge its location. We protect those interests of the individual that we consider essential to being human, to human nature, from being submerged, even by the common good. Those moral/legal fences that so protect individual humans are called rights and are based on plausible assumptions regarding what is essential to being human.

It is this notion to which society is looking to generate the new moral ideas necessary to address the treatment of animals in today's world, where cruelty is not the major problem but where such laudable, human welfare goals as efficiency, productivity, knowledge, medical progress, and product safety are responsible for the vast majority of animal suffering. People in society are seeking to "build fences" around animals to protect their interests and natures from being totally submerged for the sake of the general welfare and are trying to accomplish this goal by creating laws. In husbandry, this occurred automatically: in industrialized agriculture, where it is no longer automatic, people wish to see it legislated.

It is necessary to stress here certain things that this ethic is not and does not attempt to be. As a mainstream movement, it does not try to give human rights to animals. Since animals do not have the same interests flowing from their natures as humans do, human rights do not fit animals. Animals do not have basic interests that demand speech, religion, or property: thus according them these rights would be absurd. On the other hand, animals have natures of their own and interests that flow from these natures, and the thwarting of these interests matters to animals as much as the thwarting of speech matters to humans. The agenda is not, for society, making animals have the same rights as people. It is rather preserving the common-sense insight that "fish gotta swim and birds gotta fly" and suffer if they don't.

This new ethic is conservative, not radical, harking back to the animal use that necessitated and thus entailed respect for the animals' natures. It is based on the insight that what we do to animals matters to them, just as what we do to humans matters to them, and that consequently we should respect that mattering in our treatment or use of animals as we do in our treatment and use of humans. And since respect for animal nature is no longer automatic as it was in traditional husbandry agriculture, society is demanding that it be encoded in law. For example, New York recently banned declawing cats (Brown 2019) and California banned the sale of cosmetics tested on animals (HSUS 2018). Harvard Law School has an Animal Law and Policy Program committed to "analyzing and improving the treatment of animals through the legal system" (https://animal.law.harvard.edu).

With regard to animal agriculture, the pastoral images of animals grazing on pasture and moving freely are iconic. As the 23rd Psalm indicates, people who consume animals wish to see the animals live decent lives, not lives of pain, distress, and frustration. It is for this reason in part that industrial agriculture conceals the reality of its practices from a naive public – witness Perdue's advertisements portraying raising "happy chickens" in a bucolic, free-range fashion when less than 1% are raised organically (Animal Outlook 2018), or the California "happy cow" ads depicting Holsteins in an idyllic setting on grassy hills when, in fact, very few dairy cows in the United States have access to pasture (von Keyserlingk et al. 2017) (pasture access improves dairy cow welfare by increasing comfort, reducing competition and boredom, and facilitating motivated behavior; Crump et al. 2019). As ordinary people discover the truth, they are shocked. When I served on the Pew Commission and other commissioners had their first view of sows in stalls, many were in tears, and all were outraged.

Just as our use of people is constrained by respect for the basic elements of human nature, people wish to see a similar notion applied to animals. Animals, too, have natures or *telos* – the "pigness of the pig," the "cowness of a cow." Pigs are "designed" to move about on soft loam, not to be in gestation crates. If this no longer occurs naturally, as it did in husbandry, people wish to see it legislated. This is the mainstream sense of "animal rights."

As property, strictly speaking, animals cannot have legal rights. But a functional equivalent to rights can be achieved by limiting human property rights. When I and others drafted the US federal laws for laboratory animals, we did not deny that research animals were the property of researchers. We merely placed limits on their use of their property. I may own my car, but that does not mean I can drive it on the sidewalk or at any speed I choose. Similarly, our law states that if one hurts an animal in research, one must control pain and distress. Thus, research animals can be said to have the right to have their pain controlled (Carbone 2019).

In the case of farm animals, people wish to see their basic needs and nature, *teloi*, respected in the systems within which they are raised. Since this no longer occurs naturally as it did in husbandry, it must be imposed by legislation or regulation. Legal codification of rules of animal care respecting their *telos* is thus the form animal welfare takes where husbandry has been abandoned. Thus, in today's world, the ethical component of animal welfare prescribes that the way we raise and use animals must embody respect and provision for their psychological needs and natures. Accordingly, 49% of American adults consider animal farming to be one of the most important social issues, 72% feel some discomfort with the animal farming industry, and 36% support banning animal farming (Ladak and Anthis 2021).

A recent essay (Bartlett 2021) considers the potential ramifications of the development of plant-based and tissue-cultured meats: "Food animals may become increasingly unnecessary if large portions of the population switch to alternatives. The ideal life for food animals is one that is comfortable, healthy, and free of pain. To compete with manufactured protein, food animal agriculture will need to move much closer to achieving this goal" and warns, "Future food animal veterinarians may find themselves serving a contracting ... industry experiencing immense economic pressure." For the sake of the veterinary profession, it is therefore essential that food animal veterinarians, veterinary specialists in animal welfare, and the AVMA exert their considerable influence to persuade industrial agriculture to phase out those systems that cause animal suffering by violating animals' natures and replace them with systems respecting their natures. Or else we diminish not only the animals but ourselves as well.

# References

American Society for the Prevention of Cruelty to Animals (ASPCA) (2016). New research finds vast majority of Americans concerned about farm animal welfare. https://www. aspca.org/about-us/press-releases/new-research-finds-vast-majority-americans-concerned-about-farm-animal (accessed 24 October 2021).

Animal Outlook (2018). Tyson challenges Perdue's ads as deceptively boasting "happy" chickens. https://animaloutlook.org/perdues-ads-deceptively-boasting-happy-chickens (accessed 18 November 2021).

Animal Welfare Committee (n.d.). Farm Animal Welfare Committee (FAWC). https://www.gov.uk/government/groups/farm-animal-welfare-committee-fawc. (accessed 24 October 2021).

Anthis, J.R. (2017). Survey of US attitudes towards animal farming and animal-free food. https://www.sentienceinstitute.org/animal-farming-attitudes-survey-2017 (accessed 24 October 2021).

Aquinas, T. (1956). *On the Truth of the Catholic Faith*. Providence, NY: Doubleday.

Ballard, J. (2019). Most pet owners say their pets are part of the family. https://today.yougov.com/topics/lifestyle/articles-reports/2019/12/13/how-americas-pet-owners-feel-about-their-furry-fri (accessed 24 October 2021).

Bartlett, P. (2021). Competing with manufactured protein: Are dark days ahead for the food animal industry? *Journal of the American Veterinary Medical Association* 259 (2): 132–134.

Bentham, J. (1996). *An Introduction to the Principles of Morals and Legislation: The Collected Works of Jeremy Bentham*. Oxford: Clarendon.

Block, K. and Amundson, S. (2020). Victory! Omnibus signed into law over weekend has major wins on horse racing, slaughter, and soring. https://blog.humanesociety. org/2020/12/victory-omnibus-signed-into-law-over-weekend-has-major-wins-on-horse-racing-slaughter-and-soring.html?credit=blog_post_122820_id11883 (accessed 24 October 2021).

Block, K. and Amundson, S. (2021). Breaking: European Parliament votes to phase out animal testing and research. https://blog.humanesociety.org/2021/09/breaking-european-parliament-votes-to-phase-out-animal-testing-and-research. html?credit=blog_post_091621_id12496 (accessed 24 October 2021).

Brambell, F.W.R. (1965). *Report of the Technical Committee to Enquire into the Welfare of Animals Kept under Intense Livestock Husbandry Systems*. London: HMSO.

Brown, E. (2019). New York State bans cat declawing. *The New York Times* 22 July.

Burns, K. (2019). Groups provide new guidance on antimicrobials. *Journal of the American Veterinary Medical Association* 254 (3): 317–319.

Carbone, L. (2019). Ethical and IACUC considerations regarding analgesia and pain management in laboratory rodents. *Comparative Medicine* 69: 443–450.

Cochrane, A. (2012). *Animal Rights Without Liberation*. New York: Columbia University Press.

Council for Agricultural Science and Technology (CAST) (1981). *Scientific Aspects of the Welfare of Food Animals*. Report #91. Ames, IA.

Crump, A., Jenkins, K., Bethell, E.J. et al. (2019). Pasture access affects behavioral indicators of wellbeing in dairy cows. *Animals* 9 (11): 902.

Francione, G. (2000). *Introduction to Animal Rights*. Philadelphia, PA: Temple University Press.

Gaskell, G., Bauer, M.V., and Durant, J. (1997). Europe ambivalent on biotechnology. *Nature* 387: 845–847.

Her Majesty's Stationery Office (HMSO) (1986). Animals (Scientific Procedures) Act. https://www.legislation.gov.uk/ukpga/1986/14/contents (accessed 5 November 2021).

Humane Society of the United States (2018). California becomes first state to prohibit the sale of cosmetics tested on animals. https://www.humanesociety.org/news/california-becomes-first-state-prohibit-sale-cosmetics-tested-animals (accessed 24 October 2021).

Kelly, R. (2021). Europe leans toward banning cages for farmed animals. https://news.vin. com/default.aspx?pid=210&Id=10212024 (accessed 3 February 2022).

Kleinhenz, M.D., Viscardi, A.V., and Coetzee, J.F. (2021). Invited Review: On-farm pain management of food production animals. *Applied Animal Science* 37 (1): 77–87.

Ladak, A. and Anthis, J.R. (2021). Animals, Food, and Technology (AFT) Survey: 2020 Update. https://www.sentienceinstitute.org/aft-survey-2020 (accessed 27 October 2021).

Leavitt, E.S. (1978). *Animals and Their Legal Rights*. Washington, DC: Animal Welfare Institute.

Lohr, S. (1988). Swedish farm animals get a bill of rights. *The New York Times* 25 October: 1.

Makowska, I.J., Vickers, L., Mancell, J. et al. (2009). Evaluating methods of gas euthanasia for laboratory mice. *Applied Animal Behaviour Science* 121 (3–4): 230–235.

National Shooting Sports Foundation (NSSF) (2019). NSSF report: Americans attitudes toward hunting, fishing, sports shooting, and trapping. https://asafishing.org/wp-content/uploads/2019/04/Americans-Attitudes-Survey-Report-2019.pdf. (accessed 24 October 2021).

Pacelle, W. (2011). *The Bond*. New York: Harper Collins.

Pew Commission on Industrial Farm Animal Production (2008). Putting meat on the table: Industrial farm animal production in America. https://www.pcifapia.org/_images/PCIFAPFin.pdf (accessed 24 October 2021).

Pierce, J. and Bekoff, M. (2018). A postzoo future: Why welfare fails animals in zoos. *Journal of Applied Animal Welfare Science* 21 (sup1): 43–48.

Regan, T. (1983). *The Case for Animal Rights*. Berkeley, CA: University of California Press.

Rollin, B. (1995). *Farm Animal Welfare: Social, Bioethical and Research Issues*. Ames, IA: Iowa State University Press.

Rollin, B. (2006). *Animal Rights and Human Morality*, 3e. Buffalo, NY: Prometheus Books.

Scully, M. (2002). *Dominion*. New York: St. Martin's Press.

Singer, P. (1975). *Animal Liberation*. New York: New York Review Press.

Singer, P. (2009). Speciesism and moral status. *Metaphilosophy* 40 (3–4): 567–581.

Stanford Encyclopedia of Philosophy (2021). The grounds of moral status. https://plato.stanford.edu/entries/grounds-moral-status (accessed 23 October 2021).

Sunstein, C.R. and Nussbaum, M.C. (eds.) (2004). *Animal Rights*. New York: Oxford University Press.

United States Department of Agriculture (USDA) (2022). Economic Research Service. Farming and farm income. https://www.ers.usda.gov/data-products/ag-and-food-statistics-charting-the-essentials/farming-and-farm-income (accessed 3 February 2022).

von Keyserlingk, M.A., Cestari, A.A., Franks, B. et al. (2017). Dairy cows value access to pasture as highly as fresh feed. *Scientific Reports* 7 (1): 1–4.

Willoughby, S. (2013). Getting rid of Colorado's spring bear hunt is right call. *The Denver Post* 11 June.

## 2

## Animal Welfare

Science, Policy, and the Role of Veterinarians

*Joy A. Mench*

## Introduction

Haven't I just read a chapter on the moral status of animals? If so, why is there also a chapter on animal welfare – aren't animal ethics and animal welfare the same thing? The answer is yes – and no. Yes, because people's perceptions of animal welfare are deeply tied to their ethical views about the moral status of animals, and hence their views about appropriate animal treatment (Fraser 2008). There is no "consensus" view about animal welfare – instead, there are many, often conflicting opinions about how animals should be housed and managed and indeed whether humans should even use animals for their own purposes.

But the answer is also no – because animal welfare is something inherent to an individual animal. The World Organisation for Animal Health (OIE) defines animal welfare as "the physical and mental state of an animal in relation to the conditions in which it lives and dies" (OIE 2021). Welfare is influenced by a multitude of factors, not just the way an animal is treated by humans. An animal's welfare exists on a continuum from poor to good and is dynamic, changing as conditions change. It is influenced both by the animal's genetic predispositions and life experiences. This makes evaluating an animal's welfare challenging, because it requires understanding the long-term effects of all the practices to which an animal is exposed and determining how these should be weighed against one another to provide an assessment of the animal's quality of life.

Regardless of these complexities, thinking about animal welfare as the experience of an individual animal creates opportunities to carry out scientific research to better understand that experience, and to use that understanding to create conditions for improving welfare. In this chapter, I focus on scientific research on animal welfare and its application via policy and technology transfer, as well as the role of veterinarians in that process. The emphasis will be on farm animal welfare, although laboratory animal welfare will be addressed briefly.

## History of Animal Welfare

The origin of animal welfare as a field of scientific study is traced to an expert committee report published in 1965, the Brambell Report (Brambell 1967). The UK government appointed this committee in response to public outcry following the publication of Ruth Harrison's book *Animal Machines* (1964). Harrison described a "new type of

*Ethics in Veterinary Practice: Balancing Conflicting Interests*, First Edition. Edited by Barry Kipperman and Bernard E. Rollin.
© 2022 John Wiley & Sons, Inc. Published 2022 by John Wiley & Sons, Inc.

farming, of production line methods applied to the rearing of animals, of animals living out their lives in darkness and immobility ... of a generation of men who see in the animal they rear only its conversion factor into food" – a type of farming she called *factory farming*. After reviewing the current state of farm animal production in the UK (and Europe), the Brambell Committee echoed Harrison's concerns about certain practices, including rearing animals under conditions of extreme confinement. The committee made two particularly influential statements: that animals have "innate behavioural urges" which have been "little, if at all, bred out in the process of domestication" and that animals have feelings (Thorpe 1969). Although accepting that some restriction of animals' behavior was necessary on farms, the committee recommended that all animals be provided at least with sufficient freedom of movement to turn around, lie down, groom normally, get up, and stretch their limbs – the "Five Freedoms."

The committee noted that many of their concerns were speculative and would need to be proven to be problems (or not) based on empirical evidence. They stressed the need for scientific studies of animal behavior and physiology, especially focused on understanding animals' feelings. In so doing, they launched the field of animal welfare science (Appleby et al. 2018). Their report also highlighted what are now considered to be the three key components of animal welfare: natural living (behavior), basic health and functioning, and affective states (feelings) (Fraser 2008).

The trajectory of scientific research on animal welfare has been strongly influenced by the Five Freedoms – not just the Five Freedoms of the Brambell Committee but the expansion of those freedoms into a set of guiding principles in the 1990s by the Farm Animal Welfare Council (FAWC), a UK government advisory body set up in response to the Brambell Report. These "new" Five Freedoms (FAWC 2012) are:

1) *Freedom from pain, injury, or disease* by prevention or rapid diagnosis and treatment.
2) *Freedom from discomfort* by providing an appropriate environment including shelter and a comfortable resting area.
3) *Freedom from fear and distress* by ensuring conditions and treatment which avoid mental suffering.
4) *Freedom from hunger and thirst* by ready access to fresh water and diet to maintain health and vigor.
5) *Freedom to express normal behavior* by providing sufficient space, proper facilities, and company of the animal's own kind.

## Farm Animal Welfare Concerns

Although it is beyond the scope of this chapter to discuss the different types of farm animal production systems and how particular freedoms might be infringed in those systems, welfare concerns include:

- Long-term restriction of movement because animals are kept in very small spaces (e.g. cages for laying hens, narrow stalls for veal calves or pregnant pigs) or are tethered.

- Stressful social conditions – e.g. disruption of the mother–young bond by early weaning or separation (dairy calves, poultry), lack of social contact for individually housed animals (pigs and calves in stalls).
- Environments that are barren of stimuli needed for animals to express highly motivated behaviors (e.g. no rooting materials for pigs, no nests for laying hens).
- The expression of abnormal behaviors, particularly behaviors that lead to injury (e.g. tail biting by pigs, feather pecking and cannibalism by poultry).
- Pain and distress from procedures routinely performed on animals (often without pain relief) to prevent injury (including due to abnormal behavior) or for other management reasons (e.g. castration, dehorning, beak-trimming, branding).
- Pain and disability due to injury or disease.
- Humaneness and timeliness of on-farm euthanasia.
- Production diseases, which arise because of genetic selection and/or management of animals for high productivity (e.g. lameness in broiler chickens, pigs, and dairy cattle; bone breakage in laying hens; mastitis in dairy cattle).
- Air quality problems (dust and ammonia in indoor environments).
- Thermal stress (in indoor and outdoor environments).
- Inadequate nutrition or hydration, due to poor equipment design or placement, diets not well matched to animals' nutritional needs, or intentional withholding of feed or water (e.g. to control weight in sows and breeding flocks for broilers).
- Discomfort or injury due to badly designed or maintained standing, walking, and lying surfaces (e.g. concrete floors for cattle, wet litter for poultry, muddy conditions outdoors).
- Distress, fear, and injury associated with human–animal interactions, including transport and slaughter.

## Scope of Animal Welfare Research

There is now a large body of animal welfare research (Fraser et al. 2013; Appleby et al. 2018). In keeping with the complex nature of animal welfare, a variety of scientific approaches have been taken. These were initially drawn from the disciplines of animal behavior (ethology) and physiology, the areas highlighted by the Brambell Committee. However, the field of animal welfare science soon expanded to include expertise from a variety of other disciplines, including veterinary medicine, comparative psychology, nutrition, neuroscience, agricultural engineering, and genetics.

An ongoing challenge has been how to assess animals' feelings, which are not directly measurable and therefore have to be inferred. Measures used include physiological responses known to be linked to affective states in humans, such as eye temperature and heart rate variability; behavioral responses like escape, avoidance, facial expressions, or vocalizations to stimuli presumed to be painful or aversive; physiological and behavioral responses to pharmacological manipulation using drugs known to affect emotional states in humans; and mood assessment using cognitive bias testing (Ede et al. 2019).

The most widely used method for assessing animals' subjective states is motivational testing (Fraser and Nicol 2018). The simplest form is preference testing, where animals are presented with various options and observed to see which they prefer (or prefer to avoid). These tests tell us what animals "want." More complex tests utilize operant conditioning techniques, requiring animals to work (e.g. by pecking a key or moving a heavy door) to obtain their preferred option or avoid their nonpreferred option. Operant conditioning tests provide information both about what animals prefer and how strong their preferences and aversions are based on how hard they are willing to work – in other words, what animals "need." Motivational tests have been used to assess a wide variety of aspects of farm animal housing and management, including air quality, light levels, bedding, social conditions, and provision of nests, perches, shade, and rooting materials. They have also been used to determine how important it is to animals to perform certain behaviors. The results of motivational research have been influential – for example, the decision to ban the use of barren conventional (battery) cages for hens in the European Union was based primarily on operant research showing that hens are highly motivated to perch and to lay their eggs in a nest (Appleby 2003).

## Improving Animal Welfare

As the pace of animal welfare science has increased, so too has public concern about the treatment of farm animals, particularly in economically developed countries. Although individuals not directly involved in food animal production may have minimal knowledge about how farm animals are raised and housed, they want reassurance that those animals are well cared for and are humanely killed (Cornish et al. 2016). Recent attention has thus focused on the practical implementation of welfare improvements, particularly via policy instruments and scientific research application.

### Animal Welfare Policy

There are two different approaches to "regulating" farm animal welfare – involuntary and voluntary. The involuntary approach involves requiring compliance with laws, regulations, ordinances, or other legal vehicles. The voluntary approach involves identifying and incorporating "best practices" for animal welfare into standards or guidelines that farmers are encouraged, but not legally required, to follow. Involuntary and voluntary regulation strategies are used to different degrees in different countries, and each approach has advantages and disadvantages. This section will focus on animal welfare policy in the United States and the European Union (EU): information about Canada, Asia, the Far East, Oceania, the Middle East, and Latin America can be found in Fraser et al. (2018), Gallo and Tadich (2018), and Thornber and Mellor (2018).

#### Involuntary Regulation

Involuntary regulation has been the primary mechanism used to assure animal welfare within the EU (Knierem and Pajor 2018; Broom 2019). Although the EU places some limits on the types of legislation that can be adopted, particularly related to ensuring freedom of trade within the EU, it has enacted substantial legislation addressing the welfare of farm animals.

EU animal welfare legislation can take the form of directives or regulations. Directives set out objectives that must be made into laws in the individual Member

States, but it is up to each state to determine whether to simply adopt the objectives or add even more stringent provisions. Regulations are EU-wide laws that must be followed by all citizens and businesses. Most animal welfare legislation has taken the form of directives, which is why there is variation among the Member States in permissible farming practices. Member States can also pass their own farm animal welfare laws, as long as only their residents are subject to those laws.

The major EU farm animal welfare directives[1] are (Simonin and Gavinelli 2019):

- Farmed animals (Directive 98/58) – specifies general farming practices (e.g. feeding, breeding, freedom of movement), reflecting the principles of the Five Freedoms.
- Calves (Directive 2008/119) – requires group housing and provision of a balanced diet, prohibits calves being permanently tethered or reared in darkness; the primary focus is dairy calves raised for veal.
- Pigs (Directive 2008/120) – requires group housing of gilts and sows (except during certain specified periods, such as while lactating) and that rooting materials be provided to all pigs; places limitations on some painful procedures, like tail-docking; specifies minimum weaning age for piglets.
- Laying hens (Directive 1999/74) – specifies the configuration of different laying hen housing systems (e.g. space allowances, enrichment materials); sets standards for certain aspects of management of hen housing systems (e.g. lighting, inspection). Banned the use of conventional ("battery") cages effective 2012.
- Chickens for meat production (Directive 2007/43) – specifies minimum space allowances for meat chickens and requires Member States to implement a system to monitor specific welfare outcomes relevant to space allowance on the farm and in the slaughterhouse.

EU regulations have been implemented for aspects of animal welfare that involve multiple Member States, like animal transport (Regulation 1/2005), as well as for humane slaughter and on-farm killing (Regulation 1099/2009).

The United States regulates the transport and slaughter of farm animals via the Twenty-Eight Hour Law and the Humane Slaughter Act (HSA), respectively. The Twenty-Eight Hour Law was first passed in 1873 but was amended and reissued in its current form in 1994 (49 USC s 80502 2012). It stipulates that animals cannot be confined in a "vehicle or vessel for more than 28 consecutive hours without unloading the animals for feeding, water and rest" [of at least five hours] during transport. Although the law was originally intended to apply to transport by rail, most farm animals are now transported by truck. The US Department of Agriculture (USDA) clarified in 2005 that the law applied to truck transport (Animal Welfare Institute n.d.). It appears, however, that it is rarely enforced given how infrequently shipments are monitored and due to a lack of clarity about enforcement authority. Although the Twenty-Eight Hour Law does not apply to poultry, long-distance truck transport of poultry is uncommon because the hatcheries, rearing houses, and processing plants in integrated broiler and turkey complexes are usually located nearby.

The HSA was first passed in 1958 and then amended in 1978 (7 USC ss 1901–1907, as amended). It requires that (except for religious slaughter): "cattle, calves, horses, mules, sheep, swine and other livestock … be rendered insensible to pain … before being shackled, hoisted, thrown, cast or cut." Approved methods for rapidly and effectively inducing insensibility are listed. As part of its enforcement of the HSA, the

USDA Food Safety and Inspection Service (USDA-FSIS) inspects loading, unloading, and holding areas to ensure humane handling. Poultry are not included in the HSA, although the USDA states that poultry receive protection via the Poultry Products Inspection Act (PPIA; PL 85-172, as amended). This Act mandates inspection of poultry at the slaughterhouse for meat quality and safety. Carcasses with bruising or injury due to handling or transport can be condemned, as can "red birds," which are birds that were inadequately cut and thus still alive when they entered the scalder for defeathering. There have been repeated attempts by animal welfare organizations to either include poultry under the HSA or expand the PPIA to explicitly address welfare concerns, including stunning, but these have been unsuccessful. Regardless, stunning (either electrical or gas) is routine at large poultry processing plants for both animal welfare and food quality reasons.

In contrast to the EU, there is no federal regulation in the United States governing the welfare of animals on commercial farms, although some states have laws that specifically limit aspects of housing or management. Farm animals may also be covered under state anti-cruelty laws, although in many states they are exempted if they are subjected to practices considered to be standard for commercial agriculture (see National Agricultural Law Center 2021 for state-by-state summaries of anti-cruelty laws). Instead, voluntary regulation has been the primary pathway used in the United States and most other countries outside of the EU.

### Voluntary Regulation

Voluntary regulation of farm animal welfare originates from several sources (Mench 2008). In the United States, many farmers follow animal welfare standards developed by their respective trade organizations (e.g. United Egg Producers, National Chicken Council, National Cattlemen's Beef Association, National Pork Producers). The other sources of voluntary regulation are market-driven programs. These can either be animal welfare labeling programs for consumers or programs that are part of the "conditions of doing business" between animal producers and their customers (food retailers and distributors).

Many large food retailers and distributors now include animal welfare as part of their corporate social responsibility programs (Amos et al. 2020). Approaches, issues addressed, and supplier requirements vary between companies. A company might stipulate that the farmer participate in an independent animal welfare labeling program or adhere to company or trade organization animal welfare standards. These retailer/distributor programs are only quasi-voluntary since farmers risk losing a major market for their products if they do not comply with a company's requirements. Retailers and distributors therefore have enormous power to shape the animal welfare landscape (More et al. 2017), not only by requiring adherence to standards but also by deciding not to purchase products from animals kept in certain kinds of housing systems.

For example, a large (and growing) number of US retailers, distributors, and food service companies have announced plans to discontinue using eggs from hens housed in cages (Graber and Keller 2020). As a result, 30% of hens in the United States as of March 2021 were housed in cage-free systems, compared with only 4% in 2010; it is estimated that nearly 70% of US flocks will need to be cage-free by 2025 to meet existing food chain commitments (United Egg Producers n.d.). Whether this is achievable given the time frame and capital required for egg producers to build new housing systems is debatable- nor is it clear whether consumers are willing to spend more for cage-free eggs, which cost more to produce (Lusk 2019).

### Enforcement

A key element of voluntary and involuntary regulation is enforcement. Involuntary regulation is enforced by government bodies. In the EU, animal welfare legislation is enforced by relevant authorities in the Member States, which must submit annual reports of inspections to the European Commission (Simonin and Gavinelli 2019). Veterinary experts from the European Commission also conduct audits in the Member States to confirm adherence. In the United States, the USDA-FSIS is responsible for enforcing the HSA, while several agencies have responsibility for enforcement of the Twenty-Eight Hour Law (Animal Welfare Institute n.d.).

Voluntary program oversight is more variable. A typical process for ensuring that standards are followed is auditing. Individual farmers can carry out first-party (internal) audits and/or be subject to second-party (semi-independent, e.g. a customer directly auditing a farmer), or third-party (independent) auditing (e.g. a customer using an independent firm to audit a farmer). Large farmers may be audited multiple times annually as part of their contracts with retailers and distributors and may have to meet an array of animal welfare and food quality/safety standards.

### Strengths and Weaknesses

Involuntary and voluntary regulation have strengths and weaknesses. These are encapsulated in another phrase used to describe these different types of regulation – public and private standards (Toschi Maciel and Bock 2013; More et al. 2017; Lundmark et al. 2018). Involuntary regulation is public – the texts of laws are publicized, they may be finalized only after public comment, they are enforced by independent governmental authorities, and there is public accountability in terms of the penalties imposed for breaking the laws. Voluntary standards are private and may lack transparency – the input into the development of the standards, the content of the standards, or the method of ensuring that the standards are met may not be made obvious to the public. In essence, consumers are being asked to trust the retailer or the trade group rather than the standards. This lack of transparency can lead to a lack of confidence if people perceive that there is a conflict of interest. There are, of course, exceptions to these generalizations. Laws can be inadequately enforced or associated with such negligible penalties that they are essentially ineffective. Alternatively, voluntary programs may have mechanisms in place to build consumer trust by making their standards publicly available, by using third-party auditors, by product labeling, and/or by releasing summaries of audit results.

While this would suggest that animal welfare is best assured via public standards, there are downsides to this approach. The process of creating involuntary regulation is often protracted, and consequently, laws tend to be inflexible once they are finally passed and an enforcement mechanism established. Therefore, involuntary standards take a long time to implement and generate only short-term or limited benefits for the animals, given the pace of scientific discovery and technological innovation related to animal welfare. Voluntary standards are more flexible and can be changed as new information is obtained, can be implemented more quickly, and (in the case of multinational retailers) can lead to global change assured by market mechanisms.

For these reasons it is becoming increasingly common to combine voluntary and involuntary regulation of farm animal welfare (Knierem and Pajor 2018). In the EU, market standards that exceed EU legal requirements are assuming increasing importance. Current trends show governance of farm animal welfare moving away from new legislation to the marketplace (Toschi Maciel and Bock 2013; Lundmark et al. 2018). The last EU farm animal welfare directive was in 2009, and the protracted nature of the regulatory process means that existing legislation mainly covers higher profile issues like close confinement housing. Many species widely farmed within the EU including trout, salmon, rabbits, ducks, turkeys, beef and dairy cattle (except for veal calves), and sheep, are not covered by EU directives (Broom 2019). There are therefore many regulatory gaps that can be (and are being) filled by market-driven governance.

Conversely, involuntary regulation is assuming increasing importance in some countries that already have well-developed voluntary programs. In the United States, there has been a recent spate of state regulations restricting use of various types of confinement housing for farm animals (Vogeler 2020). Californians passed a sweeping ballot initiative in 2018, with provisions to begin in 2020 and 2022 (CDFA 2018). This law effectively bans the most highly confined housing systems for egg-laying hens, swine, and calves, and applies not only to animals raised within the state but also to animal products produced elsewhere and sold in California. This will have a ripple effect because California is a major market for animal products produced in other states where these housing systems are still permitted. Animal welfare organizations in the United States have been effective not only in exerting pressure on retailers via shareholders' resolutions and direct consumer campaigns, but in utilizing state ballot initiatives to pass farm animal welfare regulations (Vogeler 2020). However, state-by-state regulation removes one of the benefits of federal regulation, as it can cause market disruption and lead to a patchwork of standards. This is problematic if the net effect is that production just moves to states with fewer (or no) animal welfare regulations.

### Research Application

Initially, much animal welfare research was focused on addressing basic questions related to the motivation of animals to perform certain behaviors, physiological responses to stress, and pain perception. As the science has evolved there has been increasing focus on how to apply research to modify housing, management, transport, and slaughter. The last two areas have considerable uptake of research findings and associated auditing programs (Grandin 2021a). Each of these constitutes a relatively short-term stressor for the animal, which makes implementing changes more straightforward than changing practices on farms. Farm environments are complex, and the animals are kept in those environments for weeks or years, often through different developmental stages during which their needs change. Modifying housing and management can be costly, so farmers only reap tangible benefits if there is a strong driver, like regulation or market pressure. Thus, increasing attention has been directed toward facilitating research application, as well as developing practical on-farm welfare assessment and improvement tools that can allow animal welfare to be assessed continuously and in real time. In addition, social science research is attempting to understand how human factors affect the adoption of research findings.

### Making Research Relevant – Epidemiology

Because of the types of questions addressed, most animal welfare research has been conducted in experimental settings, where scientific treatments can be applied, and data collected, in a systematic and controlled way. Experimental settings are often poor approximations of commercial farming operations. First, they are often much smaller, housing dozens or hundreds of animals rather than the thousands or tens of thousands of animals kept on many commercial farms. Second, they may lack the kind of sophisticated environmental and management controls (related to things like ventilation and food and water delivery) seen on many intensive farms, which can cause important differences between the two settings. In addition, many animal welfare problems are multifactorial. For example, the incidence and severity of lameness in broiler chickens can be affected by genetics, nutrition, lighting, stocking density, litter management, and/or the presence of infectious organisms in the breeding flock, hatchery, or growing facility (Mench 2018). It is almost impossible to systematically vary and evaluate the interactions of so many factors in an experimental setting, or at least not within a reasonable time frame.

To increase the potential for research findings that improve animal welfare, experimental studies need to be complemented by research carried out on farms and during commercial transport and slaughter. Therefore, more animal welfare studies are using an epidemiological approach, collecting data from multiple sites (e.g. farms, slaughterhouses) and analyzing the data to assess patterns. Unlike an experimental study, an epidemiological study cannot demonstrate cause and effect. However, by taking advantage of the normal variation that occurs across different sites it can accomplish two important things: (i) determine the actual incidence of welfare problems in the "real world"; and (ii) pinpoint the risk factors for those problems, as well as the conditions and practices that are associated with a lower incidence. In this way, epidemiological studies can help identify "best management practices" that can form the basis for animal welfare standards and auditing programs. Epidemiological methods have now been used to study a wide range of welfare problems (Mench 2018).

### Technology Application

On-site animal welfare research is being facilitated by the development of automated data collection technologies. Many large intensive farms have some automated monitoring, typically of feed and water delivery, thermal conditions, and air quality. Farmers are also increasingly adopting "smart farming" (precision livestock monitoring) technologies. Smart farming utilizes an integrated suite of sensor and computing technologies to monitor various aspects of production, which can include animal health status, growth and/or reproduction, and animal and human (caretaker) behavior, as well as environmental factors. Thus, outcomes important for animal welfare can be monitored continuously in real time (Berckmans 2017), which can be particularly important for large flocks or herds where it is difficult for workers to assess every individual animal daily. It also makes it simpler to collect behavioral data, which are extremely time-consuming to collect in person (and logistically difficult to do well when flocks or herds are large).

Automated technologies have been used to collect a variety of behavioral and health/physical condition data on farms (van Erp-van der Kooij and Rutter 2020). Integrated automated data collection can reveal important (and sometimes unexpected) links between different aspects of animal welfare and production. An example is the optical flow system developed in the UK to determine the prevalence of lameness on commercial broiler farms (Dawkins et al. 2021). This system utilizes cameras and computing technology to evaluate the movement of a flock of birds through the house. Flock movement patterns have been found to be useful not only to assess lameness and foot problems but also infection with *Campylobacter*, a foodborne pathogen of high importance. Flow patterns in very young broilers (one to four days of age) predict later flock mortality, a critical economic measure for farmers.

### Social Science Research

Improving animal welfare depends upon animal owners or caretakers changing their behavior on behalf of the animal (Whay 2007). It is therefore critical to have a better understanding of the drivers of that behavioral change (and conversely the barriers to change). Economics is obviously an important driver for farmers, which is why there has been considerable uptake of research findings related to livestock handling, transport, and slaughter, since these are often linked to improved meat quality and/or a reduction in labor requirements (Grandin 2021b). The benefits of implementing research on housing and management on-farm have often been more obscure to farmers in the absence of regulatory or market mandates. Research methods derived from the social sciences are proving important to understand factors relevant to farmers' adoption of new animal welfare practices. These have been found to encompass not just cost considerations, but social pressure, nonuse values (empathy and "doing the right thing" for the animals), technical knowledge and skills, and input of trusted advisors, particularly veterinarians (Balzani and Hanlon 2020).

An illustration of the way in which social science approaches can improve welfare comes from work done at Bristol University. The goal of the project (Baker and Weeks 2020) was to reduce severe feather pecking behavior in laying hen flocks in the UK. Feather pecking is an abnormal behavior that spreads through a flock and can lead to hens having large areas of their bodies denuded of feathers. This affects their ability to maintain their body temperature and exposes skin to injury. Feather pecking may also escalate to cannibalism (pecking and tearing the flesh), which causes pain and can result in high flock mortality. Damage due to feather pecking and cannibalism is the reason that hens are beak-trimmed, a procedure that causes at least short-term pain and can affect the hen's ability to perform behaviors like preening effectively. While it would be desirable to end beak-trimming (it has been banned in some EU countries and is not permitted under some voluntary programs), for good flock welfare the problem of feather pecking still needs to be resolved by determining its underlying causes and making appropriate management changes.

Since it is difficult to observe feather pecking directly, a first step was to develop a practical feather scoring system that could be used by farmers to monitor their flocks (AssureWel n.d.a). Epidemiological studies were conducted to assess the incidence of feather loss on UK egg farms, as well as the risk factors for feather pecking (Lambton et al. 2010). Based on this research, a benchmarking tool was devised (AssureWel n.d.b) so that farmers could compare their self-assessed rates of feather loss to those on other farms, and a management package was produced outlining strategies that could potentially be used to reduce feather pecking (Lambton et al. 2013).

Because many farmers were reluctant to make widespread management changes, social science methods were used to assess the barriers to implementing change (Palczynski et al. 2016). Based on this study's recommendation that providing farmers with "ownership" of the problem and its solutions could be useful in overcoming the barriers, a trained facilitator was engaged to work with the farmers to create action plans that were uniquely suitable for their farms (Baker et al. 2020). This resulted in 80% of farmers making changes, even if those changes required capital investment. A similar approach has been used to reduce rates of lameness on dairy farms in the UK (Whay et al. 2021).

### Operationalizing the Five Freedoms for Research Application

Although the Five Freedoms have been a useful framework for scientific inquiry and policy development, they are mainly aspirational ethical statements – no animal (or human) ever completely achieves these freedoms throughout their life. To operationalize the Five Freedoms for practical use, several new frameworks for welfare assessment and improvement have been proposed, including the Twelve Criteria, the Five Domains, and the OIE General Principles.

The Twelve Criteria (Keeling et al. 2013) were proposed as part of Welfare Quality (Blokhuis et al. 2013), an EU-funded project focused on creating practical animal welfare assessment schemes for use on-farm and in slaughterhouses. A major goal was to incorporate animal-based measures into the assessment. Animal-based measures are outcomes that are direct indicators of animal welfare, such as injury rates, body condition, or performance of particular behaviors. The Five Freedoms are expressed as four general principles: good feeding, good housing, good health, and appropriate behavior. These are then expanded into Twelve Criteria that can be used as the basis for generating measurement methods and metrics for evaluation of animal welfare:

- Good feeding – absence of prolonged hunger, absence of prolonged thirst.
- Good housing – thermal comfort, comfort around resting, ease of movement.
- Good health – no painful management procedures, no disease, no injuries.
- Appropriate behavior – expressing social behavior, expressing other behavior, good human–animal relationship, positive emotional state.

Using these criteria, the Welfare Quality project developed metrics for on-site welfare assessment of pigs, chickens, and cattle (Welfare Quality n.d.) that can be used in audits. The Five Domains Model (Mellor et al. 2020) also categorizes welfare concerns into groupings: nutrition, physical environment, health, and behavioral interactions (which includes animals' behavioral interactions with their physical environment, other animals, and humans). This model explicitly relates each of these domains to positive and negative affect, which in turn influence the fifth domain – the animal's mental state. Mellor (2017) has suggested ways that this model can be applied to define programmatic goals and facilitate welfare assessment.

The OIE has also formulated general principles to serve as a basis for the development of animal welfare standards and auditing programs (Fraser et al. 2013). The OIE's framework for animal welfare includes the Five Freedoms as an expression of "society's expectations for the conditions animals should experience when under human control" (OIE 2021). The general principles reflect the Five Freedoms, but also provide more specific guidance about the goals – for example, that the physical environment should be suited to the animal's species and breed to minimize the risk of injury and the transmission of diseases or parasites, or that genetic selection should always take animal welfare and health into account. In conjunction with the new OIE animal welfare standards (see the section titled "OIE"), these principles will become important globally as the basis for animal welfare regulation.

## Laboratory Animal Welfare Concerns

Most animal welfare research has been conducted on farm animals, although the number of papers on companion animals and animals used in biomedical research (laboratory animals) is steadily increasing (Walker et al. 2014). Similar trends are evident with respect to research approaches and application, such as the use of epidemiological studies to determine benchmarks, risks, and potential amelioration strategies as well as the development of animal-based scoring systems (Butterworth et al. 2018), and the use of automated technologies for in situ collection of animal health and behavior data. The regulation of laboratory animal welfare in the United States also involves a mixture of involuntary and voluntary standards (Vasbinder et al. 2014).

The US federal law covering animals used in biomedical research, testing, and teaching (as well as exhibition) is the Animal Welfare Act (AWA). The AWA was enacted in 1966, and has been amended several times, with the most recent revision in 1985 (7 USC ss 2131–2159). In general, the AWA lays out standards for animal housing, care, and treatment. It also requires each institution that uses animals to establish a local committee, the Institutional Animal Care and Use Committee (IACUC) to oversee all facets of animal use, including by reviewing and approving proposed experimental procedures before they are carried out. The USDA Animal and Plant Health Inspection Service conducts regular inspections to enforce the AWA, and major noncompliance can result in financial penalties. While the Five Freedoms are certainly relevant to the welfare of laboratory animals, the main ethical principles underlying the regulation of laboratory animal welfare are the Three Rs (Russell and Burch 1959) – where possible, the *replacement* of animals with nonanimal models or the use of species less likely to experience suffering; the *reduction* of the number of animals used to the minimum necessary to achieve the stated scientific goals; and *refinement* by using methods and practices that minimize animal suffering and improve welfare.

Unlike the regulation of animal research in many other countries where all vertebrate animals are covered, only certain vertebrates are included in the AWA provisions: dogs, cats, nonhuman primates, guinea pigs, hamsters, rabbits, and "other warm-blooded animals." Birds and purpose-bred rodents are specifically excluded from coverage, as are farm animals used in agricultural research. While there are no published statistics, it is estimated that purpose-bred rats and mice make up at least 93% of research animals in the United States (Grimm 2021), meaning that most animals used are not covered by AWA oversight.

There is another federal "regulatory" mechanism for animal research that includes *all* vertebrate animals, the Public Health Service (PHS). PHS oversight is based on two documents – the *Guide for the Care and Use of Laboratory Animals* (known as "the *Guide*") and the *Public Health Service Policy for Humane Care and Use of Laboratory Animals* (known as "*PHS Policy*"). The *Guide* was first published in 1964 as a set of voluntary professional standards covering the housing, care and treatment of verte-brate animals used in biomedical research. It was last revised in 2011 (NAS 2011). In 1985, the Health Research Extension Act made adherence to the *Guide* and the *PHS Policy* (which lays out ethical responsibilities consistent with the Three Rs; PHS 2015) mandatory. An important limitation is that the law only applies to animals used in federally funded research projects, rather than to all animals at the institution. Like the AWA, the *Guide* has very detailed provisions for animal housing, care, and treat-ment, and requires oversight by an IACUC. Enforcement is via the National Institutes of Health Office for Protection from Research Risks (OPRR). The OPRR does not regu-larly inspect institutions but can impose significant financial penalties when noncom-pliances are discovered.

In terms of involuntary regulation, institutional and legal oversight is limited to spe-cies listed in the AWA, in addition to any vertebrate animals used for biomedical research, teaching, or testing as part of a federally funded project. In practice, how-ever, many institutions choose to extend these protections to all vertebrate animals used for these purposes at their institution, regardless of funding source or species. In addition, many institutions that use farm animals for agricultural research also pro-vide oversight for those animals using the *Guide for the Care and Use of Agricultural Animals in Research and Teaching* (*Ag Guide*), a voluntary standard developed by a consortium of professional societies representing animal agricultural scientists (American Dairy Science Association® et al. 2020).

One more voluntary layer of oversight exists – the Association for the Assessment and Accreditation of Laboratory Animal Care International (AAALAC), established in 1965. More than 700 programs in North America are AAALAC accredited (https://www.aaalac.org). AAALAC requires institutional oversight of *all* research, testing, and teaching animals within the certified unit. AAALAC conducts third-party certifi-cation visits of accredited units every three years and uses the *Guide* and *Ag Guide* as primary standards.

## Role of Veterinarians in Improving Animal Welfare

Historically, US veterinarians have had authority with respect to farm animal welfare via enforcement of the HSA, Twenty-Eight Hour Law, and PPIA regulations, as well as state anti-cruelty laws (Hoenig and Coetzee 2018). Given the importance of animal health to animal welfare, veterinarians should have been deeply involved in the evo-lution of farm animal welfare research, technology transfer, and application. Until recently, however, this involvement has been far less than warranted, particularly in the United States (Hoenig and Coetzee 2018). There are probably multiple reasons for this. First, the recommendations in the Brambell Report fostered a strong link between animal behavior and animal welfare. This stimulated the growth of the dis-cipline of applied ethology, but ethology was not emphasized in veterinary training. Second, practicing livestock and poultry veterinarians may have found (and still find) themselves in an ethically and professionally difficult position, trying to support their farmer clients while also imposing unwanted requirements on them or asking them to make potentially costly changes to the housing and management of their animals (see Chapter 12).

It is notable that the situation unfolded differently in the case of laboratory animals, where the role of veterinarians in providing leadership for animal welfare is clearly delineated in the AWA regulations. However, laboratory animal veterinarians initiated animal welfare oversight activities even prior to federal regulation (American Association for Laboratory Animal Science [AALAS] n.d.). In 1950, veterinarians organized the Animal Care Panel (ACP), now known as the American Association for Laboratory Animal Science. The ACP produced the first edition of the *Guide* in 1963, which at that time was a set of voluntary standards available for adoption by research institutions. Specialist training was made available to veterinarians via the incorporation of the American College of Laboratory Animal Medicine (ACLAM) in 1957, only the third specialty board to be recognized by the American Veterinary Medical Association (AVMA). The goal of ACLAM was to provide veterinary training and experience not only in the health of laboratory animals, but in their care.

Whatever the reasons for the difference between veterinary involvement in animal welfare activities in the farm and laboratory animal sectors, the historical trajectory of farm animal welfare research led ethologist Jeff Rushen to state that "we have tended to rely too much on physiological, immune and behavioral measures of welfare, and have not given sufficient weighting to health problems, which are some of the major threats to farm animal welfare" (Rushen 2003). He felt that the underrepresentation of veterinarians on research teams led to an underestimation of the importance of health problems as a source of animal welfare problems. Fortunately, this situation has been changing rapidly, with initiatives by the AVMA and the OIE as well as the research trends described earlier and the increasing importance of voluntary standards and auditing programs.

## AVMA and the Veterinary Oath

The AVMA established an Animal Welfare Committee in 1981. The committee's work is guided by eight principles that encompass both ethical responsibilities and practical guidance about animal care, which state that the "veterinary profession shall continually strive to improve animal health and welfare through scientific research, education, collaboration, advocacy, and the development of legislation and regulations" (AVMA n.d.a). The committee has developed dozens of animal welfare policies with topics ranging from painful practices like beak-trimming and dehorning to housing for egg-laying hens and pregnant sows (AVMA n.d.b).

The AVMA also created an Animal Welfare Division in 2006, and in 2010 approved a revision to the Veterinary Oath that identified animal welfare "as a priority for the veterinary profession" (AVMA 2010). Recently, the AVMA issued a joint statement with the Federation of Veterinarians of Europe and the Canadian Veterinary Medical Association on the roles of veterinarians in promoting animal welfare: "There are both societal and professional expectations for veterinarians to provide leadership in animal welfare ... [and that veterinarians] have a duty to take advantage of multiple opportunities to advocate for animal welfare" (AVMA et al. n.d.). It goes on to list key attributes of veterinarians with respect to animal welfare advocacy, as well as advocacy opportunities. In 2012, the AVMA recognized the American College of Animal Welfare (ACAW) as a veterinary specialization. The goal of the ACAW is to educate veterinarians to an advanced level in "all aspects of animal welfare science and ethics", and approximately 60 veterinarians (B. Kipperman personal communication 2021) are now board-certified in animal welfare through ACAW (https://www.acaw.org).

## OIE

The OIE has been the standards-setting body for intergovernmental animal health since 1924. In 2002, it broadened its mandate to include animal welfare, stating that animal health is a key component of animal welfare. The OIE's animal welfare initiative is described in Escobar et al. (2018). The OIE has adopted 14 sets of standards, most focusing on farmed animals. These standards cover transport of animals by land, sea, and air; slaughter of animals for human consumption and killing for disease control purposes; control of stray dog populations; the use of animals in research and education; welfare of working equids; animal welfare and broiler chicken, beef and dairy cattle production systems; and transport and killing of farmed fish. To help implement the standards, the OIE encourages each member country to nominate individuals from the country's veterinary services to serve as animal welfare focal points.

Although the OIE standards are intended for global application, their impact is likely to be most significant in developing economies in which involuntary and voluntary regulation of animal welfare is weak or absent. Veterinarians are taking a leading role in coordinating expertise, providing training and capacity building, and facilitating OIE animal welfare standards implementation. The OIE has assisted in the development of Regional Animal Welfare Strategies and produced a tool to help identify gaps and weaknesses in local veterinary services to encourage increased investment in those services (Escobar et al. 2018).

### Standards and Auditing

Provisions related to animal health are essential elements of farm animal welfare standards. Typically, standards require that farmers have an established veterinary–client–patient relationship, and that the consulting veterinarian develop an animal health plan that includes information about sourcing of animals, vaccination and other aspects of preventative care, administration of drugs, and procedures to be followed in case of disease or recurring injury. Standards also typically have guidance about biosecurity procedures, animal handling, painful procedures (e.g. castration, dehorning), and on-farm euthanasia and depopulation. Veterinarians are thus key participants in any standards-setting process, whether those standards are written on behalf of trade groups or as part of third-party labeling programs. Animal health research is also needed to provide the underpinnings for evidence-based standards. Hoenig and Coetzee (2018) discuss some of the areas of research (usually carried out by multidisciplinary teams that include veterinarians) that have contributed to understanding and improving farm animal welfare in the United States, including evaluating the effects of analgesic drugs and other pain management strategies; validating biomarkers for pain and distress; developing housing and management interventions to reduce health problems like lameness; developing and refining euthanasia and depopulation methods to ensure humaneness; and developing tools and management strategies to mitigate the negative effects of the mandated reduction in use of medically important antimicrobials on animal health.

Another recent change that highlights the need for veterinary input is the movement toward the use of outcome-based standards for auditing animal welfare (Butterworth et al. 2018). Initially, most animal welfare standards were input-based – that is, they stipulated the resources and management that animals were to be provided, for example, the amount of space and the configuration of the housing facility. However, as farms were audited it became apparent that applying resource-based standards did not always result in improved welfare. Hence, standards and auditing programs are evolving toward allowing farmers more freedom to innovate and using outcome-based measures to assess the effectiveness of those innovations. The focus has been mainly on animal-based measures, where the welfare of the animal is assessed directly rather than using the resources as a proxy. This is the approach taken in the OIE standards. Rather than being prescriptive, the OIE standards provide a list of potential animal-based measures, including a range of health and physical condition measures that can be used to evaluate the impacts of housing and management practices. Veterinarians have multiple roles to play as animal-based standards evolve, by validating measurement methods, conducting epidemiological studies to determine the on-farm incidence of health and physical condition problems, and training farmers and auditors how to use animal-based measures to assess and improve welfare.

## The Future of Veterinary Involvement in Animal Welfare – Concluding Remarks

As public interest in animal welfare intensifies, people will increasingly look to veterinarians to provide expertise and guidance about various issues, from day-to-day aspects of animal management to the development and implementation of public policy. For veterinarians to assume a leadership role will require a different approach to veterinary training and a rethinking of the competencies and values of veterinarians with respect to becoming "advocates" for animal welfare (see Chapter 7). An animal's welfare has three components: basic health and biological functioning, natural behavior, and affective states. These components may sometimes align with one another, but other times do not. For example, the health status of an animal under conditions of close confinement may be better because of a greater ability to control, diagnose, and treat illness, but that comes at the cost of the animal's normal behavior (and the aspects of its affective state related to unfulfilled behavioral wants and needs). Because of their training, veterinarians often prioritize health over the other components of welfare. Kipperman (2015) has argued this prioritization is reflected in the AVMA animal welfare policies related to confinement housing, and results in veterinarians lagging behind society's views of animal welfare rather than providing credible leadership.

Societal perspectives regarding the moral status of animals (and the ways in which they influence scientific research) are continually evolving (see Chapter 1). There has been an expansion of welfare concerns to include fish and invertebrates (Mikhalevich and Powell 2020; Franks et al. 2021), and the UK government recently recognized

lobsters, octopuses, and crabs as sentient beings (DEFRA 2021). There is also a movement toward adopting a more encompassing view of what animal welfare means, to
include not just reducing pain and suffering but providing "good" welfare – meaning
environments and stimulation that create positive experiences for animals (Lawrence
et al. 2019). The influential animal welfare scientist Marian Dawkins (2006) has argued
that good welfare can be operationalized by asking only two questions: is the animal
healthy, *and* does it have what it wants?

Broadening veterinary education is a key element in ensuring that veterinarians can
adopt an integrated view of animal welfare and exercise a leadership role. In 2017, the
AVMA Model Animal Welfare Curriculum Planning Group (Lord et al. 2017) issued a
report recommending additions to the veterinary curriculum to provide adequate
training in animal welfare. Recommendations included providing core instruction in:
animal welfare concepts; scientific and sociological components; welfare assessment
techniques; role of veterinarians, and contemporary social issues. It is notable that the
proposed curriculum includes instruction in ethics, public perception, animal behavior, motivation, and affective states.

## Note

**1** There are other EU directives that have at least some provisions related to animal
welfare; these are discussed in Broom (2019).

## References

American Association for Laboratory Animal Science (AALAS) (n.d.). AALAS timeline.
https://www.aalas.org/about-aalas/history/timeline (accessed 4 February 2022).

American Dairy Science Association®, the American Society of Animal Science, and the
Poultry Science Association (2020). *Guide for the Care and Use of Agricultural Animals
in Research and Teaching*, 4e. Champaign, IL: https://www.asas.org/docs/default-
source/default-document-library/agguide_4th.pdf?sfvrsn=56b44ed1_2 (accessed 7
December 2021).

American Veterinary Medical Association (AVMA) (n.d.a). AVMA animal welfare
principles. https://www.avma.org/resources-tools/avma-policies/avma-animal-welfare-
principles (accessed 3 February 2022).

American Veterinary Medical Association (AVMA) (n.d.b). Animal welfare policy
statements. https://www.avma.org/resources/animal-health-welfare/
animal-welfare-policy-statements.

American Veterinary Medical Association (AVMA) (2010). Veterinarian's Oath revised to
emphasize animal welfare commitment. https://www.avma.org/javma-
news/2011-01-01/veterinarians-oath-revised-emphasize-animal-welfare-commitment
(accessed 4 February 2022).

American Veterinary Medical Association (AVMA), the Federation of Veterinarians of
Europe (FVE), and the Canadian Veterinary Medical Association (CVMA) (n.d.). Joint
AVMA-FVE-CVMA statement on the roles of veterinarians in promoting animal

welfare. https://www.avma.org/resources-tools/avma-policies/joint-avma-fve-cvma-roles-veterinarians-promoting-animal-welfare (accessed 3 February 2022).

Amos, N., Sullivan, R., and Rhys Williams, N. (2020). The business benchmark on farm animal welfare report 2020. https://www.bbfaw.com/media/1942/bbfaw-report-2020.pdf (accessed 7 December 2021).

Animal Welfare Institute (n.d.). A review: The Twenty-Eight Hour Law and its enforcement. https://awionline.org/sites/default/files/uploads/documents/20TwentyEightHourLawReport.pdf (accessed 7 December 2021).

Appleby, M.C. (2003). The European Union ban on conventional cages for laying hens: History and prospects. *Journal of Applied Animal Welfare Science* 6: 103–121. https://doi.org/10.1207/S15327604JAWS0602_03.

Appleby, M.C., Olsson, I.A.S., and Galindo, F. (2018). *Animal Welfare*, 3e. Wallingford, UK: CABI.

AssureWel (n.d.a). Feather loss. http://www.assurewel.org/layinghens/featherloss.html.

AssureWel (n.d.b). Feather loss benchmarking tool. http://www.assurewel.org/layinghens/howisyourfeatherlossmeasuringup.html (accessed 28 December 2021).

Baker, P. and Weeks, C. (2020). *Maintaining Feather Cover in Laying Hens*. London: Laying Hen Welfare Forum.

Baker, P.E., Stokes, J.E., and Weeks, C.A. (2020). Enabling behaviour change in laying hen farmers using motivational interviewing. *Proceedings* 73. https://doi.org/10.3390/IECA2020-08830.

Balzani, A. and Hanlon, A. (2020). Factors that influence farmers' views on farm animal welfare: A semi-systematic review and thematic analysis. *Animals* 10: 1524. https://doi.org/10.3390/ani10091524.

Berckmans, D. (2017). General introduction to precision livestock farming. *Animal Frontiers* 7: 6–11. https://doi:10.2527/af.2017.0102.

Blokhuis, H., Miele, M., and Blokhuis, H.J. (eds.) (2013). *Improving Farm Animal Welfare: Science and Society Working Together. The Welfare Quality Approach*. Wageningen, the Netherlands: Wageningen Academic Publishers.

Brambell, F.W.R. (1967 reprinted). Report of the technical committee to enquire into the welfare of animals kept under intensive livestock husbandry systems. Command Report 2836. London: Her Majesty's Stationary Office. http://edepot.wur.nl/134379 (accessed 7 December 2021).

Broom, D.M. (2019). Animal Welfare in the European Union. https://op.europa.eu/en/publication-detail/-/publication/74df7b49-ffe7-11e6-8a35-01aa75ed71a1/language-en (accessed 22 December 2021).

Butterworth, A., Mench, J.A., Wielebnowski, N. et al. (2018). Practical strategies to assess (and improve) animal welfare. In: *Animal Welfare*, 3e (eds. M.C. Appleby, I.A.S. Olsson, and F. Galindo), 232–250. Wallingford, UK: CABI.

California Department of Food and Agriculture (CDFA) (2018). Animal Care Program. Proposition 12, Farm Animal Confinement. https://www.cdfa.ca.gov/AHFSS/Prop12.html (accessed 3 February 2022).

Cornish, A., Raubenheimer, D., and McGreevy, P. (2016). What we know about the public's level of concern for farm animal welfare in food production in developed countries. *Animals* 6: 74. https://doi.org/10.3390/ani6110074.

Dawkins, M. (2006). A user's guide to animal welfare science. *Trends in Ecology & Evolution* 21: 77–82. https://doi.org/10.1016/j.tree.2005.10.017.

Dawkins, M.S., Wang, L., Ellwood, S.A. et al. (2021). Optical flow, behaviour and broiler chicken welfare in the UK and Switzerland. *Applied Animal Behaviour Science* 234: 105180. https://doi.org/10.1016/j.applanim.2020.105180.

Department for Environment, Food and Rural Affairs (DEFRA) (2021). Lobsters, octopus, and crabs recognized as sentient beings. https://www.gov.uk/government/news/lobsters-octopus-and-crabs-recognised-as-sentient-beings (accessed 7 December 2021).

Ede, T., Lecorps, B., von Keyserlingk, M.A.G. et al. (2019). Scientific assessment of affective states in dairy cattle. *Journal of Dairy Science* 102: 10677–10694. https://doi.org/10.3168/jds.2019-16325.

Escobar, L.S., Jara, W.H., Nizam, Q.N.H. et al. (2018). The perspective of the World Organisation for Animal Health. In: *Advances in Agricultural Animal Welfare: Science and Practice* (ed. J.A. Mench), 169–182. Oxford, UK: Woodhead Publishing.

Farm Animal Welfare Council (FAWC) (2012 archived). Five Freedoms. https://webarchive.nationalarchives.gov.uk/20121010012427/www.fawc.org.uk/freedoms.htm (accessed 7 December 2021).

Franks, B., Ewell, C., and Jacquet, J. (2021). Animal welfare risks of global aquaculture. *Science Advances* 7: eabg0677. https://doi.org/10.1126/sciadv.abg0677.

Fraser, D. (2008). *Understanding Animal Welfare: The Science in Its Cultural Context.* Oxford, UK: Wiley Blackwell.

Fraser, D. and Nicol, C.J. (2018). Preference and motivation research. In: *Animal Welfare*, 3e (eds. M.C. Appleby, I.A.S. Olsson, and F. Galindo), 213–231. Wallingford, UK: CABI.

Fraser, D., Duncan, I.J.H., Edwards, S.A. et al. (2013). General principles for the welfare of animals in production systems: The underlying science and its application. *The Veterinary Journal* 198: 19–27. https://doi.org/10.1016/j.tvjl.2013.06.028.

Fraser, D., Koralesky, K.E., and Urton, G. (2018). Toward a harmonized approach to animal welfare law in Canada. *Canadian Veterinary Journal* 59: 293–302.

Gallo, C.S. and Tadich, T.G. (2018). Perspective from Latin America. In: *Advances in Agricultural Animal Welfare: Science and Practice* (ed. J.A. Mench), 197–218. Oxford, UK: Woodhead Publishing.

Graber, R. and Keller, J. (2020). Infographic: Retailers' cage-free egg pledges. https://www.wattagnet.com/articles/39998-infographic-retailers-cage-free-egg-pledges (accessed 3 February 2022).

Grandin, T. (ed.) (2021a). *Improving Animal Welfare: A Practical Approach*, 3E. Wallingford, UK: CABI.

Grandin, T. (2021b). The effect of economic factors on the welfare of livestock and poultry. In: *Improving Animal Welfare: A Practical Approach*, 3e (ed. T. Grandin), 300–313. Wallingford, UK: CABI.

Grimm, D. (2021). How many mice and rats are housed in US labs? Controversial study says more than 100 million. https://www.science.org/content/article/how-many-mice-and-rats-are-used-us-labs-controversial-study-says-more-100-million (accessed 7 December 2021).

Harrison, R. (1964). *Animal Machines.* London: Vincent Stuart Ltd.

Hoenig, D.E. and Coetzee, J.F. (2018). Perspectives on the emerging role of US veterinarians in education, policy, politics, and research. In: *Advances in Agricultural Animal Welfare: Science and Practice* (ed. J.A. Mench), 145–166. Oxford, UK: Woodhead Publishing.

Keeling, L., Evans, A., Forkman, B. et al. (2013). Welfare Quality principles and criteria. In: *Improving Farm Animal Welfare: Science and Society Working Together. The Welfare*

*Quality Approach* (eds. H. Blokhuis, M. Miele, and H.J. Blokhuis), 91–114. Wageningen, the Netherlands: Wageningen Academic Publishers.

Kipperman, B.S. (2015). The role of the veterinary profession in promoting animal welfare. *Journal of the American Veterinary Medical Association* 246: 502–504. https://doi.org/10.2460/javma.246.5.502.

Knierem, U. and Pajor, E.A. (2018). Regulation, enforcement and incentives. In: *Animal Welfare*, 3e (eds. M.C. Appleby, I.A.S. Olsson, and F. Galindo), 349–361. Wallingford, UK: CABI.

Lambton, S.L., Knowles, T.G., Yorke, C. et al. (2010). The risk factors affecting the development of gentle and severe feather pecking in loose housed laying hens. *Applied Animal Behaviour Science* 123: 32–42. https://doi.org/10.1016/j.applanim.2009.12.010.

Lambton, S.L., Nicol, C.J., Friel, M. et al. (2013). A bespoke management package can reduce levels of injurious pecking in loose-housed laying hen flocks. *The Veterinary Record* 172: 423–423. https://doi.org/10.1136/vr.101067.

Lawrence, A.B., Vigors, B., and Sandøe, P. (2019). What is so positive about positive animal welfare? – A critical review of the literature. *Animals* 9: 783. https://doi.org/10.3390/ani9100783.

Lord, L.K, Millman, S.T, Carbone, L. et al. (2017). A model curriculum for the study of animal welfare in colleges and schools of veterinary medicine. *Journal of the American Veterinary Medical Association* 250(6):632–640.

Lundmark, F., Berg, C., and Röcklinsberg, H. (2018). Private animal welfare standards – opportunities and risks. *Animals* 8: 4. https://doi.org/10.3390/ani8010004.

Lusk, J.L. (2019). Consumer preferences for cage-free eggs and impacts of retailer pledges. *Agribusiness* 35: 129–148. https://doi.org/10.1002/agr.21580.

Mellor, D. (2017). Operational details of the Five Domains model and its key applications to the assessment and management of animal welfare. *Animals* 7: 60. https://doi.org/10.3390/ani7080060.

Mellor, D.J., Beausoleil, N.J., Littlewood, K.E. et al. (2020). The 2020 Five Domains model: Including human–animal interactions in assessments of animal welfare. *Animals* 10: 1870. https://doi.org/10.3390/ani10101870.

Mench, J.A. (2008). Farm animal welfare in the U.S.A.: Farming practices, research, education, regulation, and assurance programs. *Applied Animal Behaviour Science* 113: 298–312. https://doi.org/10.1016/j.applanim.2008.01.009.

Mench, J.A. (2018). Science in the real world – benefits for researchers and farmers. In: *Advances in Agricultural Animal Welfare: Science and Practice* (ed. J.A. Mench), 111–128. Oxford, UK: Woodhead Publishing.

Mikhalevich, I. and Powell, R. (2020). Minds without spines: Evolutionarily inclusive animal ethics. *Animal Sentience* 5. https://doi.org/10.51291/2377-7478.1527.

More, S.J., Hanlon, A., Marchewka, J. et al. (2017). Private animal health and welfare standards in quality assurance programmes: A review and proposed framework for critical evaluation. *The Veterinary Record* 180: 612–612. https://doi.org/10.1136/vr.104107.

National Agricultural Law Center (2021). States' Animal Cruelty Statutes. https://nationalaglawcenter.org/state-compilations/animal-cruelty (accessed 7 December 2021).

National Academy of Sciences (NAS) (2011). *Guide for the Care and Use of Laboratory Animals*. Washington, DC: National Academy Press.

OIE (2021). What is animal welfare? https://www.oie.int/en/what-we-do/animal-health-and-welfare/animal-welfare (accessed 28 December 2021).

Palczynski, L., Buller, H., Lambton, S. et al. (2016). Farmer attitudes to injurious pecking in laying hens and to potential control strategies. *Animal Welfare* 25: 29–38. https://doi.org/10.7120/09627286.25.1.029.

Public Health Service (PHS) (2015). Public health service policy on humane care and use of laboratory animals. https://grants.nih.gov/grants/olaw/references/phspolicylabanimals.pdf (accessed 7 December 2021).

Rushen, J. (2003). Changing concepts of farm animal welfare: Bridging the gap between applied and basic research. *Applied Animal Behaviour Science* 81: 199–214. https://doi.org/10.1016/S0168-1591(02)00281-2.

Russell, W.M.S. and Burch, R.L. (1959). *The Principles of Humane Experimental Technique*. London: Methuen and Company.

Simonin, D. and Gavinelli, A. (2019). The European Union legislation on animal welfare: State of play, enforcement, and future activities. In: *Animal Welfare: From Science to Law* (eds. S. Hild and L. Schweitzer), 59–69. Paris: La Foundation Droit Animal, Éthique et Sciences. https://www.fondation-droit-animal.org/documents/AnimalWelfare2019.v1.pdf (accessed 7 December 2021).

Thornber, P.M. and Mellor, D.J. (2018). Perspective from Asia, Far East and Oceania, and the Middle East. In: *Advances in Agricultural Animal Welfare: Science and Practice* (ed. J.A. Mench), 183–196. Oxford, UK: Woodhead Publishing.

Thorpe, W.H. (1969). Welfare of domestic animals. *Nature* 224: 18–20.

Toschi Maciel, C. and Bock, B. (2013). Modern politics in animal welfare: The changing character of governance of animal welfare and the role of private standards. *The International Journal of Sociology of Agriculture and Food* 20: 219–235. https://doi.org/10.48416/IJSAF.V20I2.193.

United Egg Producers (n.d.). Facts and stats. https://unitedegg.com/facts-stats (accessed 3 February 2022).

van Erp-van der Kooij, E. and Rutter, S.M. (2020). Using precision farming to improve animal welfare. *CAB Reviews* 15. https://doi.org/10.1079/PAVSNNR202015051.

Vasbinder, M.A., Hawk, C.T., and Bennett, B.T. (2014). Regulations, policies, and guidelines impacting laboratory animal welfare. In: *Laboratory Animal Welfare* (eds. K. Bayne and P. Turner), 17–28. Amsterdam: Elsevier. https://doi.org/10.1016/B978-0-12-385103-1.00003-8.

Vogeler, C.S. (2020). Politicizing farm animal welfare: A comparative study of policy change in the United States of America. *Journal of Comparative Policy Analysis: Research and Practice* 23: 526–543. https://doi.org/10.1080/13876988.2020.1742069.

Walker, M., Diez-Leon, M., and Mason, G. (2014). Animal welfare science: Recent publication trends and future research priorities. *International Journal of Comparative Psychology*. 27: 80–100. https://escholarship.org/uc/item/1vx5q0jt (accessed 7 December 2021).

Welfare Quality (n.d.). Assessment protocols. http://www.welfarequality.net/en-us/reports/assessment-protocols (accessed 3 February 2022).

Whay, H.R. (2007). The journey to animal welfare improvement. *Animal Welfare* 16: 117–122.

Whay, H.R., Mullan, S., and Main, D.C. (2021). Improving animal care and welfare: Practical approaches for achieving change. In: *Improving Animal Welfare: A Practical Approach*, 3e (ed. T. Grandin), 314–336. Wallingford, UK: CABI.

## 3

# Animal Ethics and the Evolution of the Veterinary Profession in the United States

*Bernard Unti*

## Historical Summary

Animal ethics, a moral concern for animals' interests and well-being, did not figure prominently in the earliest years of veterinary medicine in the United States. With notable exceptions such as Benjamin Rush's 1807 statement about ethical values (Rush 1808), the humane treatment of animals was largely absent from veterinary discourse in the United States before the 1860s. Instead, the primary focus of veterinary leaders was to establish the profession's status, legitimacy, and educational institutions. In the years following the Civil War, veterinarians found viable livelihoods and asserted their authority in a range of matters bearing on the treatment and care of animals, working closely with local, state, and federal government and other stakeholders. Collaborating with the newly formed societies for the prevention of cruelty to animals on public health, safety, and humane concerns, veterinarians began to engage more meaningfully with matters of ethical importance.

The creation of the Bureau of Animal Industry (BAI) within the federal government in 1884 marked the advent of an influential veterinary establishment. The BAI championed a centralized, professional, and scientific approach to the management of animals as resources and the nationwide protection of human health and economic interests tied to animal production. The BAI's primary focus was its responsibility to the American public to establish the safety of the human food supply by ensuring the health of domestic animals used for food and fiber.

At the dawn of the twentieth century, the transition from horsepower to mechanized transportation and the emergence of a modern industrial economy created apprehensions about the future of veterinary medicine and prompted new shifts in practice and focus. By the middle decades of the twentieth century, changing attitudes toward animals and the influence of a revitalized animal protection movement presented other challenges. As the twentieth century closed, continuing social, demographic, technological, and economic transformations triggered additional changes, making animal ethics ever more important for individual veterinarians and veterinary educational institutions.

Contemporary veterinary medicine is a profession whose members provide care to animals, domestic and wild; help to manage the health and welfare of animals raised for food and other purposes; protect public health by working to safeguard the food

*Ethics in Veterinary Practice: Balancing Conflicting Interests*, First Edition. Edited by Barry Kipperman and Bernard E. Rollin.
© 2022 John Wiley & Sons, Inc. Published 2022 by John Wiley & Sons, Inc.

supply; and contribute to preventing the spread of zoonotic diseases and illness. The nexus between animal health, animal welfare, and human welfare has never been stronger. Given the heightened moral concern for animals now evident throughout American society, veterinarians have ethical, social, political, scientific, and practical responsibilities beyond what even the profession's most foresighted pioneers could have dreamed.

## The Quest for Legitimacy, Status, and Identity (1700–1880)

Before the advent of organized veterinary medicine, the care of animals in North America was rooted in folk treatments and procedures undertaken by do-it-yourselfers and lay practitioners including farriers (horse shoers), blacksmiths, cow leeches, stock raisers, farmers, medicine hawkers, and assorted "quacks" (Smithcors 1963). By the late eighteenth century, expanding livestock populations and concern about disease outbreaks that threatened domestic animals prompted calls for professional education. Benjamin Rush (1745–1813), physician and signer of the Declaration of Independence, was one of the earliest proponents of the study of animal disease in the United States. In an 1807 address, Rush spoke of the need to attend to "the health of those domestic animals which constitute a part of our aliment, in order to prevent our contracting disease by eating them." Rush included a moral argument, too, affirming the human obligation to treat animals kindly and lessen their miseries. He cited the works of David Hartley (1705–1757), a pioneer of utilitarian philosophy who had written on animal intelligence; John Hildrop (d. 1756), author of a book arguing that animals had immortal souls; the Genesis-derived concept of stewardship; and the common principle that the service of animals warranted them due consideration (Rush 1808; Blaisdell 1990; Unti 2002).

Individuals like Rush and the English veterinarian William Youatt (1839) were exceptions, however, in their focus on humane principles. Given its practical and utilitarian origins in agricultural practice and the care and husbandry of working animals, veterinary medicine lacked a focus on humane ethics in its early years. A rudimentary ethics emerged with the establishment of the first veterinary colleges and the long transition of veterinary practice from farriery and other tradesman's occupations to an authentic scientific profession. To the extent that it existed at all, veterinary ethics centered on business practices, sound production and husbandry procedures, and public health responsibilities rather than humane concern for animals.

There were few professionally educated veterinarians in the country at this time and those identifying themselves as practitioners included a few individuals trained in Europe and the UK as well as the farriers, farmers, medical doctors, tonic salesmen, and other self-taught specialists who treated horses and cattle. Anyone interested in learning about veterinary care could do so through the frequently reprinted books of English veterinarians like Edward Mayhew and Youatt, or from the more popular advice manuals that circulated widely. Some works offered sensible suggestions pertaining to improved sanitation in stables, isolation or destruction of diseased horses, and proper feeding and nutrition. However, suggested remedies also included extreme "heroic" measures still used in human medicine at the time, like bleeding, blistering, emetics, and lead or mercury-based compounds. As was the case in human medicine, veterinary diagnostics remained poor (Youatt 1839; Mayhew 1865; McShane and Tarr 2007).

In the mid-nineteenth century, cities were full of animals, encompassing domestic, semidomesticated, and undomesticated species. Urban horse populations rapidly expanded and cattle, dairy cows, pigs, sheep, and chickens, along with corrals, dairy stalls, feedlots, ranches, and slaughterhouses, were dispersed throughout cities. Such animals existed primarily to satisfy the needs of humans and the demands of a burgeoning urban industrial order. As a result, animals were incorporated into the metropolitan economy during the years leading up to the Civil War. This provided professional opportunities and made possible full-time careers in the veterinary field. Veterinarians provided care for the most economically valued animals to safeguard their health and the profits of their owners (Teigen 2000; Unti 2002; Robichaud 2019).

Veterinary medicine was a largely urban profession treating the equine populations of America's growing cities and the number of veterinarians in practice was small. Calls for practitioners with better training prompted the founding of private urban veterinary colleges and short-lived schools opened in Massachusetts, New York, and Philadelphia in the 1850s. The epizootics that occurred after the Civil War catalyzed the further growth of veterinary institutions. By 1879, of the first 6 veterinary colleges founded in the United States, just 4 were in operation, but between 1879 and 1900, 19 new schools opened (Smithcors 1963; Greene 2008).

The profession's ranks filled out under the dynamic leadership of foreign-born educators who pushed for a science-based discipline, a focus on public health, educational institutions with rigorous admissions standards, and government support for education and research. The era's most prominent veterinarians included Alexandre Liautard (France) and James Law (Scotland), who would both help to educate some of the most important figures in the field (Smithcors 1963; Dunlop and Williams 1996; Murnane 2008).

Liautard (1835–1918), founder of the American Veterinary College and Hospital (1875–1899), was the driving force behind the formation of the United States Veterinary Medical Association (USVMA). He also edited the *American Veterinary Review*, the most important manifestation of the developing profession, from 1877 to 1915. On a monthly basis, the journal presented a digest of articles and abstracts from foreign journals, accounts of cases, news concerning local associations, licensure and veterinary practice acts, and editorials. American authors contributed articles on a range of topics, mostly featuring clinical observations rather than reports of experimental work (Smithcors 1963).

By the mid-1860s, the call for professionally trained veterinary scientists gained urgency in light of recurrent and severe outbreaks of disease in cattle, hogs, sheep, and horses, which resulted in massive animal losses. With respect to the nation's urban equine population, the Great Epizootic of the 1870s, an equine influenza outbreak that crippled transportation and commerce in major cities along the eastern seaboard, marked an important juncture. As part of their response, municipal health boards began to value, assume, and employ veterinary authority. Veterinarians affiliated with these boards had the power to condemn diseased and unsound animals and to impose quarantine rules for reducing transmission of glanders and other illnesses (Unti 2002; McShane and Tarr 2007; Murnane 2008; Freeberg 2020).

The emergence of organized animal protection in the 1860s provided a direct stimulus to the consideration of ethics in veterinary medicine. Animal protection was a movement dedicated to improving the treatment of animals on moral grounds. After Henry Bergh launched the American Society for the Prevention of Cruelty to Animals (ASPCA) in 1866, societies for the prevention of cruelty to animals proliferated throughout the United States, pursuing an ambitious agenda involving the mitigation and elimination of pain and suffering, by educating the public and raising social expectations about the importance of proper care for animals, including those whose owners could not afford veterinary services. Its founders were influential, wealthy, and passionate about their cause.

To some extent, the underdeveloped character of American veterinary medicine in this period left the dissemination of veterinary knowledge and counsel to humane organizations. They positioned themselves as sources of information and action concerning animal care, training, and veterinary health matters, especially in relation to urban horse populations. Most animal protectionists, like most veterinarians, lived and worked in cities, and their welfare concerns were almost entirely tied to problems arising from the rapid incorporation of animals into the urban environment. They were active in debates about the effects of street salting on horses' hooves and legs, the treatment of glanders and farcy, the removal of exhausted, injured, or dead animals from the streets, and the training and care of balky, uncooperative work horses. Moreover, societies for the prevention of cruelty to animals were strong boosters of professional veterinary education (Unti 2002; Jones 2003).

Law, Liautard, and other veterinarians were advisers in matters that came within the ambit of humane organizations, testifying in cruelty cases, investigating the adulterated milk trade (which relied on cows fed exclusively on grain mash from distilleries and breweries), participating in efforts to regulate the sale of horses in local markets, and speaking out about streetcar cruelties and other concerns. Occasionally, too, as Law did in *The Farmer's Veterinary Adviser* (1876), they condemned "barbarous surgery," "reckless and destructive drugging," "absolute and painful poisoning," and "cruel and injurious vivisection" by unqualified practitioners, an indictment of irresponsible treatment on humane grounds (Smithcors 1963). The ASPCA supported a measure to exclude quacks from veterinary practice in 1878, and ASPCA founder Henry Bergh was a speaker at Liautard's American Veterinary College. In Philadelphia, the Pennsylvania SPCA and the University of Pennsylvania School of Veterinary Medicine had important benefactors in common (Loew 2001; Unti 2002).

Veterinarians and humane advocates who worked together experienced an interesting complementarity. Veterinarians had an unsentimental and clinical view toward animals, generally focusing on their utilitarian value, while humane advocates tended to emphasize sentimental feelings. This did not in itself create great tension. Veterinarians discovered that the broader embrace of an ethic of concern for animals promised benefits to the profession and its status, while understanding that it came with a certain cost. Humanitarians' unyielding focus on the alleviation of pain and suffering in animals presented a moral and practical challenge for a profession that, like human medicine, had largely neglected such concern.

For their part, animal advocates learned to appreciate the value of practical arguments and frequently sounded the note of human self-interest in taking better care of animals, stressing the probability that kind treatment would bring rewards in the form of animals' longer years of usefulness, health, and/or enhanced market value. It was not a heartfelt argument but rather one that acknowledged the realities of a world in which animals were going to be widely used and abused. This realism manifested itself in all aspects of animal protection work and was evident in the pamphlets that humane societies produced about the handling and treatment of horses and other draft animals. It buttressed the case for improved cattle cars, too, as humanitarians emphasized the elimination of "shrinkage" – the severe loss of stock and animal flesh during transportation to market (Unti 2002; Greene 2008).

There were exceptions to the comity between veterinarians and humane advocates. Many veterinarians accepted or strongly favored vivisection, the experimental use of animals, while humane advocates supported its restriction or abolition. Some veterinarians also carried out procedures like docking (the amputation of horses' tails as a whim of fashion) to which animal protectionists objected. In addition, the profession's gender biases did not always conduce to harmonious relations with the women who predominated within the nineteenth century humane movement (Unti 2002).

Veterinarians were not always in perfect alignment with one another, either. There was an uneasy relationship between veterinarians focused on practical relief of animal suffering and illness (like those who worked in equine practice) and those devoted to bacteriology, laboratory science, and the treatment of livestock herds – a division partly generational and partly ideological. As germ theory emerged as a transformative medical paradigm, educators like Liautard became strong champions, seeking to center veterinary science and practice on the essential challenges of disease control within animal husbandry (McShane and Tarr 2007; Greene 2008).

This emphasis helped to define the mission of veterinary schools associated with public universities. The establishment of 10 state-supported veterinary schools between 1879 and 1918 was decisive in solidifying the professional status of the practicing veterinarian, and in spelling the end of the private colleges that had been the norm for several decades. USVMA meetings were frequent occasions for spirited debate over curriculum standards, entrance requirements, and length of study. State schools were concerned about losing students due to the lower entrance requirements and shorter terms of the private schools. Private schools feared the growing prestige of their new competition, with good reason. The state schools were backed by steady funding, and gatekeeping measures placed both the BAI and the USVMA (rechristened the American Veterinary Medical Association [AVMA] in 1898) in a stronger position to shape and ensure the strength of their curricula and the caliber of their graduates. The state schools, moreover, attracted instructors who could pursue original research as well as teaching, in an atmosphere of freedom and stability that few could attain at the private institutions (Smithcors 1963, 1975; Miller 1981; Loew 2001).

The establishment of worthy institutions of higher learning was essential to the ambitious agenda of leading veterinary educators. In an 1878 report to the Pennsylvania Board of Agriculture, reprinted in the *American Veterinary Review*, Law sought to lift the sights of the field and the broader society to the larger question of animal diseases communicable to humankind. In its way, it was an ethical project, one designed not only to enhance the profession but to serve the public interest as a matter of the highest moral responsibility. Law argued for specialized qualifications in public health, proposing "a new style of practitioner, more comprehensively educated and equipped than either physician or veterinarian" (Law 1878). In the same year, Liautard, citing the threat of zoonotic diseases, urged the inclusion of veterinarians on local and state boards of health and the establishment of a national "Veterinary Sanitary Bureau" to which state authorities should report. An increasing number of states began establishing the official position of state veterinarian to oversee agricultural and other interests involving animals (Smithcors 1963).

## The Advent of a Veterinary Regime (1880–1925)

In her sociological study of veterinary medicine's origins, Joanna Swabe applied the concept of a veterinary "regime" encompassing "the social practices and institutionalized behaviors that have emerged in response to the problem of maintaining animal resources and protecting human health and economy" (Swabe 1999). This concept is useful for framing the developments associated with the profession's acceptance of germ theory and the establishment of bacteriology as a discipline, the growing influence of university-based veterinary schools, and the creation of a federal bureaucracy devoted to veterinary science and its application to the management of America's food supply. All these developments reinforced veterinarians' claim to authority and status and strengthened the institutions where the new science was taking hold.

By the 1880s, the nationalization and professionalization of American public health was well underway, and local and state public health agencies, the Department of Agriculture, and, ultimately, the US Public Health Service, were all recruiting veterinarians. With the formation of the BAI in 1884, the power of the federal government reinforced veterinarians' status and scientific authority. Now they became central players in the national effort to control and eradicate animal disease, regulate animal transportation, and ensure proper inspection of the meat supply (Smithcors 1975; Unti 2002; Jones 2003).

Daniel Salmon was the natural choice to head the BAI for he had gained notable attention with his investigation of fowl cholera and was a champion of the germ theory. During two decades of service as the BAI's chief, he helped to inaugurate the federal meat inspection system, led efforts to eradicate outbreaks of hoof-and-mouth disease and bovine pleuropneumonia, organized a framework for the control of Texas tick fever and hog cholera, established modern quarantine requirements for imported animals, and more. Salmon took a broad view of the profession's contributions to the study of animal disease. He thought its primary achievements included its roles in elucidating contagious infection, the development of aseptic surgery, the emergence of scientific disinfection, and the use of bacterial products, vaccines, animal extracts, and antitoxins for the treatment of animal disease (Smithcors 1963).

Many of these professional advances came in the wake of growing anxieties within and outside of government that inadequate safeguards to contain and eliminate the spread of contagious disease would lead other countries to prohibit the importation of American animals and animal products. Import restrictions by Great Britain based on concern over contagious pleuropneumonia in cattle in 1878 and by several European nations anxious about trichinae in pork products in 1889 brought things to a head. With the support of meat packers, livestock producers, and other stakeholders, the US Congress passed a Federal Meat Inspection Act in 1890. Additional legislation in 1891 and 1895 to address antemortem and postmortem veterinary inspections and export certification processes would be required to reassure America's trade partners (Smithcors 1963, 1975).

Via the BAI and other entities, veterinarians trained in microbiology could distinguish themselves as responders to severe outbreaks of animal disease. Limited funding and other restraints made the early years difficult, but the agency's success in eradicating outbreaks of pleuropneumonia in the west strengthened public confidence as did its work on Texas tick fever, hog cholera, and bovine tuberculosis, and its successful production of tetanus and diphtheria antitoxin. Veterinarians were claiming their place within a growing web of scientific professions and practices in a rapidly modernizing America (Smithcors 1975; McShane and Tarr 2007).

Salmon made a good-faith effort to cooperate with humane organizations in the enforcement of the Twenty-Eight Hour Law (1873), which required that carriers involved with interstate shipping of cattle must unload the animals every 28 hours to provide them with 5 hours of rest, watering, and feeding. The law was the result of an organized campaign by humanitarians concerned about the hardship and suffering endured by domestic livestock in railroad transit from the western range to midwestern and eastern slaughter plants, and anxiety about the effects of fever, disease, and poor welfare conditions on the animals and ultimately the meat produced from their slaughter (Unti 2002).

From the start, the law was poorly enforced and the BAI, whatever its will to achieve compliance, was understaffed and politically overmatched by the railroad and shipping interests. By 1905, they would succeed in watering down the law through political lobbying and other pressure. Moreover, the veterinary regime embodied in the BAI and related agencies defined animal welfare in terms of enhanced productivity and freedom from disease rather than standards of humane treatment, and this limited the agency's resolve to address concerns raised by animal protectionists. Nonetheless, Salmon would frame his career "as a contest against cruel and useless forms of treatment for very common diseases of animals," and veterinary historian J.F. Smithcors sought to give the agency's work a moral cast with his suggestion that Salmon and his colleagues had overcome a fundamental problem – the general indifference of society – members of the public, officials, and livestock owners, among others, to the need for a trained focus on disease threats in agriculture (Smithcors 1963; Unti 2002).

Ironically, given his dedicated service, Salmon was a victim of the scandals triggered by Upton Sinclair's work *The Jungle* (1906). In this explosive exposé, Sinclair highlighted the exploitation and harsh treatment of immigrant workers in Chicago's slaughtering district. But its real impact was in stoking up public anxiety about health violations and unsanitary practices in the meatpacking industry. Bad conditions were prevalent, especially in smaller establishments. The ensuing Federal Meat Inspection Act of 1906 brought about reforms that many veterinarians within and outside of the BAI had been recommending for years, including more inspectors and a broader scope of inspection (Smithcors 1963, 1975).

The profession's substantial orientation toward agriculture between 1880 and 1925 was evident in the most common avenues for veterinary employment apart from equine practice. These included the US Army; the BAI; state, county, and district agencies; municipal meat and dairy operations requiring inspectors; disease commissions; universities; and livestock-related practice. In this period, veterinarians served mainly as stewards of public health and the economic interests of livestock agriculture.

While animal ethics gained only limited purchase within the veterinary profession's educational, policy, and practice agenda in this era, the early decades of the twentieth century produced dramatic changes with lasting implications for ethics as well as practice. Henry Ford's perfection of the gasoline-powered automobile would transform veterinary medicine, leading veterinarians to reinvent themselves for an era in which the motor vehicle replaced the horse as the principal means of transportation and conveyance. The attending shifts in focus and activity powerfully shaped the profession's engagement with questions of ethics and the status of animals.

## Veterinary Practice and Policy in the Era of Animal Ethics (1925–2000)

Bernard Rollin (1943-2021) suggested that positivism (the idea that scientific knowledge is the only authentic knowledge) effectively distanced veterinary medicine for much of its history from ethics (Rollin 1999). Even so, veterinarians who supported the work of organized animal protection in the nineteenth and early twentieth centuries were part of a larger ethical reorientation that Rollin described as a transition from the realm of personal ethics to that of social consensus ethics (see Chapter 4). In the ensuing years, the question of animals' treatment, once widely considered a matter of purely personal ethics, gradually, steadily, and definitively evolved into a widespread social consensus that cruelty was wrong. This developing consensus, moreover, reinforced a longstanding principle that there was a legitimate social interest in how others treated animals, including their own animate property (Unti 2002).

Beginning in the mid-twentieth century, thinkers and advocates including Rachel Carson, Rosalie Edge, Mohandas Gandhi, Joseph Wood Krutch, and Albert Schweitzer began to assert claims for a deeper commitment to animals. By the 1980s, scholars including Carol J. Adams, Brigid Brophy, Michael W. Fox, Mary Midgley, Tom Regan, Roslind Godlovitch, and Peter Singer helped to establish the status of animals as an important subject of philosophical and public debate. This provided energy and vision for a strongly resurgent animal protection movement in the 1980s (Nash 1989; Fraser 1999).

Veterinarians have not universally viewed rising public interest in animal welfare as a positive thing, and their professional associations have sometimes had a hard time keeping up with evolving societal ethics. Perhaps the greatest institutional challenge for veterinary medicine in the twentieth century came with the emergence of intensive confinement agriculture, which made veterinarians technical managers of herd health. To the extent that many veterinarians defined themselves as the protectors of the livestock economy in the interests of human health, it came at a cost, for they increasingly found themselves essentially in service to animal use industries and not necessarily free to shape the moral and ethical debate over such use.

Veterinarians also had to maintain a balancing act quite different from peers in the medical profession. Satisfying the needs of clients for professional service on the grounds of economic or other interests on the one hand, and addressing humane and ethical concerns on the other, created dilemmas for practitioners in a host of scenarios relating to animal use in laboratories, agricultural facilities, circuses, rodeos, zoos, racetracks, performance, sport, and other venues. In all these situations veterinarians confronted potential conflicts of interest over the needs of animals versus the needs of the client/operator (Rollin 1999; Jones 2003) (see Chapter 7).

Significant changes in animal use patterns beginning in the early twentieth century carried great implications for veterinary medicine and set the stage for some of these tensions. As a primary effect, the gradual decline of the equine population due to mechanization slowed the profession's growth. The private veterinary colleges, some of which had operated hospital clinics, went out of business, their prospects for servicing the horses of the urban industrial economy diminished. A massive decline in school enrollment occurred following World War I; the total number of veterinary students in North American schools fell 75% between 1914 and 1924 (Jones 2003). The steadiest channel of employment remained that associated with livestock and public health, an avenue of opportunity powerfully shaped by the BAI. In 1908, the agency employed over 800 veterinarians, some 7% of the total number in the United States. By 1921 the agency provided full-time employment for 1500 veterinarians (10% of the whole profession) and part-time employment for countless others (Jones 2003).

The veterinary profession's expansion to small animal medicine was not seamless, as standards of practice and responsibility did not generally meet those in better established areas of focus. Major hospitals for small animals were rare in the early twentieth century. Among university veterinary schools, only Cornell and the University of Pennsylvania had them. Moreover, while affluent citizens could afford the services of a private veterinarian for dogs, cats, and other small animal pets, such care remained outside the financial reach of many people. Nonetheless, a growing number of veterinarians began to move into small animal practice, as petkeeping became more popular and a pet-oriented consumer culture emerged (Jones 2003; Grier 2006; Teigen 2012). J.C. Flynn, an early advocate for companion animal practice and professionalism in caring for dogs and other small animals, joined with others to support that goal, founding the American Animal Hospital Association in 1933 (Smithcors 1963).

Humane societies too, were shifting their focus from the horse toward companion animals and especially toward the animal control challenges posed by the stray dog and cat populations, the promotion of pet adoptions, and the need for companion animal veterinary care in their communities. Several of the largest humane organizations, including the ASPCA and the Massachusetts SPCA, built impressive animal hospitals during the first decades of the twentieth century and established themselves as leaders in innovation and practice (Unti 2002).

As small animal practice came into its own in the 1920s, veterinarians grew unhappy with animal protection groups' shift toward providing animal care. In 1928, the AVMA passed a resolution reflecting its concern with the encroachment of humane society services upon private practices, and the issue came out into the open as representatives of the profession and organized animal protection attempted to reconcile their differences (Smithcors 1963; Unti 2002).

The perception that humane societies were in competition with veterinary practitioners created tensions that would last well into the post-World War II era. The battle between the two communities focused on the operation of full-service veterinary clinics providing medical care at reduced rates to the public. In 1959, veterinarians sought to halt the operation of spay/neuter clinics by humane societies, and in a highly publicized case from the 1980s, a civil suit brought by a Michigan veterinary association drew support not only from the AVMA but from individual practitioners in 30 states. The battle spilled into the realm of federal and state legislation and even to petitions for an Internal Revenue Service ruling regarding taxation status (Unti 2002, 2004). Shelters and rescue groups have long sought to persuade veterinarians to see that spay/neuter initiatives tend to boost overall demand for veterinary services rather than infringe upon the work and income streams of private practices. All actions that inculcate a wider sense of responsibility for pets, they have argued, lead pet owners to visit and consult veterinarians more over the lifespans of their animal companions (Arluke and Rowan 2020).

Other tensions beset the relationship between veterinarians and humane advocates. For a long time, national, regional, and local animal protection societies avoided the appointment of veterinarians to their boards of directors, fearing that they would use their influence in such roles to ward off threats to the veterinary profession and to veterinarians' professional and financial interests rather than pursue the welfare of animals. Conflicting perspectives on the use of animals in research, testing, and education were also divisive. Finally, veterinarians by and large accepted the premise that the use of animals for food, fiber, research, fashion, and sport, to name a few purposes, is morally unproblematic, making for an uneasy relationship with the growing number of animal advocates who took a different view (Smithcors 1963; Unti 2004).

Veterinary medicine faced another fundamental challenge in this period, a strong and lasting bias against women in the profession. Their purported emotionality and the conviction that women would abandon practice to raise families were among the reasons cited. They began to enter veterinary colleges during the first decades of the twentieth century, and the first woman to hold an official AVMA position, secretary of the Section on Small Animals, took office in 1937. But women's inclusion and acceptance as professionals proceeded unevenly for many decades. Moreover, gendered values were an explicit part of the profession's ethical dilemma. According to one female graduate who experienced it firsthand at mid-century, the masculinist ethos that dominated veterinary medicine operated "to devalue the qualities of empathy and compassion or at least to situate them as inappropriate to scientific medicine" (Smithcors 1963; Lawrence 1997).

The reorientation of the profession around companion animal medicine in the post-World War II period restored veterinarians' confidence in the future. The 1940s and 1950s saw the founding of eight new schools. A few more emerged in the 1970s along with the advent of veterinary specialties and their allied organizations and interest groups (Smithcors 1975). Beginning in the 1980s, veterinary medicine found itself in an unprecedented situation – an animal-centered profession in an era of broad reconsideration of the human–animal relationship. The continuing expansion into new specializations and the growing social interest in animals brought ethics into greater focus and created pressure on veterinarians to engage cruelty to animals as a broader social concern and a subject of public policy, and to demonstrate leadership in this arena. The presence of a vibrant social movement devoted to animal rights and welfare also raised the stakes, for its adherents were determined to influence ethical discussion concerning the treatment of animals within veterinary medicine (Tannenbaum 1995; Rollin 1999).

Before Franklin Loew, Jerrold Tannenbaum, and Bernard Rollin began to address the topic, veterinary ethics concerned itself with matters like appropriate signage, business practices, drug and alcohol abuse, and other operational issues of professional practice. Loew highlighted the advent of an authentic veterinary ethics, one focused on "the real, and really difficult, questions in veterinary medicine. These questions have to do with the veterinarian's responsibilities to the patient, to the client, and to the public good. They have to do with the moral status of animals. And they raise issues central to the nature of humans and animals" (Loew 2001).

Much of the debate in this era centered on the ethical dilemma inherent to the veterinary oath, adopted by the AVMA House of Delegates in 1954 and revised in 1969, 1999, and 2010. The central question was whether the veterinarian owed a primary loyalty or duty to the human client or the nonhuman patient, and it was tied to the larger challenge for veterinarians in the marketplace. The dependence of veterinarians upon their clients, individual and corporate, has often made it difficult for organized veterinary medicine to take unfettered stands on humane treatment. For much of its history, professional veterinary medicine had been closely tied to the commercial interests of owners, which it has generally identified with the common good, regardless of the welfare implications for animals. The profession and its associations would spend the last decades of the twentieth century and the first decades of the twenty-first catching up (Tannenbaum 1995; Rollin 1999; Jones 2003). The present version of the Oath still does not provide guidance regarding the primary allegiance of the veterinarian (AVMA n.d. Oath).

A remarkable internal challenge developed within the field in the 1980s with the emergence of individual veterinarians and veterinary organizations influenced by the animal rights ethic who contested conventional morality and practice in veterinary medicine. Organizations like the Association of Veterinarians for Animal Rights and since 2007 the Humane Society Veterinary Medical Association frequently challenged the AVMA by identifying practices its members believed veterinarians and their professional associations should condemn. High-profile fights ensued over the use of animals in a few contexts. One of the most heated had to do with terminal surgery exercises in veterinary education (Tannenbaum 1995; Rollin 1999; Walsh 2008) (see Chapter 18).

The 1980s were a decisive decade for animal ethics and the veterinary profession in other respects. Both the 1985 Animal Welfare Act amendments in the United States and the 1986 Animals (Scientific Procedures) Act in the UK advanced new standards for the alleviation of pain and distress (ASPA 1986; AWA 2015). For the first time, the Animal Welfare Act contained provisions bearing on the conduct of experimental research and the Animals (Scientific Procedures) Act delineated an important role for the veterinarian (Rollin 1999). The introduction of a veterinarian to manage animal research operations at the Mayo Clinic in the 1930s marked the origin of the laboratory animal veterinarian (Smithcors 1963), but this field really came into its own in the 1980s. Larry Carbone combined his professional duties in laboratory animal care and his PhD studies in history and philosophy of science to articulate a bold vision for the veterinarian's role and responsibility in the laboratory setting, making the case that veterinarians had a moral charge to serve actively as advocates for animals and to some degree as ethicists (Carbone 2004) (see Chapter 11).

The AVMA and many state veterinary associations have had a somewhat beleaguered history in relation to many of the ethical fights that emerged around the treatment and use of animals. The policy agenda of the animal protection movement has prompted these fights, disputes that have frequently spilled into the AVMA House of Delegates and into public debate. In the 1980s, the AVMA opposed federal legislation to restrain doping practices in horseracing. In the 1990s, there were conflicts over ear cropping and tail docking, guardianship, mandatory spay/neuter, use of random source animals in research, and the steel jawed leghold trap (Rollin 1999). In the 2000s, struggles broke out over the intensive confinement of farm animals and several other issues, frequently putting the AVMA at odds with humane advocates. The AVMA supported the legalization of horse slaughter for human consumption, refused to condemn pâté de foie gras production, lagged on the push to ban the abuse of downer cows in the livestock industry, and defended forced molting, the egg industry's routine practice of restricting sources of light and starving egg-laying hens to extend their laying cycle. The organization supported the confinement of veal calves for years and fought against a 2002 ballot measure in Florida to require that breeding pigs be given enough room to turn around and extend their limbs. It refused to support the passage of Proposition 2 in California (2008), the Prevention of Farm Animal Cruelty Act, to phase out extreme forms of farm animal confinement. In 2009, the AVMA criticized the Pew Commission report, which condemned the injudicious use of subtherapeutic antibiotics in industrial farm animal production.

A significant development over the last half-century has been the election of veterinarians to political office. The moral leadership of veterinarians as pro-animal welfare politicians, especially in the United States Congress, has proven decisive. Senator John Melcher (D-MT) championed important revisions to the Animal Welfare Act's coverage of laboratory animals in the mid-1980s, and in subsequent years, Senator Wayne Allard (R-CO), Senator Jon Ensign (R-NV), Rep. Kurt Schrader (D-OR), and Rep. Ted Yoho (R-FL) were strong advocates for animal welfare. In 2017 Sonny Perdue (R-GA), veterinarian, state legislator, and onetime Georgia governor, became the first veterinarian to serve in a Cabinet position, as Secretary of Agriculture.

With the support and influence of elected officials with a background in veterinary medicine, the profession has maintained a strong stake in legislation concerning global bioterrorism, enhanced protection of the food supply, zoonotic disease transmission, veterinary workforce and loan repayment concerns, and disaster preparedness and planning, in addition to animal welfare.

Challenges with the AVMA and professional organizations notwithstanding, relations between the veterinary community and the animal protection movement have improved in many respects. The advent of shelter medicine as an accepted specialization has been good for the profession, bringing veterinarians closer to the needs of local shelters and to communities hindered by inadequate services, offering new career paths as shelter veterinarians and executive directors, and making them better informed and more effective as spokespersons. Many humane organizations have set aside their reluctance to appoint veterinarians as board members. At least two have served as heads of major national animal organizations, and countless others as staff members, managers, and executives (Miller and Zawistowski 2004; Unti 2004).

Cooperation in disaster relief and response has also brought veterinary and animal welfare interests together. In the aftermath of Hurricane Katrina in 2005, the burden of providing critical care and shelter support to animals displaced and/or left behind in New Orleans and other communities, the difficulty of evacuating people who would not leave their pets behind, and the need for close cooperation between veterinary, humane, and conventional responders reshaped disaster response. Among other things, it produced an outstanding public policy outcome in the passage of the PETS Act, which mandated the inclusion of pets in disaster planning at all levels. Social marketing research focusing on post-Katrina responses to animal overpopulation and related concerns in the Gulf Coast region also demonstrated the public credibility and authority of veterinarians as spokespersons and knowledge holders – bringing renewed attention to the social value of their "Aesculapian authority" (Rollin 1999; Grimm 2014).

A century-old problem, the delivery by humane organizations and other entities of low- and/or no-cost veterinary services, remains an occasional source of tension. There are still veterinarians who view this as an infringement of their professional rights and a form of unfair and illegal competition (Arluke and Rowan 2020). Recent evidence disputes this assertion, as a simulation of the effect of low-cost clinics concluded that these would increase the market for veterinary services and enhance the profits of the full-service practices (Haston and Pailler 2021). The humane movement and its shelter and rescue community need veterinarians to provide spaying and neutering services, share information, treat, and prevent disease, support public health measures, and claim a larger role in public education. Almost all service and community initiatives sponsored by animal organizations rely on cooperation with veterinarians to achieve their goals, and the strong exposure of several generations of veterinary students to the goals and needs of local societies, through shelter medicine training or clinical rotations in programs focusing on underserved communities, has built greater trust and understanding. Acceptance and participation in such activities have become part of the normative experience and education of younger veterinarians.

Consequently, veterinarians are playing a role in an emerging social campaign centered on access to veterinary care and services (see Chapter 10). The resulting initiatives seek to raise the standards of animal care and welfare in disadvantaged communities while reinforcing the strong emotional bonds that people everywhere have with their companion animals. This work has brought much-needed attention and sensitivity to issues of race, class, exclusion, and poverty, as it becomes clear that those living in depressed or underserved communities may feel intimidated by animal health care providers and alienated from their services. Private practice fees set for middle- and upper-income clients often deter less wealthy pet owners from going to a veterinarian. In addition, some people are not able to transport their animals to a practice or may have ambivalence about sterilization and other procedures. As a result, many pets in these communities have never visited a veterinarian (Arluke and Rowan 2020).

The emergence of animal law has also influenced the profession (see Chapter 5). In some areas, the evolution of law has helped veterinarians by bringing them more directly into the arena of the broader social ethic. For example, mandatory reporting of suspected cases of abuse has become common, as legal requirements have drawn veterinarians into a new role as healthcare professionals responsible for intervention whenever they suspect domestic violence involving animals or people (see Chapter 20). Nearly two dozen states have a requirement that veterinarians report such concerns. The mandate for reporting known or reasonably suspected abuse and other responsibilities may fall not just upon the veterinarian but upon other staff members in a particular practice as well (Arkow 1994; Patronek 1997; Wisch 2020).

Some developments in the law, however, have created anxiety within the profession. Many veterinarians have long been wary about the legal concept of guardianship and noneconomic damages for harms to animals, and their vocal ambivalence has led courts to assess the subject of damages in veterinary malpractice and liability cases more carefully as a result. Whatever the future holds, it is likely that legal proposals bearing on the practice of veterinary medicine, especially those advanced by animal protection organizations and other stakeholders outside of the field, will continue to generate concern and receive scrutiny from professional societies like the AVMA (Barghusen 2011; Nolen 2011).

## The Twenty-First Century Landscape of Veterinary Medicine (2000–)

The advent of animal-focused ethics, in an era in which interest in the human–animal bond has been growing stronger, has had a transformative impact on the veterinary profession. While the profession has often favored utilitarian perspectives over ethical principles relating to the treatment of animals, continuing shifts in patterns of animal use and rapidly evolving attitudes have pushed the social balance much further along the continuum toward humanitarian values when it comes to animals' treatment. The pressure on veterinarians to confront cruelty to animals as a moral and social obligation is substantial, along with the expectation that the veterinarian is well-placed to do something positive to eliminate unnecessary suffering and take a stand in favor of affirmative duties toward animals. This extends even to animal suffering resulting not from the intentional or inadvertent cruelty of individuals, but from the routinely sanctioned practices of industrialized agriculture, research and testing, and other activities (Tannenbaum 1995; Rollin 1999).

In 2010, responsive to long-running debate on the subject, the AVMA amended the Veterinarian's Oath to signal a more direct commitment to animal welfare. The revisions (in italics) read: "Being admitted to the profession of veterinary medicine, I solemnly swear to use my scientific knowledge and skills for the benefit of society through the protection of animal health *and welfare*, the *prevention and* relief of animal suffering, the conservation of animal resources, the promotion of public health, and the advancement of medical knowledge" (AVMA n.d and AVMA Oath). The oath's revision was a complicated process and has not solved every difficulty in the field. But it does represent a very important reconceptualization of animal health and welfare as extending beyond mere physical health (see Chapter 2), an acknowledgment of animals as more than just goods of production.

Ongoing debates on the revision of the Veterinarian's Oath coincided with another marker of heightening focus on animal welfare in the field: the effort to establish and secure AVMA recognition (in 2012) of the American College of Animal Welfare (ACAW) (https://www.acaw.org). The ACAW promotes and certifies a veterinary specialization in animal welfare, and its diplomates (61 at present) demonstrate detailed knowledge of and special competence in animal welfare across all species.

The emergence of ethics as a serious concern within veterinary medicine and practice has been decisively influenced by the profession's relationship with organized animal protection. At times that relationship, now more than 150 years old, has been positive, promising, and productive. Yet, the advocacy, actions, and policy agenda of a movement expressly devoted to animals' status, interests, and protection – one that consistently raises serious questions about animals' treatment in certain contexts – have also produced ambivalence and tension. Animal protection values have underpinned moral criticisms of a range of veterinary practices. Perhaps more importantly, they have raised questions concerning the larger purposes of veterinary medicine and society's expectations for practitioners. In its turn, veterinary medicine has progressed, exerting its own impact and influence on the treatment of animals and on discussions of their moral status, and has helped to shape and reshape the working imperatives and assumptions of the humane movement.

Currently, 64% of veterinarians in the United States are female (AVMA 2020). The influence of this demographic shift in the profession is still unfolding, not simply in respect to the worldwide increase in the number of women graduating from veterinary schools and moving into practice, but because of increased recognition of gendered perspectives on the status and treatment of animals in society. The implications of these perspectives for veterinary medicine are an important topic for future study (Jones 2000; Irvine and Vermilya 2010; Bonnaud and Fortané 2020). Will the expanded influence of women in the profession portend an enhanced empathy and concern for animal welfare in the future? How will we recognize its effects and how will we measure its impact in respect to practical outcomes in practice and policy?

Given their prominence in the nineteenth and twentieth centuries, there are uncertainties about the future of food animal veterinarians. But the intersecting histories of human and animal health suggest that there will be continuing opportunities for them. Recent studies have emphasized the importance of veterinarians' broadening role in maintaining a safe and sustainable global food supply (Cáceres 2020; Council on Agricultural Science and Technology 2020). With the threat of agroterrorism, animal diseases that spread globally, and multi-drug-resistant pathogens, such veterinarians are going to require additional skills, the capacity to access data and updates on animal disease outbreaks anywhere in the world, and a strong knowledge of epidemiology, forensics, and emergency preparedness (Kelly 2005). Biosecurity priorities will redefine food animal practice as a professional focus, and new responsibilities will place greater ethical burdens upon veterinarians as participants in global networks designed to ensure food safety and security by confronting large-scale public health threats.

With those who work in the medical fields, in emergency and disaster response, and in law enforcement, veterinarians are now part of a broader set of "helping professions" whose members are routinely exposed to challenging levels of moral and occupational stress (see Chapter 22). This is a natural development given the higher value afforded to pets and other animals and rising societal expectations, but it also signals the need for new skills and understanding within the profession concerning resiliency, self-care, and renewed examination of common workplace practices. The fact that veterinary medicine is a stressful occupation also raises the question of whether a clearer ethical landscape around difficult issues such as pain and distress in animals (see Chapter 19) would help to mitigate or reduce veterinarians' stress (Rollin 1999).

The contemporary veterinary profession faces several challenges in respect to ethics. These include the re-envisioning of disease treatment and prevention as an ethics-driven animal welfare concern, the development of successive generations of practitioners with heightened ethical understanding and leadership competencies, and the further integration of veterinary practice and ethics into the One Health framework that brings together animal, human, and environmental health. Today, veterinary ethics as a discipline encompasses both professional ethical concerns (see Chapter 6) and the broad-ranging field of animal ethics. It is more commonly taught within veterinary schools and has gained greater influence within clinical practice. In many respects, its development has closely paralleled that of medical ethics, with important distinctions determined by law, economics, and social sanction of customary uses of animals.

In their turn, greater gender and racial diversity, changes in the structure and economics of veterinary practice, and continuing shifts and trends in animal use and related social attitudes and habits have further reinforced the role of ethics within the field and transformed the identity and status of veterinarians (Bonnaud and Fortané 2020). Since its formal origins in North America in the mid-nineteenth century, the character of veterinary medicine has changed, its social, political, and cultural significance has grown, and its engagement with animal ethics has continued to expand the profession's practical contributions to animal welfare and its broader role in illuminating and shaping the human–animal bond.

## References

American Veterinary Medical Association (AVMA) (n.d.). Veterinarian's Oath. https://www.avma.org/KB/Policies/Pages/veterinarians-oath.aspx (accessed 7 September 2021).

American Veterinary Medical Association (AVMA) (2020). US veterinarians 2020. https://www.avma.org/resources-tools/reports-statistics/market-research-statistics-us-veterinarians (accessed 25 August 2021).

Animal Welfare Act (2015). Chapter 54 – Transportation, sale, and handling of certain animals. https://www.govinfo.gov/content/pkg/USCODE-2015-title7/html/USCODE-2015-title7-chap54.htm (accessed 7 September 2021).

Animals (Scientific Procedures) Act (1986). Animals (Scientific Procedures) Act. https://www.legislation.gov.uk/ukpga/1986/14/enacted (accessed 7 September 2021).

Arkow, P. (1994). Child abuse, animal abuse, and the veterinarian. *Journal of the American Veterinary Medical Association* 204 (7): 1004–1007.

Arluke, A. and Rowan, A. (2020). *Underdogs: Pets, People, and Poverty*. Athens, GA: University of Georgia Press.

Barghusen, S. (2011). Noneconomic damage awards in veterinary malpractice: Using the human medical experience as a model to predict the effect of noneconomic damage awards on the practice of companion animal veterinary medicine. *Animal L* 17 (13): 14–57.

Blaisdell, J.D. (1990). Benjamin Rush and the humane treatment of animals. *Veterinary Heritage* 13 (1): 14–29.

Bonnaud, L. and Fortané, N. (2020). Being a vet: The veterinary profession in social science research. *Review of Agricultural, Food and Environmental Studies* 102 (2): 125–149.

Cáceres, S.B. (2020). The roles of veterinarians in meeting the challenges of health and welfare of livestock and global food security. *Veterinary Research Forum* Summer 3 (3): 155–157.

Carbone, L. (2004). *What Animals Want: Expertise and Advocacy in Laboratory Animal Welfare Policy*. New York: Oxford University Press.

Council on Agricultural Science and Technology (2020). Impact of recruitment and retention of food animal veterinarians on the US food supply. https://www.cast-science.org/wp-content/uploads/2020/03/CAST_IP67_Vet-Students.pdf (accessed 20 December 2021).

Dunlop, R.H. and Williams, D.J. (1996). *Veterinary Medicine: An Illustrated History*. St. Louis, MO: Mosby.

Fraser, D. (1999). Animal ethics and animal welfare science: Bridging the two cultures. *Applied Animal Behaviour Science* 65 (3): 171–189.

Freeberg, E. (2020). *A Traitor to His Species: Henry Bergh and the Birth of the Animal Rights Movement*. New York: Basic Books.

Greene, A.N. (2008). *Horses at Work: Harnessing Power in Industrial America*. Cambridge, MA: Harvard University Press.

Grier, K. (2006). *Pets in America: A History*. Chapel Hill, NC: University of North Carolina Press.

Grimm, D. (2014). *Citizen Canine: Our Evolving Relationship with Cats and Dogs*. New York: Public Affairs Books.

Haston, R.B. and Pailler, S. (2021). Simulation of the effect of low-cost companion animal clinics on the market for veterinary services. *American Journal of Veterinary Research* Dec 1. https://doi.org/10.2460/ajvr.21.08.0116.

Irvine, L. and Vermilya, J.R. (2010). Gender work in a feminized profession: The case of veterinary medicine. *Gender & Society* 24 (1): 56–82.

Jones, S.D. (2000). Gender and veterinary medicine: Global perspectives. *Argos: Bulletin van Het Veterinair Historisch Genootschap* 23 (Fall): 119–123.

Jones, S.D. (2003). *Valuing Animals: Veterinarians and Their Patients in Modern America*. Baltimore, MD: Johns Hopkins University Press.

Kelly, A. (2005). Veterinary medicine in the 21st century: The challenge of biosecurity. *ILAR Journal* 46 (1): 62–64.

Law, J. (1878). A plea for veterinary surgery. *American Veterinary Review* 2 (1): 158–175.

Lawrence, E. (1997). A woman veterinary student in the fifties: The view from the approaching millennium. *Anthrozoos* 10 (4): 160–169.

Loew, F.M. (2001). Veterinary bioethics: Medical research and livestock agriculture as though the animal mattered. *Veterinary Bioethics in the 21st Century*. Tuskegee, AL: Tuskegee Institute.

Mayhew, E. (1865). *The Illustrated Horse Doctor Being an Accurate and Detailed Account of the Various Diseases to Which the Equine Race are Subjected*. London: J.B. Lippincott.

McShane, C. and Tarr, J. (2007). *The Horse in the City: Living Machines in the Nineteenth Century*. Baltimore, MD: Johns Hopkins University Press.

Miller, E. (1981). Private veterinary colleges in the United States, 1852–1927. *Journal of the American Veterinary Medical Association* 178 (6): 583–593.

Miller, L. and Zawistowski, S. (eds.) (2004). *Shelter Medicine for Veterinarians and Staff*. Oxford: Blackwell Publishing.

Murnane, T.G. (2008). James Law, America's first veterinary epidemiologist and the equine influenza epizootic of 1872. *Veterinary Heritage* 31 (2): 33–37.

Nash, R.F. (1989). *The Rights of Nature: A History of Environmental Ethics*. Madison, WI: University of Wisconsin Press.

Nolen, S. (2011). After more than a decade, has guardianship changed anything? *Journal of the American Veterinary Medical Association* 18 March: 820–824.

Patronek, G. (1997). Issues for veterinarians in recognizing and reporting animal neglect and abuse. *Society & Animals* 5: 267–280.

Robichaud, A. (2019). *Animal City: The Domestication of America*. Cambridge, MA: Harvard University Press.

Rollin, B. (1999). *An Introduction to Veterinary Medical Ethics: Theory and Cases*. Ames, IA: Iowa State University Press.

Rush, B. (1808). An introduction to a course of lectures upon the duty and advantages of studying the diseases of domestic animals. In: *Memoirs of the Philadelphia Society for Promoting Agriculture*, 1, l–lxv. Philadelphia, PA: Jane Aitken.

Smithcors, J.F. (1963). *The American Veterinary Profession: Its Background and Development*. Ames, IA: Iowa State University Press.

Smithcors, J.F. (1975). *The Veterinarian in America: 1625–1975*. Wheaton, IL: American Veterinary Publications.

Swabe, J. (1999). *Animals, Disease and Human Society: Human–Animal Relations and the Rise of Veterinary Medicine*. London: Routledge.

Tannenbaum, J. (1995). *Veterinary Ethics: Animal Welfare, Client Relations, Competition and Collegiality*. St. Louis, MO: Mosby.

Teigen, P. (2000). Nineteenth-century veterinary medicine as an urban profession. *Veterinary Heritage* 23 (1): 1–5.

Teigen, P. (2012). Dogs, consumers, and canine veterinarians. *Veterinary Heritage* 35 (2): 45–53.

Unti, B. (2002). The quality of mercy: Organized animal protection in the United States, 1866–1930. PhD Thesis. American University.

Unti, B. (2004). *Protecting All Animals; A Fifty-Year History of the Humane Society of the United States*. Washington, DC: HSUS.

Walsh, M. (2008). The emergence of animal rights in veterinary medicine. *Veterinary Heritage* 31 (2): 37–39.

Wisch, R. (2020). Table of veterinary reporting requirement and immunity laws. Animal Legal and Historical Center. https://www.animallaw.info/topic/table-veterinary-reporting-requirement-and-immunity-laws (accessed 20 December 2021).

Youatt, W. (1839). *The Obligation and Extent of Humanity to Brutes, Principally Considered with Reference to the Domesticated Animals*. London: Longman, Orme, Brown, Green, and Longmans.

# 4

# Introduction to Veterinary Ethics

*Barry Kipperman and Bernard E. Rollin*

The appeal of ethics and the demand for ethical accountability have never been stronger and more prominent – witness the forceful assertion of rights by and for people, animals, and nature – yet an understanding of ethics has never been more tentative, and violations of ethics and their attendant scandals in business, science, government, and the professions have never been more conspicuous. There is probably more talk of ethics than ever; more endowed chairs, seminars, conferences, college courses, books, media coverage, and journals devoted to ethical matters than ever before. Yet, ironically, most people probably believe that they understand ethics far less than their predecessors did. Commonality of values has given way to plurality and diversity: traditions are being eroded.

In such a world it is exigent to understand the logical geography of ethics, and to possess the tools with which to negotiate reasonably what is often tortuous and slippery terrain. This is especially true for professionals, because to maintain their autonomy, professions must anticipate and accord with changing ethical thought. Our ensuing discussion will provide a conceptual map of the nature and role of ethics, and of veterinary ethics. Attempting to analyze difficult ethical cases or to debate complex ethical issues without such a map is analogous to attempting to do surgery without an understanding of the basic concepts of anatomy, anesthesia, and asepsis: one can do it, but one literally doesn't know what one is doing and cannot, therefore, adapt to the unexpected. Conversely, once a person has mastered the relevant basic concepts, they can go well beyond what they had hitherto done by rote.

We are not saying that one cannot behave ethically without mastering the conceptual map we shall present. After all, few people make a study of ethics. Most of us just behave properly in an automatic way. Many of our ethical decisions are obvious, straightforward, and routine: we don't overcharge a gullible client; we don't attempt to steal another veterinarian's patients; we don't prescribe useless medication, etc. What we often cannot do, without a conceptual map and a reflective stance on ethics, is see the subtleties in variegated dimensions posed by complex cases: we tend to react to one obvious component and ignore others. Just as it takes training and practice and a conceptual map of medical possibilities to learn differential diagnosis of disease, it takes training and practice to dissect all the ethical nuances of many complex situations.

Detecting ethical questions is, in some ways, like detecting lameness. *Prima facie*, ordinary people not particularly knowledgeable about veterinary medicine would think that anyone can tell when a horse is lame and which leg is affected. In fact, when actually confronted with a lame horse, inexperienced laypeople, and even veterinary

*Ethics in Veterinary Practice: Balancing Conflicting Interests*, First Edition. Edited by Barry Kipperman and Bernard E. Rollin.
© 2022 John Wiley & Sons, Inc. Published 2022 by John Wiley & Sons, Inc.

students, can at best detect that something is wrong (and sometimes not even that) but they can rarely pinpoint the problem. This is exactly analogous to the activity of identifying ethical problems. People (sometimes) know something is problematic, but they have trouble saying exactly what the problem is.

The study of ethics provides a way of forcing people, on ethical matters, to go beyond their mindset and expectations: indeed, that is why many people find it discomfiting. Of course, one can free oneself from the shackles of myopic perspective by seeking out people with strongly divergent opinions as discussion partners; we often recommend veterinarians orchestrate discussion of ethical matters with their hospital teams where they can hear a wide variety of viewpoints. But this alone will not fully assure a deepened perception in the absence of an understanding of what we have called the "logical geography" of ethical or moral questions. Hearing different opinions is not enough; one must also understand the criteria by which one judges and critically assesses divergent opinions, else one runs the risk of creating a Babel of incommensurable ethical voices – a chorus of individual opinions with no way to generate the consensus that viable ethics requires in a workplace or community, and no method for changing others' opinions in a rational way. So, it is to an examination of the nature of ethics to which we must now turn.

As Plato noted, what we assume about right and wrong, good and bad, justice and injustice, fairness and unfairness, constitutes the most important assumptions we make as individuals and as societies including the professions. One sometimes encounters skepticism about philosophical ethics from people who assert that ethics is "just opinion" or "isn't based on facts" and therefore can't be rationally criticized or rationally taught.

Ethics is useful to:

- Understand, justify, and clarify your own and others' positions.
- Improve awareness of the complexity of ethical issues.
- Be able to construct rational arguments.
- Develop a personal and professional identity.

The art of ethical resolution, on both a social and a personal level, is the art of finding a middle way between apparently irreconcilable differences. Before veterinarians can resolve ethical issues, they must be able to identify and dissect out all the relevant ethical components. This is not always easy given the human predilection to perceive with one's expectations. Nor do most people have the time to engage in extensive dialogue to garner a multiplicity of perspectives on a given case. For these reasons, it is valuable to have a procedure for zeroing in on the relevant ethical components.

## Veterinary Ethics

The main emphasis of veterinary education seems to be the mastery of techniques and facts. Until very recently, virtually no emphasis has been placed in veterinary curricula on the moral and social dimensions of veterinary medicine. The educational process is far too reductionist and mechanistic. The practice of veterinary medicine is taught as if it were value neutral, and it is assumed that students will simply pick up the moral and social implications of what they do when they are in practice. What in fact happens is that these problems are ignored. Indeed, veterinarians are literally starved for ethical discussion. In a recent report, 95% of veterinary students felt that veterinary ethics should be taught in the veterinary curriculum (Kipperman et al. 2020). Almost all veterinarians are "closet moral philosophers" whose philosophical interest is evident whenever they are given the opportunity to "come out of the closet."

Too many schools fail to teach ethics, so practitioners and organized veterinary medicine get blindsided by concerns they do not see coming. Recent studies found that only 51% of US small animal practitioners reported having received ethics training (Kipperman et al. 2018), and only 29% of North American veterinarians received instruction in resolving conflicts about what is best care for patients (Moses et al. 2018). Veterinary educators should be teaching ethics throughout veterinary school curricula so that graduates are sensitized to the issues they will encounter as veterinarians. For example, we know that animal welfare issues are of increasing concern for the social ethic. We also know that society looks to veterinary medicine for answers. Thus, cognizance of animal welfare issues and recommendations for their resolution should be a top priority for organized veterinary medicine and veterinary practitioners.

Like all professionals, veterinarians are enmeshed in a web of moral duties and obligations that can and often do conflict. Veterinarians have obligations to their clients, to their peers in the profession, to society, to themselves, and finally, veterinarians have obligations to animals. Let us examine each of these in more detail.

Veterinarians have moral duties to their clients. For example, they have obligations to keep contracts, to tell the truth, to discuss options and obtain informed consent, to maintain confidentiality, etc. When stated in the abstract, these are self-evident truisms but in real life, these maxims are not so clear. For example, some veterinarians believe they are not morally obliged to euthanize a healthy animal if the client has refused to consider other options. Others believe that it is not necessary to tell the truth if the truth is very painful, as, for example, when an elderly couple asks if their terminal animal could have been saved if they had brought it in when they first observed symptoms instead of "hoping it would go away." Some veterinarians argue that one should not explain all therapeutic options to a client if one believes the client will automatically choose the cheapest, not the best, option. Other practitioners believe they should impose their values on their clients who ask them, "What would you do, Doctor?"

Similar problems arise when one considers one's obligations to peers. Veterinarians are obliged to protect the profession and treat other veterinarians in a collegial way. But how does this relate to the colleague who is incompetent? Although society expects all professionals, including veterinarians, to self-regulate in a way that accords with the social ethic, the profession, like all professions, feels inclined to band together and protect its own – which of course creates ethical conflict. Are you obliged to risk your position within the veterinary community by exposing a colleague engaged in blatantly unethical behavior that everyone else chooses to ignore?

And what of a veterinarian's obligation to society? Society seems to expect veterinarians to lead in animal welfare. Yet it seems to many veterinarians that fulfilling these social obligations can well mean betrayal of their clients. As examples, the American Veterinary Medical Association (AVMA) rarely criticizes aspects of confinement agriculture (see Chapter 1) or breeding of unhealthy animals (see Chapter 10) that society finds increasingly objectionable – indeed, they often feel compelled to defend it! In many states, veterinarians are not mandated to report suspected animal abuse. Yet strong public health arguments can be made in favor of a moral obligation to report animal maltreatment (see Chapter 20).

The veterinarian's obligation to themselves may seem straightforward, but here too there are problems. Every practitioner confronts the problem of people who cannot afford treatment (see Chapter 8). How much can, or should you, as a professional, do for free or at cost? Conversely, should a veterinarian advise tests or treatments because they will be compensated based on the generated revenues?

Finally, we must turn to the veterinarian's obligations to animals. Veterinarians are often put in the position of attempting to advocate for the interests of patients whose desires are uncertain and whose consent they cannot directly acquire. Additionally, veterinarians need the consent, commitment, and financial support of animal owners to use their skills to help animals. Do I euthanize a healthy animal because a client requests it? Do I respect a client's wish not to euthanize a suffering animal? Should I provide care that is likely to not be helpful to a suffering animal because the client will not consider humane euthanasia? How important is controlling animal pain, especially if the client declines suitable analgesia? What is my obligation to individual animals when my job is herd health? What of the claim that there is something morally odd about keeping animals healthy only to slaughter them? Then there is the fundamental question of veterinary ethics: to whom does the veterinarian owe primary obligation, the animal, or the owner (see Chapter 7)?

Practically speaking, veterinary ethics allows us to apply animal welfare science that provides information regarding what we *could* do to or for animals and address difficult questions about how we *should* treat animals including questions such as:

- *What* are we doing now?
- What *should* we be doing?
- *Why* should we be doing it?

## The Anatomy of Making Ethical Decisions

Before one can resolve ethical problems, one must recognize all the relevant ethical questions and components of a challenging situation. When evaluating a situation, one should routinely ask: does it contain elements of obligation to client, peers, animals, society, or self? One then adduces all the relevant ethical principles that could be applied to the situation or its elements and, if necessary, appeals to ethical theories for ordering and prioritizing the principles. It is important to recall that principles do not change with differing situations – principles are like wrenches in one's ethical toolbox. What does change in different situations is *which* principles apply to the case. In this way one is certain to have at least thought about all possible domains of ethical concern. Let us suppose that one has dissected a given situation into its morally relevant components. What happens next? Can we give a rational account of how one comes to a reasonable resolution? Equally important, what happens when two parties, both well intentioned, disagree about how ethical matters are to be resolved?

There are two very different senses of "ethics" that are often confused and conflated and that must be distinguished to allow for viable discussion of these matters. The first sense of ethics we shall call Ethics$_1$. In this sense, ethics is the set of principles or beliefs that govern views of right and wrong, good and bad, fair and unfair, just and unjust. Whenever one asserts that "killing is wrong," or that "discrimination is unfair," one is explicitly or implicitly appealing to Ethics$_1$, moral rules that one believes ought to bind society, oneself, and/or some subgroup of society, such as veterinarians.

Under Ethics$_1$ falls a distinction between social ethics, personal ethics, and professional ethics. Of these, social ethics is the most basic and most objective, to be explained shortly. People, especially scientists, are tempted sometimes to assert that unlike scientific judgments, which are "objective," ethical judgments are "subjective" opinion and not "fact," and thus they are not subject to rational discussion and adjudication. Although it is true that one cannot conduct experiments or gather data to decide what is right and wrong, ethics, nevertheless, cannot be based upon personal whim and caprice. If anyone doubts this, let that person go out and rob a bank in front of witnesses, then argue before a court that in their ethical opinion, bank robbery is morally acceptable if one needs money.

The fact that ethical judgments are not validated by gathering data or doing experiments does not mean that they are simply a matter of individual subjective opinion. If one thinks about it, one will quickly realize that in real life very little socially important ethics is left to one's subjective opinion. Consensus rules about rightness and wrongness of actions that have an impact on others are in fact articulated in clear social principles, which are in turn encoded in laws and policies. All public regulations, including laws against insider trading and murder, are examples of consensus ethical principles "writ large" in Plato's felicitous phrase, in public policy. This is not to say that, in every case, law and ethics are congruent. We can all think of examples of things that are legal yet considered immoral (tax dodges for the ultra-wealthy) and of things we consider perfectly moral that are illegal (parking one's car for longer than two hours in a two-hour zone).

But, by and large, there must be a close fit between our morality and our social policy. When people attempt to legislate policy that most people do not consider morally acceptable, the law simply does not work. Those portions of ethical rules that we believe to be universally binding on all members of society and socially objective, are part of the *social-consensus* ethic. A moment's reflection reveals that without some such consensus ethic, we could not live together: we would have chaos and anarchy, and a functioning society would be impossible. This is true for any society that intends to persist – there must be rules governing everyone's behavior, and they must be objectively encoded in laws. Do the rules need to be the same for all societies? Obviously not – we all know that there are endless ethical variations across societies. Does there need to be at least a common core in all these ethics? That is a rather profound question we shall address later. For now, we only need to agree that there exists an identifiable social-consensus ethic in our society by which we are all bound.

Now, the *social-consensus* ethic does not regulate all areas of life that have ethical relevance – certain areas of behavior are left to the discretion of the individual, or, more accurately, to their *personal* ethic. Such matters as what one reads, what religion one practices or does not practice, and how much charity one gives and to whom are all matters left in our society to one's personal beliefs about right and wrong and good and bad. This has not always been the case; all these examples, during the Middle Ages, were appropriated by a theologically based social-consensus ethic. And this illustrates a very important point about the relationship between *social-consensus ethics* and *personal ethics*; as a society evolves and changes over time, certain areas of conduct may move from the concern of the social-consensus ethic to the concern of the personal ethic, and vice versa.

An excellent example of a matter that has moved from the concern of the social ethic, and from the laws that mirror that ethic, to the purview of the personal ethic is the area of sexual behavior. Whereas once laws constrained activities like homosexual behavior, adultery, and cohabitation, these are now increasingly left to one's personal ethic in Western democracies. With the advent during the 1960s of the view that sexual behavior that does not hurt others is not a matter for social regulation but rather, for personal choice, social regulation of such activity withered away. Some years ago, the mass media reported, with much hilarity, that there was still a law on the books in Greeley, Colorado, a university town, making cohabitation a crime. Radio and TV reporters chortled as they remarked that, if the law were to be enforced, a good portion of the Greeley citizenry would have to be jailed! Homosexual preferences are also rapidly moving away from social or legal condemnation – witness the increasing social and legal acceptance of gay marriage.

On the other hand, many areas of behavior once left to one's personal ethic have since been appropriated by the social ethic. When we were growing up, paradigm cases of what society left to one's personal choice were represented by the kind of person to whom one chose to rent or sell one's property and whom one hired for jobs. The prevailing attitude was that these decisions were your own damned business. This, of course, is no longer the case. Federal law now governs renting and selling of property and hiring and firing to prevent discrimination.

As such examples illustrate, conduct becomes appropriated by the social-consensus ethic when how it is dealt with by personal ethics is widely perceived to be unfair or unjust. The widespread failure to rent to, sell to, or hire minorities, which resulted from leaving these matters to individual ethics, evolved into a situation viewed by society as unjust, and this led to the passage of strong social-ethical rules against such unfairness. The treatment of animals in society is also moving into the purview of the social-consensus ethic, as society begins to question the injustice that results from leaving such matters to individual discretion.

The third component of Ethics$_1$, in addition to social-consensus ethics and personal ethics, is *professional* ethics. Members of a profession are first and foremost members of society – citizens – and thus are bound by all aspects of the social-consensus ethic not to steal, murder, break contracts, etc. However, professionals – be they physicians, attorneys, or veterinarians – also perform specialized and vital functions in society. These roles require special expertise and training and involve situations that ordinary people do not encounter. The professional functions that physicians and veterinarians perform also warrant special privileges: for example, dispensing medications and performing invasive procedures. Democratic societies give professionals some leeway and assume that, given the technical nature of professions and the specialized knowledge their practitioners possess, professionals will understand the ethical issues they confront better than society does. Thus, society generally leaves it to such professionals to set up their own rules of conduct. The social ethic offers general rules, creating the stage on which professional life is played out, and the subclasses of society comprising professionals are asked to develop their own ethic to cover the special situations they encounter. Consequently, professional ethics occupies a position midway between social-consensus ethics and personal ethics because it neither applies to all members of society nor are its main components left strictly to individuals.

The failure of a profession to operate in accordance with professional ethics that reflect and are in harmony with the social-consensus ethic can result in a significant loss of autonomy by the profession in question. One can argue that recent attempts to govern healthcare by legislation are a result of the human medical community's failure to operate in full accord with the social-consensus ethic. When hospitals turn away poor people, or when insurance companies fail to provide coverage for pre-existing conditions, or when pediatric surgeons fail to use anesthesia on infants, they are not in accord with social ethics, and it is only a matter of time before society will appropriate regulation of such behavior.

In veterinary medicine, growing societal awareness of the irresponsible use and dispensing of pharmaceuticals, including use of antimicrobials in farm animals for growth promotion (which led to pathogen resistance to these drugs, creating a risk to humans), threatened the privilege of veterinarians to prescribe drugs in an extra-label fashion, i.e. in a way not dictated by the manufacturer. In 2016, Food and Drug Administration officials removed all over-the-counter access to antimicrobials that are both used in human medicine and given to livestock in feed or water. Those drugs now can be given only with veterinarian approval for disease-related reasons (Burns 2019).

## Ethics$_1$ and Ethics$_2$

Thus far we have looked at Ethics$_1$ – the set of principles that govern people's views of right and wrong, good and bad, fair and unfair, just and unjust – and found that it can be further divided into social-consensus ethics, personal ethics, and professional ethics. Now, we must consider a less familiar, secondary notion. Ethics$_2$ is the logical, rational study and examination of Ethics$_1$, which may include attempting to justify the principles of Ethics$_1$, seeking out inconsistencies in the principles of Ethics$_1$, drawing out Ethics$_1$ principles that have been previously ignored or unnoticed, engaging the question of whether all societies ought ultimately to have the same Ethics$_1$, and so on. This secondary sense of ethics, Ethics$_2$, is a branch of philosophy. Whereas we learn Ethics$_1$ from parents, teachers, churches, movies, peers, magazines, newspapers, and mass media, we rarely learn to engage in Ethics$_2$ in a disciplined, systematic way unless we take an ethics or philosophy class. In one sense this is fine – vast numbers of people are diligent practitioners of Ethics$_1$ without ever engaging in Ethics$_2$. On the other hand, failure to engage in Ethics$_2$ – rational criticism of Ethics$_1$ – can lead to incoherence and inconsistencies in Ethics$_1$ going unnoticed, unrecognized, and uncorrected. Although not everyone needs to engage in Ethics$_2$ on a regular basis, there is value in at least some people monitoring the logic of Ethics$_1$, be it social-consensus ethics, personal ethics, or professional ethics. Such monitoring helps us make ethical progress.

## Ethical Theories

Ethical theories determine what falls within the arena of moral deliberation (see Chapter 1). Ethical theories can also serve to decide between conflicting ethical principles. So let us now look at how individuals can rationally make ethical decisions and how they can rationally convince (or attempt to convince) others with whom they have putative disagreement. First, one must attempt to define all ethically relevant components of the situation. Assuming that the situation is thus analyzed, and the answer is not dictated by the social ethic, what does one do next? Let us here take a hint from the philosopher Ludwig Wittgenstein and ask ourselves how we learned about right and wrong, and good and bad. As children, we might, for example, reach over to steal our brother's chocolate pudding and be told by our mother, "No! That is wrong!" This is how we learn that certain actions are wrong, or that they are right. As we get older, we gradually move from learning that forcibly taking the chocolate pudding away is wrong on this occasion to the generalization that taking it on any occasion is wrong, to the more abstract generalization that taking something from someone else without permission is wrong, to the even more abstract notion that stealing is wrong. In other words, we ascend from particulars to generalizations in our moral beliefs, just as we do in our knowledge of the world, moving from "Don't touch this radiator," to "Don't touch any hot objects," to "Hot objects cause burns if touched."

Let us call the ethical generalizations that we learn as we grow, moral principles. Although we originally learn such moral principles primarily from our parents, as we grow older, we acquire them from many and varied sources – friends and other peers, teachers, churches, movies, books, radio and television, newspapers, magazines, etc. We learn such diverse principles as "It is wrong to lie," "It is wrong to steal," "It is wrong to hurt people's feelings." Eventually, we have the mental equivalent of a closet full of moral principles that we (ideally) pull out in the appropriate circumstances. So far this sounds simple enough. The trouble is that sometimes two or more principles fit a situation yet patently contradict one another.

For example, we have all learned the principles not to lie and not to hurt others' feelings. Yet these may stand in conflict in social-ethical situations, as when a coworker asks, "What do you think of my new hairdo?" and you think it is an aesthetic travesty, or when a client asks the veterinarian if their dog is "The cutest you have ever seen?" Veterinarians, like all professionals, face conflicting principles – indeed, one need go no further than the Veterinary Oath to see a clear conflict. For example, there is certainly a tension between the injunction to advance medical knowledge and the injunction to ameliorate animal suffering, as scientific knowledge often advances by creating animal suffering.

When faced with such conflicts, many of us simply do not notice them. The key to resolving such contradictions lies in how one prioritizes the principles in conflict. Obviously, if they are given equal priority, one is at an impasse. So, we need a higher-order theory to decide which principles are given greater weight in which sorts of situations to keep us consistent in our evaluations so that we do the same sort of prioritizing in situations that are analogous in a morally relevant way. In ethics, one begins with awareness that things are wrong or right, moves to principles, and then ascends to a theory that prioritizes, explains, or provides a rationale for both having and applying the principles. Theories can also help us identify ethical components of situations wherein we intuitively surmise there are problems but cannot sort them out. Both personal and social ethics must be based in some theory that prioritizes principles to assure consistency in behavior and action. Having such a theory helps prevent arbitrary and capricious actions.

Whatever theory we adhere to as individuals, we must be careful to assure that it fits the requirements demanded of morality in general: it must treat people who are relevantly equal equally; it must treat relevantly similar cases the same way; it must avoid favoring some individuals for morally irrelevant reasons; and it must be fair and not subject to whimsical change.

A society needs some higher-order theory underlying its social-consensus ethic. Such a need is immediately obvious as soon as one realizes that every society faces a fundamental conflict of moral concerns – the good of the group, state, or society versus the good of the individual. It is obvious in almost all social decision-making, be it the military demanding life-threatening service from citizens or the legislature redistributing wealth through taxation. It is in society's interest to send you to war – it may not be in yours, as you risk being killed. It is in society's interest to take money from the wealthy to support social programs or, more simply, to improve quality of life for the impoverished, but it arguably does not do the wealthy individual much good.

How does the ethic operative in our and other democratic societies resolve the tension between the individual and society? In our view, the United States has developed the best mechanism in human history for maximizing both the interests of the social body and the interests of the individual. Although we make most of our social decisions by considering what will produce the greatest benefit for the greatest number, a utilitarian/teleological/consequentialist ethical approach, we skillfully avoid the tyranny of the majority or the submersion of the individual under the weight of the general good. We do this by considering the individual as inviolable. Specifically, we consider those traits of an individual that we believe are constitutive of their nature – what Aristotle called *telos* – to be worth protecting at almost all costs. We take the interest flowing from this view of nature as embodied in individuals and build protective legal/moral fences around them that insulate those interests even from the powerful, coercive effect of the general welfare. These protective fences guarding individual fundamental interests against the social interests are called *rights*.

Construction of such ethical theories has occupied philosophers from Plato to the present. It is beyond the scope of this chapter to examine all the diverse theories that have been promulgated. But it is valuable to look at some of the different systems that have been synthesized in the theories underlying our own social-consensus ethic. What is our social-consensus ethic and what is the theory underlying it? It is basically the ethic encoded and articulated in the US Constitution and the laws historically derivative therefrom and, with some variation, in laws in other Western democratic societies. To understand this ethic, we need to contrast the major historical opposing ethical theories.

Ethical theories tend to fall into two major groups: those stressing goodness and badness, i.e. the results of actions; and those stressing rightness and wrongness, or duty, i.e. the intrinsic properties of actions that may be morally acceptable or forbidden. The former is called *consequentialist* or *teleological* theories (from the Greek word *telos*, meaning "result," "end," or "purpose"). The latter are termed deontological theories (from the Greek word *deontos* meaning "necessity" or "obligation"). In other words, what one is obliged to do. The most common deontological theories are theologically based, wherein action is obligatory because commanded by God.

In essence, then, the theory behind our social ethic represents a middle ground or hybrid between utilitarian and deontological theories. On the one hand, social decisions are made, and conflicts resolved by appeal to the greatest good for the greatest number. But in cases where maximizing the general welfare could oppress the basic interests of individuals, general welfare is checked by a deontological theoretical component, namely respect for the individual's nature – *telos* – and the interests flowing therefrom, which are in turn guaranteed by rights.

Now, let's examine different ethical perspectives regarding our moral obligations to animals. In practice, these theories are not mutually exclusive, and one may choose to utilize a combination of these approaches to address ethical problems.

### Contractarianism

This theory links being a moral agent with being a moral object. According to this view, only those capable of acting morally, i.e. rational creatures, are deserving of moral concern. In contractarian theory, we operate as a moral community based on self-interest. Contractors are not ultimately motivated by concern for the hardships of others and are not willing to accept personal risk or inconvenience so that others might benefit (Regan 2001). Moral laws and principles are products of convention, or of social contract, and only rational beings can participate in a social contract or, indeed, in any agreement at all. The social contract is an agreement among rational individuals to treat others a certain way provided they are themselves treated the same way in return. Humans can enter into contracts with each other and, if we break a contract with someone, they may retaliate. Therefore, we are motivated to treat them well, and vice versa.

Since animals are incapable of entering into such agreements, lacking both reason and language and not being moral agents, they are not objects of moral concern. We must treat them well only insofar as it benefits ourselves or other people with whom we do have contracts. Therefore, we can use animals for any purpose we like, provided this does not upset or jeopardize our relationships with people. Our duties to animals are therefore indirect if it benefits humans, such as prohibitions to cruelty or maltreatment to protect animal owners and society. This view is anthropocentric (human-centered).

There are many questions that can be raised about this theory. It does not seem to provide us with legitimate grounds for excluding animals from the scope of moral concern. It does not follow that just because only rational agents can set up or be party to the rules, only such agents are protected by the rules. Why is agency morally relevant? It is also hard to see why animals differ in a morally relevant way from all sorts of humans who can't rationally enter into or respect contracts: future generations of humans, infants, children, the mentally disabled, and the comatose. If the contractarian argues that we have no obligations to these sorts of humans, the theory becomes wildly implausible in its failure to account for our basic moral intuitions about such people. And if the contractarian wishes to include these humans as entities to whom we have obligations, then they must admit that entities become moral objects in virtue of characteristics other than the rational ability to enter into contracts – characteristics like the ability to suffer or to have needs. If that is the case, then all animals must be covered by moral rules, since they also have these characteristics. The idea that animal suffering is morally acceptable provided no human being is affected, is inadequate.

Finally, it is not clear that animals are not rational! Darwin (1892) concluded that earthworms possess rudimentary intelligence and that they show plasticity in their behavior and the ability to learn from experience. Köhler's (1925) classic illustration of a chimpanzee moving a box to climb onto to access bananas is an elementary example of presumed tool use demonstrating instrumental reasoning involving interventions of one's environment.

## Utilitarianism

Utilitarianism emphasizes the *consequences* of actions and is most famously associated with nineteenth-century philosophers Jeremy Bentham (1748–1832) and John Stuart Mill (1806–1873). In its simplest version, utilitarianism holds that one acts in given situations according to what produces the greatest happiness for the greatest number, wherein happiness is defined in terms of pleasure and absence of pain. The twentieth-century philosopher Peter Singer (1946–) contends that fulfilling preferences or desires (such as expressing natural behaviors) is most important (Singer 1999). The ultimate objective is to optimize welfare (see Chapter 2). Killing animals is acceptable provided that overall welfare is not diminished. All affected interests or stakeholders who are sentient, including animals, are to receive equal consideration. This does not mean we must treat chickens the same as humans, but we must attempt to weigh both interests equally.

All potential courses of action and their consequences must be considered. In situations wherein principles conflict, one decides which course of action to take by calculating which is likely to produce the greatest net benefit. Some refer to this theory as "The end [consequence or outcome] justifies the means [actions]." This theory is commonly utilized to support the use of animals in biomedical research and the practice of population medicine for food animals where the interests of a few individuals are deemed less important than the overall welfare of the herd or flock (see Chapter 12). Utilitarianism is conducive to individuals and organizations who believe that using animals for human benefit is acceptable theoretically but strive to promote animal welfare (Regan 2001) such as via legislative reforms.

In the trivial case of someone asking what you think of her new hairstyle that you find repulsive but where you do not wish to hurt her feelings, telling a white lie will likely produce no harm, whereas telling the truth will result in bad feelings, so one ought to choose the former course of action. Adherence to such a theory resolves conflict among principles like "Do not lie" and "Do not hurt anyone's feelings" by providing a higher-order rule for decision-making.

There are problems with a utilitarian basis for animal ethics. Basing ethics on maximizing pleasure and minimizing pain presupposes the commensurability of all forms of pleasure and suffering. How can such disparate forms of negative experiences as isolation from mother, hot-iron branding, neglect, beating, being deprived of food and water, and being denied interaction with conspecifics or the full range of positive experiences be neatly laid out on a homogeneous scale, measured, and compared in any consistent way? For example, how does one compare physical pain with psychological distress?

Utilitarianism may require that certain moral rules be violated to bring about the best consequences. For example, people in an overloaded lifeboat may calculate that more people would survive if they prevented other people from climbing aboard, even if those refused help will drown. It seems to follow from utilitarian principles that if some act produces more pleasure than pain, however heinous the act, it is morally acceptable. For example, if a bank robber were to tell you that if you shot a teller, they would spare the lives of everyone else in the bank, then murder would be acceptable.

Focusing on "the greatest good for the greatest number" can involve minority oppression of individual rights for the benefit of the majority.

There are many other philosophical objections to accepting utilitarianism as a basis for all ethics, including animal ethics. The requirement to consider all outcomes as they may affect all stakeholders makes application of this theory onerous and time-consuming. This theory assumes that the potential outcomes of our actions are predictable or known. The chief problem with grounding animal ethics on a utilitarian foundation is that utilitarianism is not universally accepted even by everyone seeking a theoretical basis for ethics, let alone by most ordinary citizens who need to accept animal ethics to make it practicable. If the given basis for animal ethics does not compel the allegiance of most people it addresses, it becomes more like religion, open to indefinite diversity, rather than being adopted by an overwhelming consensus.

## Animal Rights

The theory of animal rights was developed by American philosopher Tom Regan (1938–2017). He argued that mammals and birds are "subjects of a life": they are more than just alive and conscious – they have beliefs, desires, and various other mental capacities that matter to them (Regan 1984). The most fundamental right is their right to have their inherent worth respected. In contrast to utilitarianism, we are to treat individuals as ends in themselves never merely as means: "The disrespectful treatment of the individual in the name of the social good, [is] something the rights view will not ... ever allow" (Regan 1985). This right sets a rigid rule that forbids the use of animals for food, clothes, experimentation, or entertainment regardless of the potential benefits to humans. Therefore, this approach is "abolitionist" by seeking to end such practices (Francione 2008). Rights advocates believe that animal welfare-based reforms are insufficient (Regan 2001).

For rights proponents, painless killing is considered an unacceptable harm that deprives animals of potential positive experiences (Regan 1984). Regarding animal agriculture, Regan (2007) asserts:

> The fundamental moral wrong here is not that animals are kept in stressful close confinement or in isolation, or that their pain and suffering, their needs and preferences are ignored or discounted. All these *are* wrong, of course, but they are not the fundamental wrong. They are symptoms and effects of the deeper, systematic wrong that allows these animals to be viewed and treated as lacking independent value, as resources for us – as, indeed, a renewable resource.

Some rights advocates suggest that even owning animals as companions is problematic and exploitative based on their legal status as property: "Animal ownership as a legal institution inevitably has the effect of treating animals as commodities" (Francione 2004). Therefore, we should, "ultimately prohibit the ownership of animals" (Francione 2004). "We can certainly choose to treat our non-human companions well, but if we do not, their property status protects our decision. We can choose to take our healthy animal to our veterinarian and have her killed because she is no longer convenient to our lifestyle" (Francione 2006). Certainly, most animal companions have limited freedoms regarding if or when they can go outside to go to the bathroom, what they eat, when and how often, and many experience surgery such as gonadectomy (see Chapter 10) to suit human preferences, which limits sexual behaviors and their capacity to reproduce. For rights proponents, subjecting an animal to medically unnecessary surgery in the absence of informed consent violates one's right to bodily integrity.

Critics of this theory argue that ascertaining inherent value is obscure, that the emphasis is on negative rights not to be harmed rather than positive rights to be provided with something good (Milligan 2015), and that animal use in biomedical research is a vital tool of medical science and therefore animal rights would have disastrous consequences for human health and longevity (Cohen and Regan 2001; Morrison 2009). Of course, a rights perspective would also fundamentally change the veterinary profession.

### Deontology

The most famous proponent of the deontological theory is the German philosopher Immanuel Kant (1724–1804). To Kant, ethics is unique to rational beings, and only humans are considered rational. Rationality around intended conduct is to be found in subjecting the principle of action you are considering to the test of universality, by thinking through what the world would be like if everyone behaved the way you are considering behaving. Kant called this requirement the Categorical Imperative.

Suppose you are trying to decide whether you should tell a white lie in an apparently innocuous circumstance such as a client's request that you find her dog to be the cutest you have ever seen. Before you lie, you must conceive of what would occur if everyone were allowed to lie whenever it was convenient to do so. In such a world, the notion of telling the truth would cease to have meaning, and thus too, would the notion of telling a lie. In other words, no one would trust anyone. Thus, universalizing a lie leads to a situation that destroys the possibility of the very act you are contemplating, and therefore becomes rationally indefensible, *regardless of the good or bad consequences*.

Deontology emphasizes good *intentions* and *motives* and is often based on duties, principles, and a system of rules such as "honesty is the best policy" and "thou shalt not kill." As opposed to utilitarianism, which contrasts good versus bad actions, deontologists would characterize actions as right or wrong. Going back to our previous example of people in the lifeboat, the deontologist would always try to save as many people as possible regardless of the consequences.

### Relational/Contextual

In this theory, the nature of the human–animal bond serves to define our duties to animals. This also is referred to as an "ethic of care," highlighting emotions such as sympathy and empathy in our relations with others (Palmer and Sandøe 2011; Ashall 2022). According to this theory, we have a greater duty to care for animals with whom we have established a *relationship*. Burgess-Jackson (1998) summarizes this view:

> Human beings have special responsibilities to the animals they voluntarily bring into their lives – precisely *because* they bring them into their lives. The act of bringing an animal into one's life – the act of forming a bond or relationship

with a particular sentient being – generates a responsibility to care for its needs. If you believe that a parent is responsible for his or her children, then, by parity of reasoning, you should believe that humans are responsible for the animals they bring into their lives.

Consequently, humans have a greater responsibility for the welfare of domestic animals who are dependent on us compared to wild animals. Some are concerned that this philosophy suggests we have minimal to no obligations to animals we don't encounter. We might be apt to take an "out of sight, out of mind" approach whereby we ignore the suffering of farm or laboratory animals who most of us will never see or meet. What are our duties to animals affected by climate change that is anthropogenic? What about community cat programs or animals in shelters? Drawing the line as to where our relationships with animals creates this ethic of care may seem ambiguous. As the interests of wild animals appear to be diminished in this paradigm, let's consider another perspective.

### Respect for Nature

For proponents of this theory, animals' value lies in their membership of a species. The interests of the individual are subordinated. Preservation of species and ecosystems is prioritized. This is a perspective commonly held by wildlife and zoo biologists and veterinarians working in those fields (see Chapter 14). Hunting as a method of depopulation, captive zoo breeding programs, and other measures intended to preserve endangered species would all be supported by proponents of this theory.

There are numerous concerns with this position. Can a species have "interests" that are distinct from its individual members? Palmer and Sandøe (2011) note the tension between the welfare of individuals and conserving species: "So, ... we could keep all the remaining individuals of a particular species in captivity in a zoo for captive breeding; this might produce welfare problems for all those individuals, but it might, none the less, be good for the *species*, allowing it to continue and perhaps to flourish in the future." Other problems with this theory are the emphasis on wild animals as being more valuable compared to domestic animals and where this demarcation should be. How should a respect for nature perspective view genetic selection for rapid growth of chickens, or genetic modification of laboratory mice? Is this what "nature" intended?

## Reminding Versus Teaching

How does ethical change in individuals, subgroups of society, and society occur? Moral judgments are not verified or falsified by reference to experiments or to new data – indeed, recognition of this fact led twentieth-century scientists to conclude erroneously that science is "value free" and "ethics free" in particular. The knowledge that ethics is not validated by gathering empirical information has led some to conclude that the only way to change anyone's ethical beliefs is by emotion and propaganda – and that reason has no role.

The best account of the subtle way in which ethical change occurs in a rational manner is given by Plato in the dialogue *Meno*. Plato explicitly states that people who are attempting to deal with ethical matters rationally cannot *teach* rational adults, they can only *remind* them. Whereas one can teach veterinary students the various parasites of the dog and demand that they know the relevant answers on a test, one cannot do that with matters of ethics, except insofar as one is testing their knowledge of the social ethic as objectified in law.

Some years ago, one of us (BER) experienced an amusing incident that underscores this point. That year I had a class of particularly obstreperous veterinary students. Throughout the course they complained incessantly that I was only raising ethical questions, not giving them "answers." One morning I came to class an hour early and filled the blackboard with a variety of maxims, such as "Never euthanize a healthy animal," "Always tell the whole truth to clients," "Don't castrate without anesthesia," and so on. When the students filed into class, I told them to copy down these maxims and memorize them.

"What are they?" they asked.

"These are the answers," I replied. "You've been badgering me all semester to give you answers: There they are."

"Who the hell are you to give us answers?" they immediately chorused.

This illustrates the first part of Plato's point, that one cannot teach ethics to rational adults the same way one teaches state capitals. But what of his claim that though one cannot teach, one can remind?

In answering this question, we can appeal to a metaphor from the martial arts. One can, when talking about physical combat, distinguish between sumo and judo. Sumo involves two large men trying to push each other out of a circle. If a 100 lb man is engaging a 400 lb man in a sumo contest, the result is a foregone conclusion. In other words, if one is simply pitting force against force, the greater force will prevail. On the other hand, a 100 lb man can fare quite well against a 400 lb man if the former uses judo: that is, turns the opponent's force against him. For example, you can throw much larger opponents simply by "helping them along" in the direction of their attack on you.

When you are trying to change people's ethical views, you accomplish nothing by clashing your views against theirs – all you get is a counterthrust. Far better to show that the conclusion you wish them to draw is implicit in what they already believe, albeit unnoticed. This is the sense in which Plato talked about "reminding."

As we spend a good deal of time attempting to explicate the new ethic for animals to people whose initial impulse is to reject it, we can attest to the futility of ethical sumo and the efficacy of moral judo. Some years ago, one of us (BER) was asked to speak at the Colorado State University rodeo club about the new ethic in relation to rodeo. When I entered the room, I found two dozen cowboys seated as far back as possible, cowboy hats over their eyes, booted feet up, arms folded defiantly, arrogantly smirking at me. I immediately sized up the situation as a hostile one.

"Why am I here?" I began by asking. No response. I repeated the question. "Seriously, why am I here? You ought to know, you invited me."

One brave soul ventured, "You're here to tell us what is wrong with rodeo."

"Would you listen?" I said.

"Hell no!" they chorused.

"Well, in that case, I would be stupid to try, and I'm not stupid."

A long silence followed. Finally, someone suggested, "Are you here to help us think about rodeo?"

"Is that what you want?" I asked?

"Yes," they said.

"Okay," I replied, "I can do that."

For the next hour, without mentioning rodeo, I discussed many aspects of ethics: the nature of social morality and individual morality, the relationship between law and ethics, the need for an ethic for how we treat animals. I queried the cowboys as to their position on the latter issue. After some dialogue they all agreed that, as a minimal ethical principle, one should not hurt animals for trivial reasons. "Okay," I said. "In the face of our discussion, go out in the hall, talk among yourselves, and come back and tell me what *you guys* think is wrong with rodeo – if anything – from the point of view of your own animal ethics."

When they came back, all took seats in the front, not the back. One man, the president of the club, stood nervously at the front of the room. "Well," I said, not knowing what to expect nor what the change in attitude betokened, "What did you guys agree is wrong with rodeo?"

The president looked at me and quietly spoke, "Everything, Doc. When we started to think about it, we realized that what we do violates our own ethic about animals, namely, that you don't hurt an animal unless you must."

"Okay," I said, "I've done my job, I can go."

He then said, "Will you help us think through how we can hold on to rodeo and yet not violate our ethic?"

## Effecting Ethical Change

Twentieth-century Anglo-American analytic philosophy was adamant about the role of philosophy in real-world matters. Being a philosopher does not allow us the luxury of escaping from the world, however attractive that may be. Philosophers can no longer justify disengagement from the mundane on the grounds that they are concerned with what ought to be, not with what is. Consequently, it is important to make these arguments count in some real and efficacious way. And to do this requires that we confront in detail the existential facts of our moral situation and realistically assess the ways in which our arguments can meaningfully intersect with practice. A good way to begin doing this is to measure the situation against all the categories we have discussed. Does the issue fall under social ethics, personal ethics, or professional ethics? Yet we cannot expect our philosophical model to serve as a blueprint for immediate social change.

There are strong constraints on the development of a new ethic for animals:

1) Any putative ethic proposed to society must be both difficult for citizens to reject and easy for them to accept, at least on a theoretical level. In Plato's terms one must aim at *reminding* rather than *teaching*.

2) Those propagating the new ethic must not seek to establish it too quickly. The great radical activist Henry Spira often remarked that all social-ethical revolutions in the history of the United States have been gradual. To expect people to suddenly abandon established cherished practices is impracticable and unrealistic.

3) One should seek a middle ground between extremes. For example, in the case of invasive experimentation on animals, the research community aggressively argued

against any change whatsoever in the use of animals in research, while radical activists argued for an immediate and abrupt cessation of animal use. The result, of course, was a stalemate, favoring the status quo.

4) Both the new ethic being offered and the suggestions for reform entailed by it must accord with common sense and must be articulable in simple, ordinary language.

David Hume (1711–1776) noted that reason is and ought to be a slave of the passions. By this he did not mean that we should simply follow our irrational emotions, but that arguments alone do not move people; one must have an emotional pull toward actualizing the results of one's reasoning. For Hume, the ultimate basis of morality was feeling; we act on our moral positions because we were born with a predisposition toward empathy, because we have been made uncomfortable by suffering. We may learn of the suffering of millions of starving people or of millions of animals. We know intellectually that this is intolerable. We know that we are morally obligated to help, yet we are at the same time strangely unmoved. The numbers are too large. The event is unconnected with our experience. The situation may seem to be beyond comprehension. But if instead we learn of a single starving child, or of a stolen or abandoned dog, we are moved to tears and action. Here is something we can grasp, empathize with, understand, and ameliorate. We can deal with individuals and, as Aristotle said in another context, only through direct awareness of individuals ascend to an empathetic grasp of generalities. It is for these reasons that our task is not complete until we have tied our ethical theories and frameworks (Tables 7.3 and 23.2) to an actual situation with which everyone can find a point of existential and empathetic contact.

It is hard to imagine anyone more suited to address important ethical concerns involving animals than veterinarians. The essential raison d'être for the veterinarian is the health and welfare of animals. Veterinarians are (or ought to be) more knowledgeable concerning animal welfare than any other group of citizens. Veterinarians are entrusted by society with Aesculapian authority, a unique power vested in those that society perceives as healers. It is in the best interests of animals for veterinary professionals to find the courage to leverage this influence. Ultimately, the question that must always loom before us is this: are the animals any better off by virtue of our efforts?

# References

Ashall, V. (2022). A feminist ethic of care for the veterinary profession. *Frontiers in Veterinary Science* 9: doi: 10.3389/fvets.2022.795628.

Burgess-Jackson, K. (1998). Doing right by our animal companions. *The Journal of Ethics* 2 (2): 159–185.

Burns, K. (2019). Groups provide new guidance on antimicrobials. *Journal of the American Veterinary Medical Association* 254: 3:317–319.

Cohen, C. and Regan, T. (2001). *The Animal Rights Debate*. Lanham, MD: Rowman & Littlefield.

Darwin, C. (1892). *The Formation of Vegetable Mould, through the Action of Worms: With Observations on Their Habits*. London: J. Murray.

Francione, G.L. (2004). Animals – Property or persons? In: *Animal Rights* (eds. C.R. Sunstein and M.C. Nussbaum), 108–143. Oxford, UK: Oxford University Press

Francione, G.L. (2006). Equal consideration and the interest of nonhuman animals in continued existence. A response to Professor Sunstein. *The University of Chicago Legal Forum* 231–252.

Francione, G.L. (2008). *Animals as Persons*. New York: Columbia University Press.

Kipperman, B., Morris, P., and Rollin, B. (2018). Ethical dilemmas encountered by small animal veterinarians: Characterization, responses, consequences, and beliefs regarding euthanasia. *Veterinary Record* 182 (19): 548.

Kipperman, B., Rollin, B., and Martin, J. (2020). Veterinary student opinions regarding ethical dilemmas encountered by veterinarians and the benefits of ethics instruction. *Journal of Veterinary Medical Education* 48: 330–342.

Köhler, W. (1925). Intelligence of apes. *The Journal of Genetic Psychology* 32: 674–690.

Milligan, T. (2015). Regan on animal rights. In: *Animal Ethics; the Basics*. 49–67. London: Routledge.

Moses, L., Malowney, M.J., and Boyd, J.W. (2018). Ethical conflict and moral distress in veterinary practice: A survey of North American veterinarians. *Journal of Veterinary Internal Medicine* 32 (6): 2115–2122.

Morrison, A.R. (2009). *An Odyssey with Animals*. Oxford, UK: Oxford University Press.

Palmer, C. and Sandøe, P. (2011). Animal ethics. In: *Animal Welfare*, 2e (eds. M.C. Appleby, J. Mench, I.A.S. Olsson et al.), 1–13. Wallingford, UK: CABI.

Regan, T. (1984). *The Case for Animal Rights*. London: Routledge.

Regan, T. (1985). The case for animal rights. In: *In Defense of Animals* (ed. P. Singer), 13–26. Oxford, UK: Blackwell.

Regan, T. (2001). *Defending Animal Rights*. Urbana, IL: University of Illinois Press.

Regan, T. (2007). The case for animal rights. In: *Ethics in Practice*, 3e (ed. H. Lafollette), 205–211. Malde, MA: Blackwell.

Singer, P. (1999). *Practical Ethics*, 2e. Cambridge, UK: Cambridge University Press.

# 5

# Veterinary Ethics and the Law

*Carol Gray and David Favre*

This chapter consist of two parts. The first half is the realm of David Favre, a professor of animal law at Michigan State University College of Law. This half examines some of those circumstances when the law intervenes in the practice of veterinary medicine requiring action or limiting options that might otherwise be available to a veterinarian. This includes a legal duty to report when a client is suspected of violating anti-cruelty or duty of care laws, and when there is a duty to report misconduct by another veterinarian. This half will be focused entirely on the law/s of the United States as the author is unfamiliar with the veterinarian laws of other countries.

The second half of the chapter is the realm of Dr. Carol Gray, a veterinarian with a PhD in law, who considers the complex issues of consent. These include when to obtain consent from a client before giving treatment to an animal, how to obtain it, and the problem of assessing whether the client is capable of providing consent. She provides information from a number of different countries to compare and contrast these issues.

## Introduction to First Half

While the primary consideration of this book concerns the ethical questions facing the veterinary profession, it is important to be aware of the legal context and constraints on the profession. The worlds of law and ethics often overlap, but not always. The legal context is actually less intrusive, dealing with fewer issues than the ethical issues that veterinarians face. But when it does speak, it trumps personal or even group ethical policy.

Some small points of clarification for the language used in this chapter. The "law" relates to adopted statutes or court decisions that set out rules of conduct and creates legal responsibilities (for example, a law might require the reporting of suspected animal cruelty). A "regulation" is a rule adopted by an agency under the authority of legislatively adopted law (for example, a regulation adopted by a Board of Veterinary Medicine might require the keeping of specific records for all acts of euthanasia). A "code" refers to a set of directions and constraints formally adopted by a professional organization. It is not a law, but if referenced in regulations, can be operational in investigations concerning unprofessional conduct. "Professional ethics" exist when a group of veterinarians agree upon an expectation of conduct by the members of the group. This may be in writing or may not (for example, it is acceptable to cut off a dog's

*Ethics in Veterinary Practice: Balancing Conflicting Interests*, First Edition. Edited by Barry Kipperman and Bernard E. Rollin.
© 2022 John Wiley & Sons, Inc. Published 2022 by John Wiley & Sons, Inc.

tail only if there is a medical reason for that specific animal). "Personal ethics" is when an individual veterinarian makes an ethical decision out of their own beliefs and experience independent of the law or existing codes.

The legal system provides boundary lines for what any individual veterinarian may believe is or is not ethical conduct. Legal requirements will trump personal and professional ethics when there is a conflict, but hopefully, more often the law supports both. There are many fewer laws about the treatment of animals than there are ethical issues that might be faced in the practice of veterinary medicine.

## Animals as Property

The property status of domestic animals is a cornerstone to considerations both of law and ethics. This ancient categorization causes conceptual difficulty. In law, it produces the question of whether there is a duty to protect animals from bad human actors or is it just dealing with bad human actors. In the world of ethics, it raises the issue of when there is an obligation to the animal that may be different than the duty to the human client.

While no one suggests that ethical duties exist toward a car, that is, a mechanic has no obligation to the car that is in his shop, everyone reading this book will accept the base statement that a veterinarian has an ethical obligation to their animal patient. The law also distinguishes animals as a unique type of property by providing criminal laws specifically adopted for their protection. Indeed, this special status was first recognized over 150 years ago with the adoption of the 1867 New York Anti-Cruelty Law (Favre and Tsang 1993). Thus, the laws consider animals through two very different lenses – that of general personal property like a table and that of living beings who can feel pain and suffer.

The status of just being property is particularly troublesome when the issue of damages for harm to an animal arises in civil court. The most common test for determining the amount of economic damages in the United States is the fair market value test:

> We have defined it [fair market value] as the amount of money which a purchaser willing, but not obliged, to buy the property would pay an owner willing, but not obligated, to sell it, taking into consideration all uses to which the property is adapted and might in reason be applied.
>
> (*Donaldson vs. Greenwood*)

Neither veterinarians nor most companion animal owners accept this, as both understand that a substantial and real bond can exist between humans and companion animals. Additionally, this bond is beneficial to humans (Favre and Dickinson 2017) and therefore should be recognized and supported by the legal system. But after two decades of trying by owners of companion animals to convince the courts, no state supreme court has allowed compensation for the human pain and suffering or loss of companionship when a companion animal is harmed or killed (*Scheele vs. Dustin* [Vermont], and *Strickland vs. Medlen* [Texas]).

The American Veterinary Medical Association (AVMA) has stated that it accepts the existence of the human–animal bond (AVMA n.d.a), but does not support awarding damages for harms to an animal beyond that of economic damages, rejecting damages for human pain and suffering or loss of companionship (AVMA n.d.b). This suggests the dominant view of this important organization is that animals are just property. This of course is in contradiction to a profession that is very willing to advise treatment for companion animals that may well be more than 10 times their economic value.

In criminal law, the property status of the animal is also an issue when a person is being charged with a crime or sentenced for having committed a crime. Are animals individuals or a member of one group? For example, if someone breaks into a house and steals five computers, they are charged with one count of theft. If someone breaks into a house and kills six cats, is that one or six crimes? Hopefully, it can be agreed that it is six crimes. This is a cutting-edge issue that was given visibility when the Supreme Court of Oregon upheld the charging of 12 crimes when 12 horses were harmed by an individual (*Oregon vs. Crow*). The criminal sentencing guidelines that exist in many states will provide for longer prison sentences if an individual is found guilty of six counts rather than one count of a crime. In sentencing guidelines, animals are not given the status of humans, but they seem worthy of being more than just a piece of property. The sentence for bashing a bike with a bat would be no different than the sentence for bashing a cat with a bat. In fact, it might be less, for the dollar value of the bike could well be much higher than the dollar value of the cat.

Animals should not be personal property at all. Professor Favre has written extensively on the need for a new property category for animals, that of "living property" (Favre 2010). By the creation of this new category, the law can refine its perception of animals and provide them greater recognition within the legal system. The creation of this new category will also support the thinking of veterinarians in establishing their ethical code of conduct toward animals, as it gives a new space for creative thinking, perhaps in the area of damages for harm to companion animals.

On the more pragmatic level it must be acknowledged that veterinarians play a significant role in determining the ownership of specific animals. Proving, in a court of law, who owns an animal is actually difficult, as relates to companion animals, as ownership within a family setting is often fuzzy at best. Who paid for the animal? Was the purchase a gift to others within the family? Is it joint ownership between all the family members? Usually nothing is written down and three years later when the child heads off to college or a job in another city, it is unclear who owns the cute cat sitting on the sofa.

When conflicts arise between family members or neighbors, it is often veterinary records that are sought to prove who has provided the care for the animal. As the state where the animal is living has no record of ownership, a veterinary record is often the best neutral third-party evidence of ownership. Of course, this is built upon the expectation that the veterinarian did make a determination of ownership when taking the animal into care. But a veterinarian is not a lawyer and does not hold a hearing for the presentations of proof on the issue of ownership. In the legal world, veterinary records can be evidence of who is the owner of an animal, but it is not final proof. Likewise, information from a chip inserted in an animal is just evidence of who is the owner, but is not conclusive proof.

## Malpractice and Ethics

The issue of veterinary ethics is front and center when a veterinarian is sued for malpractice concerning the treatment of an animal. The law provides the place, the context, the procedure, the judge and jury, and lawyers to aid both parties to the lawsuit, but veterinarians create the substance of the dispute and testify as to the appropriate standards to use in making a judgment about the activity in question. A veterinarian is liable for civil damages under a claim of malpractice (professional negligence) only if their actions fall below the standard of care expected as a minimum within the veterinary community (*Barney vs. Pinkham*). The jury makes the final determination, but the information provided to the jury is by expert witnesses of veterinarians who practice within the community. This is not best care or average care, but least acceptable care (Block 2018). This legal threshold should be approximately the same level as that which by ethical analysis the action or inaction is unacceptable to the veterinary community and noted as unprofessional. It is also presumable that conduct below this level of care is of concern to any state administrative board with the power over the veterinarian license.

A key point is that the law itself does not prescribe where the boundary is located between acceptable and unacceptable conduct, only the profession itself can do that. This is developed within each state and sometimes on a regional basis within a state, or by specialty within the profession. Those who hold themselves out as horse specialists will be judged as to acceptable practices by other horse specialists, not the average dog and cat practitioner, nor the lawyer in the courthouse.

Now, what makes it interesting is that in a court proceeding, if the lawyers have done their jobs, there will be experts on opposing sides. This may represent a dispute within the community about where to draw the line, or just individual veterinarians who would draw the line at different places. Note that it is the jury of nonveterinarians who will decide which of the expert testimony to accept. A large number of civil cases involving veterinarians can be found at https://www.animallaw.info/cases/topic/veterinarian-issues.

## Administrative Actions Against Veterinarians

An individual must have a state-issued license to practice veterinary medicine. This gives the state licensing board jurisdiction to revoke a license of an individual if the standards of the profession have been violated. It is within the power of these state boards to sanction or punish the licensee up to the permanent revocation of the license. While the structure and power of the board is similar in the 50 states, the statement of legal standards that will be used by the agencies vary greatly. Also note that other countries may have different structures than what is presented here. As a lawyer, this author is rather amazed by the haphazard or nonexistent standards that the various state administrative boards use to judge the actions of veterinarians.

The Michigan Board of Veterinary Medicine has no such document, not one page of rules of conduct. The legislature has no comprehensive law, and the Board has not adopted detailed regulations on the level of ethics expected of veterinarians. Other states have taken different paths.

The Alabama State Board of Veterinary Medical Examiners, not the legislature, adopted regulations (Alabama State Board) with 20 items of general concern to the Board. The last specifically list grounds for disciplinary action, including:

(h) The employment of fraud, misrepresentation or deception in getting a license.
(i) Adjudication of insanity or incompetency.
(j) Chronic inebriation or habitual use of drugs.
(k) The use of advertising or solicitation, which is false, misleading or deceptive.
(l) Conviction of a felony or other public offense involving moral turpitude.

But, concerning the treatment of animals, only the following sentence is provided:

(m) Incompetence, gross negligence, or other malpractice in the practice of veterinary medicine.

All of the words in this last section are general legal terms, but no court is involved, and the terms are undefined in the regulations for the context of professional veterinarian practice. Thus, the Board has authority to consider individuals under the standard of malpractice, but there is no definition of the word, or examples, or guidelines as to what constitutes "incompetence, gross negligence, or other malpractice." This leaves individuals vulnerable. It will be difficult to know in advance if an action or inaction, which the individual may consider ethical, is in compliance with what the Board of Veterinary Medical Examiners considers professional.

The State of New Hampshire took a different approach. They relegated the issue of defining professional misconduct to an outside organization: "Conduct which violates the Principles of Veterinary Medical Ethics of the AVMA as revised April 2016 shall constitute unprofessional or dishonorable conduct pursuant to RSA 332-B:14, II(c)" (New Hampshire Board of Veterinary Medicine n.d.) (it is not clear that this delegation of the creation of legal standards to a private party is lawful).

This brings us to the one national code of ethics (AVMA Principles of Veterinary Medical Ethics) as adopted by the AVMA, a private nonprofit organization that veterinarians can join. It has no authority over the licensing of veterinarians. There is no mechanism for enforcement of this code by this organization, but obviously it can be used as a set of standards, either formally as in New Hampshire or informally by other state agencies. It is the most comprehensive statement of the general ethical obligations of veterinarians in practice. It should be pointed out that only a modest amount of this code deals with the treatment and well-being of the animals in their clinics. It has been suggested that professional codes of conduct serve as pivotal instruments of self-regulation, serving three essential functions: (i) regulate members of a profession and ensure high standards of practice; (ii) protect and reassure the public; and (iii) provide a framework that will guide practitioners in their decision-making (Magalhães-Sant'Ana et al. 2015). Many veterinarians see these codes as guidelines rather than as strict regulations that must be followed.

## Legal Duty to Report Owners/Clients

One ethical question is what to do if a veterinarian becomes aware of facts suggesting that an owner may have mistreated an animal to such a degree that may constitute a violation of the state anti-cruelty laws or the duty of care laws. To report a client runs counter to the obligations of client confidentiality. It has been observed that veterinarians often are reluctant to do such reporting (Kogan et al. 2017; Joo et al. 2020) citing lack of training in recognizing and reporting abuse, uncertainty regarding whether abuse occurred, and a desire to educate rather than report clients (see Chapter 20 for a fuller discussion of the ethical duties to report abuse and neglect) (Case Study 5.1).

---

**Case Study 5.1**

A pit bull, not previously seen, is brought in for treatment of a skin condition. In the process of an initial examination, a series of wounds on the face and shoulder of the dog is observed. These have a high probability of being bite marks from other dogs, suggesting the dog had been in a formal dog fight or perhaps used as a practice fight animal. When the owner is asked about this, he says that it must be from what the neighbor cat did. However, the nature of the wounds denotes something else is more likely.

In all states, dogfighting is a serious crime with potential felony punishments available. Is there an ethical duty to report the individual to appropriate authorities in this case? Is there a legal duty to report the individual? Report to whom? Can the dog be kept at the clinic premises? Can the client be charged for the visit? Should someone in the clinic take pictures of the dog? (Yes, a great idea.) Should someone go get the license plate number of the car that brought the animal to the clinic? In so doing, will the veterinarian violate their ethical and perhaps legal obligations of client confidentiality?

---

There is a diversity of approaches among the 50 states on these issues (for a table reporting all state laws on the topic, see: https://www.animallaw.info/topic/table-veterinary-reporting-requirement-and-immunity-laws) (Animal Rescue League 2018). Fourteen states are silent on this specific topic. Other states do not require veterinarians to report animal abuse, but rather allow veterinary professionals to take such action. This is called voluntary or permissive reporting and is seen in states such as Georgia, Maryland, and Maine. Essentially, these laws or regulations give veterinarians the authority to break patient–client confidentiality and report abuse.

Some states have laws that require reporting by veterinary professionals, while other states make it a duty in their veterinary rules of professional responsibility. In other words, a veterinarian may face disciplinary action with the veterinary licensing board in a state or even license revocation if they fail to report suspected abuse. About 20 states place a mandatory duty upon state-licensed veterinarians (and sometimes vet techs) to report suspected animal cruelty to the proper authorities including California, Colorado, Illinois, Minnesota, Oklahoma, and West Virginia. Usually, this consists of reporting the abuse to local law enforcement agencies. The Arizona statute is a good example of a broad mandate:

> A veterinarian who reasonably suspects or believes abuse, cruelty or neglect or animal fighting shall report to law enforcement within 48-hours after treatment or examination. The report shall include the breed and description of the animal and the name and address of the owner or person who sought the examination or treatment.
>
> *(Arizona Statutes)*

Usually, the duty to report is paired with a release from civil liability for making the report: "Veterinarian who files a report as provided in this section shall be immune from civil liability with respect to any report made in good faith" (Arizona Statutes). Otherwise, the veterinarian might be liable in an action of defamation for suggesting the client had engaged in criminal activity. This is referred to as a grant of immunity. For example, some of the key statutory language in Michigan is:

> A veterinarian or veterinary technician who in good faith reports to a peace officer, an animal control officer, or an officer of a private organization devoted to the humane treatment of animals an animal that the veterinarian or veterinary technician knows or reasonably believes to be abandoned, neglected, or abused is immune from civil or criminal liability for making the report.
>
> *(Michigan Statutes A)*

This language covers both civil and criminal issues, and all the law requires is that the report is in good faith. This term in the law means that the action is based upon factual information that reasonably leads the individual to believe there is a violation of the law. Even if it is later determined that there was not a violation of the law, the act of reporting is still protected. This would not cover making statements on Facebook or other social media, and so liability could still arise.

In addition to reporting requirements in state laws, administrative regulations may concern reporting of animal cruelty. For example, under Kansas' Rules of Professional Conduct for Veterinarians, the failure by a veterinarian to report to proper authorities the cruel or inhumane treatment of animals is grounds for disciplinary action. Oklahoma has a similar provision in its Rules of Professional Conduct for Veterinarians (2021). The AVMA also encourages veterinarians to report suspected abuse (AVMA n.d.c).

A significant manual created by the Kirkpatrick Foundation and Animal Folks is available and includes explanations of law and supporting materials so a veterinarian can develop protocols that can guide actions when faced with animal neglect, cruelty, or abuse (Kirkpatrick Foundation and Animal Folks 2018).

## Legal Duty to Report Other Veterinarians

Another topic where the law may intrude upon the ethical choices that an individual may make is that of what to do when a veterinarian becomes aware of unprofessional conduct by other veterinarians. What to do is a difficult personal decision, and usually the person with the information would rather not do anything, for a number of reasons. However, if the profession is to be self-policed then someone has to step forward and raise a concern with the licensing agency (see Chapter 6 for a more thorough discussion of this topic).

The duty to report is stated clearly in the AVMA Code of Ethics (AVMA Principles n.d.d):

> 3. A veterinarian shall uphold the standards of professionalism, be honest in all professional interactions, and report veterinarians who are deficient in character or competence to the appropriate entities.

In those states that have incorporated the AVMA Code by either law or regulation, then the personal ethical decision about what to do has been superseded by the legal obligation to report. The failure to report itself could be considered a failure of professionalism, or unprofessional conduct. What is unclear is just how much information or evidence must be known to a veterinarian before the threshold of legal duty is crossed.

## Where the Law Supports Ethical Decisions

In a number of difficult circumstances, a veterinarian will have to make a decision to treat or not treat an animal or perhaps to euthanize an animal when the veterinary–client–patient relationship (VCPR) has not been formally created. Society has decided that the well-being of the animal is of first priority and by law has delegated the decision to the veterinarian facing the question even when the owner is not present to consent.

Consider the state of Michigan law that provides a legal waiver against claims of professional negligence in respect to emergency treatment or euthanasia when an owner cannot be found (but not for gross negligence or willful and wanton misconduct in providing treatment to an animal) (Michigan Statute B; Case Study 5.2).

---

**Case Study 5.2**

A cat is hit by a car and brought by the driver to the nearest veterinarian. With no license or information on the collar of the cat, the veterinarian scans for an identification chip and does not find one. After examination, it is discovered that two legs are broken in multiple places, the ribs have been crushed so that there is high likelihood of organ damage, and the animal is unconscious and breathing roughly. The projected cost of immediate treatment is $3000 with only a slight chance of the animal surviving. The veterinarian decides the humane thing to do is euthanize the animal and does so immediately. A week later the true owner appears and claims he would have gladly paid whatever the cost to try to save the animal and that it was negligent to proceed to euthanize without waiting for a few days so the true owner could be found and make the necessary decision.

---

The prior Michigan Statute provides the veterinarian a full defense to any lawsuit filed by the owner. The veterinarian can just focus on the issues of care for the animal before them. This case study also illustrates one set of circumstances under which it is acceptable to proceed without consent from the animal's owner, which leads neatly into the next section where the requirement for informed consent to veterinary treatment is developed.

## Ethical and Legal Requirement to Obtain Informed Consent

In human medicine, consent from the patient traditionally protected the physician from a charge of battery, or unlawful physical contact with another human being. This charge is rare in modern medical practice, but a lack of informed consent is often invoked in claims of medical negligence (Furrow et al. 2018). In veterinary medicine, the animal patient cannot give consent and, as discussed earlier in this chapter, is regarded as property. Therefore, consent in veterinary medicine protects the veterinarian from a charge of trespass to goods, or interference with another person's property, but could a lack of informed consent also underpin claims of negligence against veterinarians? Requirements for consent to be "informed" vary between jurisdictions, so it is perhaps useful to journey around these differing professional ethical guidelines to try to distill the essence of what informed consent should look like and to discern alternative roles for consent in the veterinary context.

### Professional Ethical Guidance in the United States

Veterinarians are required to obtain consent from an animal owner before providing treatment. The requirement may be both ethical and legal. Ethical guidance is found in the AVMA's Principles of Veterinary Medical Ethics (AVMA Principles n.d.d), which requires veterinarians to "respect the rights of clients," while advising that veterinarians have a "responsibility to inform the client of the expected results and costs, and the related risks of each treatment regime." Although not specifically labeled as consent, the latter advice requires veterinarians to provide clients with the information that would underpin informed consent. Veterinary treatment requires a VCPR, which can be terminated by either party at any time, except in emergencies. The decision of whether to establish or decline a VCPR depends on the discussion of "clinical findings, diagnostic techniques, treatment, likely outcome, estimated cost and reasonable assurance of payment" (AVMA Principles n.d.d), with all but the last named also being required components of informed consent discussions. Therefore, although the AVMA's professional ethical guidance does not refer to "informed consent" per se, the required content of the discussion between veterinarian and client to establish a VCPR aligns with consent conversations.

As discussed earlier in this chapter, whether the Principles are used, and how they are used, are decisions for individual state agencies. Similarly, the Model Veterinary Practice Act (AVMA 2019) provides a template for state legislation, stating that "consent should be obtained and recorded in the medical record prior to initiating any treatment." Of course, how individual states incorporate the AVMA recommendations varies: for example, the Pennsylvania State Board (2021) expands on consent as follows:

> Veterinarians shall explain the benefits and reasonably anticipated significant potential risks of treatment options to clients. When the client or client's agent is present, veterinarians shall document, by signature, the client's consent for euthanasia and other treatments that have significant potential risks.

Thus, at least ethically, the United States appears to have adopted the doctrine of informed consent to veterinary treatment. The AVMA, however, has taken a rather hesitant approach to defining consent. In May 2007, it approved a policy on informed consent (AVMA 2007a). Shortly afterwards, in November 2007, it released a statement to the effect that it had discontinued the use of the term "informed consent" in matters relating to veterinary medicine, replacing it with "owner consent" (AVMA 2007b). The case that prompted this change in terminology, *Lawrence vs. Big Creek Veterinary Hosp.*, included a statement by the court that the informed consent doctrine as it applied to medical care also mandated the veterinarian's duty of care. This case seemed to panic the AVMA, as it released its statement discontinuing the use of "informed consent" very soon afterwards. References to consent, in the Model Act and in the Principles, still appear without any accompanying requirement for it to be "informed," although there are references to the "informed client." Furthermore, the Model Veterinary Practice Act (AVMA 2019) explains that in 2019, the term "owner" was removed from "owner consent" in recognition that it is not always the owner who gives consent for treatment. Nevertheless, throughout this section, I will assume that any requirement for consent should be "informed consent" and will therefore use this term throughout.

## Comparative Professional Ethical Guidance on Consent

In contrast to the United States, the Canadian Veterinary Medical Association (CVMA) adopts the term "informed owner consent." Its Principles of Veterinary Medical Ethics stipulate the content of a consent discussion in the section on Professional Responsibilities to Clients:

> The decision to accept or decline treatment and related costs should be based on adequate discussion of clinical findings, diagnostic techniques, treatment, likely outcome and estimated costs.
>
> *(CVMA 2016)*

Informed consent is included under "duties to clients" in the Federation of Veterinarians of Europe's (FVE) European Veterinary Code of Conduct: "Veterinarians shall, as far as reasonably possible, ensure informed consent is obtained from clients before treatments or procedures are carried out" (FVE 2019).

The necessity for informed consent is confirmed in the UK Royal College of Veterinary Surgeons (RCVS) Code of Professional Conduct: "Veterinary surgeons must communicate effectively with clients ... and ensure informed consent is obtained before treatments or procedures are carried out" (RCVS 2021) and in the Australian Veterinary Association's (AVA) Code of Professional Conduct, which states that the client's prior informed consent should be obtained for any treatment "if readily available" (AVA 2020). The Veterinary Council of New Zealand's (VCNZ) Code of Professional Conduct (VCNZ 2020) additionally requires veterinarians to check the client's understanding, ability, and authority to give consent, advises tailoring information to the individual client, treating consent as a continuing process rather than a single event, and is probably the most comprehensive ethical guidance on what constitutes informed consent.

Only UK and New Zealand ethical guidance cover in detail who, apart from veterinarians, can be responsible for receiving consent from clients: the former includes registered veterinary nurses and student veterinary nurses who have had training (RCVS 2020), while the latter includes nurses and receptionists but limits their involvement to "common procedures" where protocols and training have been made available (VCNZ 2020).

Examination of a sample of international professional ethical guidance reveals the weight given to the autonomy of the client, which is unsurprising in view of the history of informed consent in human medicine.

## The Ethical Basis of Consent – Autonomy

### Human Medicine and Patient Autonomy

Consent to treatment has been a requirement of physicians' treatment of patients for many years, with early legal references to consent emerging in the 1950s/1960s. Previously, it was assumed that physicians would act in the best interests of their patients: this included hiding facts from patients that may upset them or prevent them from having beneficial treatment (Beauchamp 2011).

The term "informed consent" first appeared in 1957, in the case of *Salgo vs. Leland Stanford, Jr. University Board of Trustees*. In the judgment of this case, the court decided that it was not enough to merely gain consent, but that the physician had to ensure that there was an accompanying "full disclosure of facts necessary to an informed consent." Subsequent cases reinforced the idea of patient-centered disclosure, for example, in *Canterbury vs. Spence* (at 787), the statement that "the test for determining whether a particular peril must be divulged is its materiality to the patient's decision: all risks potentially affecting the decision must be unmasked," was modified by setting the standard to the information required by the "reasonable person." Thus, risk disclosure involved giving the patient information about "material risks" that would be required by a "reasonable person" making a decision about treatment.

The legal definition of consent was influenced by the new field of bioethics, which placed emphasis on patient autonomy or the right to choose what happened to one's own body (Faden et al. 1986). Gradually, medicine and medical treatment moved from a paternalistic ("doctor knows best") ethic to one based on patient self-determination. Autonomy is only one of the four principles of biomedical ethics (Beauchamp and Childress 2019), the others being beneficence (acting for the "good" of the patient), nonmaleficence (not doing any harm to the patient), and justice (equal treatment of all patients): some argue, however, that the greater weighting given to autonomy is undeserved (Brazier 2006; Caplan 2014). An autonomy-based consent features in more recent medical negligence litigation, with failure to disclose risks regarded as a breach of patient autonomy. The "reasonable patient" standard for risk disclosure was taken to a "particular patient" standard in the Australian case of *Rogers vs. Whitaker*, and in the UK, which was relatively late to accept the "doctrine of informed consent," in the case of *Montgomery vs. Lanarkshire Health Board*. Human medicine has moved to a "particular patient" standard of information disclosure, which means that the information given must be based on what that particular patient needs to know, but has a similar journey taken place in veterinary medicine?

## Veterinary Medicine – Whose Autonomy?

Perhaps it is obvious that we cannot simply transpose the "patient autonomy" of human medicine to "client autonomy" in veterinary medicine, as the client is not the patient. Neither can we adopt the template of "proxy" consent given by parents on behalf of their children. Children have rights and are regarded as legal subjects, while animals are still regarded as their owner's property, as discussed earlier. Nevertheless, the owner's autonomy, unlike the autonomy of adult patients in medicine, is constrained by legal provisions protecting animal welfare. For example, an adult human patient has the right to refuse potentially life-saving treatment, a right enshrined in the Declaration of Lisbon: "A mentally competent adult patient has the right to give or withhold consent to any diagnostic procedure or therapy" (World Medical Association [WMA] 2015). Conversely, a client's refusal to allow necessary veterinary treatment may contravene animal welfare legislation. Many state animal protection laws regard failure to seek veterinary attention as cruelty; for example, in Maine's Animal Welfare Statute, it is clearly stated that "(n)o person owning or responsible for confining or impounding any animal may fail to supply the animal with necessary medical attention when the animal is or has been suffering from illness, injury, disease, excessive parasitism or malformed or overgrown hoof" (Maine Revised Statutes 2019, chapter 17, s 1036).

In most jurisdictions, veterinarians are already required to prioritize the welfare of the animal patient when providing treatment (AVMA Principles n.d.d; FVE 2019). Taking this to the next level of maximizing the animal's interests in the contextual situation requires the veterinarian to advocate for these interests (see Chapter 7 for discussion of veterinary advocacies). This could be achieved by only offering treatment that will have a positive effect on welfare: for example, not offering the "do nothing" option. Such consent could be described as one based on beneficence rather than autonomy. Alternatively, in this scenario, the veterinarian could be considered to be exercising professional or Aesculapian autonomy (Rollin 2002). Taken to its extreme, professional autonomy may involve only offering the veterinarian's "preferred" treatment option, for example, a particular method of surgery or treatment that fits with the veterinarian's individual expertise. However, in terms of fairness or justice, the offering of "reasonable treatment options" would appear ethically preferable to offering a single treatment.

## Requirements for Valid Consent

### Ownership and Agency

The person involved in giving consent for veterinary treatment is usually the owner of the animal. Although the use of the term "owner" is controversial, bringing with it the concept of the animal as property, it replicates the terminology used in most legislation. The animal owner may be replaced in the decision-making role by someone providing care for the animal: this individual then becomes the owner's "agent" when considering consent to treatment. In veterinary practice, agency includes those with whom the owner has a contract for the provision of boarding or training services (for example, kennel or stable proprietors, or trainers of sporting animals) but also friends and family of the animal owner. In view of the above, I will therefore use the term "client" to describe the person providing consent to veterinary treatment.

### Capacity

To give consent, the client must be judged to have "capacity" to make decisions based on the information provided. Capacity is legally defined as the ability to understand information relevant to a decision, to retain that information, to use or weigh that information as part of the process of making the decision, and to communicate the decision (Mental Capacity Act 2005). Clients may have capacity to make some decisions but not others. In situations where a client appears to lack capacity to make a decision and therefore to give valid consent, the advice given to veterinarians is sparse.

Professional ethical guidance from the AVMA does not mention capacity: neither do AVA nor CVMA Codes of Professional Conduct. RCVS guidance advises "Where it appears a client lacks the mental capacity to consent, veterinary surgeons should try to determine whether someone is legally entitled to act on that person's behalf, such as someone who may act under a valid lasting power of attorney or enduring power of attorney" (RCVS 2020, s 11.32). Similar advice is given by the VCNZ, which also encompasses those who may be too young to give consent: "If the owner is less than 16 years of age or has limited capacity to provide consent, veterinarians should consider whether someone else can assist in providing informed consent" (VCNZ 2020, s 2.1).

### Age Limits on Giving Consent

In addition to ascertaining capacity, the veterinarian may also need to verify the client's age. How old does a child have to be to give consent for the treatment of a pet? Many codes of professional conduct rely on a legal age for consent, with most deciding on 18 years of age as the cut-off below which veterinarians should seek consent from a parent or guardian. For example, the RCVS guidance includes this recommendation on the basis that a person under the age of 18 cannot enter into a financial contract (in many, though not all, jurisdictions). Therefore, if obtaining consent from someone between 16 (the lower age limit for animal ownership in the UK) and 18, the RCVS advises that the signature of a parent or guardian should be obtained to guarantee payment of financial obligations (RCVS 2020, ss 11.27–11.29).

## Components of Consent

### Information Requirements

The information that should be provided to clients to ensure consent is truly "informed" varies among jurisdictions. For example, a comprehensive list composed from UK medical and veterinary guidance is outlined in Table 5.1.

As these requirements may vary between jurisdictions, it is sufficient to say that if all the listed components are included, then the consent received can be considered as "informed." When considering risk disclosure, a common concern is how many risks need to be disclosed for a particular procedure? Veterinarians may be concerned that

**Table 5.1** Components of informed consent (based on Gray 2019).

| | |
|---|---|
| Diagnosis and prognosis | Right to seek a second opinion |
| Options for treatment | Costs involved in treatment(s) |
| Nature and purpose of treatment(s) | Any conflicts of interest |
| Potential benefits of treatment(s) | Potentially beneficial treatments available elsewhere |
| Risks of treatment(s) | Advice on lifestyle that may moderate the disease process |
| Likelihood of success | Potential follow-up treatment |
| Personnel involved in care, including any students | Inviting questions/checking for concerns re diagnosis, treatment and costs |
| Right to refuse to take part in teaching and/or research | |

they must mention every single risk, no matter how rare, and that disclosing too much information may scare the client and reduce the likelihood that they will pursue the procedure. The terminology used by the RCVS in its supporting guidance on communication and consent may help: its advice is to discuss "both common and serious risks" with the client (RCVS 2020, s 11.2b). Any risks that are common to the proposed treatment (for example, the risk of postoperative wound infection with most surgical procedures) or that would be regarded as serious (for example, the small but devastating risk of death with general anesthesia) should be discussed. To these should be added any risks over which the client raises concerns (for example, soundness for future sporting performance).

### Options for Treatment

Professional ethical guidance on consent varies between two extremes: it may require that the client is offered all "reasonable treatment options" (RCVS 2020, s 11.2) or that "(a)ttending veterinarians are responsible for choosing the treatment regimen for their patients" (AVMA 2019, s 2.3). If taking the former approach, it is wise to define the term "reasonable" when applied to treatment options. Reasonable treatment options would include evidence-based treatments available at the practice, in view of current personnel and equipment, and the offer of referral to another practice if an alternative treatment, unavailable at the current practice, would be in the animal's best interests. The question of how far clients should be prepared to stretch themselves financially to cover the costs of veterinary treatment is controversial. Yeates and Main (2010) suggest that they should be prepared to cover the costs of "reasonably necessary" treatment. "Reasonable" suggests that there are limits to owners' obligations to fund treatment: such a proviso is necessary as more complicated and expensive surgeries become available for animals.

### Financial Aspects of Treatment

Veterinary healthcare, like human healthcare in many jurisdictions, is a private form of medicine and therefore requires payment. The information required for a valid contract is similar to that required for informed consent. The ability and willingness to pay for an animal's treatment (including the purchase of insurance coverage) are solely the client's decision, with this aspect of decision-making regarded as a form of financial autonomy that must be respected. Clients can choose costly, innovative, and complicated surgery for their pets or can refuse to fund even basic treatment. However, this is not an unrestrained autonomy. The veterinarian may refuse to carry out the treatment requested by the client (for example, in the United States, by refusing to enter into a VCPR). Additionally, some veterinarians do not offer all clients the "ideal" options for treatment (Kipperman et al. 2017), a strategy that may not fulfill the conditions of informed consent. In other words, professional autonomy may prevail over the client's financial autonomy. For example, a veterinarian may choose not to crop a dog's ears (in countries where this is still legal) even though a client requests this and is willing to pay for it. Furthermore, as treatment progresses, the client must be involved in ongoing discussions regarding consent and fees.

## Documenting Consent Decisions

The contractual aspect of consent to veterinary treatment extends to the consent form, which can act as evidence of a financial contract provided that costs are clearly listed. However, like any other contract, it can be voided if the terms are too vague. Good practice requires that the client is provided with written evidence of the discussion that has taken place between veterinarian and client about proposed treatments, risks, and benefits, usually with the client signing a consent form. However, the presence, or production, of a signed consent form does not in itself confirm the validity of any associated consent (Maclean 2009). In this sense, consent in human and veterinary medicine are similar. Nevertheless, a well-designed consent form can provide a substantial foundation for veterinarian–client discussions, although most forms seem designed to provide authorization for treatment rather than to substantiate or facilitate client comprehension.

The veterinary healthcare consent process could therefore be regarded as a mixture of a consent process for treatment and a contract for payment for this treatment. The information provided and agreed by both parties must fulfil the minimum required for valid consent, but there also needs to be clear discussion and recording of costs. Many model consent forms include space for client and patient details, the proposed treatment(s), reference to generic risks of treatment and/or anesthesia, financial obligations, and, finally, the signature of the client. There is often no space for documenting any additional information, treatment options, or patient-specific risks. Indeed, a study of UK consent forms found that they lacked space to properly document the accompanying discussion (Gray 2020). Either current consent forms need to be radically redesigned, or other methods of documenting consent need to be explored.

Oral consent is often obtained for veterinary treatment, or for additional treatment while a patient is hospitalized. The accompanying conversation will often cover the required components of consent. With the increase in technological capacity and familiarity with its use in the veterinary context, future consent conversations could be recorded (with client consent), the recordings attached to clinical records and stored as evidence of consent.

## Limitations to Informed Consent

In the following scenarios, suggested actions are based on an amalgamation of "best practice" as described in the latest guidance on consent from several jurisdictions. However, it remains advisable that any veterinarian faced with a similar situation should check local professional ethical guidance and legislation for any differences.

### Emergency Situations

---

**Case Study 5.3**

A middle-aged dog is rushed into the clinic following an impact with a car. His mouth is bleeding, he is breathing heavily, and his left hind limb is severely traumatized. The owner is extremely upset, having seen the accident, and is crying and hyperventilating. How should consent be obtained in this scenario?

---

In Case Study 5.3 the first task is to prioritize patient welfare. This may proceed with agreement from the owner, for example, through the signing of an emergency authorization form to instigate life-sustaining treatment and analgesia. Meanwhile, a member of the veterinary team could look after the owner, trying to reassure them that everything is being done for their dog. When the owner seems better able to take part in a consent discussion, the options for treatment can be discussed and a VCPR set up if the owner wishes to proceed with treatment.

### Owner Lacks Capacity

---

**Case Study 5.4**

A cat with severe vomiting, dehydration, and slight weight loss is brought in by a kind-hearted neighbor of the owner, an elderly man in his 90s. When you phone the owner to ask for consent to treatment, the man denies having a cat, becomes abusive, and hangs up. The neighbor reports that he is "a little bit crazy" but he has managed to look after himself and the cat, until this latest illness. She thinks that he may have a son living nearby.

---

In Case Study 5.4 the first task is to admit the cat and start nonspecific treatment for vomiting and dehydration. As we have been unable to gain consent from the owner, we can rely on there being a waiver of liability for any adverse outcome. We then need to find someone with whom we can set up a VCPR. We could instigate attempts to contact the owner's son, hopefully to get him to take on responsibility for both the cat and his father. If the son cannot be contacted, then help from a community social worker could be sought.

### Owner Is Overwhelmed

---

**Case Study 5.5**

A woman in her early 20s brings in her small dog who had a luxating patella repaired at another veterinary hospital. The dog is still very lame. You are willing to take over the case, so you contact the previous practice to discuss the repair. The hospital tells you that the owner would not make a decision herself; she relied on the veterinarian to tell her what to do, and when the repair failed, she blamed the veterinarian for the decision to anchor the patella with a groove-deepening procedure and stabilizing sutures. The dog's owner now tells you to "do whatever you think is best – don't overwhelm me with information."

---

In the scenario described in Case Study 5.5 you can refuse to perform any further investigations or surgery unless the client is willing to participate in a discussion regarding the options for treatment, the risks involved with each option, and the costs. It is important that enough time is set aside for this discussion. Scheduled office visits of 10–15 minutes (Shaw et al. 2008; Robinson et al. 2014) do not allow sufficient time for consent discussions, and the ideal timing of consent discussions for elective procedures is in advance of the day of surgery. Careful scheduling of such visits is therefore essential. In this case, if the client has booked to see you in the middle of a busy day, rebooking the consent appointment would be appropriate: in the meantime, you can provide written information and diagrams (which can be useful to aid understanding) for the client to review. You can advise her that you will be happy to guide her decision, but she must ask any questions that she has after reviewing the information, she must share what is important to her, and what her ideas of a disastrous outcome and a good outcome would be, before you are prepared to recommend a way forward.

### Innovative Treatment

---

**Case Study 5.6**

You have just attended a continuing education course on the use of stem cells in fracture repair and arthrodesis. An ideal candidate for this procedure has just arrived in clinic. You are eager to try out your newly learned technique. The patient is a much-loved rescue dog with a severely hyperextended carpus, which has not responded to rest and splinting. The owner's funds are limited. You want to perform carpal arthrodesis with stem cells inserted to encourage bony growth between the prepared joint surfaces. You will harvest stem cells from the patient's pelvis.

---

With the example in Case Study 5.6, you need to ensure that you have the client's consent to the use of what is a new technique for your practice and for you as a surgeon. You should offer alternatives such as your usual approach to this injury (a standard arthrodesis procedure). You should emphasize the benefits and risks involved in pioneering a new treatment for the practice, ensure that the client is aware of the novelty of this technique for both you and your practice, and offer the option of referral to an orthopedic surgeon who has greater experience in using this technique.

## How Effective Is Informed Consent in Veterinary Practice?

Most of the literature on veterinary consent provides normative guidance on what *should* be included in a consent conversation (Fettman et al. 2002; Flemming et al. 2004; Passantino et al. 2011). Empirical studies of the consent process are rare. One study, conducted at a large veterinary referral hospital, found that although most clients felt adequately informed, two-thirds were confused about the purpose of the consent form, with 33% thinking that consent forms protected the veterinary surgeon, and 20% thinking that their main purpose was to protect the hospital (Whiting et al. 2017). In an analysis of consent forms used in UK veterinary practices, the forms examined were used to define treatment, to convey the risks associated with the proposed treatment, to evidence the financial contract, and to authorize treatment (Gray 2020). Research into consent discussions is even rarer. Although a study observing consent discussions for elective neutering procedures revealed that these contained most of the information that constitutes informed consent, the substance of these discussions was not documented on an accompanying consent form (Gray 2019).

If the literature does not indicate the effectiveness of consent in practice, the number of complaints regarding consent received by professional regulators might reveal the extent of the problem. Numbers of cases are difficult to access, although one paper suggests that a failure to obtain consent is not a reason per se for disciplinary action by many US state veterinary medical boards (Babcock et al. 2014). However, in a UK study of RCVS disciplinary cases in a 12-month period, 6 out of 20 cases involved a charge of failure to obtain informed consent (Gray 2021).

Alternatively, failure of consent in veterinary practice may be demonstrated through analysis of litigation. The professional liability insurance arm of the AVMA suggests in its 2020 newsletter that "claims related to issues around informed consent also increased" (AVMA-PLIT 2020).

Turning to cases, *Gonzalez vs. South Texas Veterinary Associates* involved a failure to inform a client about the risks to her cat of administering a feline leukemia vaccine, known to have serious side-effects, including the development of cancer. There are few other veterinary examples where failure to obtain informed consent is grounds for an original claim in negligence or malpractice. Nevertheless, the potential recognition that informed consent is part of the "duty of care" of a veterinarian increases the likelihood of its use as a basis for future claims and reinforces its importance as a foundation for veterinary treatment.

## The Purposes of Informed Consent

The acquisition of consent to the treatment of an animal patient requires careful balancing of respect for the client's wishes and protection of the best interests of the animal patient. To enable the client to reach a decision that also incorporates the wider interests of the animal requires the veterinarian to provide information about the risks, benefits, side-effects, costs, and long-term outcomes of each of the reasonable treatment options. These treatment-related aspects can then be combined with the client's knowledge of the individual animal's temperament and preferences to produce a genuinely "best interests"-based decision. The purposes of informed consent in veterinary treatment can therefore be defined as threefold: it should protect the patient from inappropriate or harmful treatment or excessive risk; it should protect the client from unexpected costs; and it should protect the veterinary professional from complaints and claims by evidencing the client's agreement to proceed. Consent is more than just a signature on a form: it requires sharing of information, ensuring mutual understanding, and collaborative decision-making. It should therefore be regarded as more of a process than a single event and should incorporate regular updating and renewal as circumstances change during the treatment of the animal patient.

# References

American Veterinary Medical Association (AVMA) (n.d.d). Principles of veterinary medical ethics. https://www.avma.org/KB/Policies/Pages/Principles-of-Veterinary-Medical-Ethics-of-the-AVMA.aspx (accessed 28 March 2021).

American Veterinary Medical Association (AVMA) (n.d.a).AVMA policy: The human-animal interaction and human-animal bond. https://www.avma.org/resources-tools/avma-policies/human-animal-interaction-and-human-animal-bond (accessed 13 March 2021).

American Veterinary Medical Association (AVMA) (n.d.b).AVMA policy: Recovery of monetary damages in litigation involving animals. https://www.avma.org/resources-tools/avma-policies/recovery-monetary-damages-litigation-involving-animals (accessed 20 April 2021).

American Veterinary Medical Association (AVMA) (n.d.c).AVMA policy: Animal abuse and animal neglect. https://www.avma.org/resources-tools/avma-policies/animal-abuse-and-animal-neglect (accessed 5 April 2021).

American Veterinary Medical Association (AVMA) (2007a). AVMA adopts policy on informed consent. https://www.avma.org/javma-news/2007-05-15/avma-adopts-policy-informed-consent (accessed 28 March 2021).

American Veterinary Medical Association (AVMA) (2007b). "Informed consent" versus "owner consent". https://www.avma.org/javma-news/2007-12-15/board-enhances-avma-visibility (accessed 28 March 2021).

American Veterinary Medical Association (AVMA) (2019). Model Veterinary Practice Act. https://www.avma.org/sites/default/files/2021-01/model-veterinary-practice-act.pdf (accessed 28 March 2021).

Animal Rescue League (2018). Reporting animal cruelty: The role of the veterinarian. https://www.animallaw.info/article/reporting-animal-cruelty (accessed 13 March 2021).

Australian Veterinary Association (AVA) (2020). Code of Professional Conduct. https://www.vsb.qld.gov.au/resources/guidelines/code (accessed 28 March 2021).

AVMA-PLIT (2020). Professional liability newsletter 39 (4). http://ektron. hubinternational.com/uploadedfiles/avma_plit/education_center/private_resources/ library/publications/q4%202020%20pl%20newsletter%20final.pdf (accessed 28 March 2021).

Babcock, S.L., Doehne, J.R., and Carlin, E.P. (2014). Trends in veterinary medical board state disciplinary actions, 2005–2011. *Journal of the American Veterinary Medical Association* 244 (12): 1397–1402.

Beauchamp, T.L. (2011). Informed consent: Its history, meaning and present challenges. *Cambridge Quarterly of Healthcare Ethics* 20: 515–523.

Beauchamp, T.L. and Childress, J.F. (2019). *Principles of Biomedical Ethics*, 8ed. New York: Oxford University Press.

Block, G. (2018). A new look at standard of care. *Journal of the American Veterinary Medical Association* 252 (11): 1343–1344.

Brazier, M. (2006). Do no harm – Do patients have responsibilities too? *The Cambridge Law Journal* 65 (2): 397–422.

Canadian Veterinary Medical Association (CVMA) (2016). Principles of veterinary medical ethics. https://www.canadianveterinarians.net/documents/principles-of-veterinary-medical-ethics-of-the-cvma (accessed 28 March 2021).

Caplan, A.L. (2014). Why autonomy needs help. *Journal of Medical Ethics* 40 (5): 301–302.

Faden, R.R., Beauchamp, T.L., and King, N.M.P. (1986). *A History and Theory of Informed Consent*. New York: Oxford University Press.

Favre, D. (2010). Living property: A new status for animals within the legal system. *Marquette Law Review* 93: 1021.

Favre, D. and Dickinson, T. (2017). Animal consortium. *Tennessee Law Review* 84: 839.

Favre, D. and Tsang, V. (1993). The development of anti-cruelty laws during the 1800's, *Detroit College of Law Review* 1.

Federation of Veterinarians of Europe (FVE) (2019). European Veterinary Code of Conduct. https://fve.org/cms/wp-content/uploads/FVE_Code_of_Conduct_2019_R1_WEB.pdf (accessed 28 March 2021).

Fettman, M.J. and Rollin, B.E. (2002). Modern elements of informed consent for general veterinary practitioners. *Journal of the American Veterinary Medical Association* 221 (10): 1386–1393.

Flemming, D.D. and Scott, J.F. (2004). The informed consent doctrine: What veterinarians should tell their clients. *Journal of the American Veterinary Medical Association* 224 (9): 1436–1439.

Furrow, B.R., Greaney, T.L., Johnson, S.H., et al. (2018). *Health Law: Cases, Materials and Problems*, 8ed. St. Paul, MN: West Academic Publishing.

Gray, C.A. (2019). The role of informed consent in the veterinary clinic: a case study in companion animal neutering. PhD thesis. University of Birmingham. https://etheses. bham.ac.uk//id/eprint/9029 (accessed 20 December 2020).

Gray, C.A. (2020). Role of the consent form in UK veterinary practice. *Veterinary Record* 187 (8): 318. 10.1136/vr.105762.

Gray, C.A. (2021). The role of disciplinary cases in effecting changes to professional ethical guidance: A case study of informed consent and the veterinary profession. *Journal of Professional Negligence* 37 (1): 21–34.

Joo, S., Jung, Y., and Chun, M.S. (2020). An analysis of veterinary practitioners' intention to intervene in animal abuse cases in South Korea. *Animals* 10 (802): 10.3390/ani10050802.

Kipperman, B.S., Kass, P.H., and Rishniw, M. (2017). Factors that influence small animal veterinarians' opinions and actions regarding cost of care and effects of economic limitations on patient care and outcome and professional career satisfaction and burnout. *Journal of the American Veterinary Medical Association* 250 (7): 785–794.

Kirkpatrick Foundation and Animal Folks (2018). Reporting animal cruelty. https://kirkpatrickfoundation.com/uploads/ok-reporting-animal-cruelty-book-web.pdf (accessed 22 September 2021).

Kogan, L.R., Schoenfeld-Tacher, R.M., Hellyer, P.W., et al. (2017). Survey of attitudes toward and experiences with animal abuse encounters in a convenience sample of US veterinarians. *Journal of the American Veterinary Medical Association* 250 (6): 688–696.

Maclean, A. (2009). *Autonomy, Informed Consent and Medical Law.* Cambridge, UK: Cambridge University Press.

Magalhães-Sant'Ana, M., More, S.J., Morton, D.B., et al. (2015). What do European veterinary codes of conduct actually say and mean? A case study approach. *Veterinary Record* 176 (25): 654.

New Hampshire Board of Veterinary Medicine (n.d.). New Hampshire Code of Adm. Rules, Vet, s 501.02. http://www.gencourt.state.nh.us/rules/state_agencies/vet100-700.html (accessed 6 March 2021).

Oklahoma Rules of Professional Conduct for Veterinarians (2021). Okla. Admin. Code s 775: 10-5-30(8)).

Passantino, A., Quartarone, V., and Russo, M. (2011). Informed consent in veterinary medicine: Legal and medical perspectives in Italy. *Open Journal of Animal Sciences* 1 (3): 128–134. 10.4236/ojas.2011.13017.

Pennsylvania State Board of Veterinary Medicine (2021). 7(e) 49Pa. Code s 31.21.

Robinson, N.J., Dean, R.S., Cobb, M. et al. (2014). Consultation length in first opinion small animal practice. *Veterinary Record* 175 (19): 486. https://doi.org/10.1136/vr.102713.

Rollin, B.E. (2002). The use and abuse of Aesculapian authority in veterinary medicine. *Journal of the American Veterinary Medical Association* 220 (8): 1144–1149.

Royal College of Veterinary Surgeons (RCVS) (2020). Code of Professional Conduct supporting guidance: Communication and consent. https://www.rcvs.org.uk/setting-standards/advice-and-guidance/code-of-professional-conduct-for-veterinary-surgeons (accessed 28 March 2021).

Royal College of Veterinary Surgeons (RCVS) (2021). Code of Professional Conduct for Veterinary Surgeons. https://www.rcvs.org.uk/setting-standards/advice-and-guidance/code-of-professional-conduct-for-veterinary-surgeons (accessed 28 March 2021).

Shaw, J.R., Adams, C.L., Bonnett, B.N., et al. (2008). Veterinarian–client–patient communication during wellness appointments versus appointments related to a health problem in companion animal practice. *Journal of the American Veterinary Medical Association* 233 (10): 1576–1586.

Veterinary Council of New Zealand (VCNZ) (2020). Code of Professional Conduct for Veterinarians: Client relationships. https://www.vetcouncil.org.nz/Web/Code_of_Professional_Conduct/Code_Of_Conduct.aspx (accessed 28 March 2021).

Whiting, M., Alexander, A., Habiba, M. et al. (2017). Survey of veterinary clients' perceptions of informed consent at a referral hospital. *Veterinary Record* 180: 20–20. https://doi.org/10.1136/vr.104039.

World Medical Association (WMA) (2015). Declaration of Lisbon on the rights of the patient. https://www.wma.net/policies-post/wma-declaration-of-lisbon-on-the-rights-of-the-patient (accessed 28 March 2021).

Yeates, J.W. and Main, D.C.J. (2010). The ethics of influencing clients. *Journal of the American Veterinary Medical Association* 237 (3): 263–267.

## Cases

*Barney vs. Pinkham*, 45 N.W. 694, (Neb. 1890)

*Canterbury vs. Spence*, 464 F.2d 772, (D.C. Cir. 1972)

*Donaldson vs. Greenwood*, 40 Wash.2d 238, 242 P.2d 1038, (1952)

*Gonzalez vs. South Texas Veterinary Associates*, WL 6729873, (2013)

*Lawrence vs. Big Creek Veterinary Hosp.*, L.L.C., No. 6-2737, 2007 WL 2579436, (Ohio App. 11 Dist. Sept. 7, 2007)

*Montgomery vs. Lanarkshire Health Board*, UKSC 11, (2015)

*Oregon vs. Crow*, 294 Or. App. 88, (2018)

*Rogers vs. Whitaker*, 175 CLR 479, (1992)

*Salgo vs. Leland Stanford, Jr., University Board of Trustees*, 317 P.2d 170, 154 Cal. App. 2d 560, (1957)

*Scheele vs. Dustin*, 998 A.2d 697, 702, (Vt. 2010)

*Strickland vs. Medlen*, 397 S.W.3d 184, 191–92, (Tex. 2013)

## Statutes

Alabama State Board of Veterinary Medical Examiners. Ala. Admin. Code r. 930-X-1-10

Arizona Statutes. Arizona Revised Statutes s 32-2239

Maine Revised Statutes 2019. Title 7. Agriculture and Animals. Pt 9. Animal Welfare. Chapter 739 Cruelty to Animals 4014 Necessary Medical Attention

Mental Capacity Act 2005 (UK), s 3.1

Michigan Statute A. Michigan Complied Law Annotated, s 333.18827

Michigan Statute B. Michigan Complied Law Annotated, s 333.18826

New Hampshire Code. New Hampshire Revised Statute, s 332-B:14

# Section 2

# Clinical Veterinary Ethics

# 6

# Professionalism

*Liz H. Mossop*

## Introduction

Consideration of any ethical dilemma in veterinary practice will necessitate regard for professionalism. While clients may be interested in the ethical viewpoint of the veterinarian caring for their animals, they are more likely to witness the overt application of this viewpoint through the veterinarian's professional behavior. Clients have been shown to desire a balance between technical competence, professionalism, and humanity in their veterinarian (Hughes et al. 2018). It is important that the veterinary profession conducts ongoing oversight of colleagues' behaviors in order to uphold standards and ensure every individual balances the competing demands of clients, animals, and the organization in which they practice. A veterinarian may lose their license to practice veterinary medicine if they are found to be demonstrating professional misconduct or falling below the standards expected of them, even if their ethical beliefs have guided this behavior. There is therefore a relationship between ethics and professionalism, which at times causes conflict for the individual and requires discussion.

## Ethics and Professionalism

A veterinarian's ability to practice appropriately and professionally is dependent on not only clinical skills and knowledge but also a willingness to engage in ethical reasoning and challenge themselves and others regarding approaches to the treatment or welfare of their animal patients (Hernandez et al. 2018). The concepts of ethics and professionalism are therefore intricately linked, and there is much debate within the literature about their meanings. Dunn (2016) is concerned that they have become conflated, particularly within an educational context where medical ethics may be "recast" as medical professionalism in order to increase relevance to students, without any real change to the curriculum. He is concerned that by teaching a professional behavior approach to medical ethics, the flexibility ethical reasoning provides is lost and that students emerge only knowing how to follow a rule book, which inevitably cannot cover all scenarios and possibilities.

In contrast, Mackenzie (2017) views medical professionalism, or professional ethics as he also calls it, as one of the "major sectors" of medical ethics. His description of medical professionalism relates to the belief systems and values of doctors, defining

*Ethics in Veterinary Practice: Balancing Conflicting Interests*, First Edition. Edited by Barry Kipperman and Bernard E. Rollin.
© 2022 John Wiley & Sons, Inc. Published 2022 by John Wiley & Sons, Inc.

what patients can expect regarding standards of care. Indeed, ethics and professionalism are often placed together within healthcare curricula and Doukas et al. (2012) argue that the teaching of ethics and humanities form the building blocks of professionalism in medical students, promoting patient-centered and critical thinking skills. Professionalism is commonly described within medical curricula as encompassing the attitudes, values, and behaviors expected of physicians (Swick et al. 1999). Buyx et al. (2008) argue that medical ethics teaching should include the teaching of moral reasoning skills, relevant ethical knowledge, and the development of "certain character traits."

It is helpful when contemplating ethics and professionalism to consider whether an individual can be ethical while being unprofessional and vice versa. A practical example helps illustrate this situation. A veterinarian encounters a dilemma around poor welfare standards on a pig farm that happens to be a very good client of the practice in which she is employed. Her ethical principles will not let her stand back and allow the mistreatment of animals to continue. She could decide to report the farm to a local news outlet – here she is acting ethically but unprofessionally. Her strong principles are maintained but she is not behaving as expected for a professional by breaking client confidentiality. Alternatively, she could be professional with her work despite violating her ethical principles to improve the animals' care, by, for example, continuing to supply antibiotics to stop infections due to tail biting, which could be prevented by providing better environmental enrichment for the pigs. Here she is acting professionally by continuing to maintain her presence on the farm and keep this important client, but unethically, as she is not acting to improve the welfare of these pigs by addressing the root cause of these issues. Of course, a compromise could also be negotiated whereby an enrichment plan for the animals' environment could be developed alongside a short-term course of antibiotics, demonstrating that ethics and professionalism are not always mutually exclusive. This scenario illustrates the relationship between ethics and professionalism.

Even though veterinarians frequently find themselves in complex ethical situations, their moral reasoning skills are not always sufficient to navigate these dilemmas, potentially contributing to high levels of moral stress and burnout (Batchelor et al. 2015; Kipperman et al. 2018; Moses et al. 2018) (see Chapter 22 for a discussion of moral stress). Veterinarians' behaviors in navigating these dilemmas is an active demonstration of their professionalism, which is therefore likely to suffer if they are unable to do so. If this is occurring frequently, it is likely to pose additional stress and increase the likelihood of a professional negligence case being brought by either a client or colleague. Hence it is clear how closely linked ethics and professionalism are. It is of concern that many veterinary curricula are not addressing this gap in development, with only 18 out of 30 accredited US veterinary schools providing ethics instruction in one survey (Shivley et al. 2016). This situation is improving as accrediting bodies include ethics teaching within required subject areas, but potentially not to the extent that is required (De Briyne et al. 2020).

It has been argued that the term veterinary ethics has caused confusion due to the tendency to apply it in an animal welfare context, worsened by the lack of professional ethics content within curricula (May 2013). May argues strongly that veterinary professional ethics is "more than etiquette" because veterinarians must understand their roles and responsibilities fully, navigate their relationships with both patients and clients, and engage in ethical reasoning in order to receive the respect and credibility that comes with membership in a profession.

Ethics and professionalism are clearly distinct concepts, but particularly when teaching veterinary students, it may be helpful to use the vehicle of professionalism – how veterinarians behave – to illustrate ethical theory. There is a strong argument that professionalism teaching should be integrated throughout a clinical curriculum including ethical theory instruction, and a delivery combination of ethicists and clinicians provides expertise and relevance (Cruess and Cruess 2008). Extending this approach to the clinical context could help with issues of moral stress in veterinarians, for example by utilizing veterinary ethical expertise to guide and inform policy and practice, working closely with clinicians.

## Professions and Professionalism

Before examining the concept of professionalism in more depth, it is helpful to consider the meaning of the word profession. While the Oxford English Dictionary (2018) defines a profession as "An occupation in which a professed knowledge of some subject, field or science is applied; a vocation or career, especially one that involves prolonged training and a formal qualification": a second definition is also included, "More widely: any occupation by which a person regularly earns a living."

The use of the term "professional" has therefore become somewhat broad, with it frequently being used synonymously with occupation and therefore losing its original meaning (Swick 2000). However, this does not detract from the importance of professionalism to those professions who identify with the first definition. When evidence of abuse of power or protectionism for this status emerges, and the changing nature of access to knowledge is considered, the concept of professionalism is perhaps even more crucial to consider.

To further understand what is meant by the term "professionalism" it is helpful to examine the work of social scientists who have been considering the role of professions in society for many years. In many cases this work is centered on the medical profession, which is identified as a foundation profession because of the pivotal role of healthcare in society. This literature tends to focus on society's relationship with professions – often called the social contract – rather than a professional's direct relationship with individuals such as the patient–doctor relationship (Cruess and Cruess 2009). The exchange within this contract is the profession's expertise and knowledge for the benefit of society, often protected by law, in return for an enhanced social standing.

While the practice of medicine has clear differences to that of veterinary medicine, the delivery of healthcare to both humans and animals has changed immeasurably in recent times. Similar challenges to both professions in the distribution of resources and dilemmas in clinical decision-making mean much of this literature can be drawn upon when considering veterinary professionalism. The somewhat nostalgic view of doctors or veterinarians as being entirely altruistic and paternalistic in their approach is perhaps unrealistic in the era of high-cost treatments and specialization (Shirley and Padgett 2006), and this situation has accelerated the discourse around professionalism.

## Human Medical Professionalism

In the past 20 years, there has been an increasing emphasis within the medical profession on defining, teaching, and assessing medical professionalism. This seems appropriate because as part of their contract with society, the public should be reassured that those entering the profession reach the standards of behavior expected of them (Buyx et al. 2008). This has always been an expectation of medical training, but previously these elements of a curriculum were delivered via the "hidden curriculum," rather than being formally included as elements of instruction (Hafferty and Franks 1994). Students were exposed to role models, rituals, and routines that they learned from often without realizing they were changing their behaviors to align with the expectations of the profession and society. The formalization of this enculturation has advanced in medical and healthcare education (Birden et al. 2013), with an increasing emphasis on reflective practice.

There are numerous definitions of medical professionalism, which are often lists of values, attributes, and behaviors that make an acceptable view of what being a doctor is or should be. While professionalism as a teachable concept is helped by a definition (Birden et al. 2013), Wynia et al. (2014) argue that this reductionist context leads to a "check list" approach to behaviors, without truly considering the broader, less individual perspective of professional standards and the "belief system" needed to underpin public trust in the actions and advice of doctors.

The discourse around medical professionalism has extended so widely that individual organizations have their own definitions and guidance. For example, the Royal College of Physicians (RCP) in the UK defines professionalism as "a set of values, behaviors and relationships that underpin the trust the public has in doctors" (RCP 2005). They set out seven roles of the doctor that help individuals to understand and interpret medical professionalism: healer, patient partner, team worker, manager and leader, advocate, learner, and teacher and innovator (Tweedie et al. 2018). Empirical work utilizing the perspective of multiple stakeholders to define medical professionalism has also generated lists of attributes. For example, Jha et al. (2006) identified seven themes: compliance to values, patient access, doctor–patient relationships, demeanor, management, personal awareness, and motivation.

There are also important cultural elements to consider around definitions of professionalism (Al-Rumayyan et al. 2017). This would perhaps be even more overt in the veterinary context, with different cultures having very diverse approaches to the status of animals in society. Indeed, the social status of veterinarians is hugely varied throughout the world, a reflection of this situation.

## Evolution of the Veterinary Profession

The veterinary profession has gone through extensive changes as it adapts to societal needs and the evolving roles animals play in our lives. The close existence of humans and animals means veterinarians contribute significantly to public health, something not always recognized by society. While animal healthcare has always been important, it took a cattle rinderpest outbreak in Europe in the eighteenth century to evolve the veterinary profession into an organized one (Dunlop and Williams 1996). This early scientific understanding of infectious disease led to the opening of the first formal veterinary school in France in 1762. The first school in the UK also had its roots in agriculture and opened in 1790. However, the profession itself was only recognized in 1844 when the Royal College of Veterinary Surgeons (RCVS) was established. In the United States, veterinary schools began establishing in the mid to late nineteenth century (Dunlop and Williams 1996). The profession began organizing formally through the American Veterinary Medical Association (AVMA) in 1863.

Changes in human–animal relationships and the perception of animals in society have led to extensive evolution to the veterinary role as the gatekeepers to animal health. Veterinarians no longer work in small, regional practices treating all species and working all hours in a "James Herriot[1]" model. The modernization of agriculture has led to increases in herd and flock size with associated reductions in the overall numbers of animal keepers. Families no longer keep a cow in the backyard for milk production – instead multinational corporations own thousands of high-producing dairy cows selling milk in bulk to supermarkets for purchase (Jones 2003). The number of veterinarians treating farm animal species has therefore reduced dramatically, but in parallel a significant increase in pet ownership has seen a rise in veterinarians treating only small animals (Leighton 2004).

Animals have moved from "barnyard to bedroom" and expectations from society are high when treating these four-legged family members. This work has become increasingly specialized and the technology and medications available are on a par with human healthcare, potentially limiting access due to the expense of these advances. This is not considered a positive by all members of the profession, as the public health aspect of the veterinarian's role has become increasingly minimized (Jones 2003; Leighton 2004). This argument is often countered by one around the importance of pets in supporting human mental health and well-being (McNicholas et al. 2005).

There is an interesting further historical perspective when considering the veterinarian as a professional. As the medical profession evolved in the eighteenth century, there were two distinct types of doctors: the university educated "professional" physician, and the hands-on surgeon "practitioner" (Mackenzie 2017). Eventually the roles merged, and all treatment of patients involved educated professionals, whether surgical or medical. Cruess and Cruess (2009) also take a historical view on the evolution of "the healer" and "the professional," with the advent of scientific knowledge empowering the development of the medical profession, with codes of ethics continuing to guide behavior throughout this evolution. The veterinary profession evolved in a similar way, with farriers extending their skills to cover basic surgery until veterinary education began formally and took over the treatment of animals surgically. These scenarios add evidence to the status of veterinary medicine as a profession: members have specific and detailed knowledge, unique to their activities, and generally self-regulate each other to a defined set of standards.

As with many professions, the social contract of the veterinary profession with society has changed as access to knowledge has increased (Cruess and Cruess 2000), and clients are increasingly demanding expert care for their animals. A relationship-centered, dialogue-based approach to the treatment of animals is increasingly sought (Pyatt et al. 2020), with the veterinarian–client–patient relationship central to all decision-making along with increasing involvement of other animal healthcare professionals. The business of veterinary practice has also changed significantly, becoming a viable economic venture with associated external financial investment and speculation (Tannenbaum 1995). These changes led the US veterinary profession to examine its purpose and function in the 1990s through a series of reports calling for professionalization of the business side of practices (Brown et al. 1999; Cron et al. 2000).

These changes to the veterinary profession are somewhat at odds with traditional views of professionalism. William Osler observed, "The practice of medicine is not a business and can never be one ... our fellow creatures cannot be dealt with as a man deals in corn and coal; the human heart by which we live must control our professional relations" (Osler 1932). While he was referring to human medicine, the same could be argued in the context of animal patients, as it is the business side of practice that causes many of the ethical dilemmas that arise daily for veterinarians (Kipperman et al. 2018).

The profession has also altered demographically, from being a white male-dominated group to a more diverse, predominantly female profession in many countries (Lloyd 2006; RCVS 2018). New graduates rightly expect a more appropriate work–life balance even though the vocational roots of the profession are still very much in existence. All these changes together increasingly cause ethical conflict and challenges to veterinary professionalism.

## Veterinary Professionalism

Veterinarians study to obtain a specific set of knowledge and skills and have the privilege of applying this knowledge to diagnose and treat animals. In return for this, they obtain a status and title – usually Doctor – and some form of self-regulation within a defined code of conduct. This is another privilege afforded to professions by society – that the best placed person to define how a veterinarian should behave is another veterinarian. The concept of veterinary professionalism is therefore important to both veterinarians and society. If the profession itself does not understand professionalism, then this social contract will be at risk, and likely the welfare of animals more generally. Professionalism should therefore be an ongoing discussion for the veterinary profession, and a key topic within veterinary education for both students and veterinarians (Mossop 2012a).

Tannenbaum (1995) describes veterinary professionalism as "five pillars," extracted from the AVMA Veterinarian's Oath (AVMA n.d.c). These are further explained as the foundations of professionalism in which veterinarians can take pride: scientific knowledge, attention to ethics, benefit to society, protection of animal health, and engagement in self-improvement. Mossop (2012b) describes a definition with a central component of balancing responsibilities – to animals, clients, employers, and society – which has many similarities with the core tenet of veterinary ethical dilemmas (Table 6.1). How veterinarians navigate these dilemmas is dependent on their ability to appropriately balance these responsibilities, with the resulting outcomes demonstrating their professionalism (see Case Study 6.1).

The concept of veterinary professionalism has received increasing attention within veterinary education, as institutions seek to ensure new graduates are equipped to navigate the challenges of veterinary work. Modern curricula are usually competency-based – that is, what graduates should know, as well as skills, attitudes, and behaviors they should be able to demonstrate (Hodgson et al. 2013; Bok 2015). Competencies may include professional behaviors, although the limited empirical definitions of professionalism have meant this may only refer to overt professional skills such as communication. The application of codes of professional conduct is frequently included,

**Table 6.1** Attributes of veterinary professionalism defined through a grounded theory approach (Mossop 2012b).

---

Honesty

Altruism

Communication skills

Personal values

Autonomy

Decision-making

Manners

Empathy

Confidence and knowing limits

Efficiency

Technical competency

---

**Case Study 6.1   A request for declawing a cat**

You are a recently graduated veterinarian working as an associate in a five-veterinarian small-animal practice. Ms. W is a long-term client at your practice, and knows the team well, especially your boss, Dr. B. Ms. W has recently acquired a new kitten, "Stanley," who is a male Persian. Stanley has settled in well to the household, and you have examined him twice during routine wellness consultations, with no health issues identified. Ms. W calls into the practice during your morning consultations and asks to talk to you about Stanley's behavior. She explains that he is scratching the furniture, which is causing damage. Ms. W's partner is particularly upset about the damage as she owns expensive antique furniture, which will now require repair at significant cost. Ms. W explains that she has searched online about the scratching and has tried shutting the cat out of the areas concerned, as well as using a water pistol as recommended by an Internet forum for Persian cat owners. Neither approach has proved effective, and her partner is now asking her to either rehome Stanley or have him declawed. This option was also suggested on the forum, and Ms. W is keen to find out about the procedure and how much it will cost. After establishing the problem, you have a brief conversation with the practice manager, who informs you that Dr. B always declaws when requested to do so.

**What should you do?**

Ethical analysis:
There are several relevant interests in this scenario: the cat, the client, the client's partner, the attending veterinarian, the practice owner and the rest of the team, the veterinary profession, and the cat-owning population. You are aware that the AVMA has a published policy on declawing (onychectomy) that discourages the procedure but states that "professional judgment is key when making a decision as to whether to declaw a cat" (AVMA 2020a). While two US states and some jurisdictions have banned the practice (AVMA 2020b), it is legal in your region.

rather than a holistic view of professionalism (Mossop and Cobb 2013). Veterinary professionals need to be able to reflect and think beyond these codes, and so many curricula also include the teaching and assessment of further professionalism attributes in order to ensure graduates recognize the complexity and challenges of veterinary practice (Bok et al. 2011). Bell et al. (2018) challenge the inclusion of competency alone in curricula design and suggest that competency, professionalism, and employability should be seen as "overlapping dimensions of the successful veterinary professional."

While veterinary ethics and professionalism teaching have become more broadly incorporated in educating veterinary students, the concept of supporting "professional identity formation" has also been described to ensure graduates are ready to enter the profession. Armitage-Chan and May (2019) define professional identity as "the set of values and priorities that are meaningful to the individual, and which guide and inform their behaviors in their professional role." This approach mitigates some of the challenges or clashes between personal and professional values, encouraging a developmental and contextual consideration of behavior and supporting workplace well-being.

## Setting Standards: The Role of Professional Regulatory Bodies

In line with the definition of a profession, veterinary professionals are held to sets of defined standards of knowledge, behaviors, and actions. These standards were developed by members of the profession as part of self-regulation and agreed upon as requirements that will uphold the reputation of veterinarians, thereby contributing to higher standards of animal welfare and care (Hern 2000). Increasingly, these standards are also influenced by lay members to mitigate any potential efforts toward protectionism. While they vary worldwide, standards commonly include conditions around educational requirements for licensure as a veterinarian, requirements for ongoing education, and ethical guidance (Hern 2000). This ethical guidance – frameworks outlining the behavior and conduct of veterinarians – is usually called a "code of conduct." These codes are usually underpinned by an oath, which is a general statement setting out a commitment to animal and public health, taken by individuals as they enter the profession.

Uniquely in the UK, this oath makes clear that animal welfare is to be the first priority of the veterinarian, potentially assisting the resolution of some ethical and professional dilemmas (Hewson 2006). In contrast to this, the AVMA's Veterinarian's Oath does not prioritize animal welfare over other interests included (AVMA n.d.c). As Rollin (1978) points out, this means a substantial dialogue is required in order to make it a more practical tool, rather than it being clear that animal welfare takes priority in all decisions. Veterinary codes of conduct commonly include themes such as definitions and framing concepts, duties to animals, clients, other professionals, competent authorities and society, professionalism, and practice-related issues (Magalhães-Sant'Ana et al. 2015).

Veterinary regulators may be state controlled or may be independent of government control. Importantly, regulators need to maintain a register of licensed practitioners and have a mechanism for removing members from this register should they not meet the required standards. This process normally involves the judgment of other registered veterinarians against the framework of a code of conduct, aligning with the concept of self-regulation.

## Regulation and Codes of Conduct in the United States

Regulation of veterinarians and veterinary technicians in the United States is at the state level, via organizations called veterinary medical boards (VMBs). Each state has specific requirements for licensing and practicing legally as a veterinarian, and subsequently can revoke veterinarians' licenses if they do not maintain the professional standards defined. For example, the California VMB states its mission as "The protection of California consumers and their animals through the regulation of veterinary medicine" (State of California n.d.). This VMB is made up of four veterinarians, one registered veterinary technician, and three lay members. The Board oversees the application of the California Veterinary Medicine Practice Act 2020, which covers regulations specific to the act of veterinary practice and further relevant regulations. A set of disciplinary guidelines (State of California 2012) is used to guide the Board's decisions regarding disciplinary actions against veterinarians, which includes a list of minimum and maximum penalties, from fines to revocation of a license to practice or closure of a premise. Violations included are very broad and cover behaviors that are likely to bring the veterinary profession into disrepute including negligence, incompetence, general unprofessional conduct, animal cruelty, and failure to report other individuals' acts of animal cruelty. Complaints leading to disciplinary procedures commonly come from members of the public but could also come from other veterinarians or animal health professionals.

The AVMA is the representative body for US veterinarians with almost 100,000 members (AVMA n.d.a). Membership in the AVMA is not compulsory for US veterinarians but all veterinarians are influenced by the work of the AVMA because of its role overseeing and accrediting veterinary schools and educational standards. The AVMA has its own Veterinarians' Oath and code of conduct for veterinarians – the Principles of Veterinary Medical Ethics (PVME) – although like many codes of conduct in other professions, it is debatable as to whether these are viewed as a rule book or as guidelines. Nevertheless, the AVMA can undertake disciplinary action against members who violate these principles (AVMA 2019).

The Veterinarian's Oath is taken by all veterinarians entering the profession from an AVMA-accredited veterinary school, and it sets out the roles and behaviors expected of veterinarians:

> Being admitted to the profession of veterinary medicine, I solemnly swear to use my scientific knowledge and skills for the benefit of society through the protection of animal health and welfare, the prevention and relief of animal suffering, the conservation of animal resources, the promotion of public health, and the advancement of medical knowledge. I will practice my profession conscientiously, with dignity, and in keeping with the principles of veterinary medical ethics. I accept as a lifelong obligation the continual improvement of my professional knowledge and competence.
>
> (AVMA n.d.c)

The nine PVME cover multiple aspects of veterinary work set out in Table 6.2.

**Table 6.2** AVMA Principles of Veterinary Medical Ethics (AVMA n.d.b).

1. A veterinarian shall be influenced only by the welfare of the patient, the needs of the client, the safety of the public, and the need to uphold the public trust vested in the veterinary profession and shall avoid conflicts of interest or the appearance thereof.
2. A veterinarian shall provide competent veterinary medical clinical care under the terms of a veterinarian-client-patient relationship (VCPR), with compassion and respect for animal welfare and human health.
3. A veterinarian shall uphold the standards of professionalism, be honest in all professional interactions, and report veterinarians who are deficient in character or competence to the appropriate entities.
4. A veterinarian shall respect the law and also recognize a responsibility to seek changes to laws and regulations which are contrary to the best interests of the patient and public health.
5. A veterinarian shall respect the rights of clients, colleagues, and other health professionals, and shall safeguard medical information within the confines of the law.
6. A veterinarian shall continue to study, apply, and advance scientific knowledge, maintain a commitment to veterinary medical education, make relevant information available to clients, colleagues, the public, and obtain consultation or referral when indicated.
7. A veterinarian shall, in the provision of appropriate patient care, except in emergencies, be free to choose whom to serve, with whom to associate, and the environment in which to provide veterinary medical care.
8. A veterinarian shall recognize a responsibility to participate in activities contributing to the improvement of the community and the betterment of public health.
9. A veterinarian should view, evaluate, and treat all persons in any professional activity or circumstance in which they may be involved, solely as individuals on the basis of their own personal abilities, qualifications, and other relevant characteristics.

## Regulation and Codes of Conduct in the UK

In contrast to the United States, veterinarians and veterinary nurses in the UK are regulated via a central professional body, the RCVS (Hern 2000). The RCVS' role is enshrined in law through the Veterinary Surgeons Act of 1966, and it is responsible for setting, upholding, and advancing standards for veterinarians in education, ethics, and clinical practice. The RCVS also accredits veterinary schools enabling graduates of recognized schools to graduate with a license to practice. The RCVS is led by a council, which has recently evolved to include more lay representation. It currently consists of 15 elected veterinarians, three appointed members from veterinary schools, two appointed veterinary nurses, and six appointed lay members.

The RCVS Code of Professional Conduct sets out the professional standards and responsibilities by which it regulates members. It includes five "Principles of Practice" (Table 6.3) and describes professional responsibilities toward animals, clients, the profession, the veterinary team, the RCVS, and the public. The code begins by stating that these professional responsibilities may conflict, creating a dilemma, and that in these situations first regard should be paid to animal welfare, which is also clear within the oath all veterinarians take on entry to the profession:

> I PROMISE AND SOLEMNLY DECLARE that I will pursue the work of my profession with integrity and accept my responsibilities to the public, my clients, the profession and the Royal College of Veterinary Surgeons, and that, ABOVE ALL, my constant endeavour will be to ensure the health and welfare of animals committed to my care.
>
> (RCVS n.d.)

**Table 6.3**  RCVS Principles of Practice from the
Code of Professional Conduct (RCVS n.d.).

1. Professional competence
2. Honesty and integrity
3. Independence and impartiality
4. Client confidentiality and trust
5. Professional accountability

The responsibilities covered within the code are diverse, from educational standards to requirements, for example, around 24-hour care, confidentiality, consent, and certification.

While the aims of both the US and UK veterinary regulators are equivalent – to ensure appropriate standards of behavior within the profession – the centralized approach in the UK contrasts with the multiple state-level VMBs in the United States. While state-level legislation with limited federal harmony is core to the US system, it could be argued that in the context of animal welfare and standards of care, this lack of consistency could lead to reduced progress in advancing these standards within the veterinary profession.

## Professional Misconduct

A reporting mechanism is required in order for a veterinarian to come under scrutiny from their regulatory body, and these are readily accessible by members of the public and colleagues. Formal processes are then followed whereby an investigation is carried out, evidence is collected, and a final judgment made – the comparison normally being derived from the code/s of conduct and what would be expected as reasonable professional behavior by other veterinarians, known as the "Golden Rule" (Tannenbaum 1995). Professional misconduct has been described as a heterogeneous phenomenon, ranging from clearly illegal acts to actions that are unprofessional and contravene codes of conduct (Gabbioneta et al. 2019). Another categorization is that of "bad cellars, bad barrels and bad apples" (Muzio et al. 2016). These boundary divisions relate to misconduct either being due to the acts of a single individual (the "bad apple"), or due to a systemic cultural issue within the profession (the "barrel") facilitating misconduct so that it becomes normalized. Muzio et al.'s (2016) third division is that of jurisdictional, geo-political, and ecological boundaries (the "cellars"), which could also act to normalize misconduct among the profession and society. Like other professionals, veterinarians may not be able to use the practice culture in which they work as their defense in a case of misconduct, because they still hold a level of individual responsibility whatever policy the practice is condoning (Clark 2007).

Sources of complaints and the reasons for investigations of misconduct of veterinarians are diverse, although there is a notable lack of extensive study of types of misconduct. A New Zealand veterinary study (Gordon et al. 2019) demonstrated that a third of client complaints related to professional behavior, and within this category, dishonesty, poor-quality care, poor communication skills, and a lack of trustworthiness were most frequently identified.

Professional regulators have a challenging role in balancing the interests of the public and acting fairly toward members of their profession. They must deal swiftly and objectively with any complaints, aware of the huge pressures such an investigation places on the individual in question (Biaggio et al. 1998). The veterinary profession has been criticized in the UK for its approach and seeming lack of consistency when dealing with cases of misconduct (Blass 2010). Equally, the profession has accused the regulator of being uncaring and unsupportive in its processes, and unclear in its expectations around professional behavior (Waters 2020). This is of real concern in a profession that suffers from significant mental health issues (Bartram et al. 2009; Nett et al. 2015). The regulators' expectations of standards of professional behavior are set out within their code of conduct, however a challenge for all professions is the difficulties of any code covering all eventualities and being flexible enough to allow professional judgment. It has been argued, for example, that codes of professional conduct for veterinarians actually constrain the "spatialities of animal care," encouraging a rational, tick box approach that does not reflect the emotions and complexity of practice (Donald 2019).

One particularly challenging aspect of misconduct is the question of professionals reporting each other when substandard practice is identified. While both the AVMA and RCVS are clear that veterinarians should report each other, self-regulating professions have always grappled with this issue, veterinarians included. While the third of the AVMA PVME (Table 6.2) provides a framework for self-regulation, the translation of this principle into a meaningful vehicle for professional accountability leaves much to be desired. Tannenbaum observes that: "Most doctors are wary of making a complaint about a colleague to a ... VMB... In years of discussing this issue with ... hundreds of veterinarians, I have never met one who has initiated a complaint about a colleague's performance" (Tannenbaum 1995).

"Occupational deviance" could lead to changes in behavior expectations over time, as veterinarians accept behaviors from each other that may be viewed by society to be in contravention of the behaviors outlined in the code of conduct (Gauthier 2001). As an example of "normalizing the abnormal" in the veterinary profession it has been noted that veterinarians observe that noisy breathing in brachycephalic breeds is "normal for the breed" (Packer et al. 2012). There are many examples in the medical profession of a lack of whistleblowing behavior by colleagues on each other leading to significant harm to patients. One such instance would be the Bristol heart baby scandal in the UK in the 1990s, where a consistent level of poor-quality care led to many unnecessary deaths of patients in a pediatric cardiac surgery unit (Quick 2008). Ultimately, an anesthetist reported this chronic example of professional misconduct, but many more babies died while the profession responded slowly to his complaints.

This event led to a much more open culture of reporting of statistics surrounding survival rates in the UK's National Health Service, something which is not the case within the veterinary profession. However, larger groups of practices are starting to adopt error reporting systems and making efforts to prevent this type of culture from developing, as the profession embraces a culture of quality improvement (Oxtoby and Mossop 2019) (see Chapter 9 for a more thorough discussion of medical errors). This will continue to be a challenge the profession has to grapple with as it evolves and changes in line with societal expectations.

## Conclusion

This chapter has explored the concept of veterinary professionalism, considering what the term means and how this relates to veterinary ethics. Although the terms ethics and professionalism are sometimes used interchangeably, especially in the context of education, professionalism is best described as the behavioral demonstration of ethical perspectives that should align with norms set out by the profession. While veterinary professionalism has many parallels with medical professionalism, there are key differences and veterinarians should not be simply considered "animal doctors," bearing in mind their impact and influence on human health. The regulation of professions is becoming increasingly challenging as society changes and expectations evolve. The veterinary profession must change in line with these expectations, and in order to maintain trust with clients it must be perceived to be responsive, accountable, and transparent in its decision-making. While a clear process for disciplinary procedures is key to maintaining this trust, a balance needs to be struck between holding veterinarians to account and allowing for the ethically complex nature of veterinary practice, which can easily lead to differing decision-making between individuals. An ongoing dialogue between society, veterinarians, and those who regulate them is therefore essential if the profession is to continue to evolve into a modern, valued, and autonomous entity that truly is able to balance the needs of animals, clients, veterinarians, and society.

## Note

1 James Herriot was the pen name of Alf Wight, a veterinarian who worked in the Yorkshire Dales, England, during the 1950s and 1960s. His books accurately reflect the role and status of veterinarians at that time in the UK – they were at the heart of every farming community and widely respected.

## References

Al-Rumayyan, A., Van Mook, W., Magzoub, M. E. et al. (2017). Medical professionalism frameworks across non-Western cultures: A narrative overview. *Medical Teacher* 39 (suppl.1): S8–S14.

American Veterinary Medical Association (AVMA) (n.d.a) We are the AVMA. https://www.avma.org/about (accessed 16 March 2021).

American Veterinary Medical Association (AVMA) (n.d.b). Principles of veterinary medical ethics of the AVMA. https://www.avma.org/resources-tools/avma-policies/principles-veterinary-medical-ethics-avma (accessed 16 March 2021).

American Veterinary Medical Association (AVMA) (n.d.c). Veterinarian's Oath. https://www.avma.org/KB/Policies/Pages/veterinarians-oath.aspx(accessed 10 October 2020).

American Veterinary Medical Association (AVMA) (2019). AVMA Bylaws – Summer 2019. https://www.avma.org/sites/default/files/2019-10/avma_bylaws.pdf (accessed 16 March 2021).

American Veterinary Medical Association (AVMA) (2020a). Declawing of domestic cats. https://www.avma.org/resources-tools/avma-policies/declawing-domestic-cats (accessed 16 March 2021).

American Veterinary Medical Association (AVMA) (2020b). AVMA revises declawing policy. https://www.avma.org/javma-news/2020-03-01/avma-revises-declawing-policy (accessed 16 March 2021).

Animal Welfare Act (2006). s 5. https://www.legislation.gov.uk/ukpga/2006/45/contents (accessed 16 March 2021).

Armitage-Chan, E. and May, S.A. (2019). The veterinary identity: A time and context model. *Journal of Veterinary Medical Education* 46 (2): 153–162.

Australian Veterinary Association (AVA) (2018). Surgical alteration of companion animals' natural functions for human convenience. https://www.ava.com.au/policy-advocacy/ policies/surgical-medical-and-other-veterinary-procedures-general/surgical-alteration-of-companion-animals-natural-functions-for-human-convenience (accessed 15 March 2021).

Bartram, D.J., Yadegarfar, G., and Baldwin, D.S. (2009). A cross-sectional study of mental health and well-being and their associations in the UK veterinary profession. *Social Psychiatry and Psychiatric Epidemiology* 44 (12): 1075.

Batchelor, C.E.M., Creed, A., and McKeegan, D.E.F. (2015). A preliminary investigation into the moral reasoning abilities of UK veterinarians. *Veterinary Record* 177 (5): 124.

Bell, M.A., Cake, M.A., and Mansfield, C.F. (2018). Beyond competence: Why we should talk about employability in veterinary education. *Journal of Veterinary Medical Education* 45 (1): 27–37.

Biaggio, M., Duffy, R., and Staffelbach, D.F. (1998). Obstacles to addressing professional misconduct. *Clinical Psychology Review* 18 (3): 273–285.

Birden, H., Glass, N., Wilson, I. et al. (2013). Teaching professionalism in medical education: A Best Evidence Medical Education (BEME) systematic review. BEME Guide No. 25. *Medical Teacher* 35 (7): e1252–e1266.

Blass, E. (2010). The failure of professional self-regulation: the example of the UK veterinary profession. *Journal of Law and Governance* 5 (4): 1.

Bok, H.G. (2015). Competency-based veterinary education: An integrative approach to learning and assessment in the clinical workplace. *Perspectives on Medical Education* 4 (2): 86–89.

Bok, H.G., Jaarsma, D.A., Teunissen, P.W. et al. (2011). Development and validation of a competency framework for veterinarians. *Journal of Veterinary Medical Education* 38 (3): 262–269.

Brown, J.P. and Silverman, J.D. (1999). The current and future market for veterinarians and veterinary medical services in the United States. *Journal of the American Veterinary Medical Association* 215 (2): 161–183.

Buyx, A.M., Maxwell, B., and Schöne-Seifert, B. (2008). Challenges of educating for medical professionalism: Who should step up to the line? *Medical Education* 42 (8): 758–764.

Clark, C. (2007). Professional responsibility, misconduct and practical reason. *Ethics and Social Welfare* 1 (1): 56–75.

Cron, W.L., Slocum, J.V., Jr., Goodnight, D.B. et al. (2000). Executive summary of the Brakke management and behavior study. *Journal of the American Veterinary Medical Association* 217 (3): 332–338.

Cruess, S.R. and Cruess, R.L. (2000). Professionalism: A contract between medicine and society. *CMAJ* 162 (5): 668–669.

Cruess, S.R. and Cruess, R.L. (2008). Understanding medical professionalism: A plea for an inclusive and integrated approach. *Medical Education* 42 (8): 755–757.

Cruess, S.R. and Cruess, R.L. (2009). The cognitive base of professionalism. In: *Teaching Medical Professionalism* (eds. R.L. Cruess, S.R. Cruess and Y. Steinert), 7–31. New York: Cambridge University Press.

De Briyne, N., Vidović, J., Morton, D.B. et al. (2020). Evolution of the teaching of animal welfare science, ethics and law in European veterinary schools (2012–2019). *Animals* 10 (7): 1238.

Donald, M.M. (2019). When care is defined by science: Exploring veterinary medicine through a more-than-human geography of empathy. *Area* 51 (3): 470–478.

Doukas, D.J., McCullough, L.B., and Wear, S. (2012). Perspective: Medical education in medical ethics and humanities as the foundation for developing medical professionalism. *Academic Medicine* 87 (3): 334–341.

Dunlop, R.H. and Williams, D.J. (1996). *Veterinary Medicine: An Illustrated History*. Maryland Heights, MO: Mosby.

Dunn, M. (2016). On the relationship between medical ethics and medical professionalism. *Journal of Medical Ethics* 42: 625–626.

Edwards, S., Bennett, P., Appleby, M. et al. (2014). Tales about tails: Is the mutilation of animals justifiable in their best interests or in ours. In: *Dilemmas in Animal Welfare* (eds. M. Appleby, P. Sandøe, and D.M. Weary), 6–27. Wallingford, UK: CABI.

Gabbioneta, C., Faulconbridge, J.R., Currie, G. et al. (2019). Inserting professionals and professional organizations in studies of wrongdoing: The nature, antecedents and consequences of professional misconduct. *Human Relations* 72 (11): 1707–1725.

Gauthier, D.K. (2001). Professional lapses: Occupational deviance and neutralization techniques in veterinary medical practice. *Deviant Behavior* 22 (6): 467–490.

Gordon, S., Gardner, D., Weston, J. et al. (2019). Quantitative and thematic analysis of complaints by clients against clinical veterinary practitioners in New Zealand. *New Zealand Veterinary Journal* 67 (3): 117–125.

Grier, K.C.K. and Peterson, N. (2005). Indoor cats, scratching, and the debate over declawing: When normal pet behavior becomes a problem. In: *The State of the Animals III* (eds. D.J. Salem and A.N. Rowan), 27–41. Washington, DC: Humane Society Press.

Hafferty, F.W. and Franks, R. (1994). The hidden curriculum, ethics teaching, and the structure of medical education. *Academic Medicine* 69: 861–871.

Hern, J.C. (2000). Professional conduct and self-regulation. In: *Veterinary Ethics* (ed. G. Legood), 63–74. London and New York: Continuum.

Hernandez, E., Fawcett, A., Brouwer, E. et al. (2018). Speaking up: Veterinary ethical responsibilities and animal welfare issues in everyday practice. *Animals* 8 (1): 15.

Hewson, C.J. (2006). Veterinarians who swear: Animal welfare and the veterinary oath. *The Canadian Veterinary Journal = La Revue Veterinaire Canadienne* 47 (8): 807–811.

Hodgson, J.L., Pelzer, J.M., and Inzana, K.D. (2013). Beyond NAVMEC: Competency-based veterinary education and assessment of the professional competencies. *Journal of Veterinary Medical Education* 40 (2): 102–118.

Hughes, K., Rhind, S.M., Mossop, L. et al. (2018). "Care about my animal, know your stuff and take me seriously": United Kingdom and Australian clients' views on the capabilities most important in their veterinarians. *Veterinary Record* 183 (17): 534.

Jha, V., Bekker, H., Duffy, S. et al. (2006). Perceptions of professionalism in medicine: A qualitative study. *Medical Education* 40 (10): 1027–1036.

Jones, S.D. (2003). *Valuing Animals: Veterinarians and their Patients in Modern America*. Baltimore, MD: Johns Hopkins University Press.

Kipperman, B., Morris, P., and Rollin, B. (2018). Ethical dilemmas encountered by small animal veterinarians: Characterisation, responses, consequences and beliefs regarding euthanasia. *Veterinary Record* 182 (19): 548.

Leighton, F.A. (2004). Veterinary medicine and the lifeboat test: A perspective on the social relevance of the veterinary profession in the twenty-first century. *Journal of Veterinary Medical Education* 31 (4): 329–333.

Lloyd, J.W. (2006). Current economic trends affecting the veterinary medical profession. *Veterinary Clinics: Small Animal Practice* 36 (2): 267–279.

Mackenzie, C.R. (2017). Ethics and professionalism 2016. *Transactions of the American Clinical and Climatological Association* 128: 75.

Magalhães-Sant'Ana, M., More, S., Morton, D. et al. (2015). What do European veterinary codes of conduct actually say and mean? A case study approach. *Veterinary Record* 176: 654.

Martell-Moran, N.K., Solano, M., and Townsend, H.G. (2018). Pain and adverse behavior in declawed cats. *Journal of Feline Medicine and Surgery* 20: 280–288.

May, S.A. (2013). Veterinary ethics, professionalism and society. In: *Veterinary and Animal Ethics: Proceedings of the First International Conference on Veterinary and Animal Ethics, September 2011* (eds. C.M. Wathes, S.A. Corr, S.A. May, S.P. McCulloch, and M.C. Whiting), 44–58. Oxford, UK: Blackwell Publishing.

McNicholas, J., Gilbey, A., Rennie, A. et al. (2005). Pet ownership and human health: A brief review of evidence and issues. *BMJ* 331 (7527): 1252–1254.

Mills, K.E., Von Keyserlingk, M.A., and Niel, L. (2016). A review of medically unnecessary surgeries in dogs and cats. *Journal of the American Veterinary Medical Association* 248: 162–171.

Moses, L., Malowney, M.J., and Wesley Boyd, J. (2018). Ethical conflict and moral distress in veterinary practice: A survey of North American veterinarians. *Journal of Veterinary Internal Medicine* 32 (6): 2115–2122.

Mossop, L.H. (2012a). Is it time to define veterinary professionalism? *Journal of Veterinary Medical Education* 39 (1): 93–100.

Mossop, L. (2012b). Defining and teaching veterinary professionalism. PhD thesis. University of Nottingham.

Mossop, L.H. and Cobb, K. (2013). Teaching and assessing veterinary professionalism. *Journal of Veterinary Medical Education* 40 (3): 223–232.

Muzio, D., Faulconbridge, J., Gabbioneta, C. et al. (2016). Bad apples, bad barrels and bad cellars: A "boundaries" perspective on professional misconduct. In: *Organizational Wrongdoing* (eds. D. Palmer, K. Smith-Crowe, and R. Greenwood), 141–175. Cambridge, UK: Cambridge University Press.

Nett, R.J., Witte, T.K., Holzbauer, S.M. et al. (2015). Risk factors for suicide, attitudes toward mental illness, and practice-related stressors among US veterinarians. *Journal of the American Veterinary Medical Association* 247 (8): 945–955.

Osler, W.O. (1932). On the educational value of the medical society. In: *Aequanimitas, With Other Addresses to Medical Students, Nurses and Practitioners of Medicine* (ed. P. Balkiston), 395–423. Philadelphia, PA: P. Blakiston's Son & Co.

Oxford English Dictionary (2018). *professionalism, n.* Oxford, UK: Oxford University Press.

Oxtoby, C. and Mossop, L. (2019). Blame and shame in the veterinary profession: Barriers and facilitators to reporting significant events. *Veterinary Record* 184 (16): 501.

Packer, R.M.A., Hendricks, A., and Burn, C.C. (2012). Do dog owners perceive the clinical signs related to conformational inherited disorders as "normal" for the breed? A potential constraint to improving animal welfare. *Animal Welfare* 21 (S1): 81–93.

Pyatt, A.Z., Walley, K., Wright, G.H. et al. (2020). Co-produced care in veterinary services: A qualitative study of UK stakeholders' perspectives. *Veterinary Sciences* 7 (4): 149.

Quick, O. (2008). Disaster at Bristol: Explanations and implications of a tragedy. *Journal of Social Welfare and Family Law* 21 (4): 307–326.

Rollin, B.E. (1978). Updating veterinary medical ethics. *Journal of the American Veterinary Medical Association* 173: 1017.

Royal College of Physicians (2005). *Doctors in Society: Medical Professionalism in a Changing World*. London: Royal College of Physicians.

Royal College of Veterinary Surgeons (RCVS) (n.d.). Code of professional conduct for veterinary surgeons. https://www.rcvs.org.uk/setting-standards/advice-and-guidance/code-of-professional-conduct-for-veterinary-surgeons (accessed 15 March 2021).

Royal College of Veterinary Surgeons (RCVS) (2018). RCVS facts. https://www.rcvs.org.uk/news-and-views/publications/rcvs-facts-2018/?destination=/news-and-views/publications/%3Fp%3D2 (accessed 15 March 2021).

Ruch-Gallie, R., Hellyer, P.W., Schoenfeld-Tacher, R. et al. (2016). Survey of practices and perceptions regarding feline onychectomy among private practitioners. *Journal of the American Veterinary Medical Association* 249 (3): 291–298.

Shirley, J.L. and Padgett, S.M. (2006). An analysis of the discourse of professionalism. In: *Professionalism in Medicine* (eds. D. Wear and G.M. Aultman), 25–41. Boston, MA: Springer.

Shivley, C.B., Garry, F.B., Kogan, L.R. et al. (2016). Survey of animal welfare, animal behavior, and animal ethics courses in the curricula of AVMA Council on Education-accredited veterinary colleges and schools. *Journal of the American Veterinary Medical Association* 248 (10): 1165–1170.

State of California (2012). Veterinary medical board disciplinary guidelines. https://www.vmb.ca.gov/forms_pubs/discip_guide.pdf (accessed 15 March 2021).

State of California (n.d.). About the board. https://www.vmb.ca.gov/about_us/board_staff.shtml (Accessed 16 March 2021).

Swick, H.M. (2000). Toward a normative definition of medical professionalism. *Academic Medicine* 75 (6): 612–616.

Swick, H.M., Szenas, P., Danoff, D. et al. (1999). Teaching professionalism in undergraduate medical education. *Journal of the American Medical Association* 282 (9): 830–832.

Tannenbaum, J. (1995). *Veterinary Ethics: Animal Welfare, Client Relations,Competition and Collegiality*, 2e. St. Louis, MO: Mosby.

Tweedie, J., Hordern, J., and Dacre, J. (2018). *Advancing Medical Professionalism*. London: Royal College of Physicians.

Waters, A. (2020). The RCVS needs to reflect on its conduct. *Veterinary Record* 187 (6): 205.

Wensley, S., Betton, V., Martin, N. et al. (2020). Advancing animal welfare and ethics in veterinary practice through a national pet wellbeing task force, practice-based champions and clinical audit. *Veterinary Record* 187 (8): 316.

Wynia, M.K., Papadakis, M.A., Sullivan, W.M. et al. (2014). More than a list of values and desired behaviors: A foundational understanding of medical professionalism. *Academic Medicine* 89 (5): 712–714.

7

# Veterinary Advocacies and Ethical Dilemmas

*Barry Kipperman*

## The Multiple Advocacies of the Veterinarian and Conflicting Interests

A fundamental ethical problem in veterinary practice is whether veterinarians should give primary consideration to the animal or to the client/animal owner (Rollin 2006a; Kipperman et al. 2018). Acknowledging this, Tannenbaum observes that veterinarians are "the servants of two masters" (1995). Rollin makes the distinction between two models of veterinarians: the pediatrician model, which is characterized by patient advocacy, and the model of the mechanic, beholden to client requests and demands regarding the disposition of their legal property (2006a).

It is assumed by animal owners and by society that veterinarians are advocates for animals. The reputation of the veterinary profession is inherently connected to its consideration and treatment of animals (Weich and Grimm 2018). Hughes et al. (2018) found that British and Australian veterinary clients considered the most important objective that veterinarians should pursue is a dedication to the well-being and quality of life of the patient. Rollin (2004) asserts that "It is ... a major part of veterinary medicine to defend the interests of animals."

One of the main impediments to animal advocacy is that veterinarians are hired by humans, not by animals (Sandøe et al. 2008). Veterinarians need to contend with clients' desires and wishes: veterinary decisions are increasingly shaped by these client-centered variables (Springer et al. 2019). In an ethnographic study of small animal veterinarians in the United States, Morris concludes that, "The role of the veterinarian is to provide a list of options for the pet owner ..., leaving nearly every decision regarding their ... patients entirely in the hands of the client" (2012). In this paradigm, the veterinarian is a medical counselor who forms a relationship with and works on behalf of the animal owner. Main acknowledges this model and asks:

> Since the client makes the decision, what contribution does the veterinary surgeon actually make? The veterinary surgeon decides what should be offered or recommended to the client. The emphasis on the client's role in the process is made very clear in the RCVS Guide to Professional Conduct, which states that "veterinary surgeons must accept that their own preference for a certain course

*Ethics in Veterinary Practice: Balancing Conflicting Interests*, First Edition. Edited by Barry Kipperman and Bernard E. Rollin.
© 2022 John Wiley & Sons, Inc. Published 2022 by John Wiley & Sons, Inc.

of action cannot override the client's specific wishes other than on exceptional welfare grounds."

*(2006)*

Consequently, veterinarians may seek to promote client autonomy in lieu of patient interests. One might believe that the fundamental responsibility of a veterinarian is to obey client decisions even to the detriment of the medical interests of patients (short of breaching cruelty laws) (Coghlan 2018). Moreover, any interventions legally and ethically require informed consent from the client.

Another obstacle discouraging the animal advocacy position is economic: the veterinarian is dependent on the animal owner who pays for veterinary services (Main 2006; Dürnberger 2020). Tannenbaum (1995) claims that veterinarians are obliged to serve client interests primarily because they are paying for such services. Consequently, a common practice philosophy is that profitability is commensurate with client satisfaction. Also, veterinarians in practice are commonly compensated based on a proportion of their revenues (Opperman 2019). Although such systems are purportedly intended to reward those seeing many patients, these also create an incentive for the veterinarian to advise costly testing, procedures, hospitalization, and surgery. Consequently, an implicit conflict of interest exists that may influence veterinary recommendations, contributing to unnecessary treatment (Rosoff et al. 2018). After sociological research of veterinary practices in the Netherlands, Swabe asserts: "The notion that profit may possibly influence veterinary decision-making ... conflicts strongly with the collective image of the ... animal doctor that we hold. In deciding the course of action to take, practical and financial considerations may well often outweigh sentiment and idealism" (2000). This conflict of interest is also perceived by clients, as 30% of pet owners agreed that veterinarians advise additional services to make money (Brown 2018).

Unfortunately, all owners do not meet their moral and legal duties to take care of their animals (Main 2006). Then, what is the responsibility of the veterinarian when they believe the decision the owner reaches is not in the animal's best interest? It can be difficult and uncomfortable for veterinarians to confront owners in these circumstances: some may not consider this as within their purview (Sandøe et al. 2008). With regard to the responsibility of the veterinarian when faced with these types of conflicts, Tannenbaum proposes an animal advocacy role, claiming that: "A [veterinarian's] ... obligation to permit a client to make the decision about care for the patient does not preclude the doctor from presenting oneself as an advocate for the animal and offering on its behalf arguments against the apparent tendencies of the client" (1995). Main also argues in support of the animal advocacy position:

> Do veterinary surgeons need to worry about causing distress (in this case, guilt) to clients concerning the cost of treatments? I would argue that ... the obligation to the animal's best interest is greater than a concern for the psychological well-being of the client. If we placed a higher value on clients' sensitivities, then our duty as animal advocates would not be fulfilled.

*(2006)*

**Table 7.1** Veterinarian interests.

| |
| --- |
| Animal |
| Client |
| Veterinarian |
| Practice owner/employer |
| Financial compensation |
| Public health |
| Referring veterinarian |
| Research/publications/teaching |

Results of a survey supported an animal advocacy posture, as 96% of Australian veterinary students agreed that their primary focus as a veterinarian should be the interests of the animals in their care (Verrinder and Phillips 2014). Morris found that many veterinarians feel compelled to advocate for the best interests of animals, just as pediatricians are expected to advocate for the best interests of children (2012). But the author concludes that adoption of this posture is rare in practice: "Because animals are legally considered property and veterinarians depend on clients for income, veterinary medicine is more client oriented than patient oriented... Because veterinarians are more likely to be subject to client demands, veterinarians are ... client-dependent professionals" (Morris 2012).

Many clients desire and select the best veterinary care for their animals. In a utopian view of veterinary practice, a model of shared decision-making occurs, in which the interests of the patient and human family are aligned and pursued (Coghlan 2018). Unfortunately, exceptions to this ideal are common in veterinary practice. Although most of the conflicts encountered by veterinary professionals involve the interests of the client and animal, a list of the factors that impact decision-making regarding patients would also include the veterinarian's interest in performing or learning procedures and professional advancement, their interest in making money, and the expectations from their employer to generate income (Table 7.1).

## Differences Between US and UK Codes of Conduct

The American Veterinary Medical Association (AVMA) Veterinarian's Oath provides no guidance in prioritization of a veterinarian's varied obligations: "I ... swear to use my scientific knowledge ... for the benefit of society through the protection of animal health and welfare, the prevention and relief of animal suffering, ... and the advancement of medical knowledge" (AVMA n.d.). In contrast, the Royal College of Veterinary Surgeons (RCVS) Oath emphasizes patient advocacy: "I will ... accept my responsibilities to ... my clients, the profession ... and that, ABOVE ALL, my constant endeavour will be to ensure the health and welfare of animals committed to my care" (RCVS n.d.).

## Types of Animal Patients

Veterinarians see patients in differing contexts with differing sets of expectations, which may influence the type and extent of care a patient may receive. As an example, a companion animal viewed as a family member who sleeps in the bed may be expected to receive a more thorough level of care compared to a guard dog, who may receive better care than a farm animal, who may be viewed as an economic asset, or a rodent in a laboratory contributing to scientific knowledge. In laboratory animal and farm animal practice, veterinary services are often intended to aid humans and society rather than the animals (Grimm et al. 2018). Even in companion animal practice, some procedures (i.e. declawing) do not promote animals' health-related interests. Huth observes these inconsistencies:

> So, being a patient in veterinary medicine ... can have different meanings with different ethical implications. While companion animals are often treated with high effort and costs to ... sustain their well-being, livestock animals are not exclusively treated with regards to their well-being but also to sustain productivity. The expectations on the part of the owner, but also social expectations differ significantly. However, in both cases the animal remains a patient ..., but they are different kinds of patients.
>
> *(2020)*

Regarding the responsibility of veterinarians toward animal patients, there are unavoidable comparisons with human medicine, especially in terms of ethical duties (Rollin 2006a). It is generally believed that physicians will (almost) always advocate for their patients, diminishing their interests and the interests of others. This norm arises from the Hippocratic Oath (Coghlan 2018). Medical decisions on behalf of children are made by parents acting as their agent, with legal engagement only when the decision is deemed to be harmful to the child's welfare (Gray et al. 2020). A recent essay suggests that companion animals are comparable with dependent children: treatment decisions are made by their owners presumably on their behalf (Gray and Fordyce 2020). Considering the obvious challenges in obtaining informed consent directly from animals and instead relying on human presumptions of their preferences (Franks 2019), comparisons with infant children may be more apt, as their desires cannot be surmised as easily (Rollin 2002; Ashall et al. 2018).

## Why the Profession of Veterinary Medicine Is Fraught with Ethical Concerns

There are a myriad of reasons that veterinary professionals are more likely to encounter ethical conflicts compared with those working in the human medical field. These disparities exist both within the profession itself, as well as between veterinary professionals and their clients, and include differences in beliefs regarding:

- The importance or value of animals
- Human responsibilities to animals

- The best interests of animals
- The primary allegiance of the veterinarian
- The influence of money on decision-making
- The legal status of animals as property.
  (modified from Morgan and McDonald 2007)

## What Is an Ethical Dilemma?

Ethical dilemmas arise when there are competing interests of perceived equal moral weight, and there is a lack of clearly defined rules to prioritize these, i.e. it is not clear what is the "right thing to do" (Morgan and McDonald 2007). Ethical dilemmas can involve the recognition of two or more choices both or all of which are believed to be equally wrong, resulting in the realization that it is impossible to "do the right thing" (Richards et al. 2020). An alternative definition may include a circumstance whereby an ethical response is clear but is difficult to act on because of anticipated undesirable consequences, such as client dissatisfaction or lost income (Morgan and McDonald 2007).

## Types of Ethical Dilemmas

Veterinary professionals in practice encounter many types of ethical dilemmas, summarized in Table 7.2.

**Table 7.2** Types of ethical dilemmas in veterinary practice (modified from Fawcett 2020).

| |
| --- |
| Financial limitations compromise patient care (Kondrup et al. 2016; Kipperman et al. 2018; Lehnus et al. 2019; Dürnberger 2020; Quain et al. 2021) |
| Futile intervention: client wishes to continue treatment despite poor animal quality of life and prognosis (Batchelor et al 2012; Moses et al. 2018; Lehnus et al. 2019) |
| Euthanasia based on economic factors or for client convenience (Batchelor et al. 2012; Rathwell-Deault et al. 2017; Kipperman et al. 2018; Dürnberger 2020) |
| Balancing interests of animal against interests of client (Tannenbaum 1995; Rollin 2006a; Kipperman et al. 2018; Moses et al. 2018; Quain et al. 2021) |
| Whether to confront or report a colleague providing incompetent or substandard care (Rollin 2006a; Crane et al. 2015) |
| Whether to report suspected animal abuse (Kogan et al. 2017; Joo et al. 2020; Dürnberger 2020) |
| Being asked to do something that feels like the wrong thing to do (Moses et al. 2018; Lehnus et al. 2019) |
| Being asked to do things that are outside of your skill set for financial or other reasons (Moses et al. 2018) |
| Disclosing bad news or medical errors (Kogan et al. 2018) |
| Whether or not to offer referral when this may provide a better outcome (Rollin 2006b) |
| Whether to perform cosmetic or convenience surgeries (Morgan and McDonald 2007; Mills et al. 2016) |

## Frequency of Encountering Ethical Dilemmas

The majority of veterinarians experience an ethical dilemma at least once per week (Batchelor and McKeegan 2012; Kipperman et al. 2018; Lehnus et al. 2019; Quain et al. 2021). Although no study has examined how often veterinarians are subject to all of the conflicts listed in Table 7.2, the most common dilemma encountered by small animal veterinarians in one study was client financial limitations compromising patient care, with a median response of a few times a week (Kipperman et al. 2018). A recent study of veterinarians and veterinary technicians also found how to proceed with clients with limited finances as the most common dilemma (Quain et al. 2021). In small animal practice, euthanasia requests perceived to be based on lack of financial means occur with a median frequency of once a month, and euthanasia requests based on perceived client unwillingness to pay for treatment occur with a median frequency of a few times a year (Kipperman et al. 2018). These findings support the premise that financial concerns of animal owners are frequent causes of ethical conflicts for veterinarians.

Female veterinarians experience ethical dilemmas more frequently than males (Kipperman et al. 2018; Chun et al. 2019). These findings are in accord with a study documenting that female small animal veterinarians were more inclined to attempt treatment of animals in the face of economic limitations than males (Kondrup et al. 2016), and with reports that female students in animal science and veterinary programs had greater empathy for animals (Hazel et al. 2011; Colombo et al. 2016). It seems logical to propose that these characteristics would make one more likely to perceive an ethical dilemma. As the majority of those entering veterinary practice in the United States and the UK are female (Association of American Veterinary Medical Colleges 2019; Institute for Employment Studies Report 2019), this propensity to perceive ethical conflicts should be particularly concerning to the profession.

More experienced practitioners are less likely to report encountering an ethical dilemma (Kipperman et al. 2018; Wojtacka et al. 2020). It is reasonable to presume that with experience a practitioner would develop improved moral reasoning skills, but a study documented no improvement in moral reasoning of veterinarians in the UK with experience, which challenges this assumption (Batchelor et al. 2015). Alternatively, experienced practitioners over time may become desensitized to circumstances that novice colleagues may find ethically problematic.

## Advocacy Behaviors of Veterinarians

There is limited scientific literature examining how veterinarians balance client and animal interests when these are at odds. In a quantitative study, 57% of small animal veterinarians described the conduct of their colleagues as prioritizing the interests of the client, and only 20% indicated that they believed other practitioners prioritize the interests of the patient (Kipperman et al. 2018). In contrast, 50% of these veterinarians reported their own behavior as prioritizing patient interests, while only 16% reported prioritizing the client's interest. Corroborating these findings, in a study by Moses et al. (2018) 60% of veterinarians revealed they prioritized the needs of clients over patients. Another report found that only 48% of veterinarians and veterinary techni-cians believed that their primary obligation was to animal patients (Quain et al. 2021). A recent report discovered that while most small animal veterinarians in Europe agreed with a patient advocacy paradigm, a client-centered orientation was more prev-alent than a patient-focused orientation (Springer et al. 2021). In another investiga-tion, 92% of veterinary students indicated that veterinarians should prioritize patient interests when the interests of clients and patients conflict, whereas 84% of students reported that veterinarians most often prioritize client interests in these circumstances (Kipperman et al. 2020).

The evidence from the studies available casts doubt as to whether veterinarians are meeting societal expectations as advocates for animals. The stark contrast between the idealism focused on animal advocacy of veterinary students and their perceptions that a client-centered paradigm prevails in practice, creates potential for disillusionment and professional burnout. From a normative perspective, these findings should also prompt the profession to consider why many of its members' behaviors do not reflect the ideals of its students. Concerted efforts to educate veterinary students and veteri-narians about ethical dilemmas unique to the profession and their roles as animal advocates are warranted. Educators should also support the veterinarians' role as ani-mal advocate and prepare students for the contrast in advocacy preferences they are apt to encounter in practice.

## The Case for a "Best Interest" or Patient Advocacy Paradigm

Numerous ethicists have proposed a "best interest" or patient advocacy model for vet-erinary medicine (Rollin 2006a; Grimm and Huth 2017; Coghlan 2018; Ashall et al. 2018; Thurner 2020). An ethics working party advised that companion animal practice be based on the principle of "in the animal's best interest," focused on two fundamen-tal criteria: aiming to restore a patient's health and respecting the patient's quality of life (Grimm et al. 2018). Another definition of a "best interest" archetype advances this commitment, asserting that an animal is a patient only if the veterinary treatment provided intends to benefit their health-related interests *for the animal's own good* and not for the purposes of others (Grimm and Huth 2017).

Coghlan (2018) takes this one step further and claims that patient advocacy should transpire, "even when advocacy may interfere with clients' plans, wishes, and inter-ests." There have been numerous instances when I had the unenviable task during the holiday season of relaying a terminal diagnosis such as widespread cancer to a client regarding a patient who was suffering. A reasonably common client response was: "Can you make him comfortable until my children are home from college in two weeks so we can all say goodbye?" This challenging circumstance offers an opportu-nity for the veterinarian to live up to Coghlan's standard by gently conveying the impact of the illness on the patient's quality of life, advocating that a more appropriate timetable for consideration of euthanasia should be measured in hours or days rather than weeks. In more explicitly characterizing this paradigm, Thurner (2020) uses the example of an animal patient with a fractured limb. The only ethically acceptable outcome is facilitating repair of the break provided there is a good chance that quality of life can be restored. A euthanasia decision based on ending suffering or for the convenience of the animal owner would not be deemed acceptable outcomes.

Coghlan implores veterinarians to pursue "strong patient advocacy" (SPA), suggesting this is a philosophy of practice:

> What distinguishes SPAs ... is the *preparedness* to engage in the full gamut of justifiable advocacy options required for preventing harm to patients. Strong patient advocacy involves a disposition and a moral stance orientated toward the goal of improved patient wellbeing and an embrace of the range of justifiable ethical means and resources veterinarians have at their disposal.
>
> *(2018)*

It has been asserted that improvements in animal welfare can only be furthered if veterinarians view animal advocacy as their primary raison d'être, and that acquiescing to the requests of animal owners may result in outcomes that may be detrimental to animal welfare (Kipperman 2017). Hernandez et al. (2018) make the welfare-based case for animal advocacy:

> Advocating for animal welfare may not be comfortable and may, at times, require courage but is necessary ... to improve human regard for animals as sentient beings. [Failure to do so] ... can lead to an inability or difficulty in speaking up about concerns with clients and ultimately, failure in their duty of care to animals, leading to poor animal welfare outcomes.

Veterinarians manifest ambivalence as they navigate ethical conflicts involving clients and patients. Having a sense of clarity regarding one's professional identity can act as a moral compass, helping to assuage the contextual inconsistencies inherent in veterinary practice. During the course of my career as an internist (often on an emotionally trying day when multiple patients had died), numerous students and interns have posed this thought-provoking question: "How do you determine whether you were a good veterinarian or had a successful day?" I tell them that defining success based on patient survival or death is unreasonable as there are so many factors influencing these outcomes that are beyond the control of the veterinarian. My response is simple: "Did I advocate for each of my patients to the best of my ability?" Or to use Coghlan's term (2018), was I a "strong patient advocate?" Let's now examine the obstacles to fulfilling this standard.

## Limitations to a "Best Interest" or Patient Advocacy Paradigm

Veterinarians cannot directly obtain the medical wishes from their patients and are dependent on the animal owner acting as the patient's agent. Therefore, pursuing a patient advocacy paradigm requires provision of informed consent to the owner, taking into account all available options for the patient including prognosis, potential benefits, risks, costs, and side effects of possible interventions (see Chapter 5 for a more thorough discussion). This is inevitably time consuming, and the limited duration of office visits in general small animal practice is a significant barrier to accomplishing this (Robinson et al. 2014; Corah et al. 2019).

Attempts to effect changes in practices regarding animal patients, such as advocating for management of patient obesity via dietary modifications, may be perceived by clients as offensive (Cairns-Haylor and Fordyce 2017). Discussing all of the available alternatives for the patient with the client, advising the option believed to provide the best chance for a positive result, and having the client regularly choose another option which the practitioner believes compromises patient outcome or prolongs poor quality of life can be emotionally draining and onerous. Consequently, pursuing a "patient best interest" model may be a metaphorical weight that becomes too heavy to lift for veterinarians over time, contributing to moral stress (see Chapter 22 for a more detailed discussion) (Springer et al. 2019). Grimm et al. (2018) argue that confronting moral stress is integral to the veterinarian's responsibility. Huth (2020) acknowledges this risk and attempts to relieve this burden on the veterinarian:

> Such [moral] distress often results from an exclusively animal-centered perspective and ethical demands for equal treatments of animals... It has a preventive effect against moral distress to be aware of the different obstacles for animal welfare and practical constraints that we [veterinarians] face... This awareness is not an abdication of responsibility but a prerequisite to acknowledging the ... limits of veterinary responsibility – particularly for effecting ethical change.

A veterinarian's capacity to pursue a "best interest" posture may reasonably be associated with their perception of autonomy within the culture and hierarchy of a particular practice. An intern, new graduate, new associate, or technician would be expected to have less independence to express their professional identity than a long-term associate or practice owner. As an example, I've had numerous colleagues tell me that they only feel comfortable referring patients to another hospital on days when their employer is not at the practice, due to intimidation. If a veterinarian feels subjected to hospital-based expectations that they are unable to overcome, this may negatively influence enactment of a "best interest" paradigm.

Veterinary care is becoming increasingly expensive (see Chapter 8 for a more detailed discussion of economic issues). The collaboration between veterinary professionals and animal owners requires discussion of the costs of tests and treatments, which may limit the viable choices. Unfortunately, pursuing a "best interest" model for small animal patients via the veterinary healthcare system is heavily reliant on the owner paying out of pocket, given the low prevalence of pet insurance (Kipperman et al. 2017). Clients may naturally be expected to select lower-cost options, especially if they do not understand why a costlier alternative may be more likely to result in a better outcome for their animal. Patient advocacy may be less ethically justifiable to pursue when a client expresses that they are unable to pay or if it is determined that such costs would be detrimental to them or their families (Coghlan 2018). Coghlan (2018) notes differing societal expectations regarding the financial obligations of animal owners compared with human parents:

> it remains true that pediatricians enjoy *comparatively* more power over good patient health outcomes than do veterinarians. ... this difference in authority is partly connected to the ... moral point: that society holds parental responsibilities to surpass client responsibilities to animal companions. For example, we might well expect parents to risk serious financial hardship ... to help their very ill children.

Clients also have the legal right to refuse well-intended veterinary counsel (Coghlan 2018). The legal status of animals as property (see Chapter 5) complicates any "best interest" paradigm as a foundation for veterinary decisions (Gray and Fordyce 2020). Gray and Fordyce have summarized the limitations of legal status and economics on patient advocacy quite nicely:

> Direct comparisons between pediatric and veterinary decision-making require specific assumptions; first, that the owner regards the animal as having intrinsic value, and second, that there is an ... acceptance of the subservience of the owner's potential "selfish interests" ... to the best interests of that animal. Because of the different ... funding arrangements for treatment that protect children and animals from harm, this "selfish interest" concept may include resolution of the dilemmas surrounding the ability or desire of the owner to fund any potential treatment.
>
> *(2020 )*

## Communication

To be an animal advocate, one must be able to effectively communicate with their human owners and caretakers to educate them, and to inspire trust and confidence in the veterinary professional as both a caring and knowledgeable figure. This can be especially challenging for new graduates (Haldane et al. 2017). An association between communication skills and client compliance with veterinary recommendations reflects my own experience and has been documented (Kanji et al. 2012). Consequently, a veterinarian may blame the client for failing to adhere to professional guidance rather than ineffective communication on the part of the practitioner.

Veterinarians appear to routinely make judgments about their clients including categorizing them as "good" or "bad" in terms of inclination to pursue treatments or pay the fees (Morgan 2009). Therefore, if a veterinarian presumed that a client could not afford diagnostic testing or would not pay for it, testing may not be offered. A study corroborates this, finding that approximately a third of small animal veterinarians indicated that they do not offer ideal diagnostic or treatment options in the list of alternatives provided to all clients (Kipperman et al. 2017).

Limiting provision of options due to classification of clients can compromise both patient advocacy and the veterinarian's capacity to promote animal welfare (Hernandez et al. 2018).

Morgan and McDonald suggest that practitioners should attempt to discern the bond clients have with their pet (2007). This may involve encouraging clients to share information regarding their emotional attachment to the patient, their mutual experiences, and the animal's role in the household (Coghlan 2018). In challenging circumstances, veterinary professionals may find it necessary to discuss their duties with clients including easing animal suffering (Morgan and McDonald 2007). It is argued that there should be limits to the extent to which veterinarians should grant client requests:

> Veterinarians should feel comfortable in drawing boundaries by indicating ... what they consider to be inappropriate solutions to a problem. ... it may be possible to develop hospital policies around issues that occur frequently... Common problem situations may be discussed during practice meetings to develop ... policies that all members of the veterinary team can support. Establishing these boundaries ... may also minimize moral stress to practitioners.
>
> *(Morgan and McDonald 2007 )*

In certain settings, negotiating with clients may be warranted to achieve the best outcome for patients. As an example, a client may not be motivated by the veterinary professional's divulged concern that the patient is gaining weight, is now overweight, and requires dietary modifications. Instead of being discouraged and giving up, the veterinary professional can instead attempt to strike a "bargain" with the client: "Mrs. S, can we agree that you'll bring Buffy by for another weight check in a month at no charge, and if she continues to gain weight, we'd agree to change her diet then?"

## Is Client Persuasion Acceptable?

Physicians and veterinarians share a formidable authority entrusted to those that society recognizes as healers (Rollin 2002). Scholars agree that such influence should be used to promote the patient's best interests and that pursuit of any other objective signifies taking advantage of that authority (Rollin 2002; Yeates and Main 2010; Shaw and Elger 2013). For example, Plato observed that one's role as a healer should not be influenced by one's role as a businessperson (Rollin 2002). A patient advocacy position should also support the idea that clients have the right to have their autonomy respected as an essential tenet of veterinary practice. This principle of recognition of autonomy in medical ethics has been the basis for the belief that it is unethical to persuade or change a patient's (or client's in veterinary medicine) decision, because doing so could represent intimidation, paternalism, or exploitation (Rubinelli 2013; Shaw and Elger 2013). Rosoff et al. (2018) dispute this assertion, suggesting that owners are not omnipotent and that veterinarians have a moral authority, which can influence client decisions regarding their animals. The challenge for veterinarians is to provide enough information to facilitate informed consent from the owner and to advocate for the patient, while not inflicting one's own beliefs that may incur approval of a degree of risk that is untenable for the client (Fettman and Rollin 2002).

Scholars (Barilan and Weintraub 2001; Shaw and Elger 2013) argue that persuasion is an integral part of medical practice. Barilan and Weintraub contend that clinicians are obligated to influence their patients:

> healthcare professionals are obliged to try to persuade their patients to accept medical advice in order to expedite medical outcome ... if a physician wishes to act with respect for the person of his or her patient, the physician must participate in a conversation in which he or she will do his or her best to persuade the patient to consent.
>
> *(2001)*

If we extend this conclusion to the profession of veterinary medicine, then veterinarians have a moral duty to encourage their clients to pursue what the clinician believes to be the best medical advice for the patient. Exerting influence may be more readily justified when clients want to be influenced. Yeates and Main (2010) observe that many clients want their veterinarian to help them make decisions by sharing their expertise and views. In this paradigm of "ethical persuasion" it would be reasonable for a practitioner to reveal their recommended course of action or to state what they would do in the same situation when clients ask "What would you do, Doctor?" One author advances this idea by contending that physicians who do not disclose their suggested plan are depriving patients of pertinent knowledge and are therefore limiting their capacity to grant informed consent (Shaw and Elger 2013).

Coghlan (2018) argues that there are limits to clinician persuasion: "Coercing or intimidating guardians ... is both illegal and wrong. ... while veterinarians may well advocate assiduously and creatively for patients, they are not typically entitled to lie to, seriously deceive, or coerce clients (except by invoking the law), even to protect their patients' vital interests."

Ultimately, the decision of when it is appropriate to influence a client must be left to the practitioner. Some veterinary ethicists contend that exerting influence is most compelling when the client makes a decision that the veterinarian deems to be unreasonable relative to the animal's best interest (Rollin 2006a; Yeates and Main 2010). As an example of when persuasion should be exercised, Rollin (2002) argues for leveraging the authority of the veterinarian when faced with requests to euthanize healthy animals:

> the only escape from moral stress in the context of demands for convenience euthanasia is to do everything in one's power to save that animal, including exerting one's Aesculapian authority as forcefully as possible. Thus, it is well within the role of veterinarian as healing professional to deploy his or her Aesculapian authority to keep a healthy animal alive.

## Ethics Instruction

Ethics education in veterinary school may improve capacity to recognize ethical conflicts and provide approaches that facilitate ethical decision-making (Hernandez et al. 2018). The need for ethics instruction for veterinarians has been examined. A survey found that only 45% of Australian veterinary students agreed that they were proficient in ethical decision-making abilities to guide views on animal ethics issues (Verrinder and Phillips 2014), and in another survey only about 25% of Australian veterinarians agreed that the behavior of colleagues is consistent with the ethics of the profession (Heath 2002). Despite these findings, training in ethics for veterinary students is not uniformly available.

Only 30% of AVMA-accredited veterinary schools in the United States that responded to a survey reported to offer a formal course in ethics (Shivley et al. 2016). Recent studies found that 51% of US small animal practitioners reported having received ethics training in their curriculum (Kipperman et al. 2018), 29% of North American veterinarians received instruction in resolving conflicts about what is best care for patients (Moses et al. 2018), and only 20% of Korean veterinarians participated in ethics training programs (Chun et al. 2019). Rawles (2000) agrees with these findings, observing that "vets … are … on an ethical high-wire, constantly balancing their concern with animal welfare against the demands of the industries, clients and practices they work for, without having been given any training in how to do this."

Regarding the effectiveness of ethics education, results are inconclusive. Only 39% of small animal veterinarians who had received ethics instruction in veterinary school agreed that such training prepared them to address ethical dilemmas (Kipperman et al. 2018). This finding differs from the opinions of most first-year Australian veterinary students, who agreed that training they received to assist them in making ethical decisions was beneficial for illuminating their own or others' positions, and for improving moral reasoning abilities (Verrinder and Phillips 2014). The most recent study on this topic found that 78% of US veterinary students from four schools reported having received training in ethical theories and approaches to address ethical dilemmas (Kipperman et al. 2020). These results were more optimistic, finding that 80% of students agreed that they feel better prepared to identify ethical dilemmas they may encounter as veterinarians as a result of their ethics training, and 55% agreed that they felt better prepared to address ethical dilemmas as a result of their ethics training.

The available evidence suggests that students are more likely to believe their ethics training has prepared them to address ethical dilemmas compared with practitioners. One explanation for this is that ethics instruction may be better at promoting ethical competencies than in the past. A report has documented the success of student-centered, case-based scenarios and discussion in ethics education (Magalhães-Sant' Ana et al. 2016). Alternatively, as students become practitioners, they may forget or fail to use the ethical principles they were taught in school. The finding that 95% of veterinary students in a recent study felt that veterinary ethics should be taught in the veterinary curriculum also corroborates the value of ethics instruction (Kipperman et al. 2020). On the basis of these findings, ethics training should be a core component of the veterinary curriculum. Postgraduate educational opportunities in ethics are warranted and may help to retain the perceived value of ethics instruction.

## Methods to Address Ethical Conflicts

Just as veterinarians are taught to use a problem-oriented or subjective, objective, assessment, and plan (SOAP) system to improve capacity to formulate a diagnostic and therapeutic plan for patient care, utilizing a systematic approach is advised to address ethical problems (Case Study 7.1). Such frameworks do not necessarily provide a right or wrong answer but are intended to guide discussion of pertinent veterinary ethical concerns and facilitate ethical problem-solving (Grimm et al. 2018). A study of small animal veterinarians discovered that gut instinct based on their personal value system was the most common method utilized to address ethical dilemmas, while guidance from written policies of state or national veterinary organizations, and consideration of varied ethical theories, were least often used (Kipperman et al. 2018). A recent study of veterinarians and veterinary technicians found that discussion with colleagues was the most commonly reported method to help address ethical dilemmas: only 25% referred to codes of conduct and 15% utilized ethical frameworks (Quain et al. 2021). It appears that veterinarians are not using step-by-step frameworks in their everyday ethical decision-making. An approach I have applied with success and teach veterinary students is shown in Table 7.3. A more elaborate methodology, the veterinary ethics tool (VET), has also been proposed (Grimm et al. 2018) (see Table 23.2).

Veterinary practitioners believe that sharing their experiences with colleagues and having ongoing ethics conversations in their workplace would be helpful (Richards et al. 2020). Yet, a recent study identified that less than half of the teams surveyed at 42 veterinary hospitals were completely satisfied with the level of discussion about ethically challenging cases (Wensley et al. 2020). When veterinary professionals are aware of ethical problems and foster discussions in a supportive setting in which practitioners can talk freely about ethical issues, an ethical culture is established (Kong 2015). This could include open-minded discussions with compatible peers as well as with veterinary ethicists (Hernandez et al. 2018). The development of "ethics rounds" and/or clinical ethics consultation/support services may help facilitate ethical problem-solving for veterinary practitioners in the future (Adin et al. 2019) (see Chapter 23).

**Table 7.3** Framework for addressing ethical dilemmas.

1. Who are the relevant interests?
What are the strengths of each interest?
How do these interests conflict?

2. What are the available choices and their potential consequences for each interest?

3. Which ethical theory best addresses this specific situation? (See Chapter 4)

4. Are there any relevant laws or codes of conduct to consider?

5. Choose a course of action or inaction.
Have I advocated for my patient/s to the best of my ability?

**Case Study 7.1    Euthanasia request: A cat with chronic illness and good quality of life**

Mrs. A is a nurse and a new client at your veterinary hospital. She presents her 12-year-old cat, Debra, for euthanasia. Hospital regulations require a consultation and examination before this procedure can be performed. Mrs. A tells you that Debra drinks water all day, eats all the time, and is losing weight. She relates that she can't bear to see Debra waste away, and she is convinced that Debra has diabetes mellitus, although no testing has been performed. Mrs. A expresses that she has no interest in treating her cat for diabetes. Examination reveals that Debra is alert, thin, and walks around and jumps on the chair in the exam room. You do not perceive that the cat is suffering. There is no hospital policy regarding declining euthanasia requests.

**What should you do?**

Ethical analysis:
The relevant interests in this ethical dilemma include the patient, the client, the attending veterinarian, the hospital team, the practice as a business entity, the veterinarian's employer, and the veterinary profession. You suspect Debra has diabetes mellitus, kidney failure, hyperthyroidism, or possibly a combination of these conditions. These diseases can usually be managed but require lifelong treatment and monitoring, which Mrs. A seems unwilling or unable to provide.

Choices include:
1) Proceed with the client's request for euthanasia.
2) Inform the client that you share her concerns regarding Debra's weight loss, but you do not believe in euthanizing animals who are not suffering and (i) provide parameters for when it is more reasonable to consider ending Debra's life, or (ii) advise she seek to have Debra adopted by another party, or (iii) advise referring Debra to another colleague.
3) Persuade the client to consider testing and treating Debra.

It is inevitable that a practicing veterinarian will experience conflicts regarding the legitimacy of euthanasia requests. Examples of what some refer to as convenience euthanasia include client requests for euthanasia based on economics, changes in personal circumstances, or lack of time, capacity, or desire to care for an animal (Batchelor and McKeegan 2012; Ogden et al. 2012; Rathwell-Deault et al. 2017). Others find this term offensive and believe that the veterinarian cannot know all the circumstances that led a client to this decision (for example, Mrs. A may have just experienced the loss of a friend or relative from chronic illness), and the veterinarian has an obligation to serve the client who pays for their services. Most veterinarians consider euthanasia of a healthy animal to be contrary to their role as animal advocate (Rollin 2006a). This case is a bit more complex, as Debra is not "healthy." It is unfortunate, but not surprising, that no hospital policy exists to address this dilemma.

Some veterinarians feel coerced or are encouraged by their employer or practice manager to perform euthanasia in settings where they disagree with this decision (Yeates and Main 2011; Morris 2012; Kipperman 2017). Supporting these findings, a study discovered that 45% of small animal veterinarians agreed that veterinarians sometimes use euthanasia as an aid or method to resolve difficult cases when this may not be in the best interest of the patient (Kipperman et al. 2018). The AVMA Guidelines for the Euthanasia of Animals (2020) are ambiguous regarding the basis of euthanasia decisions, noting "Impacts on animals may not always be the center of the valuation process, and there is disagreement on how to account for conflicting interspecific interests."

Although a contractarian approach to this case may support pursuing euthanasia as it is apt to satisfy the client and the economic interests of the practice, there may be pernicious long-term consequences such as moral stress incurred by the professional team that complies with this euthanasia request (Morris 2012; Kipperman et al. 2018). Proceeding with this request may also create tension if there is disagreement between the views of the attending veterinarian and the paraprofessional and technical team. One could attempt to rationalize a decision to perform euthanasia on the premise that it may spare Debra from suffering at some point in the future. Of course, one could then apply this reasoning to the euthanasia of any animal patient! A euthanasia decision may also reflect poorly on the perception of the veterinary profession vis-á-vis animal advocacy. An animal rights view would not condone a euthanasia decision, as this outcome is not deemed to be in Debra's best interest at this time as suffering has not been detected, and this option would deprive Debra of future positive experiences. A deontological perspective based on good intentions, duties, and principles would also likely not countenance a euthanasia decision. A utilitarian position must consider all interests and potential consequences and is the most complex to consider.

While 80% of small animal veterinarians in a recent study indicated having declined a euthanasia request, these decisions were uncommon, with a median frequency of every few years (Kipperman et al. 2018). The most common reason cited for reluctance to decline euthanasia requests was fear that the client may seek other options that could worsen the animal's welfare. The second most common reason cited for reluctance to decline euthanasia requests was the difficulty in doing so once a client had reached this decision (Kipperman et al. 2018). The AVMA Guidelines for the Euthanasia of Animals (2020) encourage discussion rather than acquiescence: "There may be instances in which the decision to kill an animal is questionable, especially if the animal is predicted to have a life worth living... In this case, the veterinarian, as ... animal advocate, should be able to speak frankly about the animal's condition and suggest alternatives to euthanasia." These findings suggest there may be benefit to training in veterinary curricula emphasizing navigating challenging end-of-life decisions and, in particular, encouraging students and veterinarians to feel comfortable advocating for alternatives to euthanasia when this may not be in an animal's interest. A patient advocacy posture requires skillful and resolute dialogue and courage to avoid a euthanasia decision.

Informing the client that you are not comfortable complying with this request based on your belief that Debra's present quality of life is still good may allay Mrs. A's concerns or may be perceived as confrontational and jeopardize your and the practice's relationship with the client, is awkward and difficult to accomplish, may elicit unflattering or derogatory comments by the client about you on social media, and may be considered to place your job and financial security at risk if your employer is displeased. Acknowledging how difficult it must be to see Debra lose weight and the fear of seeing her condition decline, and providing parameters for when euthanasia should be considered, is a reasonable course of action that respects both Mrs. A's feelings and Debra's interest in enjoying the remainder of her life. What if you were to provide discrete criteria regarding symptoms of illness that justify euthanasia in the future, but Mrs. A. does not recognize or chooses not to act when such symptoms arise? Engaging in behavior that you believe to be dubious or wrong (in this case, euthanasia) on the assumption that someone else (the client) *may* do something that results in a worse outcome for the animal (not returning when Debra's condition worsens, causing suffering) is an insufficient premise on which to base ethical decisions. We are responsible for our own choices, not for the decisions and actions of others. You as the attending veterinarian have to live with the consequences of *your* actions.

Proposing adoption by another party would sever the bond the patient has with the owner and would likely be perceived as impugning Mrs. A's commitment to Debra. Moreover, a geriatric cat with a chronic medical condition/s may not be considered highly adoptable. Advising that Mrs. A see another veterinarian may serve to convince her that a euthanasia decision is inappropriate only provided that another colleague also would not proceed with euthanasia. If your colleague were to consent to this request, Mrs. A would be more likely to feel resentment about your unwillingness to accommodate her and perceive you were insensitive to her emotional state. Perhaps for this reason, I have experienced colleagues defending euthanasia decisions reasoning that "If I don't do it, someone else will." Some practitioners may be reluctant to shift this responsibility on to another colleague (Morris 2012). Offering testing to discern the cause of Debra's symptoms and prognosis is reasonable, but expecting Mrs. A to consent to a complete battery of testing and treatment seems unlikely under the circumstances.

Attempting to identify the reasons for Mrs. A's reluctance to treat Debra could be quite valuable, as some of these barriers (such as fear of needles) may be irrelevant if the cat is hyperthyroid, and other obstacles (such as administration of subcutaneous fluids) can potentially be surmounted via creative measures such as having a veterinary technician come to the home to give injections. Ideally, meeting with your employer, hospital manager, and paraprofessional team to discuss available options and their potential consequences is most likely to result in a decision that can be agreed upon as satisfactory or that achieves the greatest net benefit. In fact, alternative solutions may be discovered. If there are significant differences of opinion regarding the best course of action despite such measures, the attending veterinarian may conclude that their professional identity is not aligned with the culture of the practice. Though disappointing in the short term, this may facilitate the veterinarian pursuing a position in another practice that better suits their ideals.

# References

Adin, C.A., Moga, J.L., Keene, B.W. et al. (2019). Clinical ethics consultation in a tertiary care veterinary teaching hospital. *Journal of the American Veterinary Medical Association* 254 (1): 52–60.

American Veterinary Medical Association (AVMA) (2020). Guidelines for the euthanasia of animals. https://www.avma.org/sites/default/files/2020-02/Guidelines-on-Euthanasia-2020.pdf (accessed 10 October 2020).

American Veterinary Medical Association (AVMA) (n.d.). Veterinarian's Oath. https://www.avma.org/KB/Policies/Pages/veterinarians-oath.aspx (accessed 10 October 2020).

Ashall, V., Millar, K.M., and Hobson-West, P. (2018). Informed consent in veterinary medicine: Ethical implications for the profession and the animal "patient". *Food Ethics* 1: 247–258.

Association of American Veterinary Medical Colleges (2019). Annual data report 2018–2019. https://www.aavmc.org/assets/Site_18/files/Data/2019%20AAVMC%20Annual%20Data%20Report%20(ID%20100175).pdf (accessed 28 October 2020).

Barilan, Y.M. and Weintraub, M. (2001). Persuasion as respect for persons: An alternative view of autonomy and of the limits of discourse. *Journal of Medicine and Philosophy* 26 (1): 13–34.

Batchelor, C.E.M. and McKeegan, D.E.F. (2012). Survey of the frequency and perceived stressfulness of ethical dilemmas encountered in UK veterinary practice. *Veterinary Record* 170: 19.

Batchelor, C.E.M., Creed, A., and McKeegan, D.E.F. (2015). A preliminary investigation into the moral reasoning abilities of UK veterinarians. *Veterinary Record* 177: 124.

Brown, B.R. (2018). The dimensions of pet-owner loyalty and the relationship with communication, trust, commitment and perceived value. *Veterinary Sciences* 5 (4): 95.

Cairns-Haylor, T. and Fordyce, P. (2017). Mapping discussion of canine obesity between veterinary surgeons and dog owners: A provisional study. *Veterinary Record* 180 (6): 149.

Chun, M.S., Joo, S., and Jung, Y. (2019). Veterinary ethical issues and stressfulness of ethical dilemmas of Korean veterinarians. In: *Sustainable Governance and Management of Food Systems: Ethical Perspectives* (eds. E. Vinnari and M. Vinnari), 193–202. Wageningen, the Netherlands: Academic Publishers.

Coghlan, S. (2018). Strong patient advocacy and the fundamental ethical role of veterinarians. *Journal of Agricultural and Environmental Ethics* 31 (3): 349–367.

Colombo, E.S., Pelosi, A., and Prato-Previde, E. (2016). Empathy towards animals and belief in animal-human-continuity in Italian veterinary students. *Animal Welfare* 25: 275–286.

Corah, L., Lambert, A., Cobb, K. et al. (2019). Appointment scheduling and cost in first opinion small animal practice. *Heliyon* 5 (10): e02567.

Crane, M.F., Phillips, J.K., and Karin, E. (2015). Trait perfectionism strengthens the negative effects of moral stressors occurring in veterinary practice. *Australian Veterinary Journal* 93: 354–360.

Dürnberger, C. (2020). Am I actually a veterinarian or an economist? Understanding the moral challenges for farm veterinarians in Germany on the basis of a qualitative online survey. *Research in Veterinary Science* 133: 246–250. https://doi.org/10.1016/j. rvsc.2020.09.029

Fawcett, A. (2020). Moral distress in veterinarians: Why ethical challenges impact wellbeing. Proceedings of VetFest 2020. https://vetfest.ava.com.au (accessed 24 September 2021).

Fettman, M.J. and Rollin, B.E. (2002). Modern elements of informed consent for general veterinary practitioners. *Journal of the American Veterinary Medical Association* 221: 1386–1393.

Franks, B. (2019). What do animals want? *Animal Welfare* 28: 1–10.

Gray, C. and Fordyce, P. (2020). Legal and ethical aspects of 'best interests' decision-making for medical treatment of companion animals in the UK. *Animals* 10 (6): 1009.

Grimm, H. and Huth, M. (2017). One Health: Many patients? A short theory on what makes an animal a patient. In: *Comparative Medicine: Disorders Linking Humans with their Animals* (ed. E. Jensen-Jarolim), 219–230. Cham, Switzerland: Springer.

Grimm, H., Bergadano, A., Musk, G.C. et al. (2018). Drawing the line in clinical treatment of companion animals: Recommendations from an ethics working party. *Veterinary Record* 182 (23): 664.

Haldane, S., Hinchcliff, K., Mansell, P. et al. (2017). Expectations of graduate communication skills in professional veterinary practice. *Journal of Veterinary Medical Education* 44 (2): 268–279.

Hazel, S.J., Signal, T.D., and Taylor, N. (2011). Can teaching veterinary and animal-science students about animal welfare affect their attitude toward animals and human-related empathy? *Journal of Veterinary Medical Education* 38: 74–83.

Heath, T.J. (2002). Longitudinal study of veterinarians from entry to the veterinary course to 10 years after graduation: Attitudes to work, career and profession. *Australian Veterinary Journal* 80: 474–478.

Hernandez, E., Fawcett, A., Brouwer, E. et al. (2018). Speaking up: Veterinary ethical responsibilities and animal welfare issues in everyday practice. *Animals* 8 (1): 15.

Hughes, K., Rhind, S.M., Mossop, L. et al. (2018). "Care about my animal, know your stuff and take me seriously": United Kingdom and Australian clients' views on the capabilities most important in their veterinarians. *Veterinary Record* 183: 543.

Huth, M. (2020). On facing different kinds of animal patients – Reflecting veterinary ethical responsibility. Über verschiedene Arten von tierlichen Patientinnen und Patienten – Reflexionen über tierärztliche Verantwortung. *Berliner und Münchener Tierärztliche Wochenschrift.* 19 May.

Institute for Employment Studies Report (2019). The 2019 survey of the veterinary profession. A report for the Royal College of Veterinary Surgeons. https://www.rcvs.org. uk/news-and-views/publications/the-2019-survey-of-the-veterinary-profession (Accessed 28 October 2020).

Joo, S., Jung, Y., and Chun, M.S. (2020). An analysis of veterinary practitioners' intention to intervene in animal abuse cases in South Korea. *Animals* 10 (5): 802.

Kanji, N., Coe, J.B., Adams, C.L. et al. (2012). Effect of veterinarian-client-patient interactions on client adherence to dentistry and surgery recommendations in companion-animal practice. *Journal of the American Veterinary Medical Association* 240 (4): 427–436.

Kipperman, B. (2017). Ethical dilemmas encountered by small animal veterinarians: Characterization, responses, consequences and beliefs regarding euthanasia. MSc thesis. University of Edinburgh.

Kipperman, B.S., Kass, P.H., and Rishniw, M. (2017). Factors that influence small animal veterinarians' opinions and actions regarding cost of care and effects of economic limitations on patient care and outcome and professional career satisfaction and burnout. *Journal of the American Veterinary Medical Association* 250 (7): 785–794.

Kipperman, B., Morris, P., and Rollin, B. (2018). Ethical dilemmas encountered by small animal veterinarians: Characterization, responses, consequences and beliefs regarding euthanasia. *Veterinary Record* 182 (19): 548. doi: 10.1136/vr.104619

Kipperman, B., Rollin, B., and Martin, J. (2020). Veterinary student opinions regarding ethical dilemmas encountered by veterinarians and the benefits of ethics instruction. *Journal of Veterinary Medical Education* 48: 330–342.

Kogan, L.R., Schoenfeld-Tacher, R.M., Hellyer, P.W. et al. (2017). Survey of attitudes toward and experiences with animal abuse encounters in a convenience sample of US veterinarians. *Journal of the American Veterinary Medical Association* 250 (6): 688–696.

Kogan, L.R., Rishniw, M., Hellyer, P.W. et al. (2018). Veterinarians' experiences with near misses and adverse events. *Journal of the American Veterinary Medical Association* 252 (5): 586–595.

Kondrup, S.V., Anhoj, K.P., Rodsgaard-Rosenbeck, C. et al. (2016). Veterinarian's dilemma: A study of how Danish small animal practitioners handle financially limited clients. *Veterinary Record* 179: 596.

Kong, W.M. (2015). What is good medical ethics? A clinician's perspective. *Journal of Medical Ethics* 41: 79–82.

Lehnus, K.S., Fordyce, P.S., and McMillan, M.W. (2019). Ethical dilemmas in clinical practice: A perspective on the results of an electronic survey of veterinary anaesthetists. *Veterinary Anaesthesia and Analgesia* 46 (3): 260–275.

Magalhães-Sant' Ana, M. and Hanlon, A.J. (2016). Straight from the horse's mouth: Using vignettes to support student learning in veterinary ethics. *Journal of Veterinary Medical Education* 43: 321–330.

Main, D. (2006). Offering the best to patients: Ethical issues associated with the provision of veterinary services. *Veterinary Record* 158: 62–66.

Mills, K.E., Von Keyserlingk, M.A., and Niel, L. (2016). A review of medically unnecessary surgeries in dogs and cats. *Journal of the American Veterinary Medical Association* 248 (2): 162–171.

Morgan, C.A. and McDonald, D. (2007). Ethical dilemmas in veterinary medicine. *Veterinary Clinics of North America: Small Animal* 37: 165–179.

Morgan, C.A. (2009). Stepping up to the Plate: Animal welfare, veterinarians and ethical conflicts. PhD thesis. University of British Columbia.

Morris, P. (2012). *Blue Juice: Euthanasia in Veterinary Medicine*. Philadelphia, PA: Temple University Press.

Moses, L., Malowney, M.J., and Boyd, J.W. (2018). Ethical conflict and moral distress in veterinary practice: A survey of North American veterinarians. *Journal of Veterinary Internal Medicine* 32 (6): 2115–2122.

Ogden, U., Kinnison, T., and May, S.A. (2012). Attitudes to animal euthanasia do not correlate with acceptance of human euthanasia or suicide. *Veterinary Record* 171: 7.

Opperman, M. (2019). Pro on ProSal. *Today's Veterinary Business.* https://todaysveterinarybusiness.com/pro-on-prosal (accessed 14 October 2020).

Quain, A., Mullan, S., McGreevy, P.D. et al. (2021). Frequency, stressfulness and type of ethically challenging situations encountered by veterinary team members during the COVID-19 pandemic. *Frontiers in Veterinary Science* 8: 647108. 10.3389/fvets.2021.647108

Rathwell-Deault, D., Godard, B., Frank, D. et al. (2017). Conceptualization of convenience euthanasia as an ethical dilemma for veterinarians in Quebec. *Canadian Veterinary Journal* 58: 255–260.

Rawles, K. (2000). Why do vets need to know about ethics? In: *Veterinary Ethics, An Introduction* (ed. G. LeGood), 15–16. New York: Continuum Publishing.

Richards, L., Coghlan, S., and Delany, C. (2020). "I had no idea that other people in the world thought differently to me": Ethical challenges in small animal veterinary practice and implications for ethics support and education. *Journal of Veterinary Medical Education* 47: 728–736.

Robinson, N.J., Dean, R.S., Cobb, M. et al. (2014). Consultation length in first opinion small animal practice. *Veterinary Record* 175: 486.

Rollin, B. (2002). The use and abuse of Aesculapian authority in veterinary medicine. *Journal of the American Veterinary Medical Association* 220: 1144–1149.

Rollin, B. (2004) The broken promise: Ethics and the human–animal bond. Part 2. *Vet Forum* February: 22–29.

Rollin, B.E. (2006a). *An Introduction to Veterinary Medical Ethics*, 2e. Ames, IA: Blackwell Publishing.

Rollin, B. (2006b). The ethics of referral. *Canadian Veterinary Journal* 47 (7): 717.

Rosoff, P.M., Moga, J., Keene, B. et al. (2018). Resolving ethical dilemmas in a tertiary care veterinary specialty hospital: Adaptation of the human clinical consultation committee model. *American Journal of Bioethics* 18 (2): 41–53.

Royal College of Veterinary Surgeons (RCVS) (n.d.). Code of Professional Conduct for Veterinary Surgeons. https://www.rcvs.orguk/setting-standards/advice-and-guidance/code-of-professional-conduct-for-veterinary-surgeons/#animals (Accessed 10 October 2020).

Rubinelli, S. (2013). Rational versus unreasonable persuasion in doctor–patient communication: A normative account. *Patient Education and Counseling* 92 (3): 296–301.

Sandøe, P., Christiansen, S.B., and Morgan, C. (2008). Role of veterinarians and other animal science professionals. In: *Ethics of Animal Use* (ed. P. Sandøe and S.B. Christiansen), 49–67. Hoboken, NJ: John Wiley & Sons.

Shaw, D. and Elger, B. (2013). Evidence-based persuasion: An ethical imperative. *Journal of the American Medical Association* 309 (16): 1689–1690.

Shivley, C.B., Garry, F.B., Kogan, L.R. et al. (2016). Survey of animal welfare, animal behavior, and animal ethics courses in the curricula of AVMA Council on Education – accredited veterinary colleges and schools. *Journal of the American Veterinary Medical Association* 248: 1165–1170.

Springer, S., Sandøe, P., Bøker Lund, T. et al. (2019). "Patients' interests first, but..." – Austrian veterinarians' attitudes to moral challenges in modern small animal practice. *Animals* 9 (5): 241.

Springer, S., Sandøe, P., Grimm, H. et al. (2021). Managing conflicting ethical concerns in modern small animal practice – A comparative study of veterinarian's decision ethics in

Austria, Denmark and the UK. *PLoS ONE* 16 (6): e0253420. https://doi.org/10.1371/journal.pone.0253420

Swabe, J. (2000). Veterinary dilemmas: Ambiguity and ambivalence in human–animal interaction. In: *Companion Animals and Us: Exploring the Relationships between People and Pets* (ed. A.L. Podberscek, E.S. Paul, and J.A. Serpell), 292–312. Cambridge, UK: Cambridge University Press.

Tannenbaum, J. (1995). *Veterinary Ethics: Animal Welfare, Client Relations, Competition and Collegiality*, 2e. St. Louis, MO: Mosby.

Thurner, E. (2020). Aiming at the patient's good? Considering legitimate and illegitimate forms of promoting health-related interests. Zum Wohle des Patienten? Über legitime und illegitime Formen der Förderung gesundheitsbezogener Interessen. *Berliner und Münchener Tierärztliche Wochenschrift*. 12 May.

Verrinder, J.M. and Phillips, C.J.C. (2014). Identifying veterinary students' capacity for moral behavior concerning animal ethics issues. *Journal of Veterinary Medical Education* 41 (4): 358–370. https://doi.org/10.3138/jvme.1113-153R

Weich, K. and Grimm, H. (2018). Meeting the patient's interest in veterinary clinics. Ethical dimensions of the 21st century animal patient. *Food Ethics* 1 (3): 259–272.

Wensley, S., Betton, V., Martin, N. et al. (2020). Advancing animal welfare and ethics in veterinary practice through a national pet wellbeing task force, practice-based champions and clinical audit. *Veterinary Record* https://doi.org/10.1136/vr.105484

Wojtacka, J., Grudzień, W., Wysok, B. et al. (2020). Causes of stress and conflict in the veterinary professional workplace – a perspective from Poland. *Irish Veterinary Journal* 73 (1): 1–9.

Yeates, J.W. and Main, D.C. (2010). The ethics of influencing clients. *Journal of the American Veterinary Medical Association* 237 (3): 263–267.

Yeates, J.W. and Main, D.C.J. (2011). Veterinary opinions on refusing euthanasia: Justifications and philosophical frameworks. Veterinary Record 168 (10): 263.

# 8

## Economic Issues

*Barry Kipperman, Gary Block, and Brian Forsgren*

## Introduction

The origins of small animal practice in the United States were associated with efforts to help animal owners who could not afford veterinary services. The Animal Medical Center in New York City was founded as the Women's Auxiliary to the American Society for the Prevention of Cruelty to Animals (Animal Medical Center n.d.). In 1910, the Auxiliary created an outpatient clinic for animals whose owners were unable to pay for medical treatment.

In a focus group study, pet owners believed that the veterinary profession should be more concerned about the welfare of animals than about the cost of care (Coe et al. 2007). Yet results of two studies revealed that most pet owners agreed that veterinary costs were higher than expected (Volk et al. 2011; AAHA 2014). This suggests there is a concerning disparity between what pet owners believe the costs of veterinary care to be versus what these are. Some reasons for rising veterinary costs include:

- Societal expectations that companion animals have access to comparable medical care to humans.
- The growth of specialist practices with sophisticated equipment and 24-hour staffing.
- As a result of better veterinary care, dogs and cats are living longer, resulting in the treatment of geriatric conditions.

Most human patients have health insurance, which insulates them from the costs of medical care. Veterinarians in practice utilize a fee-for-service model of income. The practices are businesses, and clients of companion animals are typically expected to leave a deposit prior to their pet receiving care and pay the balance of the fees when the patient leaves the hospital. The repercussions of this model are summarized by Rosoff et al.:

> Unlike human medicine, veterinary medicine has no safety net that ensures that patients receive needed care, and thus the role of money ... very much dictates the treatment received. Since only a small ... minority of owners purchase health insurance for their animals, veterinary medicine's payment structure leaves owners liable for the full cost of veterinary care. Thus, the ability to receive treatment is intimately tied to both the ability and the willingness of the

*Ethics in Veterinary Practice: Balancing Conflicting Interests*, First Edition. Edited by Barry Kipperman and Bernard E. Rollin.
© 2022 John Wiley & Sons, Inc. Published 2022 by John Wiley & Sons, Inc.

owner to pay for it. Some owners can't afford to get the care they believe their pet needs. (2018)

A report assessing the implications of this economic model discovered that 28% of pet-owning households indicated they had been unable to access veterinary care for one or more of their pets at least once in the past two years (Access to Veterinary Care Coalition 2018). Studies have concluded that cost was the largest barrier to veterinary care (AAHA 2017; Park et al. 2021). Morris (2012) observed that small animal veterinarians negotiate with clients to evaluate their inclination to pay for needed care, and to avert economic euthanasia (where the cause of the animal's death is owner inability or unwillingness to afford care rather than a poor prognosis), veterinarians bargain with animal owners for less costly treatment options. These types of discussions place the professional in the role of financier rather than healer, a position that many are unprepared and disinclined to assume: "Negotiations that involve bargaining with owners over treatment costs to avoid euthanasia are particularly unsavory for most veterinarians" (Morris 2012). Substantiating the limitations of this model, 72% of veterinarians agreed that the for-profit business model is not meeting the needs of all pets (Access to Veterinary Care Coalition and the Center for Applied Research and Evaluation 2018). (Case Study 8.1).

---

**Case Study 8.1   Economic limitations to life-saving surgery**

Molly is a six-month-old dog seen for vomiting for three days, progressive lethargy, and declining appetite. You advise blood testing and radiographs to discern the cause and provide an estimate of $500 including your consultation. Molly's owners request that you perform testing in an incremental fashion. You start with abdominal radiographs, which reveal segmental dilation of small intestinal bowel loops, consistent with intestinal obstruction, most likely due to ingestion of a foreign object. You discuss this finding with the owners and inform them that surgery will be necessary to resolve this problem. Without surgery, there will be a progressive decline in Molly's condition and death. The estimated cost for surgery and postoperative care is $5000. You provide an 85% chance of complete recovery and a 15% chance of perioperative complications. The owners respond that if you cannot make Molly well for less than $1000, "we will have to put her down." You offer a financial line of credit program per hospital protocol: the owner's application is declined. The hospital has no other policies regarding addressing clients and pets with financial limitations.

**What should you do?**

Ethical analysis:
The relevant interests in this ethical dilemma include Molly, the client, the attending veterinarian, the hospital team, the practice as a business entity, and the veterinary profession.

Choices include:

1. Pursue non-hospital-based funding options for care.
2. Submit to the owners' request for euthanasia in light of Molly's poor quality of life.
3. Have the hospital subsidize care and:

a) return Molly to the owner after recovery; or

b) mandate that the owner relinquish Molly to the practice.

Molly has an interest as a sentient being in experiencing good quality of life and avoiding suffering. Is it in Molly's best interest to die when the odds of complete recovery with intervention are very high, the remedy is readily available, and she is so young? Molly's owner has an emotional interest in restoring Molly's health but may experience feelings of guilt if she cannot afford the surgery. A euthanasia decision may foster a potentially negative view of the profession by the client as emphasizing profits over patients. The owner may choose to allocate the fewest economic resources toward Molly's care so that such costs would not harm them or their family.

The attending veterinarian has an interest in using their knowledge to improve Molly's health and welfare, and to accrue a reasonable income for services provided. This must be weighed against the duty to respect owner autonomy and the responsibility to provide informed consent to facilitate owner decisions. A euthanasia decision based primarily on economic limitations may contribute to moral stress and burnout, and the veterinarian may also experience pressure from their employer to do as the owner wishes, to satisfy the client. Acquiescing to the owners' request for euthanasia ends Molly's suffering and is therefore consistent with the American Veterinary Medical Association (AVMA n.d.c) Veterinary Oath ("relief of animal suffering") and the AVMA (n.d.b) Principles of Veterinary Medical Ethics ("A veterinarian shall be influenced ... by ... the needs of the client") and is acceptable based on the legal status of animals as property.

The practice owner has an interest in being profitable to ensure the hospital can afford the equipment and staff to properly care for its patients, and therefore the practice is not obligated to divert its own resources at a financial loss to save patients. The practice also has an interest in preserving its reputation among the pet-owning public as well as to safeguard the mental health of its employees.

Pursuing non-hospital-based funding may allow subsidization of Molly's surgery, which may satisfy the client and benefit the hospital's reputation. But there is no assurance that you will be able to procure funding, or the extent of subsidization may be incomplete. Declining euthanasia requests carries the risk of upsetting the client and may create the perception that the client is being judged, with potential negative consequences for the practice. Finally, procuring funding for this problem does not address recurrence of vulnerability due to economic limitations for a future illness Molly may incur.

Offering that the hospital subsidize Molly's surgery provides many benefits including knowing that this likely saves Molly's life, improves the morale of the professional team, and should result in a high level of owner satisfaction, with positive public relations for the practice. But this requires approval from the practice owner, and is not a viable long-term business strategy for the hospital, as the need for economic relief for all patients far surpasses the hospital's capacity to perform pro bono work. What if the word gets out that your practice is the "place to go" for those that can't afford veterinary care? The ethical principle of justice suggests that if the hospital is willing to intervene in this way, then the hospital should do so for all patients with a good prognosis who cannot afford life-saving surgery. Is this expectation reasonable? If so, is this strategy sustainable? This option also does not address recurrence of vulnerability due to economic limitations for a future illness Molly may incur.

If the practice requests transfer of ownership on the premise that this may find Molly a new owner who can afford her future veterinary care, this may be perceived as impugning Molly's present owner and have unfavorable repercussions for the practice via social media ("Don't take your pet to Dr. X, she'll take your animal away from you"). This may negatively impact the economic viability of the practice. Finally, this burdens the practice owner or manager with finding a suitable home for Molly. Should the practice allow any employee to adopt her? Should the practice screen the financial capacity of any prospective new owner to ensure history does not repeat itself? Is this legal, feasible, or desirable?

The veterinary profession must consider difficult questions regarding its role in providing care for animals with economic need. Tannenbaum (1995) has noted some of the concerns with confronting this problem:

> Do I [the veterinarian] have ... an ethical obligation to reduce my customary fee [or allow installment payments] for clients who may not be able to afford the best care I can provide...? [If so], ...would it be appropriate ... to ask [clients] to prove their inability to pay...? ... given that I cannot afford to help all clients, how do I decide which clients to help?

The financial limits pet owners place on veterinary care reflect their perception of the value of animals and economic realities. In order to pay for veterinary care, should clients be expected to forego their interests (Morgan and McDonald 2007)? This raises the question of whether pet ownership should be limited based on capacity to pay for veterinary care (Access to Veterinary Care Coalition and the Center for Applied Research and Evaluation 2018):

> One view is that pet ownership is a privilege and not a right, and only those who can afford proper care should own a pet. An opposing view is that all people, regardless of ... ability to afford proper care, have the right to own a pet. While it may be logical that someone should not have a pet if they cannot provide veterinary care, it is difficult to defend denying companionship with pets. Consequently, pets will continue to live with families with limited means.

While 95% of veterinarians in one report agreed that "all pets deserve some level of veterinary care," the majority of veterinarians did not believe that everyone should be allowed to own a pet (Access to Veterinary Care Coalition and the Center for Applied Research and Evaluation 2018). These sentiments are likely indicative of the detrimental impacts of economic limitations experienced by veterinary professionals. Rollin argued that pet ownership should be regulated to mitigate the negative effects that a lack of economic resources has on the welfare of dogs and cats (2006). Such regulations could mandate the acquisition of pet insurance or proof of financial means as a prerequisite for ownership. The majority of small animal veterinarians in one study opposed such measures (Kipperman et al. 2017).

## How Often Do Veterinarians Encounter Economic Limitations to Care?

Client financial limitations compromising patient care has been documented as the most common ethical dilemma encountered by small animal veterinarians (Batchelor and McKeegan 2012; Kipperman et al. 2018; Moses et al. 2018; Quain et al. 2021). In a study of US small animal veterinarians, 57% reported that economic limitations of clients adversely affected their ability to provide the quality of care they would like at least once or multiple times per day (Kipperman et al. 2017). A recent report found that 64% of veterinarians and veterinary technicians faced difficult decisions about client finances at least weekly (Quain et al. 2021). In another study of small animal veterinarians, euthanasia requests perceived to be based on lack of financial means occurred with a median frequency of once a month, and euthanasia requests where the respondent believed this decision was due to client unwillingness to pay for treatment, with a median frequency of a few times a year (Kipperman et al. 2018).

## Consequences of Economic Limitations

Consequences of economic limitations for animals and veterinary professionals include a decrease in the number of visits to the veterinarian, delayed presentation to the veterinarian so the animal is seen when illness is more advanced, decline in quality of patient care, economic euthanasia, professional income limitations, and moral stress (see Chapter 22).

Veterinarians have the desire and capacity to heal their patients, and to have that capability be repeatedly denied because of economic limitations is inevitably disheartening; 77% of small animal veterinarians reported that the economic limitations of clients were either a moderate or primary contributor to their burnout (Kipperman et al. 2017). For caring practitioners, the moral stress incurred by economic constraints may have debilitating consequences such as career disenchantment and premature transition out of clinical practice, demoralization, or desensitization to the plight of patients and blaming clients as an adaptive mechanism.

From a client's perspective, being denied access to the best care available for their animal over money may elicit feelings of guilt and a negative perception of the veterinary profession as placing economic considerations above patients. This can result in resentment toward the veterinarian and the profession (Sandoe et al. 2016). The reason most frequently cited among pet owners for leaving a practice was cost of care (Brown 2018).

Veterinarians in practice learn quickly that client complaints commonly relate to money. Frequent criticisms on websites that review hospitals include spending money on diagnostic testing when results are inconclusive or normal, or on treatments that are not successful. Veterinarians may feel the greatest pressure when clients "invest" in animals that die. Some clients will accuse the veterinarian of exploiting the patient for income, knowing the outcome would be poor. This can have a profoundly detrimental effect on a veterinarian's willingness to recommend costly and risky procedures that may benefit patients.

In a recent study of small animal internal medicine specialists, the most common reason cited for client complaints was the cost of care and 43% considered changing their career because of complaints made against them (Bryce et al. 2019). Another study concluded that complaints about fees arose in the context of serious complications or patient deaths that the veterinarian had not predicted (Gordon et al. 2019). Multiple investigations have concluded that client complaints about cost of care are a common source of psychological stress for veterinarians (O'Connor 2019; Bryce et al. 2019).

Despite many advances in the veterinary profession in the past few decades, on the issue of economic limitations, little progress has been made. If no action is taken by the profession to change this, veterinarians are likely to hear the following statements from clients over the course of their careers:

"If you only cared enough, you would do the work without profit" (Bonvicini 2009).
"You're a veterinarian; you're supposed to love animals" (Bonvicini 2009).
"You're going to let him die over $1000?"

## Options for Addressing Economic Limitations

The majority of veterinarians report using the following methods to address economic limitations (Access to Veterinary Care Coalition and the Center for Applied Research and Evaluation 2018):

1. Offer a variety of treatment options.
2. Payment options such as installment plans.
3. Provide services for reduced fees or no charge.
4. Other financial resources such as pet health insurance and credit services.

The options most frequently offered by small animal veterinarians to clients with economic limitations included credit services (66% of practitioners), hospital-based payment plans (18%), acceptance of postdated checks (11%), and pro bono or discounted services (5%) (Kipperman et al. 2017). Most veterinarians in one study agreed that pet owners should be required to supply verification of income before receiving veterinary care at reduced fee or at no cost (Access to Veterinary Care Coalition and the Center for Applied Research and Evaluation 2018).

As of the end of 2020, almost 3.5 million pets in North America were insured (NAPHIA 2021). Based on a conservative estimate of 145 million companion animals in the United States (AVMA n.d.a), the prevalence of insurance is about 2%. A study substantiates this, as 76% of North American small animal veterinarians estimated that less than 5% of their clients had pet health insurance (Kipperman et al. 2017). By comparison, 58% of dogs and 36% of cats in the United Kingdom are insured (Statista 2019a and b) and in Sweden, 80% of dogs and 25% of cats are insured (Konkurrensverket 2018).

## Effects of Client Awareness of Veterinary Care Costs and Pet Health Insurance on Patient Care

Before a recommendation can be made regarding what veterinarians should do to mitigate economic limitations, the potential benefits associated with improved client education regarding future veterinary care costs and pet health insurance must be known. In a report examining these issues, most small animal veterinarians felt that increased client awareness of potential future veterinary care costs would have a positive effect on financial stress and money-saving behavior of clients, the veterinary–client relationship, and professional stress and job satisfaction (Kipperman et al. 2017). Approximately three-quarters of practitioners believed an increase in client awareness of potential future veterinary care costs would have a positive effect on their ability to provide the medical care they feel is in the best interest of their patients.

Most small animal veterinarians also believe that increased adoption of pet health insurance would have a positive effect on financial stress for clients, the veterinary–client relationship, economic euthanasia, professional stress and job satisfaction, and their ability to provide the desired medical care for their patients (Kipperman et al. 2017). A recent study concluded that dog owners with pet health insurance spent significantly more money on veterinary visits (Williams et al. 2020).

Gastric Dilatation-Volvulus (GDV) is a life-threatening condition of older dogs. Diagnosis is inexpensive, and there is an 87% chance of recovery with surgery (Song et al. 2020), but emergency surgery and hospitalization can cost at least $5000. A retrospective study of dogs with GDV presenting to emergency clinics found that euthanasia decisions were primarily due to costs; only 10% of insured dogs were euthanized before surgery and noninsured dogs were seven times more likely to be euthanized (Boller et al. 2020). The authors concluded that pet health insurance is very successful in preventing preoperative euthanasia.

These studies suggest significant benefits to all parties involved in the practice of veterinary medicine from greater awareness among owners of the costs of veterinary care and pet health insurance.

## Discussion of Veterinary Care Costs and Pet Health Insurance

Discussion of veterinary care costs is fundamental to patient care, client satisfaction, and practice success (Bonvicini 2009). Pet owners may be distrustful because of the tension they perceive between veterinary medicine as a healing profession and veterinary medicine as a business (Coe et al. 2007). Communicating about the costs of veterinary care with emotional clients in a manner that will be perceived as caring can be challenging and is a source of anxiety for many veterinary professionals (Coe et al. 2007). Morris (2012) concluded that veterinarians experience guilt regarding the costs of care and that "veterinarians often hate talking with clients about money."

Results of a survey indicate that pet owners are generally not satisfied with the extent of discussions regarding costs provided by small animal veterinarians, and many stated that they received little information about pet health insurance from their veterinarian (Coe et al. 2007). Results of another study found that only 29% of companion animal veterinary visits included a discussion of actual costs (Coe et al. 2009). Moreover, costs were discussed in only 42% of visits in which diagnostic testing was recommended.

A recent investigation found that 67% and 71% of small animal veterinarians in the UK and Denmark, respectively, frequently or always discuss insurance with pet owners (Springer et al. 2021). By comparison, only 31% and 23% of Canadian and US small animal veterinarians discussed potential future veterinary care costs and pet health insurance, respectively, with over half of their clients (Kipperman et al. 2017). Reasons most frequently cited for not discussing these topics were lack of time and the belief that it would not change client behavior or financial preparation (Kipperman et al. 2017). Yet, most of these veterinarians believed that there should be an increase in efforts to improve client awareness and adoption of pet health insurance (Kipperman et al. 2017). In fact, a recent report concluded that providing pet owners with information about the costs of disease can increase their willingness to purchase pet insurance (Verteramo Chiu et al. 2021).

It is difficult to reconcile the documented benefits associated with improved client education regarding potential future veterinary care costs and pet health insurance with the small proportion of Canadian and US veterinarians who report that they routinely discuss these topics with their clients.

## An Ethical Argument for Discussing Costs of Care with Clients

Neutering of small animal patients is customary in the United States, and virtually all general practitioners address this topic with the majority of their clients (Kipperman et al. 2017). Let's pursue an ethical argument using neutering as a basis for routinely discussing costs of care with clients.

When animal welfare scientists make decisions regarding where to invest limited resources in addressing welfare concerns, four criteria are often considered (Smulders 2009):

1. The number of animals affected.
2. Duration of effect.
3. Is the problem reversible?
4. Impact on quality of life.

Hypothetically, if we did not routinely neuter dogs and cats, it is estimated that 20–60% of these animals would develop mammary cancer or become ill from pyometra (uterine infection) (Kustritz 2007; Howe 2015). These diseases typically affect older animals, which may be reversible with treatment or may be fatal. Based on the data presented in this chapter, it is reasonable to assume that at least 20% of all owned companion animals are subject to economic limitations to care. But unlike mammary cancer and pyometra, susceptibility to economic limitations is lifelong, affecting both young and old animals. Economic limitations to care may be reversible or may have fatal outcomes. A strong case can be made that these two issues have comparable welfare impacts on companion animals, but at this time the profession uniformly discusses neutering with clients and does not discuss economic preparation.

Who should conduct these conversations (see Script)? Veterinarians have a substantial influence on owner decisions with regard to their pet's care. In one study, the veterinarian was identified as the most vital source of knowledge regarding pet care by 70% of pet owners (Sprinkle 2019), and another report found that 65% of consumers purchased pet health insurance because a veterinarian advised it (AVMA Veterinary Economics Division 2015). Potential drawbacks of addressing this issue are that clients may perceive the veterinarian as mercenary; clients may be dissatisfied with insurance company policies over which the practitioner has little control; or the client may not comply or prepare. Additionally, it is conceivable that a veterinarian's awareness that a patient has insurance could lead to overuse of diagnostic tests or overtreatment (Springer et al. 2022).

Script: "Winston is a cute little guy, and I'm honored to be on your and Winston's healthcare team. We've discussed several important measures for ensuring that Winston lives a long, happy, and healthy life including regular veterinary visits and vaccinations. If Winston gets sick, our profession can provide care comparable to human medicine, including access to specialists and 24-hour monitoring. A serious illness can cost thousands of dollars, whether at this hospital or another I may refer you to. I want to help you prepare for an illness or injury while Winston is young and healthy, by giving you some resources including information about health insurance (which I recommend), so that our decisions about Winston's medical care can be based primarily on what is best for Winston, and not so much on what things cost. Do you have any questions?"

If the veterinary profession believes in the value of neutering to prevent reproductive diseases and vaccinations to prevent infectious diseases, why would we not prioritize preventing the harmful impacts of economic limitations? If there were an infectious disease afflicting millions of our patients, there would be clamor within the profession for a vaccine. Veterinarians should view the issue of economic limitations to care with the same degree of concern we would for a disease endangering animal health. Veterinarians hold proprietary knowledge about the costs of veterinary care that is unavailable to pet owners. It is time for a new paradigm in which practitioners reliably provide their clients with information and options to help them prepare for the costs of veterinary care for their animal companions. The potential benefits to animals, clients, and the profession outweigh an individual veterinarian's interest in avoiding difficult discussions. Efforts to alleviate client economic limitations would also be financially beneficial to veterinarians.

## Actions to Address Economic Limitations

Despite a practitioner's best efforts toward preventing economic limitations, these are still inevitable. A pivotal means of addressing economic limitations in practice is to establish a written hospital policy. Research has yielded differing conclusions regarding the prevalence of such policies. While 82% of US small animal veterinarians indicated that their hospitals had policies to address economic limitations of clients (Kipperman et al. 2017), only 9% of veterinarians in a Danish study had access to a written policy (Kondrup et al. 2016).

Having a policy in place better ensures a consistent approach toward financially limited clients, thereby averting potential for unfairness in distributing limited economic resources (Tannenbaum 1995). Such policies make it clear that the practice acknowledges the importance of this problem, encourage management to be aware of available resources including rescue groups, and reduce the emotional burden on the veterinarian to decide who should receive assistance and via which sources. We encourage all veterinary students to inquire whether a practice they are considering working for has such a policy.

## Addressing Economic Limitations: A Specialist's Perspective – Gary Block

### Factors Contributing to Rising Costs in Referral Practice

The number of tertiary care veterinary hospitals in the United States has increased dramatically in the past three decades. These referral and emergency practices often cater to a unique subset of clients given the type of care they can provide. The higher costs associated with equipping and staffing 24-hour referral practices are not surprisingly reflected in the fees charged and bills over $5000 are not uncommon. As noted earlier in this chapter, the most common client complaint against veterinarians involves the cost of care (Bryce et al. 2019). The likelihood of such complaints being leveled against veterinary specialists may be higher given the sums of money people often spend and because of the misconceived assumption that these costs should always translate to a successful patient outcome.

Numerous parallels exist between human medicine and specialty veterinary care, including rapid growth in spending over the past two decades and increased spending on end-of-life care (Einav et al. 2017). Although tertiary care facilities are often capable of providing advanced diagnostics and treatments including endoscopy, radiation, magnetic resonance imaging (MRI), interventional radiology, cataract surgery, and chemotherapy, the costs associated with providing these services can be prohibitively expensive. In an examination of the similarities between ethical dilemmas faced in tertiary care veterinary hospitals and human medicine, some have noted that "technological advances [may be] outpacing the ability to consider their prudent implementation" (Rossoff et al. 2018).

The rate of veterinary consolidation has been increasing over the past 20 years. Veterinary corporations control more than 4000 practices in the United States and over one-third of the small animal market by total revenue (Hargrove 2020). During this period and continuing to the present, veterinary prices have increased faster than the consumer price index (Davidow 2018). Given that private equity and venture capital firms are in the business of making money and have understandably targeted larger revenue-producing specialty practices, one may reasonably ask about the impact of consolidation on the ability of pet owners to afford specialty-level care. Although human medicine may provide some indication of an association between hospital consolidation and the increasing cost of care, it remains to be determined if such a link exists in veterinary medicine. It is of concern that veterinarians who have sold their practices to corporate consolidators frequently report that one of the first changes instituted by the new owners was a significant increase in fees (personal communications).

### Options for Addressing Economic Limitations

The need to find ways to help clients afford advanced care is more frequent, more acute, and, given the cost of care, often more daunting than ever before. Expanding payment options for pet owners is an important way to increase access to specialty-level care. While checks, credit cards, and cash will continue to make up the bulk of collected fees, there is an increasing percentage of clients who need other options to afford often life-saving care for their pets. Despite an increasing number of financial tools available to help clients, many veterinarians are not taking advantage of them. Only 65% of veterinarians made clients aware of payment options and only 51% provided information on alternative financial resources when faced with situations where traditional payment options were not feasible (Access to Veterinary Care Coalition and the Center for Applied Research and Evaluation 2018).

Some of the increasingly utilized financing options for veterinarians include independent credit services such as CareCredit[®] (CareCredit.com) or ScratchPay (scratch-pay.com), hospital-administered extended payment plans, and accepting postdated checks. More active promotion of pet insurance can be the difference between a pet obtaining specialty care and economic euthanasia. As long as the current third-party payer insurance model doesn't morph into something resembling the human medical care insurance model where insurance companies often dictate care, there is no reason veterinarians should avoid embracing pet insurance. Other less commonly utilized payment options include creating hospital-administered financial assistance funds, utilizing companies such as VetBilling (vetbilling.com) that allow practices to outsource collections from clients who get approved for payment plans, and crowd-funding options such as GoFundme[®] (gofundme.com) and Waggle (waggle.org). Waggle is more transparent than some GoFundme[®] campaigns and is dedicated exclusively to veterinary care while allowing the veterinarian to approve which clients they would like to add to the Waggle platform. Given the time and expense involved in setting up an IRS-recognized nonprofit, some practices have taken advantage of the American Veterinary Medical Foundation Veterinary Charitable Care Fund (vccfund. org), which can be used as an umbrella 501(c)(3) for charitable donations and disbursement of funds to qualifying clients.

Veterinarians should also familiarize themselves with regional, state, and federal financial assistance programs that can often provide funds for specific breeds and animals with specific medical conditions. For a continually updated list of such programs, the reader can visit https://www.speakingforspot.com and https://www.humanesociety. org/resources/are-you-having-trouble-affording-your-pet. Rather than veterinary staff searching for financial assistance for clients in need, this information can be provided to the client with the understanding that they need to take on some of the responsibility for finding help for their pet.

Another option for helping pets obtain specialty-level care is to enroll them in subsidized clinical research trials. This may be a good option when the cost of recommended care at a referral hospital is prohibitively expensive. Many specialty practices currently participate in such trials and veterinary schools often have multiple clinical trials open that provide significant stipends or reduced cost for enrolled pets. The AVMA Animal Health Studies database (https://www.avma.org/FindVetStudies) is a clearinghouse of clinical veterinary trials and most veterinary schools have continually updated websites that publicize clinical trials that are currently recruiting patients.

Regardless of the number and types of efforts veterinary practices undertake to increase the ability of their clients to afford care, it is critical that a hospital have a well-articulated, uniformly administered, easily accessible financial assistance algorithm that everyone from the receptionists to the doctors understand and find acceptable. In the absence of such protocols, veterinary professionals may be more inclined to assist emotional clients (Kondrup et al. 2016) rather than patients with the greatest need or with the best prognosis. A clear sequence of steps should be consistently followed, which should help ensure that the funds are equitably and impartially administered based on previously identified criteria. Figure 8.1 is an example of an algorithm that the author has created for his own referral and emergency hospital when veterinarians are faced with a pet owner unable to afford an initial estimate.

## How Philosophy of Practice Can Influence Affordability of Care

General practitioners have a critical responsibility in helping clients decide whether their pet should be referred to a specialty or emergency hospital. Referring veterinarians should appropriately counsel their clients on the anticipated costs associated with referral. Too often, pets are presented only for the owner to find out that needed care is prohibitively expensive. Referring a patient only to have it end up getting care that could have been provided by their family veterinarian, or worse, one who is euthanized immediately after the initial evaluation at the referral hospital, represents a failure of communication between all involved.

One of the most important and often neglected responsibilities of those working in specialty and emergency practices is being able to distinguish between "what we *can* do and what we *should* do." With the knowledge and equipment to provide life-saving and life-prolonging care, some veterinarians in specialty practices tend to "treat

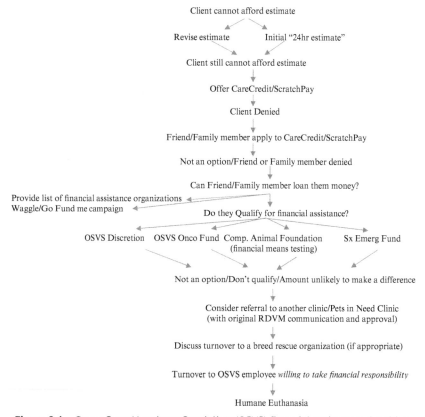

**Figure 8.1** Ocean State Veterinary Specialists (OSVS) financial assistance algorithm.

the disease and not the patient." Geriatric patients with multisystemic illnesses, animals with poor to grave prognoses, and situations where clients have unreasonable expectations all require the veterinarian to marshal their wisdom, experience, and honesty to have conversations with the client about whether euthanasia may be in the pet's best interest. This is particularly true in situations where pet owners with limited finances are faced with a poor prognosis. Holding out false hope or overemphasizing the patient who "beat the odds" in the past represents a failure to adhere to some of the most basic principles of informed consent and bioethics. Being familiar with commonly accepted criteria for determining quality of life and being comfortable bringing up both the concept and practical realities associated with euthanasia are critical skills for veterinarians in specialty and emergency practice. Helping these owners navigate through a complex web of options for care in a way that is effective and efficient and considers the needs of the pet and pet owner is part of the "art" of veterinary medicine.

Specialists must also be familiar with less expensive options that may still provide benefit to the patient even if such care might not be considered "gold standard." Educating owners as to various options, and the risks, benefits, and costs associated with each, will allow them to make a truly informed decision. With the profusion of expensive equipment in referral hospitals, doctors in specialty practice must take care to avoid the temptation to use this equipment to justify its cost rather than because it is medically appropriate. This approach to medicine does a disservice to our clients, may unnecessarily increase the costs of care, and has the potential to undermine the public's trust in our profession.

Similarly, not performing tests if it won't change the way you treat your patient should be the mantra of every veterinarian, but some specialists fall victim to running diagnostics under the guise of "being thorough" or because they feel pressured to practice defensive medicine. This latter concern may not be surprising based on research that found that 72% of board-certified veterinary internists changed the way they practiced medicine to avoid a client complaint against them (Bryce et al. 2019). The often-recommended "minimum database" is sometimes used to justify testing prior to the specialist thoughtfully engaging about the case and actively engaging with the client about the appropriate diagnostic approach for their pet (Kipperman 2014). In situations where a pet owner explicitly notes financial concerns or limitations, veterinarians must always aspire to use the client's funds judiciously. Spending money on initial diagnostics or "screening tests" to the extent that it financially constrains subsequent efforts to provide definitive treatment to the patient is a failure in fidelity and imagination by the veterinarian.

While there are many ways for veterinarians to help clients afford veterinary care, the factor that plays the greatest role is what a specific hospital charges for its services. In a capitalist market, for-profit businesses must collect fees to remain financially solvent. But how hospitals set their fees and what they consider an acceptable profit margin can vary widely and, as a result, the percentage of clients able to afford specialty care can vary widely as well. It is not the place for the author to dictate how a privately run business should determine an acceptable profit margin other than to say that the AVMA Principles of Veterinary Medical Ethics dictate that "benefit to the patient should transcend personal advantage or monetary gain" (AVMA n.d.b). As such, veterinarians must never lose sight of the trust our clients place in us and that this trust extends not only to our competence but an assumption that maximizing profit will not be the primary motivator when we are entrusted with someone's beloved pet.

## Consequences of the Status Quo

While burnout and compassion fatigue are issues for all veterinarians (Ouedraogo et al. 2021), specialists and those in emergency practice may be particularly prone to suffering from psychological distress because none of the patients we treat are healthy and our clients come to us burdened with emotions including anxiety, fear, anger, and sadness. Compounding these stressors, pre-existing long-term relationships between pet owners and veterinarians that would facilitate understanding and trust are often lacking in pets referred for evaluation. Client financial limitations, inability to afford needed care, and economic euthanasia are inherently more common in specialty and emergency practice by the very nature of the patients we treat. Having the equipment and skill to perform advanced diagnostics, therapies, and life-saving procedures, but having to make trade-offs daily with respect to what is in a pet's best medical interests and a client's ability to pay for this care, take an emotional toll on those working in referral practices. Dr. Melanie Bowden succinctly captures this painful reality in a 2020 TED talk when she notes that "There is nothing more soul-crushing in life than having the skills and ability to help something helpless and you can't do it because someone can't afford treatment" (Bowden 2020).

While financial limitations will continue to loom large over pet owners' ability to afford veterinary care, veterinarians in specialty practice can make several organizational, financial, and philosophical changes to how we practice and interact with clients to help make specialty care accessible to as many pet owners as possible. These recommendations are not simply abstract exhortations, as their adoption will sometimes make the difference between a patient living or dying.

## Addressing Economic Limitations: A General Practitioner's (GP) Perspective – Brian Forsgren

The Veterinary Oath has no asterisk indicating that a veterinarian's obligation to animal health and welfare is limited to those that have resources to afford care. Caring for animals and the human–animal bond is an implicit part of our role in society. The economic issues we face are admittedly daunting. I will try to offer some ideas that may be helpful to those interested in the ethical and societal obligations inherent in being a caregiver.

My practice was devoted to providing care to communities with limited resources. Poor people have animals. The welfare of those animals is in peril due to economic restrictions. While realism relative to the cost of animal ownership is rarely in the mind of the consumer, the escalating costs of veterinary care makes pet ownership a very real financial obstacle. One could argue that such a system creates a neglect-based type of animal cruelty.

I imagine my task in this text is akin to being a veterinary caregiver alchemist. How can we turn lead into gold? Or referring to the problem at hand, provide care when resources are limited?

If one considers the philosophical aspects of the idea of an alchemist, the process is not a simple formula. The metaphor is applicable to the struggles of a caregiver facing overwhelming odds in situations that seem untenable. The key is to persevere and rejoice in the process of trying to do the right thing. The right thing may not be the perfect thing. But it's better than denying care or looking the other way. Think in terms of "above all, do something."

The remarkable experiences that I enjoyed can be attained by the willing. I can guarantee that you can "do good and do well." The journey is not that complex if you have a vision and a dedication to that philosophy. It helps to connect to like-minded people. You need to be economically realistic. You joined this profession for a balanced relationship between empathy and economics. Try to maintain or regain that balance. Philosophy and ethics go hand in hand. A driving force in your life should be based in the ideals that inspired you to become a caregiver. Business is an important piece to the picture. It is a distant second to being a caregiver. Finding the way to "do well" is not that distant from "doing good."

To do the right thing is an ideal that requires a great deal of thought and dedication. There is a required discipline to making the right choices beyond self-interest. Society holds the veterinary profession in high esteem. Our image is that of a caring doctor. Maintaining that public perception is important and challenging. Our responsibility is maximizing animal health and welfare. Traditional case management can go hand in hand with the new age wizardry that is available. GPs, and those in specialty and academic settings need collaboration, communication, and the recognition of a common cause as a healthcare delivery system.

In human medicine perhaps the best example of such a dynamic is the 1986 enactment of the Emergency Medical Treatment and Labor Act (EMTALA) (American College of Emergency Physicians n.d.). This legislation ensures public access to emergency services regardless of the ability to pay. As the story goes (and a tawdry tale it is) indigent patients seeking care at all the hospitals in the area were universally referred to a community hospital in Parkland, Texas (in the fictional work *House of God* (Shem 1978), such actions are whimsically referred to as "turfing"). The situation became so blatantly abusive that eventually a tipping point came to pass. The Parkland situation became the genesis for the creation of the EMTALA. Legislators were forced to act driven by the unethical approach of the human medical community toward indigent patients.

Society expects that a medical profession be responsive to the needs of *all* its members. The veterinary profession's failure to respond to the needs of all society's animals represents an ethical breach to our social contract as caregivers.

As veterinary medicine parallels human medicine in advancements in technology and patient care, it is important to realize what machinery is driving this progress (Pellegrino et al. 1992):

> We should never forget that medicine is big business. Its activities are for profit, ... and include ... medical instrumentation; production and distribution of drugs, some of which can lower the quality of life and even endanger it; the management of medical institutions and schools; and finally, research and development of biotechnologies. These activities, however necessary are NOT AIMED at improving quality of life; they are aimed at maximization of profit.

As members of a caring profession, we should be aware of the implications of such forces and how such a framework impacts our patients, our practices, and our sense of who we are. Is "the tail wagging the dog" from an economic perspective? Where is Socrates when we need him? Whatever happened to the idea of getting into the profession to help animals?

Before we get too depressed, let's consider a view of our caregiving opportunities through a realistic lens.

Allow me to propose a simplified overview of a small animal practice's caseload:

1. Preventive care – vaccines, parasite control, spay/neuter.
2. Life stage care – pediatrics, early adult, geriatric, and end of life.
3. Sick animal care/emergency care/urgent care.

The capacity to manage a great proportion of those "sick animal" opportunities is key to a rewarding sense of self-worth. Self-image and an institutional core purpose went hand in hand in my approach to develop a practice model. Access to care and cost-effective management of sick animals became a major focus of my clinic's responsiveness to the community's needs.

A practice strategy emerged that went beyond financial self-interest. It is important to realize that such a model does not preclude financial success: it enhances success. I attribute a great deal of the success of my practice's model to the idea that *we* (all my veterinary staff and employees) were the clinic that would respond to the veterinary needs of the entire community.

Our approach was not to create a client demographic base solely with a focus on those who could pay. With what I may describe as an "open door" policy driving our operational model, we flourished.

The key ingredient was to get the animal in front of the doctor. That simple step can put the process in motion. Barriers were reduced. People and sick animals showed up.

Managing those cases was the biggest challenge, but also offered the most gratification. At this juncture, a problem develops. Is the clinician confident enough in prescribing treatment without support from imaging and laboratory testing? Once a differential diagnosis is established, we all enjoy confirmation from the lab or radiology. When that support is not feasible, an experienced clinician must continue down a treatment path with minimal or no confirmatory testing. Basically, a decision is made as to what the most likely etiology is. A treatment plan is instituted.

The key to treatment without diagnostic confirmation is the capacity for re-evaluation of the patient. The most effective way to encourage re-evaluation is to develop a no charge or much reduced recheck category within your fee structure.

Consider the management of a typical clinical presentation (Case Study 8.2):

---

**Case Study 8.2    Puppy with gastrointestinal signs and limited owner resources**

A four-month-old mixed breed puppy is presented for anorexia, vomiting, and diarrhea. The owner is a single mother who works two jobs. The babysitter reports that the puppy has been chewing on everything in sight including the baby's bottles. Further questioning reveals that the dog frequently gets into the garbage.

A boyfriend gave the owner the dog claiming the pup "had all his shots." The owner has had the dog for three months. This is her first visit to the vet. The puppy has received no vaccinations.

Physical examination reveals: temperature = 100.5/mild dehydration/lethargy/ gassy, slightly painful abdomen/rectal exam reveals blood, mucus, and tapeworm segments.

Differential diagnosis includes:

1. foreign body obstruction;
2. gastroenteritis;
3. parasitic enteritis;
4. parvoviral enteritis;
5. some combination of the above.

The owner is adamant that she can't spend any money on this dog right now. Her boyfriend is in county lockdown for two more weeks. When he gets his welfare check, she assures you he will be glad to pay for any charges.

A real-world approach to this multipronged dilemma could entail the following steps:

1. Initiate a treatment plan of antiemetics, subcutaneous fluids, parasite control, 24-hour NPO (nil per os) then bland diet (if parvo is high on your differential list, consider the Colorado State University [CSU] outpatient treatment protocol; CSU 2013). Initial fees can be charged with the hope the owner can pay what they can at this visit, or in the future. The "above all do something" approach.
2. Run a minimum of tests. Take abdominal radiographs to rule out a foreign body, submit a fecal flotation and/or parvo test, and follow an outpatient approach as outlined in option 1.

The key is to establish without any doubt that the puppy must be returned for a follow-up exam in 24 hours if symptoms persist. The author would put this client on a *must call back* list for the following day.

If symptoms of illness persist despite these measures:

3. Clinical progress dictates the path ahead. Daily outpatient therapy with progressive improvement and resolution is the best-case scenario. Continued deterioration including animal and client suffering can warrant euthanasia. Avoiding "economic euthanasia" is preferable.

In some cases, the client can retain ownership and acquire assistance from a reliable rescue organization. Or the rescue group may request transfer of ownership to them with the hospital providing the needed care in both cases. Such scenarios are best managed by the funding group and the client. The financial burden to the clinic is minimized with this approach.

A constant part of a GP's world is the cost factor. The traditional modality that allows management of the vast majority of cases a GP faces is the history and physical exam, the clinician's experience and intuition, the gravity of the symptoms relative to the potential differential diagnoses, and the client's ability to afford supportive testing. This dynamic is less problematic within academic/specialty settings as clients that go to these clinics are often preselected for economic commitments. The real-world management of cases is clear to the GP who faces resource limitations.

Such an operational model worked well in my practice. The clients appreciated us, the veterinary community referred their "financially challenged" clients to us, and the staff were aware that the practice stood for something beyond legal tender. The clinic lived up to the expectations of the community. The "lost causes" would arrive at our doors. Managing those cases was certainly a source of stress, but that sort of stress is much more readily handled than the cognitive dissonance generated by ignoring the pain and suffering of those animals caught up in a system based primarily on financial self-interest.

A key point being the greater a practitioner's skills, the more clinical cases you manage, the greater your emotional and financial rewards. You can make an enormous difference, feel better about who you are, and win more battles than you lose. When you lose you will have experienced a learning curve that makes you a better caregiver. Caregiver. Be that.

Integrating that ethos into a practice may be challenging if that practice mentality has a profit motive that vastly outweighs the caregiver empathy motivation. There needs to be a balance. The infrastructure of a practice's core purpose must be focused on community needs to balance empathy and economics. The greatest swing and miss in practice philosophy is to preach money, money, money to the caring folks who populate our veterinary care teams. Such a strategy eviscerates those people's souls.

So how can a practitioner in a resource-deprived scenario do better?

Spectrum of care (Brown et al. 2021) is a philosophy of practice intended to address the caregiving and financial complexity we face by offering all available options consistent with evidence-based medicine. This includes making clinical diagnoses based on history and physical examination and then *treating. Then* follow up. The key to spectrum of care management is timely re-evaluation. If the patient gets better, you *may* have been correct in your presumptive diagnosis and treatment. If the animal does *not* respond, then you are obligated to restart the diagnostic process with a more exhaustive evaluation and then move through the available diagnostic options or a new clinical trial.

We are here for the animals, not the other way around. Without that ethical piece to our professional identity, a caregiver can get lost. Let's not be lost. Let's be thoughtful, empathetic, socially responsible, and empowered. Serve the animals, the owners, and the community. Feel good about who you are. The future is not written. It awaits new authors.

# References

Access to Veterinary Care Coalition and the Center for Applied Research and Evaluation (2018). Access to veterinary care: Barriers, current practices, and public policy. University of Tennessee. https://pphe.utk.edu/wp-content/uploads/2020/09/avcc-report.pdf (accessed 17 December 2020).

American Animal Hospital Association, AAHA (2014). Reversing the decline in veterinary care utilization: Progress made, challenges remain. Partners for Healthy Pets. https://www.partnersforhealthypets.org/Uploads/iv4kcp3e.juc/VetCareUsageStudy_WhitePaper_July2014.pdf (accessed 16 December 2020).

American Animal Hospital Association (AAHA) (2017). New research from AAHA reveals changing pet owner perceptions of veterinary hospitals. https://www.aaha.org/publications/newstat/articles/2017-03/new-research-from-aaha-reveals-changing-pet-owner-perceptions-of-veterinary-hospitals (accessed 5 January 2021).

American College of Emergency Physicians (n.d.). EMTALA fact sheet. https://www.acep.org/life-as-a-physician/ethics--legal/emtala/emtala-fact-sheet/ (accessed 17 December 2020).

American Veterinary Medical Association (AVMA) (n.d.a). 2017–2018 U.S. pet ownership and demographics sourcebook. https://www.avma.org/resources-tools/reports-statistics/us-pet-ownership-statistics (accessed 15 December 2020).

American Veterinary Medical Association (AVMA) (n.d.b). Principles of Veterinary Medical Ethics. https://www.avma.org/KB/Policies/Pages/Principles-of-Veterinary-Medical-Ethics-of-the-AVMA.aspx (accessed 10 October 2020).

American Veterinary Medical Association (AVMA) (n.d.c).Veterinarian's Oath. https://www.avma.org/KB/Policies/Pages/veterinarians-oath.aspx (accessed 10 October 2020).

American Veterinary Medical Association (AVMA) (2015). Veterinary Economics Division. Department of Agricultural Economics. Consumer preferences for pet health insurance. Schuamburg, IL: Mississippi State University.

Animal Medical Center (n.d.). About us. https://www.amcny.org/meet-amc/about-us (accessed 16 December 2020).

Batchelor, C.E.M. and McKeegan, D.E.F. (2012). Survey of the frequency and perceived stressfulness of ethical dilemmas encountered in UK veterinary practice. *Veterinary Record* 170: 19.

Boller, M., Nemanic, T.S., Anthonisz, J.D. et al. (2020). The effect of pet insurance on presurgical euthanasia of dogs with Gastric Dilatation-Volvulus: A novel approach to quantifying economic euthanasia in veterinary emergency medicine. *Frontiers in Veterinary Science* 7: 590615. doi:10.3389/fvets.2020.590615.

Bonvicini, K.A. (2009). Talking to clients about money. *Trends Magazine* 3: 61–66.

Bowden, M. (2020). What being a veterinarian really takes. TED talk. https://www.ted.com/talks/melanie_bowden_dvm_what_being_a_veterinarian_really_takes (accessed 18 May 2021).

Brown, B.R. (2018). The dimensions of pet-owner loyalty and the relationship with communication, trust, commitment and perceived value. *Veterinary Sciences* 5 (4): 95.

Brown, C.R., Garrett, L.D., Gilles, W.K. et al. (2021). Spectrum of care: More than treatment options. *Journal of the American Veterinary Medical Association* 259 (7): 712–717.

Bryce, A.R., Rossi, T.A., Tansey, C. et al. (2019). Effect of client complaints on small animal veterinary internists. *Journal of Small Animal Practice* 60 (3): 167–172.

Coe, J.B., Adams, C.L., and Bonnett, B.N. (2007). A focus group study of veterinarians' and pet owners' perceptions of the monetary aspects of veterinary care. *Journal of the American Veterinary Medical Association* 231: 1510–1518.

Coe, J.B., Adams, C.L., and Bonnett, B.N. (2009). Prevalence and nature of cost discussions during clinical appointments in companion animal practice. *Journal of the American Veterinary Medical Association* 234: 1418–1424.

Colorado State University (CSU) (2013). Outpatient treatment protocol of parvoviral enteritis. http://csu-cvmbs.colostate.edu/documents/parvo-outpatient-protocol-faq-companion-animal-studies.pdf (accessed 22 September 2021).

Davidow, B. (2018). The impact of consolidation on price and quality. *The Veterinary Idealist*. https://vetidealist.com/impact-consolidation-price-quality/ (accessed 20 December 2021).

Einav, L., Finkelstein, A., and Gupta, A. (2017). Is American pet health care (also) uniquely inefficient? *American Economic Review: Papers and Proceedings* 107 (5): 491–495.

Gordon, S.J.G., Gardner, D.H., Weston, J.F. et al. (2019). Quantitative and thematic analysis of complaints by clients against clinical veterinary practitioners in New Zealand. *New Zealand Veterinary Journal* 67 (3): 117–125.

Hargrove, M. (2020). Power hour: Practice sales. Western Veterinary Conference, Las Vegas, NV (16–19 February).

Howe, L.M. (2015). Current perspectives on the optimal age to spay/castrate dogs and cats. *Veterinary Medicine: Research and Reports* 6: 171.

Kipperman, B. (2014). The demise of the minimum database. *Journal of the American Veterinary Medical Association* 244 (12): 1368–1370.

Kipperman, B.S., Kass, P.H., and Rishniw, M. (2017). Factors that influence small animal veterinarians' opinions and actions regarding cost of care and effects of economic limitations on patient care and outcome and professional career satisfaction and burnout. *Journal of the American Veterinary Medical Association* 250 (7): 785–794.

Kipperman, B., Morris, P., and Rollin, B. (2018). Ethical dilemmas encountered by small animal veterinarians: Characterization, responses, consequences and beliefs regarding euthanasia. *Veterinary Record* 182 (19): 548 doi:10.1136/vr.104619.

Kondrup, S.V., Anhoj, K.P., Rodsgaard-Rosenbeck, C. et al. (2016). Veterinarian's dilemma: A study of how Danish small animal practitioners handle financially limited clients. *Veterinary Record* 179: 596.

Konkurrensverket (2018). Battre konkurrens om fler byter djurforsakring. https://www.konkurrensverket.se/globalassets/publikationer/rapporter/rapport_2018-6.pdf (accessed 13 January 2021).

Kustritz, M.V.R. (2007). Determining the optimal age for gonadectomy of dogs and cats. *Journal of the American Veterinary Medical Association* 231 (11): 1665–1675.

Morgan, C.A. and McDonald, D. (2007). Ethical dilemmas in veterinary medicine. *Veterinary Clinics: Small Animal* 37: 165–179.

Morris, P. (2012). *Blue Juice: Euthanasia in Veterinary Medicine*. Philadelphia, PA: Temple University Press.

Moses, L., Malowney, M.J., and Boyd, J.W. (2018). Ethical conflict and moral distress in veterinary practice: A survey of North American veterinarians. *Journal of Veterinary Internal Medicine* 32 (6): 2115–2122.

North American Pet Health Insurance Association (NAPHIA) (2021). State of the pet insurance industry in North America. https://naphia.org/industry-data/ (accessed 10 January 2022).

O'Connor, E. (2019). Sources of work stress in veterinary practice in the UK. *Veterinary Record* 184: 19.

Ouedraogo, F.B., Lefebvre, S.L., Hansen, C.R. et al. (2021). Compassion satisfaction, burnout, and secondary traumatic stress among full-time veterinarians in the United States (2016–2018). *Journal of the American Veterinary Medical Association* 258 (11): 1259–1270.

Park, R.M., Gruen, M.E., and Royal, K. (2021). Association between dog owner demographics and decision to seek veterinary care. *Veterinary Sciences* 8: 7. https://doi.org/10.3390/vetsci8010007.

Pellegrino, E.D., Mazzarella, P., and Corsi, P. (1992). *Transcultural Dimensions in Medical Ethics*. Hagerstown, MD: University Publishing Group.

Quain, A., Mullan, S., McGreevy, P.D. et al. (2021). Frequency, stressfulness and type of ethically challenging situations encountered by veterinary team members during the COVID-19 pandemic. *Frontiers in Veterinary Science* 8: 647108. doi:10.3389/fvets.2021.647108.

Rollin, B. (2006). *Animal Rights and Human Morality*, 311. Amherst, MA: Prometheus Books.

Rosoff, P.M., Moga, J., Keene, B. et al. (2018). Resolving ethical dilemmas in a tertiary care veterinary specialty hospital: Adaptation of the human clinical consultation committee model. *American Journal of Bioethics* 18 (2): 41–53.

Sandoe, P., Corr, S., and Palmer, C. (2016). Companion animals and the future. In: *Companion Animal Ethics* (eds. P. Sandoe, S. Corr, and C. Palmer), 252–269. Wheathamstead, UK: UFAW.

Shem, S. (1978). *House of God*. New York: Richard Marek Publishers.

Smulders, F.J.M. (2009). A practicable approach to assessing risks for animal welfare-methodological considerations. In: *Welfare of Production Animals: Assessment and Management of Risks* (eds. F.J.M. Smulders and B. Algers), 239–275. Wageningen, the Netherlands: Wageningen Academic Publishers.

Song, K.K., Goldsmid, S.E., Lee, J. et al. (2020). Retrospective analysis of 736 cases of canine gastric dilatation volvulus. *Australian Veterinary Journal* 98: 232–238. doi:10.1111/avj.12942.

Springer, S., Sandoe, P., Grimm, H. et al. (2021). Managing conflicting ethical concerns in modern small animal practice – A comparative study of veterinarian's decision ethics in Austria, Denmark and the UK. *PLoS ONE* 16 (6): e0253420. https://doi.org/10.1371/journal.pone.0253420.

Springer, S., Lund, T.B., Grimm, H., et al. (2022). Comparing veterinarians' attitudes to and the potential influence of pet health insurance in Austria, Denmark and the UK. *Veterinary Record*: e1266. https://doi.org/10.1002/vetr.1266.

Sprinkle, D. (2019). Competing in the omnichannel era: A customer perspective on veterinary services. Proceedings of the United Veterinary Services Association Member Webinar Abingdon, MD. (12 June).

Statista (2019a). Proportion of dog owners taking preventative healthcare measures to protect their dog's health in the United Kingdom in 2019, by key measures. https://www.statista.com/statistics/299866/dog-owners-health-measures-in-theunited-kingdom-uk/ (accessed 10 January 2022).

Statista (2019b). Proportion of cat owners taking preventative healthcare measures to protect their cat's health in the United Kingdom in 2019, by key measures. https://www.statista.com/statistics/299885/cat-health-measures-in-the-unitedkingdom-uk/ (accessed 10 January 2022).

Tannenbaum, J. (1995). *Veterinary Ethics: Animal Welfare, Client Relations, Competition and Collegiality*, 2. St. Louis, MO: Mosby.

Verteramo Chiu, L.J., Li, J., Lhermie, G. et al. (2021). Analysis of the demand for pet insurance among uninsured pet owners in the United States. *Veterinary Record* 18 April. https://doi.org/10.1002/vetr.243.

Volk, J.O., Felsted, K.E., Thomas, J.G. et al. (2011). Executive summary of the Bayer veterinary care usage study. *Journal of the American Veterinary Medical Association* 238 (10): 1275–1282.

Williams, A., Williams, B., Hansen, C.R. et al. (2020). The impact of pet health insurance on dog owners' spending for veterinary services. *Animals* 10 (7): 1162.

# 9

# Medical Errors

*Jim Clark and Barry Kipperman*

## Introduction

"First, do no harm" is a frequently cited tenet of the medical profession, often incorrectly attributed to the Hippocratic Oath (Shmerling 2015). It serves as a reminder that medical practitioners should, at all costs, avoid harming their patients. The reality, however, is that every individual devoted to the medical care of patients, whether human or animal, will occasionally make mistakes, and some of these mistakes will unfortunately harm our patients.

The original version of the Hippocratic Oath suggests that physicians should, "abstain from all intentional wrong-doing and harm." By including the word "intentional," this is a far more realistic goal, and one that all medical professionals should aspire to, while also accepting that we are imperfect and will occasionally make mistakes despite our best intentions.

A number of terms have been used to describe different types of conditions related to patient safety, which are summarized in Tables 9.1 and 9.2. Some published definitions for the same terms differ or even conflict.

**Table 9.1** Definitions of types of events related to patient safety (modified from Wallis et al. 2019).

| Term | Definition |
| --- | --- |
| Unsafe condition | Circumstances or conditions that increase the probability of a patient safety event |
| Near miss | An incident that could have had adverse consequences but did not reach the patient |
| Harmless hit | An error that reached the patient but did not cause harm |
| Medical complication | An unfavorable evolution of a disease, condition, or therapy |
| Adverse event/ outcome | Unanticipated harm caused by the medical treatment rather than the disease process itself |
| Medical error | An action or omission with potentially negative consequences for the patient that would have been judged wrong by peers at the time it occurred, independent of whether there were negative consequences (Wu et al. 1991) |
| Sentinel event | Any unanticipated event in the healthcare setting resulting in death or serious physical or psychological injury not related to the natural course of the illness (Wikipedia n.d.) |

*Ethics in Veterinary Practice: Balancing Conflicting Interests*, First Edition. Edited by Barry Kipperman and Bernard E. Rollin.
© 2022 John Wiley & Sons, Inc. Published 2022 by John Wiley & Sons, Inc.

**Table 9.2** Circumstances associated with different types of events related to patient safety.

| Term | Reached patient? | Harmed patient? | Team member(s) and/or system at fault? |
|---|---|---|---|
| Unsafe condition | No | No | Possibly |
| Near miss | No | No | Yes |
| Harmless hit | Yes | No | Yes |
| Medical complication | Yes | Yes | Yes or no |
| Adverse event/outcome | Yes | Yes | Yes or no |
| Medical error | Yes | Yes or no | Yes |
| Sentinel event | Yes | Yes | Yes or no |

The following example (Case Study 9.1) demonstrates different types of patient safety events.

---

**Case Study 9.1   Patient safety events in a german shepherd with osteosarcoma**

After developing lameness in his right front limb, "Prince," a nine-year-old neutered male german shepherd, was diagnosed via radiographs and a bone biopsy with osteosarcoma, an aggressive and painful bone cancer. After consulting with their veterinarian, the clients elected for amputation of Prince's diseased limb followed by chemotherapy.

1. *Unsafe condition*: A veterinary team member noticed that some hospitalized patients weren't clearly identified by cage cards and patient identification bands. Because she was concerned this could lead to an error of mistaken patient identity, she brought the issue up at a staff meeting.

2. *Near miss*: Not realizing that two german shepherd dogs with similar appearances were in the hospital, and failing to check the cage card, a technician anesthetized "Champ" rather than "Prince" for surgery. She clipped the hair from the right front leg and prepared the limb for surgical removal. Before Champ was transferred into the operating room, however, a kennel worker noticed the error and the procedure was aborted.

3. *Harmless hit*: Prior to his surgery, Prince was scheduled to receive an analgesic injection. Due to a miscalculation, he received a 1.5 times overdose of the medication. The error was quickly recognized and reported to the veterinarian, who determined that this was not a safety concern for Prince and did not require any change in his treatment plan.

4. *Medical complication*: After being hospitalized on the morning of his scheduled surgical procedure, Prince became acutely painful on his right forelimb and could no longer bear any weight. Recheck radiographs showed that the bone, weakened by the cancer, had fractured. This event, termed a "pathologic fracture" is a recognized complication associated with osteosarcoma. In this case, there was no error on the part of the staff or hospital. In other situations, however, complications may be due to errors, and/or may be due to the medical intervention itself.

5. *Adverse event/outcome*: Near the end of the surgical procedure, Prince abruptly went into cardiopulmonary arrest. Cardiopulmonary cerebral resuscitation was unsuccessful. A detailed analysis of his medical care revealed no known cause for his sudden death. In this case, there was no error on the part of the staff or hospital. In other types of adverse events, there is an error. Note that although adverse events are caused by a medical intervention, this does not necessarily mean that an error occurred.

6. *Medical error and sentinel event*: Near the end of the surgical procedure, Prince abruptly went into cardiopulmonary arrest. Cardiopulmonary cerebral resuscitation was unsuccessful. A detailed analysis of his medical care revealed that the pop-off valve in the anesthetic circuit had been left fully closed, which resulted in excessive pressure causing respiratory arrest, which then led to cardiac arrest. The error was the fault of an inexperienced technician, who had taken over because her colleague called in sick that day. The system and equipment were also at fault.

As demonstrated by this example, there are many ways that patient safety can be compromised. It would be difficult to overstate the importance of medical errors given their potentially devastating impact on patients, family members, and healthcare team members. A study in the human medical field found that more than 250,000 patient deaths per year in US hospitals are attributable to medical errors, making medical errors the third leading cause of death in the United States (Mamary and Daniel 2016). The World Health Organization (WHO) estimates that 14% of hospitalized patients in higher income countries will experience an adverse event when hospitalized (Gartrell and White 2021). According to one source, 83% of physicians surveyed had experienced an adverse event or near miss at some point in their career (Harrison et al. 2014). In another study involving physicians in internal medicine, pediatrics, family medicine, and surgery, 92% reported being involved in a medical error or near miss (Waterman et al. 2007).

The veterinary profession is well behind the human medical profession in establishing systems to track, report, and productively address medical errors (Wallis et al. 2019). Reliable data on the actual incidence of medical errors in the veterinary profession are scarce. A survey of 606 veterinarians showed that 74% indicated being involved with at least one adverse event or near miss in the preceding 12 months (Kogan et al. 2018). In another study of 108 recent veterinary graduates in the UK, 78% admitted making a mistake since entering practice (Mellanby and Herrtage 2004).

In a study from three companion animal teaching/multi-specialty private practice hospitals using a voluntary reporting system, approximately five medical errors occurred per 1000 patient visits (Wallis et al. 2019). Forty-five percent of errors did not cause patient harm, however 15% resulted in severe harm. The frequency of serious errors causing permanent harm or death was less than 2% of reported incidents. Following an adverse event, however, more than 82% of patients had temporary harm. As these results were based on self-reporting, they almost certainly underestimate the true incidence and severity of errors.

In addition to causing harm to patients, medical errors are harmful to members of the medical staff. The emotional impact on healthcare team members in the human medical field has been investigated and described (Waterman et al. 2007; Harrison et al. 2015). In one study among US and UK physicians, approximately one-third reporting an adverse event or near miss indicated feeling that their work performance or personal life had suffered (Harrison et al. 2015).

## Causes of Errors

The intent of identifying the causes of veterinary medical errors should be to seek better understanding, not to assign blame. Additionally, understanding causation is an essential step toward learning from our mistakes and making changes to reduce the likelihood of recurrent errors. Though often well intentioned, discussion of *preventing* medical errors is misguided, as it perpetuates the expectation that medical caregivers should be infallible. The terms *error reduction* or *error mitigation* are more accurate and appropriate. Some experts in the human medical field have argued that even the term "error" is antagonistic in a medical setting and perpetuates a culture of blame (Rodziewicz et al. 2021). Rather than focusing on individual failings, the trend in human healthcare has been to target improvements in delivery systems to reduce the probability of errors and mitigate their effects (Rodziewicz et al. 2021).

Extensive research has been performed in the human medical field seeking the causes of medical errors and attempting to classify them (World Alliance for Patient Safety 2005; Anderson and Abrahamson 2017; Clapper and Ching 2020). Broadly, errors may be due to individual factors and/or system/environmental factors. Individual cognitive deficits by healthcare team members may cause errors of commission (wrong action) or omission (failure to take action). Communication lapses, either due to miscommunication or a failure to communicate, are another broad category of errors.

Causation of medical errors is often multifactorial and is best understood by examining the entire system (Figure 9.1). Studies in human healthcare indicate that

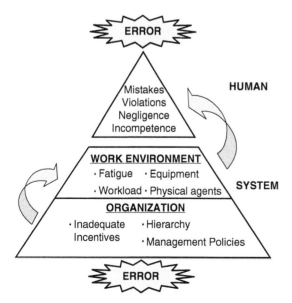

**Figure 9.1** Influence of system factors on human deficiencies in causing error (Kalra 2004).

medical errors arise not only through individual acts of negligence or incompetence by practitioners but also as a result of system complexities (Kalra 2004). Both veterinary and human medical environments are complex, dynamic, and subject to cost and time constraints. Additionally, there is substantial variation in different healthcare facilities in the expertise of staff members, levels of staffing, equipment available, complexity of medical cases, quality of leadership, and organization size. When seeking to identify the causes of medical errors, it is essential to consider the broader context of the organization and to recognize that many errors have multiple root causes. Often errors in the *system*, rather than by sole individuals, are responsible for adverse events.

According to research of US human medical malpractice claims, the 10 most common errors were: (i) technical medical error; (ii) failure to use indicated tests; (iii) avoidable delay in treatment; (iv) failure to take precautions; (v) failure to act on test results; (vi) inadequate monitoring after a procedure; (vii) inadequate patient preparation before a procedure; (viii) inadequate follow-up after treatment; (ix) avoidable delay in diagnosis; and (x) improper medication dose or method of use (Clapper and Ching 2020).

Communication deficits have been identified as a common cause of errors in the human medical field. According to a 2007 report by The Joint Commission on Accreditation of Healthcare Organizations, communication failures were the leading cause of patient harm in healthcare (The Joint Commission 2007). The importance of communication failures as a cause of medical errors in human healthcare has recently been called into question. A systematic review of research articles related to medical errors did not support the assertion that a majority of errors are caused by miscommunication (Clapper and Ching 2020). Instead, errors of omission or commission were by far the most common, with communication errors causing just 10% of all errors. Accurate identification of the causes of errors is challenging, as many errors go unreported and reporting nomenclature and protocols vary widely.

Relatively few studies have been performed in the veterinary field investigating error occurrence or causation. In a three-year multi-center study conducted in the United States, drug errors were the most commonly reported (>54%) error type (Wallis et al. 2019). These errors were categorized as wrong patient, wrong drug, wrong route, wrong time, or wrong dose. Giving the wrong dose was the most common form (>40%) of medication error. Communication errors were the second most common (30%) error type. Communication errors were categorized as a failure of transmission (illegible handwriting, poor medium for transmitting information), a failure of the source (missing or incomplete information), or receiver failure (information forgotten or incorrectly interpreted). This study revealed that 39% of communication errors were transmission errors, 35% source errors, and 21% were receiver errors.

In two studies on veterinary errors, communication deficits caused or contributed to 30% of voluntarily reported errors at three US practices and 5% of coded insurance claim cases in the UK (Oxtoby et al. 2015; Wallis et al. 2019). An analysis of client complaints against New Zealand veterinarians revealed that communication between the veterinarian and client underpinned many of the regulatory notifications and complaints (Gordon et al. 2019).

Another study investigating causes and types of errors was based on claims made to the largest veterinary insurer in the UK (Oxtoby et al. 2015). Among 225 coded cases, causes included: cognitive limitation (51%), owner contribution (15%), lack of technical knowledge or skill (14%), productivity/time pressure (7%), failure of communication (5%), and other factors (individually <5%). As this study was based on insurance claims, an important limitation is that the findings regarding error types and causation may not reflect their actual distribution in practice. It's likely that clients are more apt to pursue a claim with some types or causes of errors than others.

Cognitive error has been identified as the leading cause of human medical mistakes (Goh 2019) and was also the leading cause of errors identified in a veterinary study (Oxtoby et al. 2015). Cognitive error may be caused by excessive reliance on cognitive biases, the mental short cuts caregivers take to facilitate decision-making. In his text *Thinking Fast and Slow*, psychologist Daniel Kahneman reveals how prevalent these largely unconscious processes are in our everyday lives (Kahneman 2011). Two different types of thinking – System 1 and System 2 – have been described and are summarized in Table 9.3. Both types of thinking are essential for our daily function, expediting decision-making in some cases and slowing it in others (Kohn et al. 1999; Kahneman 2011).

Experienced medical caregivers tend to utilize System 1 thinking more often than less experienced colleagues. While this saves time and improves efficiency in practice, these shortcuts can sometimes lead to errors in thinking through medical cases. Diagnostic errors constitute a substantial portion of preventable medical mistakes, largely due to faulty clinical reasoning (Kohn et al. 1999). Often the culprit is excessive reliance on cognitive biases. Common biases in medical work include diagnosis momentum bias (failure to re-examine an existing diagnosis), availability bias (remembering a similar recent presentation), confirmation bias (overweighting evidence that supports an initial hypothesis), and search satisfying bias (stopping at the first plausible explanation) (Gartrell and White 2021). Effective clinical reasoning requires the intentional and courageous practice of rigorously examining assumptions and differing perspectives to inform better decisions and reduce the likelihood of medical errors.

Veterinarians and physicians often have demanding work schedules. A study of human medical interns showed elevated medical error rates among those sleeping less than six hours per night, working more than 70 hours per week, and who were acutely

**Table 9.3** System 1 vs. System 2 thinking.

| System 1 thinking | System 2 thinking |
| --- | --- |
| Pattern recognition | Analytical |
| Unconscious/reflexive | Deliberate |
| Faster | Slower |
| Little effort | Significant effort |
| Increases with experience | *May* decrease with experience |
| *Extremely valuable* | *Extremely valuable* |

or chronically depressed (Kalmbach et al. 2017). Stress and fatigue have been documented to cause performance deficits and sleep deprivation has been identified as one of the main concerns in the practice of medicine. Stress has been recognized as a cause of errors affecting patient safety in veterinary practice (Oxtoby et al. 2015). Long, continuous working hours and sleep deprivation are incompatible with enhancing quality care and patient safety (Dinges et al. 1997; Shine 2002).

Another characteristic of medical practice is that caregivers are frequently interrupted as they go about their work, and these interruptions increase the risk of error. In a study of human nurses at two hospitals, the occurrence and frequency of interruptions were significantly associated with the incidence of procedural failures and clinical errors (Westbrook et al. 2010). In fact, each time a nurse was interrupted while preparing and administering medications resulted in a 12% increase in procedural failures and a 13% increase in clinical errors. Interruptions occurred in more than half of all medication administrations.

A subsequent study was performed to assess the effectiveness of a "do not interrupt" intervention with human nurses in Australia, which included donning a vest to indicate they were involved in an important task and should not be interrupted (Westbrook et al. 2017). Although a significant reduction in interruptions was achieved, nurses reported the intervention was cumbersome and less than half would support making this hospital policy. Interventions need to account for those interruptions that are necessary and integral to the medication administration process and target the reduction of interruptions that are unnecessary to the immediate safety critical task (Westbrook et al. 2017).

Yet another potential cause of errors in medical practice is the prevalence of power differentials among members of the healthcare team (Weller et al. 2014). Some doctors may distance themselves physically and/or figuratively from other members of the team performing nursing or client service tasks, creating communication barriers. By virtue of their position, and sometimes behavior, doctors are often viewed as having greater power than other members of the healthcare team. This power dynamic may reduce the likelihood of a nondoctor, or any less experienced member of a healthcare team, questioning directives, even when they sense a potential error.

Lack of adequate training or supervision undoubtedly also contributes to the occurrence of medical errors. In a survey of recent veterinary graduates, 82% said they "frequently or always" worked unsupervised (Mellanby and Herrtage 2004). Many veterinary practices are small businesses that lack formal onboarding procedures. Practices vary in the emphasis they place on ongoing training, and in what opportunities are available for members of the team.

## Responding to Errors

When an error occurs, the initial focus is understandably and appropriately on efforts to mitigate harm to the patient and their family. Except in the case of fatal errors, immediate medical steps to care for affected patients should be a priority. Once the immediate patient care has been initiated, the following steps are often helpful:

1. If the owner is present and witnessed the event, you should immediately communicate with them.
2. If the owner isn't immediately present, pause and take a deep breath. If you are directly involved in a serious error, it's normal and understandable that emotions may arise that could make it difficult for you to function normally. If possible, discuss the situation with a colleague and ask for their support. This might include their taking over care of the patient so you can focus on other things and/or offering advice on how to proceed with the patient and client.
3. Unless you own the practice, it is advisable to immediately notify the owner and/or hospital administrator and seek their advice.
4. Make some quick notes. This is not the time for a detailed analysis: instead, capture the initial facts of the event, including the time frame and names of any individuals who were involved in any way, even as just witnesses to the event. When time permits (but relatively soon after the event) it is essential to record detailed notes in the patient medical record, including communications with the client.
5. It may be appropriate to contact your professional liability insurance carrier. Some agents have extensive experience with these situations and can offer helpful advice. Remember, however, that *you* need to feel comfortable with how the situation is handled.
6. As discussed throughout this text, it's important to consider the ethical implications of the event to guide how you should respond.
7. Take a little time to review and mentally rehearse how you will communicate with the client.
8. Share the news with the client following the guidelines discussed in the section on "Communicating About Errors." This should be a two-way conversation and include suggestions for a plan going forward.
9. For all sentinel events, complete a structured sentinel event investigation, which should include a root cause analysis.
10. Implement changes to reduce the risk of the event occurring again.

Choosing to disclose medical errors can be scary. A tension exists between the moral duty to acknowledge a mistake and the resulting harm vs. the desire to protect oneself from the potentially serious repercussions of admitting errors. There is growing encouragement and progress in the medical field, however, to develop compassionate and effective incident reporting systems (King et al. 2006). Reporting allows caregivers to honor their values and ethical beliefs, has the potential to rebuild trust and retain clients, and may reduce the likelihood of legal action or veterinary medical board complaints.

Unfortunately, studies in human and veterinary medicine indicate that there is widespread underreporting of near misses, adverse events, and errors. According to a study in the UK, "Research studies have validated an epidemic of grossly underreported preventable injuries due to medical management" (Barach and Small 2000). Another paper suggested that underreporting in the human field ranges from 50% to 90% (Oxtoby and Mossop 2019). According to another source, less than 10% of errors in the human medical field are reported (Anderson and Abrahamson 2017). Why is underreporting so prevalent in the human medical field? The 10 most frequently cited impeding factors were: professional repercussions, legal liability, blame, lack of confidentiality, negative patient/family reaction, humiliation, perfectionism, guilt, lack of anonymity, and absence of a supportive forum for disclosure (Kaldjian et al. 2006).

A survey of 606 veterinarians explored reporting of adverse events and near misses (Kogan et al. 2018). When asked if they had disclosed an adverse event to a client within the past 12 months, 77% reported doing so, with the most common justifications being that it was the ethically correct thing to do, wanting to foster client trust, and that it was clinic policy. The majority of those who reported an adverse event to their client reported feeling satisfied with the result. Of veterinarians who experienced one or more adverse events in the prior 12 months, 29% failed to disclose it to their client, with 79% failing to report one or more near miss. The most common reasons cited for not disclosing an adverse event were wanting to avoid needlessly upsetting the client, being afraid of damaging their relationship with the client, and being afraid the client would be angry or upset.

Given this strong evidence of widespread underreporting of errors and near misses, it's clear that there are multiple powerful impediments. In a practice setting, a multipronged approach will be most effective in overcoming these barriers and must be supported by the leaders of the practice through both words and actions. We advise that every veterinary practice develop policies and procedures for responding to medical errors. Practice policies on the handling of errors and near misses should be discussed proactively, rather than reactively. Reporting will improve when there is a culture of support, opportunities for anonymous disclosure, and where response is focused on learning rather than assignment of blame or punishment.

Consulting with trusted professional colleagues, friends, and family can be helpful following the decision to acknowledge and address errors. In a survey of veterinarians, 92% who experienced an adverse event reported discussing it with someone, most commonly colleagues, family, or friends (Kogan et al. 2018). Among respondents with a supervisor, 81% indicated they reported the event to their supervisor, suggesting that 19% did not report. Among those who disclosed an event, 64% reported receiving empathy from their colleagues. Sadly, this suggests that more than one-third of practitioners did not receive support from their colleagues (Kogan et al. 2018).

Applying a standardized ethical framework (see Table 7.3) upon discovery of errors is helpful in determining a course of action that considers the interests of all stakeholders and will allow caregivers to honor their values. After conducting an ethical analysis and communicating with the client, the next step is often conducting an investigation of the adverse event, error, or near miss. Use of a structured event investigation process is helpful. A root cause analysis is an iterative technique seeking to identify underlying causes or contributory factors that led to an unfortunate outcome. A simple and helpful approach is referred to as the "5 whys." The investigator begins by describing the most obvious cause for the adverse event and then repeatedly asks why that, and additional contributing events, occurred.

For example: A patient received a medication overdose. *Why?* Beth gave the wrong dose. *Why?* The dose was incorrect on the treatment sheet. *Why?* When Larry created the treatment sheet, he wrote the wrong dose. Beth isn't familiar with this drug, so didn't realize the error. *Why?* Larry was distracted when he created the treatment sheet and had trouble remembering the doctor's verbal dosing instructions. Beth hasn't been trained on this drug. *Why?* The hospital was understaffed as two team

**Table 9.4** The DISCLOSE medical error reporting tool (King et al. 2006).

| Category | Description |
| --- | --- |
| Drugs | Dosage, timing, route, omitted doses, allergies, reactions, wrong drug, wrong patient |
| Iatrogenic | Complications from procedures, treatments |
| System issues | Delays, missed treatments, order entry |
| Communication | Identification issues, confusion over orders, failure to give information |
| Lab/tests | Lost/mislabeled specimens/films, results not reported, delays, improper studies |
| Oversights | Judgment issues, missed diagnoses, deviations from standard of care |
| Staff | Nursing, respiratory, consultants, transport |
| Equipment | Delays in equipment, wrong equipment, failures, supply problems |

members were out sick. Larry isn't trained on creating treatment sheets, nor Beth on use of this drug as our training program doesn't include these tasks. We also don't have a call-in list to fill shift vacancies.

The DISCLOSE error investigation/reporting tool is widely used in the human medical field and is easily adapted to the veterinary profession (Table 9.4).

Once the investigation of the adverse event, error, or near miss has been completed, it's important to share and learn from this information. The goal should not be to assign blame, though in the case of repeated errors of the same type by the same individual, action must be taken to protect the safety of patients. This might include additional coaching, greater supervision, a change in position or responsibilities, or termination. Far more often, the appropriate action is to support those individuals who were involved and collectively agree on changes in protocols indicated by the analysis with the goal of improving patient safety in the future. In other words, the focus shifts from looking backward to looking forward.

Creating standard operating procedures (SOPs) can be another helpful approach to reducing errors. A SOP for a condition or procedure should include: (i) the name of the condition/procedure; (ii) which team members are qualified to provide care; (iii) helpful definitions; (iv) specific steps for testing and/or treatment; and (v) known risks or hazards to mitigate. Clearly defining important specific steps can be facilitated by the use of checklists. Surgical checklists such as the WHO Surgical Safety Checklist and Surgical Patient Safety System (SURPASS) are promising tools for decreasing patient morbidity and mortality (Treadwell et al. 2014). Successful checklist implementation includes enlisting support from leaders, training staff on use, and adapting the checklist to incorporate team feedback.

As medication administration errors (MAEs) are among the most common types of errors in practice, specific attention should be paid to reducing the likelihood of these events. A tried-and-true reminder for anyone administering medications is to first review the "Five Rights of Medication Administration" (Craven and Hirnle 2008):

- Right patient
- Right time and frequency
- Right dose
- Right route
- Right drug.

Another approach is to require that medications are double-checked by a second team member before administration. This is a standard practice for many high-risk drugs in the human medical setting. Unfortunately, a recent study of physicians found that double-checking was not associated with lower rates of MAEs or decreased harm to patients (Koyama et al. 2020). The authors concluded that the considerable resources required for double-checking medications might not be warranted.

Effective communication regarding patient care and client expectations is also essential in minimizing and mitigating medical errors. The simple practice of "closed loop communication," where the receiver restates the message (for example, a medication dose or treatment plan) to ensure clarity and understanding, can reduce miscommunication and errors. Another simple intervention is the requirement that all medication orders from doctors be written down, rather than delivered verbally. As doctors are notorious for illegible handwriting, use of digital medical records and treatment sheets can be very helpful. Improving communication during transfers of care between caregivers has been shown to be of particular importance, with miscommunication contributing to increased errors (Clapper and Ching 2020).

As discussed previously, deficiencies in clinical reasoning are cited as another major cause of medical errors. Improved metacognitive skills – the ability to think about one's thinking – among healthcare team members would undoubtedly reduce the incidence of medical errors related to diagnosis and treatment (Mamede et al. 2008). In teaching clinical reasoning skills to veterinary students at the University of California, Davis, one of the authors (JC) developed a simple acronym "REFLECT" to promote improved clinical decision-making:

1. **R**ecognize assumptions: consider and question assumptions about the patient and etiology.
2. **E**xplore alternatives: investigate alternative etiologies and diagnoses.
3. **F**ight bias: intentionally resist common biases, including availability and confirmation bias.
4. **L**ook for patterns: view data both individually and collectively.
5. **E**valuate pros and cons: weigh pros and cons before initiating therapy.
6. **C**onsider worst case: consider what might be the greatest risk to patient safety.
7. **T**urn to others: seek input from colleagues.

Improving the culture and communication within a practice and healthcare team is another worthwhile strategy to reduce the incidence of medical errors. If nondoctors on the team don't feel empowered or welcomed to raise potential concerns related to patient care and safety, more errors are likely to occur. Conversely, when doctors treat other members of the healthcare team as respected colleagues, team members are more likely to feel comfortable asking questions and raising concerns.

Every veterinary practice would be wise to proactively develop policies and procedures for responding to medical errors that can guide decision-making in the face of these unfortunate events. Although members of the medical team will always feel badly about adverse events, it will help if they can feel good about how these incidents are handled by their employer.

## Applying Ethics to Errors: The Ethics of Lying in Veterinary Practice

Veterinarians have multiple obligations – to animals, clients, society, themselves, and to colleagues (American Veterinary Medical Association [AVMA] Oath, AVMA Principles; AVMA n.d.b, n.d.a). Ethicists have argued that the primary duty of the veterinarian is to the animal (Rollin 2006; Ashall et al. 2018; Coghlan 2018; Weich and Grimm 2018). Some refer to this role as animal advocacy, where the veterinarian utilizes all available resources to promote the course of action that is most likely to provide the best outcome for the patient regardless of costs or concerns about the psychological well-being of the client (Fettman and Rollin 2002; Main 2006; Coghlan 2018). Veterinarians in practice also have a fiduciary duty to serve the animal owner because the client is paying them (Tannenbaum 1995). A pivotal means of fulfilling this responsibility is to provide informed consent (see Chapter 5 for a more detailed discussion) (Fettman and Rollin 2002; Flemming and Scott 2004; Ashall et al. 2018). The goal of informed consent is that owners be provided adequate information so they can make the best decision for their animal and for themselves (Fettman and Rollin 2002).

In some situations, a veterinarian may be conflicted between the ethical and legal mandates to provide informed consent and the desire to ensure the client's or patient's well-being by minimizing harm and suffering. For example, if a client inquires, a veterinarian may choose not to divulge the full extent of a patient's pain to spare their feelings. In other circumstances such as the admission of errors, a veterinarian may resort to dishonesty, lying, or nondisclosure. "To lie is to make an assertion that one knows to be false with the purpose of inducing another to believe that it is true" (Tannenbaum 1995). "Honesty is more than not telling a lie or telling the truth when a client specifically requests information." Failing to inform a client about something they could not know, whether a client specifically asks or not, can also be dishonest (Tannenbaum 1995).

Veterinary medicine is viewed by the public as an honest and ethical profession (Kedrowicz and Royal 2020). A study in the UK revealed that a larger proportion of clients than small animal veterinarians considered honesty to be a very important attribute to what constitutes "a good vet" (Mellanby et al. 2011). Clients in New Zealand placed great importance on the honesty and trustworthiness of the veterinarian (Gordon et al. 2019). Lying is in violation of the AVMA Principles of Veterinary Medical Ethics, which state that a veterinarian shall be "honest in all professional interactions" (AVMA.n.d.a).

### Philosophy and Deception

The belief that deception is harmful and immoral has been promulgated by theologians such as St. Augustine, who claimed that "'every lie is a sin,'" and philosophers such as Immanuel Kant, who argued that "'The greatest violation ... is lying'" (Gaspar et al. 2015). Deontologists (see Chapter 4 for a more thorough discussion of ethical theories) maintain that one should never lie and therefore favor unconditional application of informed consent (Kant 1785; Richard et al. 2010). Utilitarian theory emphasizes morality based on positive net outcomes; the ethical acceptability of lying depends upon its consequences, and the obligation to tell the truth can be outweighed by the duty not to hurt others (Tannenbaum 1995; Richard et al. 2010). Professional conduct such as using euphemisms, being ambiguous or evasive, omitting facts, and lying can be morally justified by the utilitarian so long as it promotes the patient's or client's well-being (Richard et al. 2010).

### Paternalism and Dishonesty

Paternalism is the predominant communication style in veterinary practice, in which the practitioner assumes that the client's values are the same as theirs and assumes the role of animal guardian (Shaw et al. 2006; Bard et al. 2017; Svensson et al. 2019). Practitioners may justify paternalism because clients often ask for their veterinarian's opinion ("What would you do if this were your animal?"), a client seems unable to reach a decision, or a client appears so emotionally upset that they are unable to understand the nature and consequences of the options being communicated (Tannenbaum 1995). Within this paradigm, a veterinarian may be inclined to pursue dishonest behavior citing the authority to make the decision on behalf of the client, reasoning that they wish to avoid confusing or overwhelming the client, not wanting to cause unnecessary stress or expense, or not wanting to eliminate hope (Palmieri and Stern 2009).

### Types and Examples of Dishonesty

A *pro-social lie* is made with the intention of misleading and benefiting another person (Levine and Schweitzer 2014). Examples of pro-social lies include:

1. Informing a client that their animal died quickly and peacefully when in fact this was not the case (Tannenbaum 1995).
2. Telling a client after a euthanasia decision has been reached that they did everything possible for the animal, when in fact the veterinarian feels that more could or should have been done, but the client previously declined their recommendations.
3. Telling a client after the death of their animal that the animal's outcome would not have been different, and that decline was unavoidable even if they had brought the animal in earlier, when the veterinarian does not believe this to be true (Tannenbaum 1995).
4. Describing patient prognosis in a more positive manner than is warranted by medical evidence (Iezzoni et al. 2012).

A *white lie* is a false statement made with the intention of misleading another about something trivial (Levine and Schweitzer 2014). Examples of white lies include a veterinarian responding affirmatively to a pet owner asking if their pet is adorable, when they do not believe that this is true. Bok (1999) has questioned whether white lies are harmless, noting the commonplace use of placebos in clinical medical practice as a source of erosion of trust. The placebo effect represents a beneficial response to a treatment that exists for reasons unrelated to the actual treatment given (Gruen et al. 2017). Studies indicate that approximately half of all physicians acknowledge prescribing a placebo (such as analgesics and antibiotics) on a regular basis, and a majority of them believe that such practices are ethically permissible (Tilburt et al. 2008; Kermen et al.

2010). One study revealed a profound placebo effect in caregiver ratings of improvement in mobility and activity in cats receiving therapies for arthritis-associated pain (Gruen et al. 2017). In veterinary medicine, therapeutic trials are common and can have unfavorable consequences for the animal patient and owner (Kipperman 2014; Kipperman et al. 2018).

One may also lie to preserve one's own *self-interest* (Levine and Schweitzer 2014). This type of lying is the most difficult to justify in that it is intended to benefit the liar to the detriment of clients and/or animals.

Examples of lies based on self-interest include:

1. Advising hospitalization of an animal overnight, but not disclosing that there is no one on site to observe the animal.
2. Failing to disclose a medical error that results in increased client cost and/or in the animal's death.
3. Not informing a client regarding the availability of referral that may provide an increased probability of a successful patient outcome, due to concern for lost income.

### Consequences of Lying

If a client were to somehow discover that their veterinarian did not disclose the truth, consequences could include loss of trust in the profession, feelings of anger and betrayal, and compromised care of the patient. Lying also carries costs for the liar such as feelings of guilt, entitlement, loss of credibility, pursuit of retribution by the client, and actions by regulatory authorities (Bok 1999; Palmieri and Stern 2009).

### Conclusion

When faced with the prospect of having to disclose medical errors to clients, a veterinarian may resort to dishonesty, lying, or nondisclosure. Lies based on self-interest are in violation of professional codes of conduct, can result in loss of trust in the veterinary profession, and may be harmful to both the animal and the client. Once a veterinary clinician recognizes the types and examples of deception, they will be in a better position to assess the ethical limits of "therapeutic privilege" as a license to deceive or withhold information from clients (Richard et al. 2010). Professional dishonesty may be reconsidered if the veterinary practitioner felt compelled to defend such decisions to peers, clients, or the veterinary medical board. Divulging medical errors to clients requires courage, empathy, and excellent communication skills. It has been our experience that disclosure, honesty, and transparency regarding medical errors result in more satisfactory outcomes for both the veterinarian and client than efforts to conceal and thwart admission of the truth.

## Communicating About Errors

In a survey of human medical patients, 98% desired some acknowledgment of even minor errors (Witman et al. 1996). This study showed that, following a moderate to severe mistake, patients were significantly more likely to consider litigation if the physician did not disclose the error (meaning they learned of the error from another source). Veterinary clients whose animals have been affected by an error want and deserve to know the cause. When veterinary clients learn of an error, they may experience two different types of disappointment: (i) with the error; and (ii) with the *handling* of the error. In the authors' experience, clients tend to be less forgiving of mistakes in the handling of the situation. Once an event has occurred, we can't change the facts, but we can influence how it's managed.

As you will be sharing unexpected bad news that may trigger a strong emotional reaction from the client, a "warning shot" may be helpful. This is a brief statement conveying concern delivered shortly before the actual bad news. For example, "Ms. Davis, I regret that I'm calling with some concerning news about Lady. May I update you on her status?" This is likely to be more helpful than opening with, "Ms. Davis, Lady has stopped breathing." On the other hand, don't significantly delay sharing important information, as this will frustrate some clients and might signal you are feeling defensive. Avoid the temptation to sugarcoat the actual situation – be frank but caring. The six-step SPIKES model (Baile et al. 2000; Shaw and Lagoni 2007) for breaking bad news can serve as a helpful guide:

1. **S – S**et up the interview: Arrange for privacy, invite significant others to attend, sit rather than stand, use good eye contact and connect with the client, manage time constraints, and avoid interruptions.
2. **P –** Patient's (client in veterinary medicine) **P**erception: Ask before you tell. For example, "What's your understanding of Benny's condition at this time?"
3. **I –** Obtain the client's **I**nvitation: Ask if the client would like you to proceed. You may also ask how much information the client desires at this time.
4. **K –** Giving **K**nowledge and information to the client: Gently share information while avoiding medical jargon. Incremental disclosure – sharing pieces of information interspersed with checking in with the client – gives the client time to absorb the information. The timeframe should be adjusted for the client rather than the clinician.
5. **E –** Address the client's **E**motions: Rather than ignoring emotions, address and validate them while expressing empathy. Use the client and pet names. Consider including an "I wish" statement. For example, "I can see how painful it is for you to hear this news, Beth. That's understandable and I'm so sorry about Pepper's decline. I wish this hadn't happened."
6. **S – S**trategy and **S**ummary: Ask if the client would like to discuss options for care. Share options, pausing often to check client understanding and feelings.

Another somewhat simpler model for sharing concerning news is the TEAM model (O'Connell and Reifsteck 2004; Institute for Healthcare 2008):

1. **T –** Be **T**ruthful: Use a warning shot and ask permission to continue.
2. **E – E**xplain and **E**mpathize: "Chunk and check" and use reflective and empathy statements. Avoid defensiveness and acknowledge client feelings.
3. **A – A**pologize: Depending on the situation, use an apology of sympathy or responsibility.
4. **M – M**anage: Be accountable and discuss handling of the situation and (if appropriate) what changes you will make in the future.

Should a doctor apologize to their patient/client after an error? This is an important question with ethical implications that has been debated for years in the human and veterinary professions. There has been an evolution regarding this topic toward the use of an apology (Bendix 2019). Although physicians have some legal protections for offering apologies to their patients in more than 39 states, veterinarians have no such protections. Liability settlements, however, are likely far lower for veterinarians than for physicians.

The author of a recent paper on veterinary medical errors in New Zealand states that insurers actively discourage apologies as an admission of liability (Gartrell and White 2021). One of the authors (JC), who co-owned several large emergency/specialty practices in California for many years and has interfaced with insurance representatives representing the AVMA and the California Veterinary Medical Association programs, has found that they consistently support disclosing errors and apologizing to veterinary clients who have suffered harm. This stance may vary, however, among other carriers or in other geographic areas. Whether recommended or not by an insurance company, our recommendation is to disclose errors and offer apologies.

There are two forms of apology: (i) an apology of sympathy, which does not acknowledge accountability for the event; and (ii) an apology of responsibility. For example, "I'm so sorry this happened" is an apology of sympathy, whereas "I'm so sorry we made this error" is an apology of responsibility. With this in mind, caregivers always have the option of offering an apology without acknowledging culpability. This may be very appropriate as an empathetic gesture before the true cause(s) of an adverse event is known, or in situations where an adverse event occurred, but there was no fault by the medical personnel. Either way, it would be wise to record in the medical record exactly what was said to the client in the way of apology.

If, however, a known error occurred, an apology of responsibility is warranted and important. A full apology should convey accountability and culpability, a promise of corrective actions, and an explanation of the circumstances that led to the mistake (Petronio et al. 2013). Apologies should not include justifications that may be interpreted as denials of fault, and there should be no requests for forgiveness within the apology, which has the effect of shifting focus from the needs of the client to those of the clinician (Petronio et al. 2013).

A groundbreaking study was initiated in 2001 at the University of Michigan Health System where they encouraged caregivers to fully disclose errors and offered compensation to patients for any harm (Kachalia et al. 2010). After full implementation of this program, the average rate of new claims and average rate of lawsuits both decreased. Average monthly costs decreased for total liability, patient compensation, and related legal costs. This multi-year study suggests that, in at least some settings, disclosing and accepting responsibility for errors may make good business sense in addition to being the right thing to do.

## Consequences of Errors

The majority of veterinary clients consider their pets to be members of the family (Cohen 2002), so the consequences of serious adverse events can be emotionally devastating. Despite efforts by members of the veterinary healthcare team to explain potential risks in advance (as required to obtain informed consent), many pet owners are still not emotionally prepared for something bad to happen to their beloved animal companion. This is understandable and requires that the disclosure and handling of these events be conducted with compassion, empathy, and respect. Even when adverse events are handled in this fashion, however, many clients will still experience a range of emotions that can include denial, anger, guilt, and profound grief.

Following the occurrence of a medical error or perceived medical error, hurt and disgruntled clients have at least three responses that strike fear into every veterinarian: (i) file a lawsuit; (ii) file a veterinary medical board complaint; and/or (iii) broadcast accusations (whether founded or not) on social media. Thus, the consequences of making an error could be financial loss, loss of the ability to continue to practice, and/or widespread public humiliation, in addition to the emotional pain of the initial event.

Malpractice lawsuits in the human medical field have been on the decline, but there were still more than 11,500 cases filed in 2018, with payouts of approximately four billion dollars in 2017 (Bendix 2019). In addition to seeking financial compensation, litigants may also seek understanding of what went wrong, who was responsible, and what will be done to prevent the error from happening again. This is especially true when communication about the event was poorly handled.

Though less common, litigation also occurs in the veterinary field and defending oneself can be a daunting and expensive process. Every practicing veterinarian should obtain good-quality professional liability protection insurance and license defense insurance. Several large veterinary organizations offer this coverage and working with agents with veterinary-specific experience may have advantages. As this coverage is often arranged and paid for by veterinary employers, it is important for veterinary associates to understand that they are *not* protected when performing veterinary work that is not associated with their place of employment. When reviewing policies, veterinarians should ensure that they retain control of whether a case will be settled or not.

While medical errors have a negative impact on patients and clients, they can also cause mental and emotional harm to members of the medical team, who should be considered as secondary victims of these events. Studies in the human medical field have shown that providers involved with medical errors have a heightened risk of burnout, lack of concentration, poor work performance, posttraumatic stress disorder, depression, and even suicidality (Robertson and Long 2018). Physicians and other providers may feel a variety of adverse emotions after medical errors, including guilt, shame, anxiety, and fear. It is thought that the pervasive culture of perfectionism and blame in medicine plays a considerable role in these negative effects (Robertson and Long 2018). In addition, studies have found that despite physicians' desire for support after committing a medical error, many physicians feel a lack of personal and administrative support. This may further contribute to poor emotional well-being (Robertson and Long 2018).

A study of mistakes by recent veterinary graduates in the UK indicated that medical errors contribute significantly to emotional burnout, and veterinarians have reported negative effects on their confidence and mental health after serious errors (Mellanby and Herrtage 2004). Another UK study revealed that making professional mistakes was second only to number of hours worked as the greatest contributor to stress, with 40% of veterinarians indicating this contributed "quite a lot" or "very much" to their level of stress (Bartram et al. 2009). Among respondents treating clinical cases, the possibility of client complaints or litigation was the greatest contributor to clinical work-related stress.

A survey of US veterinarians indicated that, following an adverse event, 77% had a short-term negative impact on their personal life and 50% had a long-term negative impact (Kogan et al. 2018). A significantly greater proportion of women than men reported short- and long-term negative impacts on both their professional and personal lives. Adverse impacts reported included diminished confidence in their abilities, reduced job satisfaction, increased feelings of burnout, reduced happiness, feeling persistently guilty, and having difficulty focusing (Kogan et al. 2018).

This evidence clearly highlights the importance of providing care, kindness, and support not just for animal patients and their families impacted by adverse events, but also for members of the veterinary healthcare team. Though research is lacking on the impact of errors on members of the veterinary team beyond veterinarians, there is little doubt that they are also significantly affected and deserve equal compassion and support.

## Healing and Moving On

Considering the pervasiveness of medical errors in veterinary practice, it is likely that nearly every member of a veterinary healthcare team will at some point be directly affected. In the authors' experience, very few practices take a proactive stance regarding medical errors and their aftermath. Policies, procedures, and systems can and should be put in place, ideally *before* they are needed. Professional barriers separating doctors from other members of the team need to be broken down; all members of the team share the common goal of patient safety. When that is compromised due to an error, all members of the team share collective responsibility and can learn from these events. If you have made mistakes in practice, you are not alone! Providing veterinary medical care is a very complex undertaking, with inherent uncertainty, limited resources, and high expectations.

Gartrell and White summarize the need for a novel paradigm:

> The veterinary profession needs a more mature approach to its handling of clinical errors... As a profession, as employers and as supervisors, we need to move away from the "blame and shame" model of response to clinical errors. As individuals we need to accept our fallibility, strive to learn compassionately from our own mistakes, but also build our own resiliency to the effects of making clinical errors. Organizational and professional communication tools can be implemented in workplaces to create a culture of safe disclosure, and discussion and reflection techniques promoting resilience.
>
> *(2021)*

Perhaps most importantly, remember to approach every adverse event or medical error situation with sensitivity and empathy for all parties affected. With open dialogue, open minds, a desire to learn from others, and adherence to ethical principles and approaches, the veterinary profession's handling of medical errors will continue to evolve in a positive direction.

# References

American Veterinary Medical Association (AVMA) (n.d.a). Principles of Veterinary Medical Ethics. https://www.avma.org/KB/Policies/Pages/Principles-of-Veterinary-Medical-Ethics-of-the-AVMA.aspx (accessed 10 October 2020).

American Veterinary Medical Association (AVMA) (n.d.b). Veterinarian's Oath. https://www.avma.org/KB/Policies/Pages/veterinarians-oath.aspx (accessed 10 October 2020).

Anderson, J.G. and Abrahamson, K. (2017). Your health care may kill you: Medical errors. *Studies in Health Technology and Informatics* 234: 13–17.

Ashall, V., Millar, K.M., and Hobson-West, P. (2018). Informed consent in veterinary medicine: Ethical implications for the profession and the animal "patient". *Food Ethics* 1: 247–258.

Baile, W.F., Buckman, R., Lenzi, R. et al. (2000). SPIKES-A six-step protocol for delivering bad news: Application to the patient with cancer. *The Oncologist* 5 (4): 302–311.

Barach, P. and Small, S.D. (2000). Reporting and preventing medical mishaps: Lessons from non-medical near miss reporting systems. *BMJ (Clinical Research Education)* 320 (7237): 759–763.

Bard, A.M., Main, D.C., Haase, A.M. et al. (2017). The future of veterinary communication: Partnership or persuasion? A qualitative investigation of veterinary communication in the pursuit of client behavior change. *PLoS ONE* 12 (3): e0171380.

Bartram, D.J., Yadegarfar, G., and Baldwin, D.S. (2009). Psychosocial working conditions and work-related stressors among UK veterinary surgeons. *Occupational Medicine* 59: 334–341.

Bendix, J. (2019). Should doctors apologize for mistakes?. *Medical Economics* 10: 17.

Bok, S. (1999). *Lying: Moral Choice in Public and Private Life*. New York: Vintage Books.

Clapper, T.C. and Ching, K. (2020). Debunking the myth that the majority of medical errors are attributed to communication. *Medical Education* 54 (1): 74–81.

Coghlan, S. (2018). Strong patient advocacy and the fundamental ethical role of veterinarians. *Journal of Agricultural and Environmental Ethics* 31 (3): 349–367.

Cohen, S.P. (2002). Can pets function as family members? *Western Journal of Nursing Research* 24 (6): 621–638. https://doi.org/10.1177/019394502320555386

Craven, R.F. and Hirnle, C.J. (2008). *Fundamentals of Nursing: Human Health and Function*, 6e. Philadelphia, PA: Lippincott Williams & Wilkins.

Dinges, D.F., Pack, F., Williams, K. et al. (1997). Cumulative sleepiness, mood disturbance, and psychomotor vigilance performance decrements during a week of sleep restricted to 4–5 hours per night. *Sleep* 20 (4): 267–277.

Fettman, M.J. and Rollin, B.E. (2002). Modern elements of informed consent for general veterinary practitioners. *Journal of the American Veterinary Medical Association* 221: 1386–1393.

Flemming, D.D. and Scott, J.F. (2004). The informed consent doctrine: What veterinarians should tell their clients. *Journal of the American Veterinary Medical Association* 224: 1436.

Gartrell, B. and White, B. (2021). Surviving clinical errors in practice. *New Zealand Veterinary Journal* 69 (Issue): 1.

Gaspar, J.P., Levine, E.E., and Schweitzer, M.E. (2015). Why we should lie. *Organizational Dynamics* 4: 306.

Goh, R.L.Z. (2019). To err is human: An ACEM trainee's perspective on clinical error. *Emergency Medicine Australasia* 31: 665–666.

Gordon, S., Gardner, D.H., Weston, J.F. et al. (2019). Quantitative and thematic analysis of complaints by clients against clinical veterinary practitioners in New Zealand. *New Zealand Veterinary Journal* 67 (3): 117–125.

Gruen, M.E., Dorman, D.C., and Lascelles, B.D.X. (2017). Caregiver placebo effect in analgesic clinical trials for painful cats with naturally occurring degenerative joint disease. *Veterinary Record* 180 (19): 473.

Harrison, R., Lawton, R., and Stewart, K. (2014). Doctors' experiences of adverse events in secondary care: The professional and personal impact. *The Clinical Medicine (Lond)* 14: 585–590.

Harrison, R., Lawton, R., Perlo, J. et al. (2015). Emotion and coping in the aftermath of medical error: A cross-country exploration. *Journal of Patient Safety* 11: 28–35.

Iezzoni, L.I., Rao, S.R., DesRoches, C.M. et al. (2012). Survey shows that at least some physicians are not always open or honest with patients. *Health Affairs* 31 (2): 383–391.

Institute for Healthcare (2008). Communication Module 12, Breaking the Silence: Disclosing medical errors. Bayer Animal Health Communication Project, New Haven, CT. https://healthcarecomm.org/veterinary-communication (accessed 24 September 2021).

Kachalia, A., Kaufman, S.R., Boothman, R. et al. (2010). Liability claims and costs before and after implementation of a medical error disclosure program. *Annals of Internal Medicine* 153 (4): 213–221.

Kahneman, D. (2011). *Thinking Fast and Slow*. New York: Farrar, Straus and Giroux.

Kaldjian, L.C., Jones, E.W., Rosenthal, G.E. et al. (2006). An empirically derived taxonomy of factors affecting physicians' willingness to disclose medical errors. *Journal of General Internal Medicine* 21 (9): 942–948.

Kalmbach, D.A., Arnedt, J.T., Song, P.X. et al. (2017). Sleep disturbance and short sleep as risk factors for depression and perceived medical errors in first-year residents. *Sleep* 40 (3): zsw073.

Kalra, J. (2004). Medical errors: An introduction to concepts. *Clinical Biochemistry* 37 (12): 1043–1051.

Kant, I. (1785). *Foundation of the Metaphysics of Morals*. L.W. Beck, translator., 1959. Indianapolis, IN: Bobbs-Merrill.

Kedrowicz, A.A. and Royal, K.D. (2020). A comparison of public perceptions of physicians and veterinarians in the United States. *Veterinary Sciences* 7 (2): 50.

Kermen, R., Hickner, J., Brody, H. et al. (2010). Family physicians believe the placebo effect is therapeutic but often use real drugs as placebos. *Family Medicine* 42 (9): 636.

King, E.S., Moyer, D.V., Couturie, M.J. et al. (2006). Getting doctors to report medical errors: Project DISCLOSE. *Joint Commission Journal on Quality and Patient Safety* 32 (7): 382–392.

Kipperman, B.S. (2014). The demise of the minimum database. *Journal of the American Veterinary Medical Association* 244: 1368–1370.

Kipperman, B., Morris, P., and Rollin, B. (2018). Ethical dilemmas encountered by small animal veterinarians: Characterization, responses, consequences and beliefs regarding euthanasia. *Veterinary Record* 182 (19): 548: 10.1136/vr.104619

Kogan, L.R., Rishniw, M., Hellyer, P.W. et al. (2018). Veterinarian's experiences with near misses and adverse events. *Journal of the American Veterinary Medical Association* 252: 586–595.

Kohn, K.T., Corrigan, J.M., and Donaldson, M.S. (1999). *To Err Is Human: Building a Safer Health System*. Washington, DC: National Academy Press.

Koyama, A.K., Maddox, C.S.S., Li, L. et al. (2020). Effectiveness of double checking to reduce medication administration errors: A systematic review. *BMJ Quality & Safety* 29 (7): 595–603.

Levine, E.E. and Schweitzer, M.E. (2014). Are liars ethical? On the tension between benevolence and honesty. *Journal of Experimental Social Psychology* 53: 107–117.

Main, D. (2006). Offering the best to patients: Ethical issues associated with the provision of veterinary services. *Veterinary Record* 158: 62–66.

Mamary, M.A. and Daniel, M. (2016). Medical error – The third leading cause of death in the US. *British Medical Journal* 353: i2139.

Mamede, S., Schmidt, H.G., and Penaforte, J.C. (2008). Effects of reflective practice on accuracy of medical diagnoses. *Medical Education* 42 (5): 468–475.

Mellanby, R.J. and Herrtage, M.E. (2004). Survey of mistakes made by recent veterinary graduates. *Veterinary Record* 155 (24): 761–765.

Mellanby, R.J., Rhind, S.M., Bell, C. et al. (2011). Perceptions of clients and veterinarians on what attributes constitute 'a good vet'. *Veterinary Record* 168: 616. 10.1136/vr.d925

O'Connell, D. and Reifsteck, S.W. (2004). Disclosing unexpected outcomes and medical error. *The Journal of Medical Practice Management: MPM* 19 (6): 317–323.

Oxtoby, C. and Mossop, L. (2019). Blame and shame in the veterinary profession: Barriers and facilitators to reporting significant events. *Veterinary Record* 184: 501.

Oxtoby, C., Ferguson, E., White, K. et al. (2015). We need to talk about error: Causes and types of error in veterinary practice. *Veterinary Record* 177 (17): 438.

Palmieri, J.J. and Stern, T.A. (2009). Lies in the doctor–patient relationship. *The Primary Care Companion to the Journal of Clinical Psychiatry* 11: 163.

Petronio, S., Torke, A., Bosslet, G. et al. (2013). Disclosing medical mistakes: A communication management plan for physicians. *The Permanente Journal* 17: 73–79.

Richard, C., Lajeunesse, Y., and Lussier, M.T. (2010). Therapeutic privilege: Between the ethics of lying and the practice of truth. *Journal of Medical Ethics* 36: 353.

Robertson, J.J. and Long, B. (2018). Suffering in silence: Medical error and its impact on health care providers. *The Journal of Emergency Medicine* 54 (4): 402–409.

Rodziewicz, T.L., Houseman, B., and Hipskind, J.E. (2021). Medical error reduction and prevention. In: *StatPearls*. Treasure Island, FL: StatPearls Publishing.

Rollin, B.E. (2006). *An Introduction to Veterinary Medical Ethics*, 2e. Ames, IA: Blackwell Publishing.

Shaw, J.R. and Lagoni, L. (2007). End-of-life communication in veterinary medicine: Delivering bad news and euthanasia decision making. *The Veterinary Clinics of North America. Small Animal Practice* 37 (1): 95–ix.

Shaw, J.R., Bonnett, B.N., Adams, C.L. et al. (2006). Veterinarian-client-patient communication patterns used during clinical appointments in companion animal practice. *Journal of the American Veterinary Medical Association* 228: 714–721.

Shine, K.I. (2002). Health care quality and how to achieve it. *Academic Medicine: Journal of the Association of American Medical Colleges* 77 (1): 91–99.

Shmerling, R.H. (2015). First, do no harm. Harvard Health Publishing. https://www. health.harvard.ed/blog/first-do-no-harm-201510138421 (accessed 5 March 2021).

Svensson, C., Emanuelson, U., Bard, A,M. et al. (2019). Communication styles of Swedish veterinarians involved in dairy herd health management: A motivational interviewing perspective. *Journal of Dairy Science* 102 (11): 10173–10185.

Tannenbaum, J. (1995). *Veterinary Ethics: Animal Welfare, Client Relations, Competition and Collegiality*, 2e. St. Louis, MO: Mosby.

The Joint Commission (2007). The Joint Commission releases improving America's hospitals: The Joint Commission's annual report on quality and safety. *Joint Commission Perspectives. Joint Commission on Accreditation of Healthcare Organizations* 27 (12): 1–3.

Tilburt, J.C., Emanuel, E.J., Kaptchuk, T.J. et al. (2008). Prescribing "placebo treatments": Results of national survey of US internists and rheumatologists. *British Medical Journal* 337: a1938.

Treadwell, J.R., Lucas, S., and Tsou, A.Y. (2014). Surgical checklists: A systematic review of impacts and implementation. *British Medical Journal Quality & Safety* 23 (4): 299–318.

Wallis, J., Fletcher, D., Bentley, A. et al. (2019). Medical errors cause harm in veterinary hospitals. *Frontiers in Veterinary Science* 6: 12.

Waterman, A.D., Garbutt, J., Hazel, E. et al. (2007). The emotional impact of medical errors on practicing physicians in the United States and Canada. *The Joint Commission Journal on Quality and Patient Safety* 33: 467.

Weich, K. and Grimm, H. (2018). Meeting the patient's interest in veterinary clinics. Ethical dimensions of the 21st century animal patient. *Food Ethics* 1 (3): 259–272.

Weller, J., Boyd, M., and Cumin, D. (2014). Teams, tribes and patient safety: Overcoming barriers to effective teamwork in healthcare. *Postgraduate Medical Journal* 90: 149–154.

Westbrook, J.I., Woods, A., Rob, M.I. et al. (2010). Association of interruptions with an increased risk and severity of medication administration errors. *Archives of Internal Medicine* 170 (8): 683–690.

Westbrook, J.I., Li, L., Hooper, T.D. et al. (2017). Effectiveness of a 'Do not interrupt' bundled intervention to reduce interruptions during medication administration: A cluster randomised controlled feasibility study. *British Medical Journal Quality & Safety* 26 (9): 734–742.

Wikipedia (n.d.). Sentinel event. https://en.wikipedia.org/wiki/Sentinel_event/URI (accessed 2 May 2021).

Witman, A.B., Park, D.M., and Hardin, S.B. (1996). How do patients want physicians to handle mistakes? A survey of internal medicine patients in an academic setting. *Archives of Internal Medicine* 156 (22): 2565–2569.

World Alliance for Patient Safety (2005). *WHO Draft Guidelines for Adverse Event Reporting and Learning Systems: From Information to Action*. Geneva, Switzerland: World Health Organization. [Google Scholar].

Wu, A.W., Folkman, S., McPhee, S.J. et al. (1991). Do house officers learn from their mistakes? *Journal of the American Medical Association* 265: 2089–2094.

# Section 3

# Ethical Concerns by Practice Type

# 10

# Companion Animals

## 1   Shelter Medicine

*Julie D. Dinnage*

Modern animal shelters provide an array of services with population control and animal welfare at the forefront (Zawistowski and Morris 2013; Miller and Zawistowski 2017). Shelters operate under the direction of a board of directors or government body and must follow the overarching mission of the organization. Attention to animal welfare and the growing importance of the human–animal bond lead to decision-making complexity in shelters. The shelter veterinarian often navigates ethical challenges involving sensitive topics (Turner et al. 2012). At the same time, the veterinarian must abide by state veterinary practice acts and stay current on standards of care (Newbury et al. 2010). Veterinarians working in shelters provide advice on both management and medical issues. Shelter veterinarians' training makes them uniquely qualified to assist organizations with ethical decisions, balancing the interests of animal populations versus the welfare of individual animals.

## Types of Shelters

Open admission shelters intake any animal in need, then make decisions about their care and outcome. Municipal shelters are often mandated by state or local laws to provide services to animals in need. A limited admission shelter (sometimes referred to as "no kill") is more selective about which animals to intake, often prioritizing highly adoptable animals: however animals in limited admission shelters may endure prolonged stays (The Humane Society 2012). Open admission shelters may have to choose between treating injured and ill animals or euthanasia due to lack of space or resources. The veterinarian should be integrally involved in these decisions, providing expert opinion to ensure the prevention or alleviation of suffering through appropriate care or, if that is not possible, by performing humane euthanasia.

## Euthanasia

Several longstanding and heated ethical dilemmas surround euthanasia – from how to perform the procedure in a humane manner (Rhoades 2002) to its utilization to control populations (American Veterinary Medical Association [AVMA] Euthanasia Guidelines 2020). Shelters that refuse to perform euthanasia have unique ethical dilemmas in ensuring they are not contributing to animals suffering in their care due

*Ethics in Veterinary Practice: Balancing Conflicting Interests*, First Edition. Edited by Barry Kipperman and Bernard E. Rollin.
© 2022 John Wiley & Sons, Inc. Published 2022 by John Wiley & Sons, Inc.

to extended lengths of stay or by burdening potential adopters by placing animals with medical or behavioral conditions. Shelter professionals who perform euthanasia must be thoroughly trained in appropriate injection techniques and safe drug and animal handling. Shelters should provide compassion fatigue training and opportunities to discuss the stressors of performing euthanasia as one means of minimizing burnout (Figley and Roop 2006).

## Adoptability

There are ethical questions surrounding what constitutes an adoptable animal and the veterinarian's perspective may differ from that of other decision makers. A key ethical responsibility has been to provide medically and behaviorally healthy animals for adoption. More recently, shelters may strive to increase live release rates (LRR). LRR is defined as the number of animals leaving a shelter by means other than euthanasia or in-shelter death. This is generally achieved through rehoming, owner reclaim, or transfer to another agency (Scarlett et al. 2017). Increasing LRR may involve preventing and treating diseases but could also result in rehoming animals with chronic medical or behavioral conditions. Consideration for the potential financial and emotional toll on an adopter should be carefully reviewed along with the potential for repeat relinquishment. Methods to dependably assess the behavioral health of shelter animals to minimize repeat relinquishment and prevent potential risk to the public due to aggressive or fearful behavior are also subject to significant debate (Patronek and Bradley 2016).

## Capacity for Care

The quality of life for animals in a shelter is closely associated with its capacity for care (Newbury et al. 2010), which can change on a day-to-day basis. Veterinarians should work with shelter leadership to regularly assess capacity for care and to operate within that capacity, including offering environmental enrichments. Ultimately, the ethical role of a shelter veterinarian involves balancing their responsibility to provide appropriate care and ensure the best possible welfare for the animals with often limited resources.

## Sterilization

Sterilization programs have been an integral part of shelter missions to control overpopulation and stop the influx of unwanted animals into shelters. State laws and/or local ordinances often mandate that animals adopted from shelters be sterilized. Pediatric sterilization has been proven safe in the short term and has long been a common practice in shelters. Later studies raised ethical and medical questions regarding age of gonadectomy and the potential link to long-term health risks, especially in certain breeds (Torres de la Riva 2013; Hart et al. 2014). The overall benefit to the community and pet population has long been the first ethical consideration. As demand for pets increases, the shelter veterinarian may face a new ethical question if delayed gonadectomy could increase long-term well-being of an individual animal.

## Animal Transport

Increasingly, areas in the United States no longer have an overabundance of unwanted pets (Rowan and Kartal 2018). Consequently, shelters may transport animals in from other geographic areas to provide a supply of desirable pets. Transport of animals, sometimes from foreign countries or different geographies, creates an ethical responsibility to prevent spread of diseases or other pathogens to nonendemic areas (Wright et al. 2020; American Heartworm Society 2021) and to ensure humane transport while abiding by all animal health regulations involving movement of animals (United States Department of Agriculture Animal and Plant Health Inspection Service [USDA-APHIS] 2020).

## References

American Heartworm Society, Association of Shelter Veterinarians (2021). Minimizing heartworm transmission in relocated dogs. https://www.sheltervet.org/assets/Brochures/sko_transport_guidelines_for_web_e.pdf (accessed 2 April 2021).

American Veterinary Medical Association (AVMA) (2020). Guidelines for the euthanasia of animals. https://www.avma.org/sites/default/files/2020-02/Guidelines-on-Euthanasia-2020.pdf (accessed 10 October 2020).

Figley, C.R. and Roop, R.G. (2006). *Compassion Fatigue in the Animal-Care Community*. Washington, DC: The Humane Society Press.

Hart, B.L., Hart, L.A., Thigpen, A.P. et al. (2014). Long-term health effects of neutering dogs: Comparison of Labrador Retrievers with Golden Retrievers. *PLoS ONE* 9 (7): e102241. doi:10.1371/journal.pone.0102241.

The Humane Society of the United States (2012). The HSUS Shelter advocate toolkit. All shelters are not alike – the important differences that can affect the mission. https://www.humanesociety.org/sites/default/files/docs/all-shelters-are-not-alike.pdf) (accessed 2 April 2021).

Miller, L.T. and Zawistowski, S.L. (2017). Animal shelter medicine: Dancing to a changing tune. *Veterinary Heritage* 40 (2): 44–49.

Newbury, S., Blinn, M.K., Bushby, P.A. et al. (2010). Association of Shelter Veterinarians. Guidelines for standards of care in animal shelters. https://www.sheltervet.org/assets/docs/shelter-standards-oct2011-wforward.pdf (accessed 4 April 2021).

Patronek, G.J. and Bradley, J. (2016). No better than flipping a coin: Reconsidering canine behavior evaluations in animal shelters. *Journal of Veterinary Behavior* 15: 66–77.

Rhoades, R.H. (2002). *Euthanasia Training Manual*. Washington, DC: The Humane Society Press.

Rowan, A. and Kartal, T. (2018). Dog population and dog sheltering trends in the United States of America. *Animals* 8 (5): 68. https://doi.org/10.3390/ani8050068.

Scarlett, J.M., Greenberg, M., and Hoshizaki, T. (2017). *Every Nose Counts. Using Metrics in Animal Shelters*. Pleasanton, CA: Maddie's Fund.

Torres de La Riva, G., Hart, B.L., Farver, T.B. et al. (2013). Neutering dogs: Effects on joint disorders and cancers in Golden Retrievers. *PLoS ONE* 8 (2): e55937. doi:10.1371/journal.pone.0055937.

Turner, P., Berry, J., and MacDonald, S. (2012). Animal shelters and animal welfare: Raising the bar. *The Canadian Veterinary Journal* 53 (8): 893–896.

United States Department of Agriculture Animal and Plant Health Inspection Service (USDA-APHIS) (2020). Import and export: Animal and animal products. https://www.aphis.usda.gov/aphis/ourfocus/importexport/animal-import-and-export/CT_Animal_Import_Export (accessed 4 April 2021).

Wright, I., Jongejan, F., Marcondes, M. et al. (2020). Parasites and vector-borne diseases disseminated by rehomed dogs. *Parasites & Vectors* 13: 546. https://doi.org/10.1186/s13071-020-04407-5.

Zawistowski, S. and Morris, J. (2013). Introduction to animal sheltering. In: *Shelter Medicine for Veterinarians and Staff*, 2e (L. Miller and S. Zawistowski), 3–13. Hoboken, NJ: John Wiley & Sons.

## 2   Outdoor Cats

*Andrew Rowan*

Discussions about outdoor cats and their management are controversial. Conservation biologists complain about the outdoor presence of domestic cats and their impact on wildlife, while animal advocacy organizations (who support the need to develop successful measures to control outdoor cats), oppose the catch-and-kill approach promoted by some conservation biologists (Marra and Santella 2017; Read et al. 2020). The veterinary profession is divided on how best to manage outdoor cats with some supporting the arguments of conservation biologists (Jessup 2004; Jessup et al. 2018) while others promote trap–neuter–vaccinate–return (TNVR) programs (Levy et al. 2014; Kreisler et al. 2019).

### Is the Outdoor Cat Situation Getting Worse or Better?

Unfortunately, good data to answer this question are scarce. Current estimates of pet cat populations in the United States vary from 58.4 million (AVMA 2018) to 94.2 million (American Pet Products Association [APPA] 2018). Given the big differences in the estimated pet cat populations produced by major pet surveys, there are no reliable estimates of the total number of outdoor (stray and feral) cats in the United States. Based on the average density of outdoor cats, Rowan et al. (2020) estimated that there could be 32 million outdoor cats in the continental United States.

In 1973, the intake of cats into US shelters was around 8–9 million (7 million were euthanized that year by shelters) (Rowan and Williams 1987). In 2019, total cat intake into US shelters was an estimated 3.8 million (PetHealth n.d.) even though the pet cat population had almost doubled since 1973. This 50+% decline in the shelter intake of cats is an indication that outdoor cat populations might be declining (NB cat euthanasia in shelters has declined by over 90% since 1973; Rowan et al. 2020).

### The Health of Outdoor Cats

Some shelters have stopped taking in unsocialized cats and euthanizing them. Instead, these cats are now being sterilized, vaccinated, and returned to field (RTF) (Johnson and Cicirelli 2014). RTF has raised concerns that outdoor cats do not thrive but the euthanasia rate of outdoor cats that are trapped, sterilized, vaccinated, and then returned to the capture site is very low. Levy and Crawford (2004) report that only 0.4% of cats were euthanized for health reasons in an outdoor cat sterilization program in Florida. However, it is widely recognized that kittens born to outdoor cats have high (70+%) mortality rates. Hence, sterilizing an outdoor cat prevents the subsequent litter production and high kitten mortality (Boone et al. 2019). It has also been reported that sterilized outdoor cats live longer than intact outdoor cats so there may be a positive welfare impact of sterilization (Tabor 1983).

## Does TNVR Work?

Conservation biologists criticize TNVR claiming that such programs do not "work" (Read et al. 2020). In contrast, cat advocates claim that TNVR programs will lead to the eventual elimination of outdoor cat colonies or, at least, a big reduction in outdoor cat numbers (Kreisler et al. 2019; Wolf et al. 2019). In examining the various publications cited by both opponents and advocates of TNVR, it is apparent that population reductions in cat colonies where TNVR has been practiced generally take at least three to five years to become evident. Several of the papers cited by opponents of TNVR as supporting the "do not work" argument described projects that lasted from one to three years at most. In addition, papers criticizing TNVR take issue with the removal of some of the cats (kittens and socialized individuals) for adoption. Such removal may account for an immediate halving of the outdoor cat population and this, it is argued, artificially increases the outdoor cat population reduction. But the longer running TNVR projects report population reductions after adjusting for the removal of cats that may be adopted (Levy et al. 2014; Kreisler et al. 2019; Wolf et al. 2019).

## Veterinary Options for Addressing the Outdoor Cat Issue

While an obvious role for veterinarians in the outdoor cat issue would be to become involved in sterilization projects, there are other recommendations that could be offered to cat-owning clients. Animal advocacy and wildlife conservation groups promote the keeping of pet cats indoors and these campaigns have had considerable success, almost doubling the percentage of cats that are indoor-only pets (APPA 2018). Therefore, veterinarians should promote maintaining cats as indoor pets but should be aware of behavioral issues that might arise. One way to address behavioral problems would be to suggest the construction of a "catio" that allows a cat outdoor access but would prevent it from catching and killing wildlife (see http://www.feralcats.com/catio-resources for examples).

If one's cat-owning clients do not want to restrict their cat's outdoor access, then a recent study from the UK has some additional options (Cecchetti et al. 2021). Households where a high meat protein, grain-free food was provided, and households where 5–10 minutes of daily object play was introduced, recorded decreases of 36% and 25%, respectively, in the numbers of animals captured and brought home by cats. Fitting Birdsbesafe collars (https://www.birdsbesafe.com/index.html) reduced the number of birds captured and brought home by 42% but had no discernible effect on the number of mammals brought home.

## References

American Pet Products Association (APPA) (2018). American Pet Products Association's 2017–2018 national pet owners survey. https://www.iii.org/fact-statistic/facts-statistics-pet-statistics#Total%20Number%20Of%20Pets%20Owned%20In%20The%20United%20States,%20By%20Type%20Of%20Animal (accessed 26 March 2021).

American Veterinary Medical Association (AVMA) (2018). *AVMA Pet Ownership and Demographics Sourcebook, 2017–2018 Edition*. Schaumburg, IL: American Veterinary Medical Association.

Boone, J.D., Miller, P.S., Briggs, J.R. et al. (2019). A long-term lens: Cumulative impacts of free-roaming cat management strategy and intensity on preventable cat mortalities. *Frontiers in Veterinary Science* 6: 238. doi:10.3389/fvets.2019.00238.

Cecchetti, M., Crowley, S.L., Goodwin, C.E.D. et al. (2021). Provision of high meat content food and object play reduce predation of wild animals by domestic cats, *Felis catus*. *Current Biology* 31: 1–5. https://doi.org/10.1016/j.cub.2020.12.044.

Jessup, D.A. (2004). The welfare of feral cats and wildlife. *Journal of the American Veterinary Medical Association* 225: 1377–1383.

Jessup, D.A., Cherkassky, D., Karesh, W.B. et al. (2018). Reducing numbers of free-roaming cats. *Journal of the American Veterinary Medical Association* 253: 977–978.

Johnson, K.L. and Cicirelli, J. (2014). Study of the effect on shelter cat intakes and euthanasia from a shelter neuter return project of 10,080 cats from March 2010 to June 2014. *PeerJ* 2: e646. doi:10.7717/peerj.646.

Kreisler, R.E., Cornell, H.N., and Levy, J.K. (2019). Decrease in population and increase in welfare of community cats in a twenty-three-year trap-neuter-return program in Key Largo, FL: The ORCAT program. *Frontiers in Veterinary Science* 1 February. https://doi.org/10.3389/fvets.2019.00007.

Levy, J.K. and Crawford, P.C. (2004). Humane strategies for controlling feral cat populations. *Journal of the American Veterinary Medical Association* 255: 1354–1360.

Levy, J.K., Isaza, N.M., and Scott, K.C. (2014). Effect of high-impact targeted trap-neuter-return and adoption of community cats on cat intake to a shelter. *Veterinary Journal* 201: 269–274. https://doi.org/10.1016/j.tvjl.2014.05.001

Marra, P.P. and Santella, C. (2017). *Cat Wars: The Devastating Consequences of a Cuddly Killer*. Princeton, NJ: Princeton University Press.

Pethealth (n.d.). PetPoint industry reports. https://www.petpoint.com/Industry_Data (accessed 20 December 2021).

Read, J.L., Dickman, C.R., Boardman, W.S.J. et al. (2020). Reply to Wolf et al: Why Trap-Neuter-Return (TNR) is not an ethical solution for stray cat management. *Animals* 10 (9): 1525. https://doi.org/10.3390/ani10091525

Rowan, A.N., Kartal, T., and Hadidian, J. (2020). Cat demographics and impact on wildlife in the USA, the UK, Australia and New Zealand: Facts and values. *Journal of Applied Animal Ethics Research* 2: 7–37.

Rowan, A.N. and Williams, J. (1987). The success of companion animal management programs: A review. *Anthrozoos* 1: 110–122.

Tabor, R. (1983). *The Wildlife of the Domestic Cat*. London: Arrow Books (Random House).

Wolf, P.J., Rand, J., Swarbrick, H. et al. (2019). Reply to Crawford et al.: Why Trap-Neuter-Return (TNR) is an ethical solution for stray cat management. *Animals* 9 (9): 689. https://doi.org/10.3390/ani9090689

## 3   Overpopulation

*Andrew Rowan*

In the 1970s in the United States, there were reports in news outlets and academic journals (including an editorial in *Science*; Feldman 1974) that drew attention to the "overpopulation" of dogs and cats and the euthanasia of millions of animals every year by animal shelters (Djerassi et al. 1973). This led to meetings that included representatives of veterinary and animal protection organizations. A *Legislation, Education and Sterilization* initiative was proposed to address the overpopulation crisis although most agreed that sterilization would not be able to mitigate the problem. However, those arguments were incorrect. Over the next 45 years, companion animal euthanasia by shelters has been reduced by over 90% (Table 10.3.1).

There are no conclusive data identifying what caused the significant declines in dog and cat shelter intake and euthanasia, but it has been argued (Rowan and Kartal 2018) that surgical sterilization of pet dogs and cats and roaming outdoor cats has been a significant factor. An AVMA (2018) survey indicated that 70% of pet dogs and 80% of pet cats in the United States were sterilized (Trevejo et al. 2011). Sterilization appears to have been a key factor in reducing the euthanasia of unwanted animals in shelters from around 13 million a year in 1973 to just over a million in 2019 (Rowan and Kartal

**Table 10.3.1**   Change in US dog and cat (D&C) populations and shelter intake/euthanasia.

|  | 1950[b] | 1973[c] | 1982[c] | 2011 | 2016 | 2019 |
|---|---|---|---|---|---|---|
| Total US dog population (millions) | 32.6 | 35 | 46 | 69.9[d] | 76.8[d] | 80[d] |
| US pet dogs and cats (millions) | 52 | 65 | 92 | 146[d] | 135[d] | 140[d] |
| Stray dogs and/or stray shelter intake (millions)[a] | 10 | 8–9 | 4–5 | 1.7[e] | 1.3[e] | 1.1[e] |
| Percentage stray dogs (of total dog population) | 30% | 22.9–25.7% | 8.7–10.9% | 2.4% | 1.7% | 1.4% |
| Stray cat shelter intake (millions)[a] |  |  |  | 2.0[e] | 1.65[e] | 1.83[e] |
| D&C shelter euthanasia (millions) |  | 13.5 | 7.6–10 | 3.4[e] | 1.5[e] | 1.2[e] |
| % D&C euthanized in shelters |  | 20.8% | 8.3–10.7% | 2.4% | 1.1% | 0.9% |

[a]The numbers for "stray" dogs refer to dogs identified as unowned strays (1950) or all dogs entering shelters in 1973 and 1982. From 2011 to 2019, the numbers for stray dogs and cats refer only to animals picked up as strays and not to animals entering the shelter as a result of being relinquished by owners or for some other reason.
[b]Marbanks 1954.
[c]Rowan and Williams 1987.
[d]AVMA dog and cat population reports (AVMA 2012, 2018) or derived from equations developed from AVMA data.
[e]Derived from PetHealth (n.d.) industry reports (https://www.petpoint.com/Industry_Data).

2018; PetPoint n.d.). Approximately two-thirds of the sterilizations have been and are currently being carried out by private veterinary practices (AVMA 2018).

The dog and cat overpopulation crisis in the 1970s coincided with surgical sterilizations becoming routine in private clinics. However, surgical sterilization sparked conflicts between the veterinary profession and animal protection organizations because the profession argued tax-exempt organizations had a financial advantage and that clients would gravitate to the shelter clinics. As more animal shelters offered surgical sterilization, organized veterinary medicine launched a variety of challenges to such clinics with varying success.

This century, surgical sterilization offered by animal protection groups has become much more common, but some state veterinary associations continue to try to control or eliminate the competition from animal shelters. These actions are perceived by the animal protection movement to be against the best interests of animals. At the same time, the Association of Shelter Veterinarians was launched this century and has grown rapidly, and one can now become a board-certified specialist in shelter medicine (Levy et al. 2020). Individual veterinarians have been a key resource in addressing the problem of too many puppies and kittens, but the opposition of organized veterinary medicine to high volume sterilization clinics operated by animal organizations has tended to be a barrier to addressing overpopulation effectively.

Another related issue that is stirring debate is the question of the impact of sterilization on the health of individual dogs and cats. Several recent reports have identified adverse consequences (increased cancer rates, joint injuries, and incontinence) in animals that have been sterilized, especially those that were sterilized prepubertally (Kutzler 2020). But sterilization can also offer health advantages (e.g. reduced rates of mammary cancer). In addition, sterilized dogs live longer than intact animals (Hoffman et al. 2013). Longevity may be a better indicator of overall health and welfare than the incidence of a few specific diseases or ill-health conditions (O'Neill et al. 2013).

Ironically, we have now reached a point in the United States where the supply of puppies may not be sufficient to satisfy demand. Around 9–10% of the dog population die each year. Therefore, we need around 8 million puppies to replace the pet dogs that die and another 800,000 to accommodate the annual increase in the overall dog population. In 2019, the Centers for Disease Control (CDC) estimated that 1.06 million dogs were imported into the country, up from 400,000 ten years earlier (CDC 2019). Therefore, we need around 7.8 million domestically sourced puppies to sustain the US pet dog population. The percentage of dogs under one year of age has dropped from 20% in 1986 to 10% today (AVMA 2018).

This trend should be of concern to the veterinary profession as fewer pet dogs will result in fewer paying clients for veterinary clinics. Veterinarians need to pay attention to pet supply–demand curves for many reasons affecting both animal well-being and their own (Bauer et al. 2016). Veterinary expertise is going to be in demand as the nation grapples with how to manage a humane and balanced supply of pet dogs and cats.

# References

American Veterinary Medical Association (AVMA) (2012). *US Pet Ownership and Demographics Sourcebook, 2012 Edition*. Schaumburg, IL: American Veterinary Medical Association.

American Veterinary Medical Association (AVMA) (2018). *US Pet Ownership and Demographics Sourcebook, 2017–2018 Edition*. Schaumburg, IL: American Veterinary Medical Association.

Bauer, A., Beck, A., Stella, J. et al. (2016). *Overpopulation or Too Many Unwanted Pets? Perspective on Concepts and Management Approaches*. West Lafayette, IN: Purdue Extension, Purdue University.

Centers for Disease Control (CDC). (2019). Guidance regarding agency interpretation of "rabies-free" as it relates to the importation of dogs into the United States. Federal Register. https://www.federalregister.gov/documents/2019/01/31/2019-00506/guidance-regarding-agency-interpretation-of-rabies-free-as-it-relates-to-the-importation-of-dogs (accessed 21 December 2021).

Djerassi, C., Israel, A., and Jochle, W. (1973). Planned parenthood for pets? *Bulletin of the Atomic Scientists* 29: 10–19.

Feldman, B.M. (1974). The problem of urban dogs. *Science* 185: 931.

Hoffman, J.M., Creevy, K.E., and Promislow, D.E.L. (2013). Reproductive capability is associated with lifespan and cause of death in companion dogs. *PLoS ONE* 8 (4): e61082. https://doi.org/10.1371/journal.pone.0061082.

Kutzler, M.A. (2020). Possible relationship between long-term adverse health effects of gonad-removing surgical sterilization and luteinizing hormone in dogs. *Animals* 10 (4): 599. https://doi.org/10.3390/ani10040599.

Levy, J., Crawford, C., and Griffin, B. (2020). Shelter medicine: A rising tide. https://ufl.pb.unizin.org/integratingveterinarymedicinewithsheltersystems/chapter/shelter-medicine-a-rising-tide (accessed 13 May 2021).

Marbanks, J. (1954). Going to the dogs (and cats). *National Humane Review* January: 7.

O'Neill, D.G., Church, D.B., McGreevy, P.D. et al. (2013). Longevity and mortality of owned dogs in England. *Veterinary Journal* 198: 638–643. https://doi.org/10.1016/j.tvjl.2013.09.020.

PetPoint (n.d.). Industry reports. https://www.petpoint.com/Industry_Data (accessed 21 December 2021).

Rowan, A.N. and Kartal, T. (2018). Dog population & dog sheltering trends in the United States of America. *Animals* 8: 68. doi:10.3390/ani8050068

Rowan, A.N. and Williams, J. (1987). The success of companion animal management programs: A review. *Anthrozoos* 1: 110–122.

Trevejo, R., Yang, M., and Lund, E.M. (2011). Epidemiology of surgical castration of dogs and cats in the United States. *Journal of the American Veterinary Medical Association* 238: 898–904.

# 4  Neutering/Gonadectomy

*Anne Quain*

Neutering (gonadectomy) involves the surgical removal of gonads. It is performed primarily to prevent companion animal overpopulation.

Other indications for gonadectomy include:

- Preventing or treating sex hormone-influenced conditions including mammary neoplasia and pyometra in females, and benign prostatic hyperplasia and prostatitis in males.
- Preventing sex hormone-driven behaviors including fighting, urine marking, and roaming.
- Preventing the perpetuation of extremes of conformation or inherited disease.

Gonadectomy is differentiated from convenience surgeries because of its benefits to the individual animal. In countries such as the United States and the UK, routine gonadectomy of companion animals not intended for breeding is synonymous with responsible pet ownership (Palmer et al. 2012; BVA 2019; AVMA n.d.c). Gonadectomy is the most common surgical procedure performed in dogs in the United States (Trevejo et al. 2011; Root Kustritz 2018), and is therefore an important source of income to companion animal practices. The AVMA has promoted surgical and nonsurgical sterilization of privately owned intact dogs and cats (AVMA n.d.a). More recent policy supports routine sterilization of all cats not intended for breeding by five months of age but offers no consensus recommendation for dogs (AVMA n.d.b).

Yet, routine gonadectomy is not considered ethical in some countries, such as Norway and Sweden, where it is only recommended for medical reasons (Wongsaengchan and McKeegan 2019). Gonadectomy raises several ethical questions, including whether it should be performed routinely, and whether current practices are ethically acceptable. To explore these questions, I will apply Professor David Fraser's "practical ethic" for animals (Fraser 2012). This is based on four principles, addressed sequentially below.

## Principle 1: Provide Good Lives for Animals in Our Care

Gonadectomy is an elective procedure, and like other procedures carried out by veterinarians, is performed without the consent of the patient. There are risks associated with anesthesia, and the potential for surgical complications, which can be minimized through careful patient screening and appropriate anesthetic and surgical techniques. The development of safe, effective nonsurgical alternatives may reduce harms associated with gonadectomy, but these are not readily available at this time (Root Kustritz 2018).

Gonadectomized animals benefit from a reduced incidence of sex hormone-associated conditions, enjoy a closer bond with their owners, and may be less likely to suffer from sexual frustration (Trevejo et al. 2011; Palmer et al. 2012; Wongsaengchan and McKeegan 2019). But, it may be argued that reproduction is an important element of a "good life" for animals, and therefore removing the ability to reproduce may be considered a harm (Palmer et al. 2012). Alternatively, one could contend that a sexually intact animal who is unable to reproduce may experience sexual frustration (Palmer et al. 2012). Whether a life where an animal can reproduce is better or worse than a life where reproduction is prevented is difficult to resolve.

## Principle 2: Treat Suffering with Compassion

Unless indicated for medical reasons, gonadectomy itself does not treat suffering. However, it is justified as a means of *preventing* suffering.

Gonadectomized animals are spared suffering associated with whelping and queening and potential complications such as dystocia. Potential offspring are spared the fate of unwanted animals, who it may be argued are more likely to experience "a life worth avoiding." Many of the diseases prevented by gonadectomy are also painful and potentially fatal.

The process of gonadectomy should incorporate appropriate pre-, peri- and postoperative analgesia to minimize surgical pain (Epstein et al. 2015), and perioperative behavioral management to minimize fear, anxiety, and stress associated with veterinary care (Bain 2020).

## Principle 3: Be Mindful of Unseen Harm

As scientists committed to lifelong learning, veterinarians must continually review practices in light of new evidence. Even where routine gonadectomy has been recommended, recent research revealing an association between gonadectomy and a higher incidence of some diseases in dogs has prompted a re-examination of such policies (Nolan 2021).

Population-level studies suggest breed and weight-related variation in vulnerability to negative consequences of gonadectomy, including joint disease (hip dysplasia, cranial cruciate ligament tear, and elbow dysplasia), some cancers (lymphoma, mast cell tumor, hemangiosarcoma, and osteosarcoma) and urinary incontinence (Hart et al. 2020a, 2020b). Some of these harms may be reduced by increasing exposure to gonadal hormones by delaying gonadectomy, particularly in male dogs. Recent research also suggests that gonadectomy does not eliminate problem behaviors and may in fact increase these behaviors (McGreevy et al. 2018; Starling et al. 2019).

## Principle 4: Protect the Life-Sustaining Processes and Balances of Nature

The extent to which gonadectomy contributes to the impact of companion animals on the environment is currently unknown. Owned and stray companion animals impact the environment negatively both through their dietary footprint (Okin 2017) and contribution to biodiversity loss (Legge et al. 2020). Gonadectomy may mitigate these harms in reducing the absolute population of companion animals, and reducing behaviors associated with predation, like roaming.

To address these principles, the veterinary profession must take a more nuanced approach to decision making around gonadectomy, taking both individual and population factors into account. Professional associations have a role in ensuring that the highest quality, current evidence is available to veterinarians to ensure that harms to animal patients, the animal population at large, and the environment are minimized, while benefits are maximized.

## References

American Veterinary Medical Association (AVMA) (n.d.a). Spaying and neutering. https://www.avma.org/resources/pet-owners/petcare/spaying-and-neutering (accessed 29 March 2021).

American Veterinary Medical Association (AVMA) (n.d.b).Elective spaying and neutering of pets. https://www.avma.org/resources-tools/animal-health-and-welfare/elective-spaying-and-neutering-pets (accessed 30 March 2021).

American Veterinary Medical Association (AVMA) (n.d.c). Dog and cat population control. Available at: https://www.avma.org/resources-tools/avma-policies/dog-and-cat-population-control (Accessed March 30, 2021)

Bain, M. (2020). Surgical and behavioral relationships with welfare. *Frontiers in Veterinary Science* 7: 519.

British Veterinary Association (BVA). (2019). BVA policy statement: Neutering of cats and dogs. https://www.bva.co.uk/media/1167/neutering-cats-dogs-policy-print.pdf (accessed 29 March 2021).

Epstein, M.E., Rodan, I., Griffenhagen, G. et al. (2015). 2015 AAHA/AAFP pain management guidelines for dogs and cats. *Journal of Feline Medicine and Surgery* 17: 251–272.

Fraser, D. (2012). A "practical" ethic for animals. *Journal of Agricultural & Environmental Ethics* 25: 721–746.

Hart, B.L., Hart, L.A., Thigpen, A.P. et al. (2020a). Assisting decision-making on age of neutering for 35 breeds of dogs: Associated joint disorders, cancers, and urinary incontinence. *Frontiers in Veterinary Science* 7.

Hart, B.L., Hart, L.A., Thigpen, A.P. et al. (2020b). Assisting decision-making on age of neutering for mixed breed dogs of five weight categories: Associated joint disorders and cancers. *Frontiers in Veterinary Science* 7.

Legge, S., Woinarski, J.C.Z., Dickman, C.R. et al. (2020). We need to worry about Bella and Charlie: The impacts of pet cats on Australian wildlife. *Wildlife Research* 47: 523–539.

McGreevy, P.D., Wilson, B., Starling, M.J. et al. (2018). Behavioural risks in male dogs with minimal lifetime exposure to gonadal hormones may complicate population-control benefits of desexing. *PLoS ONE* 13: e0196284.

Nolan, R.S. (2021). When should we neuter dogs? It depends. *Journal of the American Veterinary Medical Association* 258: 446–449.

Okin, G.S. (2017). Environmental impacts of food consumption by dogs and cats. *PLoS ONE* 12: e0181301.

Palmer, C., Corr, S., and Sandøe, P. (2012). Inconvenient desires: Should we routinely neuter companion animals? *Anthrozoos* 25: S153–S172.

Root Kustritz, M.V. (2018). Population control in small animals. *The Veterinary Clinics of North America. Small Animal Practice* 48: 721–732.

Starling, M., Fawcett, A., Wilson, B. et al. (2019). Behavioural risks in female dogs with minimal lifetime exposure to gonadal hormones. *PLoS ONE* 14: e0223709.

Trevejo, R., Yang, M., and Lund, E.M. (2011). Epidemiology of surgical castration of dogs and cats in the United States. *Journal of the American Veterinary Medical Association* 238: 898–904.

Wongsaengchan, C. and McKeegan, D.E.F. (2019). The views of the UK public towards routine neutering of dogs and cats. *Animals:* 9: 138.

## 5   Conformational Disorders: Brachycephaly
*Anne Quain*

Conformational disorders occur when an animal's shape and structure negatively impact its health and welfare. Perhaps the most concerning conformational disorder is brachycephaly in dogs. Brachycephaly, or foreshortening of the facial skeleton, is a mutation selected for in over 20 breeds, including the French bulldog, Pug, and British bulldog, who have the most extreme forms (Packer et al. 2015b).

Despite well documented health problems, brachycephalic breeds are increasing in popularity in countries including the United States, the UK, and Australia (Fawcett et al. 2018), with owners prioritizing appearance over the health of the breed (Packer et al. 2017). In the United States, 7 brachycephalic breeds are in the top 29 most popular breeds and the French bulldog is now the second most popular breed (American Kennel Club 2021).

Brachycephalic dogs are predisposed to a range of health conditions including brachycephalic obstructive airway syndrome (BOAS) (Packer et al. 2015a, 2015b; O'Neill et al. 2020). Their shortened noses result in air turbulence, leading to BOAS symptoms such as noisy breathing and an incapacity to breathe or exercise normally. Objective measurements have determined that 50% of pugs and French bulldogs and 45% of bulldogs have clinically significant signs of BOAS (Ladlow et al. 2018). Upper respiratory disorders were the cause of death for 17% of dogs with extreme brachycephalic conformation compared with 0% for all other breeds of dogs (O'Neill et al. 2015). Brachycephalic breeds have shorter lifespans compared with nonbrachycephalic dogs (median longevity 8.6 years and 12.7 years, respectively) (O'Neill et al. 2013).

Over half (58%) of owners of dogs with BOAS reported their dog did not have a breathing problem (Packer et al. 2012), while 71% of owners considered their brachycephalic dog in very good health or the best health possible, despite awareness of their dog's health issues (Packer et al. 2019). It appears that many prospective and current owners of dogs with extreme brachycephalic conformation are unaware of the enormity of the costs borne by these dogs or are in denial of their consequences.

From a utilitarian perspective, it is difficult to justify breeding animals to meet human aesthetic preferences (a relatively trivial benefit) knowing that they suffer lifelong health and welfare compromise (a significant cost).

One of the ethical challenges presented by animals bred for extreme conformation is how to ensure that veterinarians do not perpetuate welfare compromise. Veterinarians may fear alienating owners of brachycephalic breeds and breeders of these animals if they "speak up" about conformation-related problems (Fawcett et al. 2018). In the author's experience, clients cite feeling "judged" or criticized for the very features they find most endearing about their animal as a reason for changing veterinarians. Some veterinarians feel that as they cannot reverse conformational disorders, the best they can do is mitigate these to provide the best welfare for their current patient.

But according to the British Veterinary Association (BVA), failure of veterinarians to "speak out about systemic welfare problems" leaves the profession open to "weak morality and, worse, complicity in animal welfare problems" (BVA 2016). It is critical that clients are fully informed, as those who recognized BOAS-associated health issues in their dog were less likely to want to own a dog of the same breed in the future (Packer et al. 2020). Clients who fail to recognize the extent of these health problems may be less likely to seek appropriate treatment for their dog (Packer et al. 2012). Extreme brachycephaly is not simply an issue to be addressed in the individual patient – it is a veterinary public health problem that also imposes emotional and financial burdens on the owners of these dogs.

Veterinarians have professional and moral obligations to prevent and, where they occur, minimize the health and welfare impacts of extreme conformation. Suggested actions include explaining that the disorder is inextricably linked to conformation, discouraging ownership of these breeds during preadoption consultations, educating owners of these dogs regarding signs of BOAS (i.e. snorting and snoring are not normal), lifestyle limitations and the need for early surgical intervention, and advise against breeding any dog with BOAS symptoms (Fawcett et al. 2018).

Professional associations can influence animal welfare legislation, breed standards, and societal norms through policies which specifically prohibit depiction of conformation that compromises animal health and welfare in advertising, publications, and social media (unless for educational purposes). Indeed, both the British and Australian veterinary associations have adopted advertising policies banning the portrayal of brachycephalic breeds (BVA 2017; Latter 2017). Professional associations can work with researchers, kennel clubs, and breed societies to improve the health of brachycephalic dogs and undertake and disseminate the findings of research about the relationship between conformation and health and welfare. The UK's Brachycephalic Working Group is an example of such a collaboration. (http://www.ukbwg.org.uk).

Veterinarians and veterinary professional organizations should actively discourage the demand for and breeding of animals with welfare-compromising conformation and promote healthy phenotypes.

## References

American Kennel Club (2021). The most popular dog breeds of 2020. https://www.akc.org/expert-advice/dog-breeds/the-most-popular-dog-breeds-of-2020 (accessed 30 March 2021).

British Veterinary Association (BVA) (2016). Vets speaking up for animal welfare: BVA animal welfare strategy. https://www.bva.co.uk/take-action/our-policies/animal-welfare-strategy (accessed 21 December 2021).

British Veterinary Association (BVA) (2017). Information on advertising policy re bulldogs, French bulldogs and pugs. http://veterinaryrecord.bmj.com/pages/wp-content/uploads/sites/50/2017/04/Vet-record-Letter-for-advertisers-amended-for-website.pdf (accessed 19 January 2018).

Fawcett, A., Barrs, V., Awad, M. et al. (2018). Consequences and management of canine brachycephaly in veterinary practice: Perspectives from Australian veterinarians and veterinary specialists. *Animals* 9: 3.

Ladlow, J., Liu, N.C., Kalmar, L. et al. (2018). Brachycephalic obstructive airway syndrome. *Veterinary Record* 182: 375–378.

Latter, M. (2017). AVA moves away from brachycephalic breeds in advertising. *Australian Veterinary Journal* 95: N4.

O'Neill, D.G., Church, D.B., McGreevy, P.D. et al. (2013). Longevity and mortality of owned dogs in England. *Veterinary Journal* 198: 638–643.

O'Neill, D.G., Jackson, C., Guy, J.H. et. al. (2015). Epidemiological associations between brachycephaly and upper respiratory tract disorders in dogs attending veterinary practices in England. *Canine Genetics and Epidemiology* 2: 10.

O'Neill, D.G., Pegram, C., Crocker, P. et al. (2020). Unravelling the health status of brachycephalic dogs in the UK using multivariable analysis. *Scientific Reports* 10: 17251.

Packer, R.M.A., Hendricks, A., and Burn, C.C. (2012). Do dog owners perceive the clinical signs related to conformational inherited disorders as 'normal' for the breed? A potential constraint to improving canine welfare. *Animal Welfare* 21: 81–93.

Packer, R.M.A., Hendricks, A., and Burn, C.C. (2015a). Impact of facial conformation on canine health: Corneal ulceration. *PLoS ONE* 10: e0123827.

Packer, R.M.A., Hendricks, A., Tivers, M.S. et al. (2015b). Impact of facial conformation on canine health: Brachycephalic obstructive airway syndrome. *PLoS ONE* 10: e0137496.

Packer, R.M.A., Murphy, D., and Farnworth, M.J. (2017). Purchasing popular purebreds: Investigating the influence of breed-type on the pre-purchase motivations and behaviour of dog owners. *Animal Welfare* 26: 191–201.

Packer, R.M.A., O'Neill, D.G., Fletcher, F. et al. (2019). Great expectations, inconvenient truths, and the paradoxes of the dog-owner relationship for owners of brachycephalic dogs. *PLoS ONE* 14: e0219918.

Packer, R.M.A., O'Neill, D.G., Fletcher, F. et al. (2020). Come for the looks, stay for the personality? A mixed methods investigation of reacquisition and owner recommendation of bulldogs, French bulldogs and pugs. *PLoS ONE* 15: e0237276.

## 6 Convenience Surgeries

*Anne Quain*

Convenience surgeries, or medically unnecessary surgeries, are those performed to benefit humans, rather than veterinary patients themselves. They include caudectomy ("tail docking"), cosmetic otoplasty ("ear cropping"), ventriculo-cordectomy ("debarking" or "devocalization"), and onychectomy ("declawing") when performed for non-medical purposes (Mills et al. 2016).

Requests for convenience surgery are ethically problematic because one stakeholder (the animal) bears the costs including the harms of hospitalization, anesthetic risk, perioperative pain, risk of complications, and potential chronic pain, without clear benefits (Bain 2020). Furthermore, procedures such as ventriculo-cordectomy and onychectomy may be viewed as a convenient means of preventing so-called problem behaviors, without addressing the drivers of those behaviors such as social isolation and lack of enrichment.

Onychectomy involves the surgical amputation of the third digital phalanges of both front feet and is performed primarily to reduce damage to property or injury to people caused by "inappropriate" scratching. Scratching is a normal feline behavior that sharpens and maintains claws, and serves as a visual and olfactory means of communication (Deporter and Elzerman 2019). Cats use their claws for balance, climbing, and self-defense (Canadian Veterinary Medical Association 2017).

However, 52–84% of cat owners reported their cat displayed "inappropriate" scratching behavior (Wilson et al. 2016; Moesta et al. 2017). Onychectomy eliminates the ability to perform normal scratching behavior by removing the claws.

For decades, onychectomy was performed routinely in cats in North America and Canada, with an estimated 21–24% of cats in the United States having undergone the procedure (Patronek 2001; Lockhart et al. 2014). In one study, 73% of veterinarians indicated that they performed onychectomy (Ruch-Gallie et al. 2016). The procedure is associated with acute and chronic pain, and increased risk of unwanted behaviors including urinating and defecating outside the litter box, excessive grooming, biting, and aggression (Martell-Moran et al. 2018).

There have been increasing calls from animal welfare organizations to ban non-medical onychectomy (Humane Society Veterinary Medical Association [HSVMA] 2010; Paw Project 2021; American Society for the Prevention of Cruelty to Animals [ASPCA] 2021). The procedure is banned or restricted in other regions and countries, including the European Union, the UK, Australia, and New Zealand, and is banned in cities including New York, Los Angeles, San Francisco, and West Hollywood (American Association of Feline Practitioners [AAFP] 2017; Cima 2020). Elective onychectomy is opposed by the AAFP and the American Animal Hospital Association. These organizations encourage veterinarians to educate cat owners about normal feline behavior and provide alternatives to onychectomy (American Animal Hospital Association 2015; AAFP 2017; Canadian Veterinary Medical Association 2017).

Alternatives include provision of suitable surfaces for scratching, regular nail trims, application of synthetic nail caps, the use of synthetic pheromones to minimize stress, and environmental enrichment (Deporter and Elzerman 2019).

In 2020, the AVMA updated its declawing policy, discouraging the procedure and supporting nonsurgical alternatives while respecting "the veterinarian's right to use professional judgment when deciding how to best protect their individual patients' health and welfare" (Cima 2020).

Performing such procedures is a source of moral conflict, challenging the concept of the veterinarian as patient advocate (Atwood-Harvey 2005). Given these concerns, can veterinarians ethically justify performance of convenience surgeries?

A veterinarian may argue that declawing is a "last resort" and that if these procedures were unavailable, some owners might elect relinquishment or euthanasia, therefore, cats will be "less worse off" if the procedure is performed (Ruch-Gallie et al. 2016). This argument is undermined by evidence that legislation prohibiting onychectomy didn't increase the risk of relinquishment for destructive behavior or other reasons (Ellis et al. 2021). "Last resort" implies that onychectomy should occur only if nonsurgical alternatives fail. But there is no consensus regarding the point at which nonsurgical alternatives are considered unsuccessful. Some owners may not be willing to invest their resources (time, money, effort) into nonsurgical options when a surgical "fix" is available (Mills et al. 2016).

A veterinarian may assert that "I acknowledge the welfare costs of onychectomy, but I will use optimal technique, including multimodal analgesia, to minimize the welfare costs to the cat, while ensuring that other stakeholders (such as the client, their landlord, the practice) benefit." But performing a convenience surgery known to be associated with acute and chronic pain, and known to eliminate the possibility of performing a natural behavior, violates the principle of nonmaleficence (doing no harm).

A veterinarian may argue that "If I don't perform the procedure, another veterinarian will." But by continuing to offer onychectomy, veterinarians signal to their clientele that feline scratching is problematic, and declawing is an acceptable solution. Offering a procedure simply to meet a demand abdicates moral responsibility. It suggests that consumer demand, rather than educated veterinarians, should set the agenda for animal welfare. This could lead to a situation where veterinarians may be seen as compromising rather than promoting animal welfare (BVA 2016).

Legislation against convenience surgeries would support veterinarians who feel pressured to perform declawing. Rather than wait for legislation, veterinary corporations are adopting policies that their veterinarians will not perform convenience surgeries (Banfield Pet Hospital 2020; VCA Hospitals 2021). Since January 2021, the AAFP only accredits cat-friendly practices that do not perform elective declawing – and previously accredited clinics must stop doing so within six months to retain accreditation (Anon. 2021).

If veterinarians are to fulfill their role as advocates for animal welfare, convenience surgeries are not ethically justifiable.

# References

American Animal Hospital Association (2015). AAHA position statements and endorsements: Declawing. https://www.aaha.org/about-aaha/aaha-position-statements/declawing/#:~:text=The%20American%20Animal%20Hospital%20Association,is%20a%20normal%20feline%20behavior.&text=Trim%20cats'%20nails%20every%20one%20to%20two%20weeks (accessed 22 March 2021).

American Association of Feline Practitioners (AAFP) (2017). AAFP position statement: Declawing. *Journal of Feline Medicine and Surgery* 19: NP1–NP3.

American Society for the Prevention of Cruelty to Animals (ASPCA) (2021). Position statement on declawing cats. https://www.aspca.org/about-us/aspca-policy-and-position-statements/position-statement-declawing-cats (accessed 25 April 2021).

Anon. (2021). Elective declawing banned in cat friendly practices. https://www.veterinarypracticenews.com/elective-declawing-banned-in-cat-friendly-practices/#:~:text=1&text=Elective%20onychectomy%20(declawing)%20procedures%20will,cats%20as%20an%20elective%20procedure (accessed 29 March 21 2021).

Atwood-Harvey, D. (2005). Death or declaw: Dealing with moral ambiguity in a veterinary hospital. *Society & Animals* 13: 315–342.

Bain, M. (2020). Surgical and behavioral relationships with welfare. *Frontiers in Veterinary Science* 7: 519.

Banfield Pet Hospital (2020). Banfield feline declaw position statement. https://www.banfield.com/pet-healthcare/additional-resources/article-library/veterinary-services/declaw-policy-statement#:~:text=Declaw%20Position%20Statement-,Banfield%20Feline%20Declaw%20Position%20Statement,normal%20digits)%20of%20any%20animal (accessed 21 March 2021).

British Veterinary Association (BVA) (2016). Vets speaking up for animal welfare: BVA animal welfare strategy. https://www.bva.co.uk/take-action/our-policies/animal-welfare-strategy (accessed 21 December 2021).

Canadian Veterinary Medical Association (2017). Partial digital amputation (onychectomy or declawing) of the domestic felid – position statement. https://www.canadianveterinarians.net/documents/partial-digital-amputation-onychectomy-or-declawing-of-the-domestic-felid-position-statement (accessed 22 March 2021).

Cima, G. (2020). AVMA revises declawing policy. *Journal of the American Veterinary Medical Association* 256: 502–504.

Deporter, T.L. and Elzerman, A.L. (2019). Common feline problem behaviors: Destructive scratching. *Journal of Feline Medicine and Surgery* 21: 235–243.

Ellis, A., Van Haaften, K., Protopopova, A. et al. (2021). Effect of a provincial feline onychectomy ban on cat intake and euthanasia in a British Columbia animal shelter system. *Journal of Feline Medicine and Surgery* 1098612X211043820.

Humane Society Veterinary Medical Association (HSVMA) (2010). Cosmetic and convenience procedures in companion animals. https://hsvma.memberclicks.net/policy_statements#cosmeticsurgeries (accessed 25 April 2021).

Lockhart, L.E., Motsinger-Reif, A.A., Simpson, W.M. et al (2014). Prevalence of onychectomy in cats presented for veterinary care near Raleigh, NC and educational attitudes toward the procedure. *Veterinary Anaesthesia and Analgesia* 41: 48–53.

Martell-Moran, N.K., Solano, M., and Townsend, H.G. (2018). Pain and adverse behavior in declawed cats. *Journal of Feline Medicine and Surgery* 20: 280–288.

Mills, K.E., Von Keyserlingk, M.A., and Niel, L. (2016). A review of medically unnecessary surgeries in dogs and cats. *Journal of the American Veterinary Medical Association* 248: 162–171.

Moesta, A., Keys, D., and Crowell-Davis, S. (2017). Survey of cat owners on features of, and preventative measures for, feline scratching of inappropriate objects: A pilot study. *Journal of Feline Medicine and Surgery* 20: 891–899.

Patronek, G.J. (2001). Assessment of claims of short- and long-term complications associated with onychectomy in cats. *Journal of the American Veterinary Medical Association* 219: 932–937.

Paw Project (2021). About the Paw Project. https://pawproject.org/about-us/about-the-paw-project (accessed 22 March 2021).

Ruch-Gallie, R., Hellyer, P.W., Schoenfeld-Tacher, R. et al. (2016). Survey of practices and perceptions regarding feline onychectomy among private practitioners. *Journal of the American Veterinary Medical Association* 249: 291–298.

VCA Hospitals (2021). New VCA policy on elective declaw procedures in cats. https://vcahospitals.com/press-center/2020-02-21 (accessed 22 March 2021).

Wilson, C., Bain, M., Deporter, T. et al. (2016). Owner observations regarding cat scratching behavior: An internet-based survey. *Journal of Feline Medicine and Surgery* 18: 791–797.

# 7  Behavioral Medicine

*Melissa Bain*

Behavioral problems, including aggression, house soiling, and separation anxiety, are among the most common causes of pet relinquishment and euthanasia (Coe et al. 2014).

## Options for Addressing Behavioral Problems

In behavior medicine, we have four options for the care of an individual pet:

1) Do nothing (*not an option*).
2) Do something.
3) Find a shelter or home that will take the pet, treat it humanely, and keep others safe.
4) Euthanasia.

### Do Something

Options vary widely, from trigger avoidance to full behavior modification. When discussing treatment options with owners, practitioners should consider what risks owners are willing to take when management fails.

Veterinarians may feel pressured by owners to prescribe medications to treat problem behaviors. Owners may rely on medications to "cure" the problem, ignoring other treatment modalities perceived to be more arduous, including management recommendations. While medications are often part of a treatment plan, by themselves these rarely effect long-term improvement. If or when medications are not effective, or if an animal causes harm to a person or other animal while on medications, the owner may blame the veterinarian.

Alternatively, withholding treatment may be detrimental to the animal's welfare. Despite their limitations, medications can offer some respite from anxiety even when behavior modification is not pursued. Veterinarians should offer referral to a veterinary behaviorist if they are unable to provide a suitable treatment plan.

### Find a New Home

Rehoming an animal with a history of a problem behavior, especially aggression or anxiety, is risky for the safety of people and other animals, as well as for the welfare of the affected animal, who may be subject to inhumane treatment or another rehoming. Animal shelters and rescue agencies may have limited resources to perform appropriate behavior modification, disclose any previous history, and/or provide support after adoption. If an owner plans to rehome a pet, they should fully disclose the problem, and request transparency from the new owner as to what course of action will be taken. Owners also must consider their liability if they rehome a pet with a history of aggression.

### Euthanasia

If an owner is not able or willing to work with the pet while keeping all involved physically and emotionally safe, or to find it a new home, then euthanasia is the only remaining option.

Some view euthanasia of a physically healthy animal as a "convenience." Aside from minor problems that don't involve anxiety or aggression, "convenience" is not an accurate term for behavioral euthanasia. Many owners agonize over this decision. It is imperative that veterinarians attempt to gather a full history, as what may appear as a "convenience request" often has other valid reasons. Some owners may not disclose all circumstances leading to this decision. The practitioner must consider the psychological health of the individual animal and the owner's ability to maintain a safe environment for people and other pets.

## Factors Affecting Prognosis and Treatment Recommendations

The animal's condition, the environment, and the owner's capacity for care all affect diagnosis, prognosis, and treatment recommendations, with moral and ethical ramifications.

### Animal Factors

Size affects an owner's ability to control their dog, as well as the increased danger it poses if it were to bite a person or another animal. Breed is related to size, and there are documented breed tendencies toward specific behaviors (Miklosi 2016).

It is important to determine the motivation for any behavior. Most cases of aggression are due to fear and anxiety. Anxiety diminishes welfare. Owners often punish aggressive behavior to protect others; however, dogs that have been punished for expressing any type of aggression, such as growling, may not display warning signs before biting (Ziv 2017).

### Environmental Factors

Children, the elderly, other at-risk people, and other pets must be kept physically and emotionally safe. The presence of these factors worsens the prognosis. Also, other pets need care and time with their owners, and management and behavior modification of the affected pet can interfere with that relationship.

Where the pet lives affects treatment options. Management recommendations for a dog with aggression are more easily followed if they live on a fenced property, thus avoiding unfamiliar people on walks, compared with if they live in an apartment, requiring the dog to be walked on leash multiple times per day. Management decisions may keep others safe while limiting the affected animal's need to socialize, causing ethical concerns.

Trigger predictability and capacity to avoid triggers are very important factors. It is challenging if owners cannot identify a trigger or if the animal reacts unpredictably, leaving them to wonder "when" it will happen. It is problematic when the triggers are unavoidable, such as petting, any type of food object dropped on the ground, looking at, or walking past the dog, especially if children reside in the house.

### Owner Factors

No one can ever truly understand how previous experiences affect an owner: therefore, an owner's ability and willingness to undertake risk is an individual decision. Some owners are unable to take any risk, while others take risks that few would or should. If an owner takes an unacceptable risk, such as not supervising interactions between a dog and a child, veterinary professionals are ethically obligated to protect the vulnerable. This can range from having a serious (and documented) conversation with the owner, to reporting the situation to authorities.

Owners are exposed to a lot of incorrect information, perhaps more so about behavior. Owners may be constrained by time and ability to effectively institute management and behavior modification. In some cases, an owner's response to the diagnosis or treatment recommendations can include guilt or shame, and it can be a challenge for veterinarians to help owners through this decision-making process. Veterinary professionals can develop relationships with counselors to help clients navigate these decisions (Canino et al. 2007).

## Conclusion

Prevention and early identification of behavior problems are the best course of action to improve both prognosis and welfare. Consequently, practitioners should ask owners at every visit about their pet's behavior. Veterinary behavior textbooks offer guidance often with downloadable questionnaires (Horwitz 2018). Reflecting the importance of timely and compassionate management of problem behaviors in pets (Ballantyne and Buller 2015), behavior is part of the standard of care for hospitals certified by the American Animal Hospital Association (Hammerle et al. 2015).

Veterinarians have a duty to promote public health. When faced with the ethical quandary of behavioral euthanasia, practitioners should approach it with compassion and concern for the safety and well-being of all involved, not just the patient. As an alternative to euthanasia or rehoming, veterinarians can encourage owners to pursue treatment, either treating the patient themselves or by referral to a behaviorist.

## References

Ballantyne, K.C. and Buller, K. (2015). Experiences of veterinarians in clinical behavior practice: A mixed-methods study. *Journal of Veterinary Behavior* 10 (5): 376–383.

Canino, J., Shaw, J., and Beck, A.M. (2007). A look at the role of marriage and family therapy skills within the context of animal behavior therapy. *Journal of Veterinary Behavior* 2 (1): 15–22.

Coe, J.B., Young, I., Lambert, K. et al. (2014). A scoping review of published research on the relinquishment of companion animals. *Journal of Applied Animal Welfare Science* 17 (3): 253–273.

Hammerle, M., Horst, C., Levine, E. et al. (2015). AAHA canine and feline behavior management guidelines. *Journal of the American Animal Hospital Association* 51 (4): 205–221.

Horwitz, D.F. (ed.) (2018). *Blackwell's Five-Minute Veterinary Consult Clinical Companion: Canine and Feline Behavior*. Hoboken, NJ: Blackwell.

Miklosi, A. (2016). *Dog Behaviour, Evolution, and Cognition*, 2e. Oxford: Oxford University Press.

Ziv, G. (2017). The effects of using aversive training methods in dogs – A review. *Journal of Veterinary Behavior* 19: 50–60.

# 8 Referrals

*Barry Kipperman*

With the growth of veterinary specialist practices, the questions of whether, when, and how to refer a patient from a general practitioner (GP) to a specialist have important ethical dimensions.

There should be little debate about the duty of *whether* to refer a patient. Rollin (2006) asserts that "If the animal will benefit, ... the veterinarian has a moral duty to refer and defer to greater expertise." The AVMA (n.d.) Principles of Veterinary Medical Ethics state, "When appropriate, ... veterinarians are encouraged to seek assistance in the form of ... referrals." The ideal reasons to refer include improved patient outcome or likelihood of survival or less invasive diagnostic or treatment options (such as laparoscopic or endoscopic biopsies instead of surgery). As most pet owners are not aware of the existence of specialists (Buechner-Maxwell and Byers 2013), the GP is considered the gatekeeper to the referral process. Consequently, he/she *in conjunction with the client* should consider if the potential benefits of referral outweigh the cost, inconvenience, and necessity to trust a clinician regarding potential life-or-death decisions that the client may have no previous relationship with.

One barrier to referral is ego and pride: for some practitioners, acknowledging that a colleague is better suited to care for a patient is difficult. Another obstacle is perceived loss of income, with the specialist seen as competition for finite revenues associated with each patient. Main notes regarding referral that "If the goal ... is to advocate the best treatment option, then the loss of clinical income for the practitioner should not be a relevant factor" (2006). Surely a live patient cared for by a colleague is more valuable to the practice than one that is deceased! Specialist availability regarding time as well as proximity can also be limiting factors to referral. Finally, given the property status of pets, practitioners have virtually no malpractice concerns or economic liability for failing to refer.

The next decision is *when* to refer. Block and Ross (2006) suggest that "Any animal that has not received a definitive diagnosis or fails to improve despite medical treatment should be considered a candidate for a second opinion." In my experience, if the duration of patient illness exceeds five days, a patient has lost 10% of its body weight, or patient survival is more likely, referral is compelling. A premature or unnecessary referral is a waste of client and specialist time and resources: these can easily be diminished via a screening phone call to the specialist. A suitably timed referral is most likely to achieve the ideal goals. Delayed referrals often have devastating consequences including poor patient prognosis and suffering, increased client costs, loss of faith in the value of specialists by clients and GPs, the perception by the specialist that the GP did not prioritize the patient's interest, and moral stress and demoralization for the specialist, who often feels they cannot disclose to the client (to adhere to professionalism) or the GP that an earlier referral would have achieved a better patient outcome or allowed the patient to survive.

The final important issue is *how* to refer. Ideally, when the GP suggests referral, they should address the goals or rationale, which often involve access to greater expertise and/or specialized equipment, express confidence in the specialist, and broach the potential costs of diagnostic testing and treatment, which often involve hundreds to thousands of dollars. GPs should never assume that a client cannot afford to see a specialist. Clients should be informed of possible diagnoses that may be discovered and tests that may be performed without tying the hands of the specialist to a specific expectation. Ensuring that the specialist receives all pertinent medical records and test results at least 12 hours prior to patient arrival maximizes the value of the consultation.

The specialist has a responsibility to communicate in a timely manner with the GP to summarize the nature of the consultation and client options and to provide daily progress reports for hospitalized patients. It is imperative that referral hospitals immediately inform the GP if a patient has died. By virtue of the client's longstanding relationship with the GP, the GP may be in a better position to help guide the pet owner faced with difficult decisions. The trust that has been built over years with the GP cannot be rivaled by the specialist, where the duration of interaction with one client is often brief. Consequently, clients should be expected to confer with their GP regarding decisions about their animal companions. The advanced knowledge of the specialist can also be a double-edged sword. While they may be the best person to treat the patient's Cushings disease, the specialist may diminish the impact of the old-age arthritis that such treatment has worsened on the pet's quality of life. The GP may be in a better position to see the patient as a whole compared with the limited expertise of the specialist.

Although "Specialists have a responsibility to educate referring veterinarians ... when they believe animals may or should have been managed differently" (Block and Ross 2006), in my experience this seldom occurs; just as GPs are careful not to offend pet owners, specialists feel the same way about referring veterinarians out of fear of losing referrals and their associated income. Unfortunately, attempts to constructively discuss what could have been done better with referring colleagues sometimes results in a punitive loss of future referrals. Professionally crafted referral letters are also an opportunity to educate the GP in a less confrontational format. When the GP and the specialist appreciate the boundaries of their respective areas of expertise, communicate well, and work as a team on behalf of the best interests of the animal, the well-being of our patients and the reputation of the profession are best served.

# References

American Veterinary Medical Association (AVMA) (n.d.). Principles of Veterinary Medical Ethics. https://www.avma.org/KB/Policies/Pages/Principles-of-Veterinary-Medical-Ethics-of-the-AVMA.aspx (accessed 10 October 2020).

Block, G., Ross, J., and Northeast Veterinary Liaison Committee (2006). The relationship between general practitioners and board-certified specialists in veterinary medicine. *Journal of the American Veterinary Medical Association* 228 (8): 1188–1191.

Buechner-Maxwell, V. and Byers, C. (2013). ACVIM member engagement and brand assessment survey corona insights survey results summary. *Journal of Veterinary Internal Medicine* 27: 1287–1287.

Main, D. (2006). Offering the best to patients: Ethical issues associated with the provision of veterinary services. *Veterinary Record* 158: 62–66.

Rollin, B. (2006). The ethics of referral. *Canadian Veterinary Journal* 47 (7): 717.

# 9 Futile Intervention

*Christian Dürnberger, Herwig Grimm*

The so-called "Supervet," the veterinarian on an English television series, is known for performing advanced and risky surgeries. His fans praise his heroic efforts: the "Supervet" treats animals when others give up. However, at the same time critics speak of pointless treatments that put undue stress on the animals and cause more harm than good. Both his supporters and detractors claim that they are representing the best interest of the animal. Undoubtedly, veterinarians have a positive duty to help animals, but at what point do they run the risk of violating the negative duty not to harm animals? This debate leads to an important issue in veterinary medicine, namely to *medical futility*: when do well-intended interventions instead cause unwarranted harm? In this essay, we focus on small animal practice.

Studies show that veterinarians are requested to provide treatment that they consider futile (Moses et al. 2018; Lehnus et al. 2019). Moses et al. (2018) found that 79% of North American veterinarians reported being asked to provide care that they considered futile. The term has its origin in the French "futile," which translates to "vain," "worthless," and "incapable of producing results." Since interventions typically *do* produce results, the key question shifts to "What is a *valued* result?" In the medical literature, futile treatments are described as interventions that are unlikely to produce any significant benefit to the patient or that are even harmful when the negative effects outweigh the beneficial ones (Angelucci 2007). Quantitative futility arises when the *probability* that an intervention will benefit the patient is extremely low; qualitative futility occurs when the *quality* of the benefits is considered to be extremely low (Pope 2017). Thereby, medical futility refers to the balance of benefit and harm of a *particular* intervention for an *individual* patient in a *specific* situation. To assess the extent to which an intervention is futile or not, medical prognoses are needed first, which always involve uncertainties. Second, assessing the *benefit* of a treatment for an individual patient goes beyond simply evaluating the physiological effects of a medical intervention. The following questions illustrate this. They are not intended as a simple to-do list but are put forward to be considered when reflecting as to whether an intervention may be futile or not.

1) *Is the decision in the best interest of the animal?* Studies show that veterinarians see themselves – among other roles – as "advocates for the animal" (Grimm et al. 2018; Springer et al. 2019; for veterinarians in livestock farming, Dürnberger 2020). If an intervention causes more harm than good, there is an "ethics of non-treating patients" (Moore 2011) that is aligned with the role of the "advocate" (Fordyce 2017) since medicine is not about *treating* but *helping* the sick. This leads to the second question.

2) *Are the goals of the treatment clear?* The specific goals of potential treatments and interventions must be made explicit in the conversation between pet owner and veterinarian, because "getting healthy" is too vague and is not realistic in many cases: "Disagreements about whether a treatment is futile may often be disagreements about the goals of treatment" (Angelucci 2007). For example, "Buster should be eating within 48 hours after starting treatment," rather than "Until Buster feels better."

3) *At what point can or should the treatment be stopped?* Some interventions such as surgery cannot readily be reversed, while chemotherapy or radiation treatments can be stopped if side effects are significant, or if the mutually desired goals have not been achieved within the agreed timeframe. Such endpoints should be discussed with clients *before* the treatment is initiated.

4) *To what extent does the decision reflect one's personal beliefs?* The questions of whether a life is still worth living, at what point suffering becomes "unnecessary," and about the boundary between adequate treatment and "overtreatment" find their source in personal beliefs – be they of the veterinarian or the pet owner – of what constitutes a good life, death, suffering, harm, etc. Since this factor cannot be totally avoided, these ideas and their role in our decision-making process should be explicitly considered.

Decisions along the fine line between futile and warranted interventions direct the future of the profession. Keeping this in mind, veterinarians are encouraged to promote discussion about futile interventions with professional colleagues. Herewith, veterinarians should be aware that futile interventions not only lead to negative effects on the individual patient, but can also offer false hope to pet owners and be seen as emotionally and financially exploitative, which can cause distrust in the veterinarian or the veterinary profession. These can also cause moral stress for the practitioner (see Chapter 22). In addition, the rapidly increasing technical possibilities paired with pet owners' increasing willingness to pursue advanced and often expensive therapies are driving forces for possible futile interventions. This means, among other things, that veterinary ethics should embrace the key idea that not everything technically feasible is morally well founded (i.e. "just because you can, doesn't mean you should"). For instance, there might be cases in which the preferable option would be palliative care instead of "aggressive" therapy.

Precisely because the widespread expectation that "doctors always and only treat sick patients" runs the risk of medical futility, it is of great importance to make transparent that nontreatment options, palliative care, and euthanasia might be positive duties in specific cases. Hence, to avoid futile interventions as a violation of the negative duty not to harm patients will require not only medical knowledge but also empathic, transparent communication with clients under stressful circumstances to navigate responsibly the boundaries between over- and undertreatment.

# References

Angelucci, P. (2007). What is medical futility? *Nursing Critical Care* 2 (1): 20–21.

Dürnberger, C. (2020). Am I actually a veterinarian or an economist? Understanding the moral challenges for farm veterinarians in Germany on the basis of a qualitative online survey. *Research in Veterinary Science* 133: 246–250. https://doi.org/10.1016/j.rvsc.2020.09.029.

Fordyce, P.S. (2017). Welfare, law and ethics in the veterinary intensive care unit. *Veterinary Anaesthesia and Analgesia* 44 (2): 203–211. https://doi.org/10.1016/j.vaa.2016.06.002.

Grimm, H., Bergadano, A., Musk, G.C. et al. (2018). Drawing the line in clinical treatment of companion animals: Recommendations from an ethics working party. *Veterinary Record* 182: 664. https://doi.org/10.1136/vr.104559.

Lehnus, K.S., Fordyce, P.S., and McMillan, M.W. (2019). Ethical dilemmas in clinical practice: A perspective on the results of an electronic survey of veterinary anaesthetists. *Veterinary Anaesthesia and Analgesia* 46 (3): 260–275. https://doi.org/10.1016/j.vaa.2018.11.006.

Moore, A.S. (2011). Managing cats with cancer. An examination of ethical perspectives. *Journal of Feline Medicine and Surgery* 3 (9): 661–671. https://doi.org/10.1016/j.jfms.2011.07.019.

Moses, L., Malowney, M.J., and Boyd, J.W. (2018). Ethical conflict and moral distress in veterinary practice: A survey of North American veterinarians. *Journal of Veterinary Internal Medicine* 32 (6): 2115–2122. https://doi.org/10.1111/jvim.15315.

Pope, T.M. (2017). Medical futility and potentially inappropriate treatment: Better ethics with more precise definitions and language. *Perspectives in Biology and Medicine* 60 (3): 423–427. https://doi.org/10.1353/pbm.2018.0018.

Springer, S., Sandøe, P., Bøker Lund, T. et al. (2019). "Patients' interests first, but …" Austrian veterinarians' attitudes to moral challenges in modern small animal practice. *Animals* 9: 5. https://doi.org/10.3390/ani9050241.

## 10  Obesity

*Barry Kipperman*

Obesity is a condition where excess body fat has developed to the point that health is adversely affected (National Institutes of Health [NIH] 1985). Dogs and cats are considered overweight when their weight is more than 10–20% above their ideal weight (German 2006) and obesity is present when a dog or cat is over 30% above its ideal weight (AVMA 2016). It is estimated that 56% of dogs and 60% of cats in the United States are overweight or obese (Association for Pet Obesity Prevention n.d.). The rise in prevalence of obesity in humans may be reflected in the companion dogs and cats with whom lifestyles are shared (Sandoe et al. 2016). Studies suggest that owners of overweight and obese dogs and cats use food as a pivotal means of interaction with their animal companions (Kienzle and Bergler 2006; Shearer 2010; White et al. 2016).

Overweight dogs and cats are at increased risk for many medical conditions, including diabetes mellitus and orthopedic disorders (Scarlett and Donoghue 1998; Lund 2005; Lund et al. 2006). Health-related quality of life is worse in dogs with obesity compared with dogs at ideal weight (German 2006; German et al. 2012). The great majority of obese companion animals will remain obese for a significant portion of, or for the remainder of their lifespan, obesity causes significant impairments to welfare and longevity (Kealy et al. 2002; Lawler et al. 2008), and it has been confirmed that dogs that successfully lose weight have significantly improved quality of life (German et al. 2012). Obesity also imposes a significant financial burden on pet owners, with one report revealing that owners of overweight dogs and cats spent more on diagnostic procedures, healthcare, and medications (Banfield 2017).

An investigation of 74 general practices in the UK involving more than 49,000 dog visits revealed that only 1.4% of all medical records contained words pertaining to overweight or obese (Rolph et al. 2014). Other retrospective studies have examined the medical records of GPs to assess the frequency of documentation of patient body weight (German and Morgan 2008) and the disclosure of overweight dogs (McGreevy et al. 2005). A recent study found that only 7% of dogs were diagnosed as obese (O'Neill et al. 2021). These studies confirm what my experience has made clear; small animal veterinarians are not reliably recognizing and discussing pet obesity with clients.

Two studies have documented that fear of alienating or jeopardizing their relationship with the client is an obstacle to confronting pet obesity (Cairns-Haylor and Fordyce 2017; Aldewereld et al. 2021). Practitioner sentiments may be altruistic (i.e. considerate of the client's emotional state), self-interested (i.e. an unwillingness to risk loss of an income source), or reluctant, due to the perceived sensitive nature of the topic. Other contributing factors to poor compliance among veterinarians in discussing obesity may include desensitization to recognizing obesity, a normalization of obesity, or a belief that client compliance in addressing their pet's obese state would fail regardless of professional concern.

If veterinarians are to fulfill societal expectations as advocates for animals, then we must summon the courage to confront overweight and obesity each time we see it (Kipperman and German 2018). This can be accomplished without stigmatizing and shaming the client or jeopardizing the client relationship. In fact, there is cause for optimism that an increased willingness and motivation by veterinarians to address weight gain can succeed in achieving weight loss. Approximately two-thirds of owners who agreed with their veterinarian's opinion that their dog was overweight were encouraged to take measures to reduce weight (Cairns-Haylor and Fordyce 2017). The strength of that motivation was associated with the information provided during the consultation.

The most successful method for encouraging pet owners to improve the health and welfare of overweight or obese animal companions is a combination of reminding them that their pet is or will become overweight, addressing the health and welfare consequences of obesity, and providing details about how to achieve weight loss (Cairns-Haylor and Fordyce 2017). The One Health perspective encourages coordinated action by human and veterinary healthcare professionals to address obesity in people and companion animals as a public health concern (Chandler et al. 2017).

Failure to recognize, discuss, and document pet obesity places the perceived interest of the practitioner in retaining clients and income above their professional duty to protect animal welfare and public health. Since making the diagnosis of obesity is straightforward and the health and welfare consequences of the disease are well known, the veterinary profession needs to take a proactive stance regarding this problem. Such an approach should prioritize prevention rather than resolution.

# References

Aldewereld, C.M., Monninkhof, E.M., Kroese, F.M. et al. (2021). Discussing overweight in dogs during a regular consultation in general practice in the Netherlands. *Journal of Animal Physiology and Animal Nutrition*. https://doi.org/10.1111/jpn.13558.

American Veterinary Medical Association (AMVA) (2016). Study: Over half of pet dogs and cats were overweight in 2015. https://www.avma.org/javma-news/2016-06-15/study-over-half-pet-dogs-and-cats-were-overweight-2015 (accessed 23 January 2021).

Association for Pet Obesity Prevention. (n.d.). Homepage. https://petobesityprevention.org (accessed 6 March 2021).

Banfield. (2017). State of pet health; obesity is an epidemic. https://www.banfield.com/state-of-pet-health/obesity (accessed 22 January 2021).

Cairns-Haylor, T. and Fordyce, P. (2017). Mapping discussion of canine obesity between veterinary surgeons and dog owners: A provisional study. *Veterinary Record* 180 (6): 149.

Chandler, M., Cunningham, S., Lund, E.M. et al. (2017). Obesity and associated comorbidities in people and companion animals: A One Health perspective. *Journal of Comparative Pathology* 156: 296–309.

German, A.J. (2006). The growing problem of obesity in dogs and cats. *Journal of Nutrition* 136 (7): 1940S–1946S.

German, A.J. and Morgan, L.E. (2008). How often do veterinarians assess the bodyweight and body condition of dogs?. *Veterinary Record* 163: 503–505.

German, A.J., Holden, S.L., Wiseman-Orr, M.L. et al. (2012). Quality of life is reduced in obese dogs but improves after successful weight loss. *Veterinary Journal* 192: 428–434.

Kealy, R.D., Lawler, D.F., Ballam, J.M. et al. (2002). Effects of diet restriction on life span and age-related changes in dogs. *Journal of the American Veterinary Medical Association* 220: 1315–1320.

Kienzle, E. and Bergler, R. (2006). Human-animal relationship of owners of normal and overweight cats. *Journal of Nutrition* 136: 1947–1950.

Kipperman, B.S. and German, A.J. (2018). The responsibility of veterinarians to address companion animal obesity. *Animals* 8 (9): 143.

Lawler, D.F., Larson, B.T., Ballam, J.M. et al. (2008). Diet restriction and ageing in the dog: Major observations over two decades. *British Journal of Nutrition* 99: 793–805.

Lund, E. (2005). Prevalence and risk factors for obesity in adult cats from private US veterinary practices. *International Journal of Applied Research in Veterinary Medicine* 3: 88–96.

Lund, E.M., Armstrong, P.J., Kirk, C.A. et al. (2006). Prevalence and risk factors for obesity in adult dogs from private US veterinary practices. *International Journal of Applied Research in Veterinary Medicine* 4: 177.

McGreevy, P.D., Thomson, P.C., Pride, C. et al. (2005). Prevalence of obesity in dogs examined by Australian veterinary practices and the risk factors involved. *Veterinary Record* 156: 695–701.

National Institutes of Health (NIH) (1985). Health implications of obesity: National Institutes of Health consensus development conference statement. *Annals of Internal Medicine* 103: 1073–1077.

O'Neill, D.G., James, H., Brodbelt, D.C. et al. (2021). Prevalence of commonly diagnosed disorders in UK dogs under primary veterinary care: Results and applications. *BMC Veterinary Research* 17: 69. https://doi.org/10.1186/s12917-021-02775-3.

Rolph, N.C., Noble, P.J.M., and German, A.J. (2014). How often do primary care veterinarians record the overweight status of dogs? *Journal of Nutritional Science* 3: e58.

Sandøe, P., Corr, S., and Palmer, C. (2016). Feeding and the problem of obesity. In: *Companion Animal Ethics* (eds. P. Sandøe, S. Corr, and C. Palmer), 117–132. Wheathampstead: Universities Federation for Animal Welfare. ISBN.

Scarlett, J.M. and Donoghue, S. (1998). Associations between body condition and disease in cats. *Journal of the American Veterinary Medical Association* 212: 1725–1731.

Shearer, P. (2010). *Literature Review: Canine, Feline and Human Overweight and Obesity*. Portland, OR: Banfield Applied Research and Knowledge Team.

White, G.A., Ward, L., Pink, C. et al. (2016). Who's been a good dog? Owner perceptions and motivations for treat giving. *Preventive Veterinary Medicine* 132: 14–19.

# 11 Access to Veterinary Care: A National Family Crisis

*Michael J. Blackwell*

Two out of three households in America have pets (APPA 2020a). These *bonded families* have at least one human and one nonhuman member (i.e. pet) in a human–animal bond relationship. As a comparison, only approximately 40% of US households have children (US Census 2020). Humans derive psychological and physiological benefits from the human–animal bond (Walsh 2009; Herzog 2011). Reported benefits include fewer doctor visits, increased physical activity, and a higher probability of reporting being happy. People with pets report lower rates of depression, stress, anxiety, and loneliness. In their *State of the Industry Report*, the APPA states that Americans spent $103.6 billion on pets in 2020 (APPA 2020b), reflecting the significant integration of pets in American society.

Not having access to veterinary care is the most significant animal welfare crisis affecting "owned" pets in the United States, negatively impacting families, veterinary service providers, and communities. Access to veterinary care means recognizing when a pet needs care, having a physically reachable veterinary service provider, and the ability to pay for the care. When veterinary care is not accessible, a pet may face prolonged illness, pain, and recovery time, or premature death, including economic euthanasia, causing emotional distress for the family. In too many instances, pets are relinquished to the animal sheltering system, breaking up the family.

Through a generous grant from Maddie's Fund®, the Access to Veterinary Care Coalition (AVCC) commissioned a national study to better understand the barriers to veterinary care experienced by pet owners (AVCC 2018). The study also sought to understand the knowledge, attitudes, and practices of veterinarians regarding access to veterinary care.

Participating households reported owning an average of 2.2 pets, with about one out of four owning only one pet. Households with lower incomes were more likely than those with higher income levels to own more than one pet. When asked about their level of agreement with the statement, "My pet is considered a member of my family," 88% of respondents agreed. One out of four (28%) households experienced veterinary care barriers, with the overwhelming barrier being financial (80%). Dogs and cats living in lower-income households and with younger pet owners are most at risk of not receiving recommended care.

Findings from the AVCC study confirm that veterinary service providers recognize the severity of the problem and want to explore ways to address it. The highest level of agreement among veterinarians was in response to the statement, "All pets deserve some level of veterinary care." Almost all respondents (95%) either agreed or strongly agreed. Nearly 9 out of 10 respondents (88%) indicated they agreed or strongly agreed that owned pets are family members. Yet, 72% of veterinarians agreed that the for-profit business model is not meeting the needs of all pets. Similarly, 87% agreed that not obtaining needed veterinary care impacts the owner's mental and emotional health.

Veterinarians take an oath (AVMA n.d.b) to use their "knowledge and skills for the benefit of society" while adhering to the Principles of Veterinary Medical Ethics (AVMA n.d.c). Historically, to reach parts of society, e.g. when the client has limited funds, veterinarians have had to modify the patient's treatment plan to avoid doing nothing to help. Having the knowledge, skills, and desire to provide care, but being unable to because of financial barriers, are ethical and moral dilemmas inherent in the practice of veterinary medicine. Repeated instances of these dilemmas can lead to compassion fatigue, burnout, and moral stress (see Chapter 22), made worse when the situation results in euthanasia over a treatable problem (Kipperman et al. 2017). Committing to doing something for a patient when there are limited options is preferable to not helping. Veterinarians must be advocates for themselves, their patients and clients, and society within a valid veterinarian–client–patient relationship (AVMA n.d.a). When advocating for multiple parties, competing priorities invariably occur. Understanding one's core values and personal mission helps ensure sound, consistent decisions that help safeguard the well-being of all parties.

Intentional efforts and better alignment of existing resources can help mitigate barriers to veterinary care. These barriers are primarily associated with the pet family's realities. Although low socioeconomics is the primary factor, there are others. Veterinary service providers have limited capacity to address adequately the financial barriers families face. However, there are often untapped resources in the community that may help (see Chapter 8). Thus, a One Health interprofessional approach, i.e. focusing on the pet's people and their ecosystem, helps reach underserved pets more effectively. The Program for Pet Health Equity (PPHE), University of Tennessee is addressing interprofessional collaborations through AlignCare (PPHE 2018), a One Health healthcare system that *aligns* the current resources of social service agencies and veterinary service providers while utilizing community funding. The alignment of these resources improves access to veterinary care for families currently underserved as well as enables social service and animal care professionals to meet their goals in serving families. Veterinary service providers alone cannot adequately solve this problem.

The paradox we face is that while it may seem logical that someone should not have a pet if they cannot provide veterinary care, it is challenging to defend denying companionship with pets. Consequently, pets will continue to live with families with limited means. To ensure all pets have access to veterinary care, a paradigm shift to include interprofessional collaborations, including social service agencies, animal welfare organizations, veterinarians, and other stakeholders, is essential.

# References

Access to Veterinary Care Coalition (AVCC) (2018). Access to Veterinary Care: Barriers, current practices, and public policy. http://avcc.utk.edu (accessed 1 June 2021).

American Pet Products Association (APPA) (2020a). Pet industry market size, trends and ownership statistics. https://www.americanpetproducts.org/press_industrytrends. asp?ftag=MSF0951a18 (accessed 1 June 2021).

American Pet Products Association (APPA) (2020b). National pet industry exceeds over $100 billion in sales for first time in industry history. https://www.americanpetproducts.org/press_releasedetail.asp?id=1239 (accessed 1 June 2021).

American Veterinary Medical Association (AVMA n.d.a). The veterinarian-client-patient relationship (VCPR). www.avma.org/resources-tools/pet-owners/petcare/veterinarian-client-patient-relationship-vcpr (accessed 1 June 2021).

American Veterinary Medical Association (AVMA n.d.b). Veterinarian's Oath. https://www.avma.org/javma-news/2004-06-01/veterinarians-oath-reaffirmed (accessed 1 June 2021).

American Veterinary Medical Association (AVMA n.d.c). Principles of Veterinary Medical Ethics. https://www.avma.org/javma-news/2015-03-01/principles-veterinary-medical-ethics-revised (accessed 1 June 2021).

Herzog, H. (2011). The impact of pets on human health and psychological well-being: Fact, fiction, or hypothesis? *Current Directions in Psychological Science* 20 (4): 236–239.

Kipperman, B.S., Kass, P.H., and Rishniw, M. (2017). Factors that influence small animal veterinarians' opinions and actions regarding cost of care and effects of economic limitations on patient care and outcome and professional career satisfaction and burnout. *Journal of the American Veterinary Medical Association* 250 (7): 785–794.

Program for Pet Health Equity (PPHE), University of Tennessee. (2018). AlignCare. https://pphe.utk.edu (accessed 21 December 2021).

US Census Bureau (2020). New estimates on families and living arrangements, U.S. Census Bureau. https://www.census.gov/newsroom/press-releases/2020/estimates-families-living-arrangements.html (accessed 1 June 2021).

Walsh, F. (2009). Human-animal bonds II. The role of pets in family systems and family therapy. *Family Process* 48 (4): 488–499.

# 11

# Laboratory Animals

*Larry Carbone*

Veterinarians swear to protect animal welfare and relieve animal suffering. How can they participate in animal research that causes so much animal suffering? On the other hand, where better to meet the challenge of their oath than in animal laboratories? Many ethical questions of animal use echo across disciplines in veterinary medicine. Other questions are specific to the use of animals in laboratories:

- Does animal research provide enough useful knowledge that cannot reasonably be obtained via alternative methods?
- What special justifications might be necessary when experiments can cause significant pain and distress to the animals?
- How should ethics oversight committees factor in uncertainty about how much an experiment might harm the animals or how much benefit is likely to result?
- If animals are sufficiently like humans to serve as useful models of human biology, are they too similar to humans emotionally for their use in experiments to be justifiable?

An assortment of formal laws and informal guidelines reflect the applied ethics of laboratory animal work. Key features of the common ethic are:

- It is sentientist: sentience grants a human or nonhuman the right to moral consideration.
- It is animal welfarist: animal pain, suffering, and well-being, rather than autonomy, telos, or a right to life are animals' interests of concern.
- It is consequentialist: significant potential benefits (usually to humans) may justify some harms to animals.
- It is speciesist: humans interests receive greater consideration than other sentient species' interests.
- It is jurisdictional: veterinarians have a defined role in overseeing laboratory animal health and welfare.

In this chapter, I review this applied ethic in the broader context of veterinary ethics and animal ethics.

*Ethics in Veterinary Practice: Balancing Conflicting Interests*, First Edition. Edited by Barry Kipperman and Bernard E. Rollin.
© 2022 John Wiley & Sons, Inc. Published 2022 by John Wiley & Sons, Inc.

# Laboratory Animal Ethics in the Context of Veterinary and Animal-use Ethics

## Species Hierarchies

Scientists, like ranchers, animal breeders, and even pet guardians, use animals in accord with society's general approval and with legal principles that allow for priority of human interests over animal interests even to the point of seriously harming animals. Within the laboratory, species hierarchies of legal and moral consideration rest on our human assessment of animals' degrees of sentience (Mellor 2019). For example, a highly sentient rat or monkey receives greater concern and protections than a fish or fruit fly. Legal coverage also depends on the individual animal's species status (e.g. endangered, "pest," domestic, etc.), on the source of funding for a laboratory, or on the goals of a research project (e.g. agricultural versus biomedical). Economic concerns and lack of public concern seem to be the basis for excluding rats and mice from legal coverage that other sentient mammals such as monkeys or hamsters receive (Carbone 2004).

## Harms Are Allowed But Must Be Justified

Under current laws, scientists may harm animals via confinement, induction of disease, or pain and distress, but they must have a strong justification proportional to the degree of harm. Killing is not generally considered a harm in the eyes of laboratory animal laws. Quite the opposite, killing or euthanasia is mandated if it is the only way to end an animal's suffering.

Even in a human-centric ethic, justification is only possible if the human interests are compelling. Different people will have different assessments of how compelling it is to seek a cure for cancer, to produce tasty meat, or to watch animals in races or rodeos. Certainty and timing of interests factor in here: whatever human interests a rodeo serves, they are present for the audience at the moment of attendance. In animal research, most benefits are potential and in the future. Data may or may not lead to medical breakthroughs, and when they do, it may still be years before their application, and people not even alive today may be the beneficiaries.

## Competence

A veterinary degree, license, or specialty certification confers certain exclusive permissions to practice, with a duty to practice competently and to assure the competence of nonveterinarians under the vet's oversight. In the laboratory, scientists and their staff may perform many tasks normally exclusive to veterinarians in other areas of practice, including major surgery, anesthesia, and pain management. A veterinarian may have only indirect responsibility for researchers' competence, by serving as a member of an institutional animal ethics committee that approves research proposals and monitors postapproval compliance. In no other area of practice are veterinary decisions made by a committee on which the veterinarian gets one vote, rather than the veterinarian in dialogue with animal owners or guardians.

### Standard of Care

The standard of providing for best-possible animal health and welfare has limits in all aspects of veterinary medicine. Cost is a universal factor in veterinary practice (see Chapter 8 for a discussion of economic issues). In the laboratory, cost, compliance, and controlled substances availability may all affect veterinary care. But the biggest challenge is that analgesic and therapeutic drugs may sometimes affect an experiment's outcome, limiting the veterinarian's ability to do what they feel is best for a given patient.

## Animal-use Ethics in Laboratories

Some aspects of laboratory animal care will seem familiar to veterinarians in other disciplines, but it helps to understand how scientists use animals to understand the veterinary and ethical issues in this field. That requires an understanding of the varied ways in which an animal may be used as a *model*.

Most animal research uses nonhuman animals to learn something about human biology. No one animal species can replicate all aspects of human biology. Some examples illustrate the breadth of laboratory animal use:

- For some people, the first image of animals in laboratories might be rabbits in restrainers for testing cosmetics and cleaners for eye injury (the Draize test) or dosing mice with compounds to find the dose that will kill 50% of a cohort (the median lethal dose [LD50] test).
- Most animal studies of SARS-Cov-2 virus (the causative agent of the Covid-19 pandemic) require an animal with human-like angiotensin-converting enzyme 2 (ACE-2) receptors on cells: such species choices include ferrets, monkeys, and hamsters (Munoz-Fontela et al. 2020). Mice engineered with the human ACE-2 receptor gene are now common in Covid labs.
- Healthy animals are used to study basic biology. To study individual brain cells' reactions to light or other inputs, a scientist may surgically place recording electrodes in a rat or a monkey's cerebral cortex.
- Scientists induce and study a wide variety of human-like injuries, illnesses, and treatments in animals and test treatments. Animals can be the beneficiaries too. This may be indirect where things we learn about human biology are applicable to other animals, in human settings or in the wild. Or more direct, as when scientists study mice, cats, dogs, or cattle with the specific goal of improving companion animal or food animal health (Bailey 2018).
- Laboratory animals may be used in hypothesis-driven experiments (i.e. research), but also as teaching models for veterinary and human medicine and as subjects in toxicology and safety testing.

There is thus a menagerie of species in laboratories, chosen through a constellation of factors – size, cost, genetics, safety, susceptibility to various microorganisms and diseases, and established knowledge in a particular field. Most animals in modern laboratories have been purpose-bred for research. United States Department of Agriculture (USDA) statistics on animal use in research in 2017–2018 totaled 780,070, including:

- 182,580 miscellaneous mammals (e.g. ferrets, voles, gerbils)
- 171,406 guinea pigs
- 133,634 rabbits
- 80,539 hamsters
- 70,797 nonhuman primates
- 63,094 pigs and sheep
- 59,401 dogs
- 18,619 cats. (USDA 2019)

These statistics do not include mice, rats, fish, or other species, with estimates of mouse and rat use in the United States ranging from as low as 15 to as high as 110 million per year (Carbone 2021).

The USDA reports animals in "pain categories." For FY 2018, about 60% of animals were in Category C (no significant pain or distress; includes euthanasia of healthy animals); about 32% were in Category D (procedures that could cause significant pain or distress, but receive anesthetics, analgesics, or other drugs for alleviation); with about 7% in Category E (significant pain or distress, but drugs withheld if they could interfere with the experiment) (USDA 2019).

Public opinion polls and current laws and regulations reflect a societal ethic that scientists should have limited license to use animals in laboratories (Ormandy and Schuppli 2014; Pew Research Center 2018). Human interests preempt animal interests in this setting but with some limits. Thus, concern for animals' welfare can require scientists to invest time, energy, and money. Highly invasive or painful studies in species people care most about (such as dogs and primates) done for trivial purposes receive the lowest levels of public support, and regulations reflect these priorities. The application of this limited license to use animals mostly takes the form of a cost–benefit analysis in which most of the costs are the animals' diminished welfare and most of the benefits are knowledge that may help current and future humans but only rarely do the experimental animals in the laboratories benefit.

For laboratory animal use to be justifiable two conditions are necessary but neither alone is sufficient:

1. Human interests must sometimes be able to take precedence over nonhuman animals' interests.
2. Animal research must produce useful, valid knowledge (Carbone 2012b; Beauchamp et al. 2019).

In other words, laboratory animal research must be rejected if human-privileging speciesism is immoral or the data from such experiments are not reliable.

The consensus among scientists is that animal research produces valuable knowledge (Nuffield Council on Bioethics 2005; Ainsworth 2006). Thousands of scientists use millions of animals with the expectation that much animal data will "translate" to human biology and medicine (Carbone 2021). Others are skeptical that animal studies are useful, or at least, are skeptical that they are as useful as scientists expect them to be (Greek and Greek 2004; Hansen and Greek 2013). Critics explain their concerns in evolutionary terms (LaFollette and Shanks 1996). While all animals, humans included, share many biological similarities, there are also many differences. Therefore, it is not always predictable which animals will be most like humans at the level necessary for extrapolation from nonhuman to human.

**Table 11.1** Stakeholders, costs, and benefits in laboratory animal ethics.

| Stakeholder | Costs | Benefits |
|---|---|---|
| Current and future generations of humans | Financial costs of research: missed knowledge when animal data do not translate to human medicine (Nuffield Council on Bioethics 2005; Beauchamp and Degrazia 2019) | Knowledge: medical advances |
| Scientists | Labor, delays, and expense of meeting animal welfare standards | Satisfaction of successful science: career benefits and prestige |
| Veterinary and animal care professionals | Career risks if advocate, or moral stress if fail to advocate for animal welfare | Career satisfaction in contributing to science and to animal welfare |
| Animals in laboratories | Suffering, pain, distress, confinement, thwarted telos | Research findings rarely benefit the individual animals in experiments |
| Future laboratory animals | As above, including animals bred to have genetically based disease | As above |
| Other animals: on farms, in homes, in the wild, etc. | Minimal | Advances in veterinary, species and ecosystem health |

There are many stakeholders, costs, and benefits associated with animal research (Table 11.1).

## Regulation of Animal Use in Research, Testing, and Education

Legal regulation of animal laboratories varies globally. Most laws focus on some sort of cost–benefit analysis and standards for minimizing animal suffering. In the United States, laboratories generally operate outside of local anti-cruelty laws, and most are regulated by some combination of laboratory-specific laws at the federal and state level.

At the federal level, two main laws cover laboratory animal welfare (Carbone 2004). The Health Research Extension Act of 1985 mandates oversight by the National Institutes of Health Office of Laboratory Animal Welfare (NIH OLAW) for institutions that receive federal research grants from the NIH or other government agencies. It covers all vertebrate animals and relies on self-regulation by institutions via annual reports and self-reports. Rather than a complex set of regulations, it relies on a guidance document from the US National Academies of Science, the *Guide for the Care and Use of Laboratory Animals* (Institute for Laboratory Animal Research 2011). The evolution of the Guide from its first edition in 1963 to the current 2011 edition reflects evolving thoughts and priorities in laboratory animal care (Animal Care Panel 1963). OLAW's mandate to assure animal welfare in federally funded research means that many animals, for example used by private pharmaceutical companies that do not receive federal research dollars, are outside its jurisdiction.

The Animal Welfare Act (AWA), first passed in 1966, has comparable standards to the Guide and OLAW, with a set of Animal Welfare Regulations that covered institutions must follow (USDA Animal Care 2019). Passed in reaction to stories of pet theft for laboratories, its early years focused on animal acquisition, husbandry, and veterinary care up to the point at which the animals start on an experiment. Since the 1980s, the AWA now has standards for how animals are used in experiments. Enforcement is via self-reports, as well as unannounced inspections, both routine and "for cause," by veterinarians with the USDA. The AWA covers most mammal species used in laboratories regardless of funding, but alone among Western nations, excludes most rats and mice, who combined likely comprise 99% of mammals in US labs (Carbone 2021). It also excludes frogs, birds, and – possibly most numerous – fish. The USDA publishes inspection reports on its website, along with annual self-reports of animal use, in three "pain categories" (USDA 2019, 2020)

Complementing the AWA and NIH rules, US and international laboratories can apply for accreditation via an independent organization, the American Association for Accreditation of Laboratory Animal Care (AAALAC) International (AAALAC International 2021a). This voluntary program includes triennial site visits by practicing laboratory animal veterinarians and research specialists as well as self-reporting. In the United States, it relies mainly on the Guide as its standard of accreditation, and its accreditation reports are confidential and not available to the public. Its coverage includes all vertebrates, as well as "higher-level" invertebrates such as cephalopods (AAALAC International 2021b).

All three oversight programs converge on the central role of an in-house animal oversight committee for institutions under their purview. Institutional Animal Care and Use Committee (IACUC) is the common name for these ethics committees in the United States: such committees are central to laboratory animal welfare oversight around the world. In the United States, the committee must include a veterinarian and a nonaffiliated member, usually a nonscientist. Under US rules, at least one veterinarian must have a seat on the committee, with no special voting priority, i.e. one member, one vote.

The main functions of these committees include self-policing and self-inspection of animal care facilities and animal use, including investigation of in-house allegations and concerns about animal treatment. Most of their time and effort goes to prospectively reviewing scientists' proposals (usually called *protocols*) to conduct animal experiments. Committees review the reasons for doing the experiments, the qualifications of the people doing the work, the choice of species, the number of animals, and the potential for pain and distress and for mitigating or preventing pain and distress.

## The Three Rs Alternatives and Six Principles of Animal Research Ethics

A long-standing set of organizing principles for scientists, veterinarians, and ethics committees is the consideration of Russell and Burch's "Three Rs" of alternatives in animal research (Russell et al. 1959). *Alternatives* is an unfortunate word choice insofar as it suggests substituting animals with something different, but in this context, its definition is broader: it refers to alternatives *in* animal research, not just alternatives *to* animal research.

*Replacement alternatives* are conceptually the most straightforward: find ways to generate research data without using animals at all. Candidates for *replacement* include studying cells in tissue culture (in vitro techniques), developing computer simulations, making better use of human epidemiological data and human volunteers, or using inanimate models in teaching (see Chapter 18 for a thorough discussion of nonanimal methods). Scientists also seek to replace so-called "higher" animals when possible, by switching from dogs to mice, or from mice to fruit flies, though the moral consistency in replacing sentient dogs with sentient mice, sometimes referred to as "relative replacement," is questionable (Tannenbaum and Bennett 2015).

*Reduction* comprises efforts to lower the numbers of animals required. This often means rethinking statistical tests to use just the number necessary for statistically valid results.

*Refinement* constitutes all the myriad ways to reduce the potential for pain and distress, and to increase positive life experiences and happiness (Carbone 2004). Scientists may seek humane endpoints, such as euthanizing animals before they develop severe disease, or they may expand their use of anesthetics and painkillers. Other refinements include replacing surgery with noninvasive manipulations or improving the housing for animals in their experiments.

Russell and Burch's framework categorizes pain and distress as direct versus contingent. For example, scientists induce direct pain in an experiment in order to study pain neurobiology; scientists in other fields perform surgeries for experiments, but pain is an unwanted, or contingent, side-effect of (for example) placing electrodes in the animal's brain. Pain, distress, and suffering can result from experimental procedures, but also from the daily housing of animals, with boredom, isolation, fighting, noise, bright lights, and cramped quarters all possible housing-related stressors.

Cost–benefit analyses in animal research weigh benefits (mostly to humans) against harms/costs (mostly to the animals). Beauchamp and DeGrazia have built on the Three Rs framework in their *Principles of Animal Research Ethics* (2019). Three of their six principles address the benefits of animal research and the other three build on the animal-harm reduction strategies of the Three Rs (Table 11.2). Consistent with longstanding practice, their animal welfare principles call for meeting animals' basic needs

**Table 11.2** Six principles of animal research ethics (Beauchamp and Degrazia 2019).

**Principles of social benefit**

The principle of no [reasonably available] alternative method

The principle of expected net benefit

The principle of sufficient value to justify harm

**Principles of animal welfare**

The principle of no unnecessary harm

The principle of basic needs

The principle of upper limits to harm

throughout their lives, not just during an actual experiment. They continue the principle that any harms to animals must be limited to those that are absolutely necessary to obtain important data, implicitly allowing that some experiments will cause pain or distress, or will confine animals or deprive them of various pleasures and freedoms (United States Interagency Research Animal Committee 1985). Their most radical-looking principle suggests setting upper limits on harm to animals, but they do allow for the current practice that proposed upper limits may be exceeded when research needs strongly justify that (Carbone 2019b).

The principles of social benefit flesh out how scientists, veterinarians, research funders, and ethics committees might better evaluate the necessity of using animals. They argue that scientists should pursue alternatives but allow that some alternatives may be so impractical or expensive as to be unreasonable or unavailable, in which case some animal use might be permissible. They contend that "net benefit" is not just hoping that studying cancer in mice may produce useful knowledge, but also the possibility that animal studies may draw resources from other potentially valuable research projects or can be misleading. "Net benefit" should account for translatability, a growing concern among scientists in various fields, as well as their critics (Garner 2014; Fernandez-Moure 2016; Mogil 2019). If animal research is to be of value, its animal data must "translate" to human biology, successfully predicting benefits and harms. For example, by the time a drug has cleared all of the years of preclinical animal studies and is ready for human clinical trials, highly translatable animal data will yield a strong chance that drug is safe and effective in people. Different readers will interpret a commonly cited statistic – that some 90% of drugs at this stage fail in human trials – differently (Kola and Landis 2004; Hay et al. 2014). Is 10% success an encouraging reflection on the value of animal studies? Is 90% failure a condemnation that animal studies are misleading? Is it a number to prompt examination of the failures in order to better animal models?

The principle of sufficient value to justify harm holds that some projects or some scientific questions are more important than others. In a medical setting, for instance, it may be of more value to conduct research on fatal brain cancers of children than on largely cosmetic conditions in adults.

These principles would work best if people with sufficient expertise and a diversity of perspectives and values simultaneously evaluated a scientist's plan in terms of the harms to animals, the potential value of the project, and the scientific quality and merit (Figure 11.1). At present in the United States, these three evaluations occur separately, in different bodies' hands and in no set sequence. Thus, an animal ethics committee or IACUC may evaluate a project's animal welfare issues before or after a funding agency evaluates the scientific merit, and neither will know the outcomes of the other's review (Carbone 2019b).

## The Ethics of Uncertainty in Laboratory Animal Use

Ethical harm–benefit review of proposed animal experiments starts with establishing several important facts. It requires technical knowledge to assess the possibility and severity of potential animal harms, to prevent or treat pain and suffering, and to

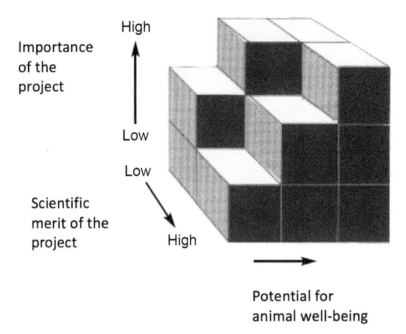

**Figure 11.1** Three dimensions for ethical animal research (modified from Bateson 1986). Ethical justification is highest when the research addresses important issues, has sound design with high likelihood of generating valid, translatable findings, and the potential for animal welfare is high. Trivial research with low merit that causes significant animal suffering is of low justifiability.

evaluate if pain mitigations, whether drugs or nursing care, will adversely affect the experiment (Peterson et al. 2017; Bleich et al. 2020). It requires a scientific evaluation of the likelihood the work will produce reliable data that can be translated to humans and other animals. With these facts in hand, a scientist or their ethics committee might then determine if the goals of the project are of sufficient value to justify any harms to the animals.

Ethics committees frequently operate in uncertainty. Animal ethics committees have a breadth of members but evaluating the merit of the proposed methods requires a panel with expertise in the particular model, to help the scientist avoid harming animals in an experiment that does not even provide clear data. Without communication among these various review bodies, the harm–benefit analysis is weak. The potential impact of the research is similarly hard to state with certainty, especially in basic science without apparent immediate application, leading some to question whether evaluation of likely benefits is possible (Niemi 2020).

If animals are at risk of suffering from experiments, then only projects with the best chances of success in pursuit of important goals should receive approval. In the face of uncertain harms and benefits, the committee faces the ethical decision of whether to err more toward precaution about harming animals, or the risk of delaying potentially valuable science.

## Veterinarians in Animal Laboratories

Veterinarians work wherever there are laboratory animals. Their numbers are small: of about 100,000 American Veterinary Medical Association member veterinarians who list their primary field of activity, only about 1100 (well under 2%) list laboratory animal care as their primary responsibility (American Veterinary Medical Association [AVMA] 2020). The size and mission of the research program often determines the numbers and specialties of veterinarians. Veterinarians may specialize in one of several roles at large institutions or may fill many roles simultaneously at large or small laboratories. Table 11.3 lists some of these roles that veterinarians play directly, or in a supervisory capacity.

The relationship between veterinarians, scientists, and animals is complex. Veterinarians have partial authority over how scientists use animals (Case Study 11.1). In laboratories covered by US laws, veterinarians are guaranteed a voting membership on the animal ethics committee, but most decisions to grant or revoke research privileges are at the committee level. In cases of individual animals' health and welfare, veterinarians have more autonomy, including the authority to prescribe treatment or euthanasia even if the scientist using the animals disagrees (Institute for Laboratory Animal Research 2011). Despite that authority for on-the-spot decisions for individual animals, in my experience, veterinarians usually have less authority over animal health and welfare problems at the group or project level, which can lead to professional and moral distress.

A common model in large programs is that scientists' research funds purchase animals and pay a daily charge to the animal care program. This *per diem* charge pays for husbandry, staffing, food, bedding, cages, enrichments, and veterinary services. Veterinarians in research are not immune from the financial challenges private practitioners face, as every health and welfare enhancement they would invest in must come from *per diem* revenues whose rates are set by administrators, not the veterinarian.

**Table 11.3** Roles of veterinarians in research laboratories.

| |
|---|
| Clinical veterinarian for individual animals |
| Colony veterinarian for mouse, fish, or other "herd health" |
| Director of animal housing/husbandry |
| Research scientist in veterinary or basic sciences |
| Director of ethics committee programs |
| Trainer for hands-on animal procedures |
| Animal welfare in-house compliance officer |
| Enrichment and behavioral management specialist |
| Pathologist |
| Anesthesia and/or surgery services for researchers |
| Adviser for scientists planning animal research projects |
| Government inspectors |

The veterinary roles in Table 11.3 can compete with each other, whether one individual is filling many of these roles, or whether members of a team of specialized veterinarians are each pursuing a specific role with its own agenda. A veterinarian running an enrichment and welfare service will seek resources such as staff time, special foods, and exercise pens that the veterinarian managing a cost-conscious animal husbandry program may resist. A clinician for rodent colonies may sometimes treat ill or injured animals but will also sacrifice individual "sentinel" animals to monitor infections within colonies (de Bruin et al. 2016). Large research programs typically have veterinarians as directors of the vivarium, and the vivarium's finances rely on having enough animals to cover its costs. In these settings, the veterinarian will have an interest in maintaining numbers of animals, though simultaneously serving on an ethics committee that should be working to reduce animal numbers. A veterinarian running an in-house compliance program will want some oversight authority to audit records and visit laboratories to critically evaluate the work of researchers and also of veterinarians who are in a clinical role. The facility's clinical veterinarians want frequent access to their animal patients and the chance to collaborate with researchers who need their expertise, but researchers can sometimes fear that veterinarians are more often police than collaborators and can become resistant to granting access to their labs.

---

**Case Study 11.1   Conflict between animal researcher and veterinarian**

A veterinarian visits a laboratory where graduate students perform abdominal surgeries on research animals to inject pancreatic tumor cells, then compare two months of chemotherapy against two months of placebo before euthanizing animals to compare tumor burdens. One animal looks thin, and the veterinarian sees that the surgical site looks infected and is coming apart (dehiscence). The veterinarian tells the scientists that they must promptly euthanize the animal, or at the least, start antibiotic and analgesic treatments. The scientists say that those drugs will interfere with their experiment, and they must keep the animal four more days to complete the experiment and they will then euthanize. They remind the veterinarian that the animal ethics committee approved the project knowing that the cancer and the chemotherapy could make the animals sick. The veterinarian knows that management of infected surgical sites was not discussed in the approval and the default action for such unplanned-for contingencies is either euthanasia or treatment under veterinary supervision.

When the veterinarian comes by two days later, the animal still looks sick, but the scientist had a new graduate student repair the surgical site using anesthesia. There remain two more days until the scheduled euthanasia for tissue analysis, and the scientists need every animal to go to that endpoint so they will have a large enough cohort for statistical analysis of their data.

**What should the veterinarian do?**

Ethical analysis:

The ethics committee conducted a harm–benefit analysis, applying the principle of sufficient value to justify harm (Table 11.2). The veterinarian was part of this deliberation and should have spoken up at the time if there were concerns about this decision. In failing to anticipate surgical site infections and problems, the veterinarian let the committee skew their harm–benefit analysis by underestimating potential harm. Under a principle of upper limits to harm, there should have been clear intervention and humane endpoints, so that animals who are suffering are treated or euthanized. The scientist should have anticipated that not all animals could be expected to survive a two-month cancer chemotherapy experiment. They are now at risk of jeopardizing the study and wasting the lives of the animals if they cannot obtain valid data. As it is, the value of this animal to the study is questionable: a second surgery and anesthesia, untreated pain, inflammation, and infection may all skew how the animal's cancer develops and how the animal responds to the treatment. Can this animal really be treated as just one data point when differing from the other animals in these serious ways? Should animals pay the price of these errors?

The committee should not have approved this study if it was under-powered (too few animals) and if commitments to humane interventions were not in place to limit harms to individual animals. The scientist, more than the committee or the veterinarian, should know that keeping this ill animal on the study is not good science. Any further suffering is unjustifiable. The scientist should have called the veterinarian at the initial dehiscence to discuss, possibly with the committee, whether treatment or euthanasia was warranted. Failing that, the veterinarian should have insisted on euthanasia or treatment at the first encounter, not just suggested, and the scientist, consistent with the Guide, should have complied (Institute for Laboratory Animal Research 2011).

The veterinarian faces some difficult choices, having participated in a poorly performed ethics committee review, and having initially trusted the scientists to follow collegial veterinary advice. The vet can leave the situation as is, knowing the animal is suffering, will continue to suffer or die, and with little prospect for generating important data for analysis. The veterinarian can jeopardize the collegial relationship with the scientists that might promote better animal welfare, either by forcing them to euthanize the animal, or threatening to report to the ethics committee. Few animals are covered by the AWA, but if this animal is one of those, the veterinarian could report this situation, openly or anonymously, to the USDA. If the veterinarian decides to believe this suffering animal could actually live long enough to generate useful data, the veterinarian and scientist may decide together to continue; both are at risk of sanction if they are discovered to be out of compliance with regulatory standards.

The veterinarian–client relationship in laboratories differs from that in private practice. In laboratories, the scientist cannot bring their animals to a different practice, nor can the veterinarian refuse to work with this client's animals. They are both employees of the same institution and regulatory standards require that veterinarians have some authority over animal health and welfare.

## Moral Distress and Laboratory Animal Veterinarians

Veterinarians can experience moral stress when they believe they know what is right but feel compelled in their practice to do something else (see Chapter 22 for a discussion of moral stress) (Rollin 2006). Among veterinarians in companion animal practice, a common example is euthanasia of a healthy animal (Hernandez et al. 2018; Kipperman et al. 2020). How might this differ in fields such as food animal or laboratory animal medicine? It is hard to say, as I find no empirical studies with this population as their focus. Veterinarians in research may have animal welfare as a high priority, but often share the scientists' prioritization of generating important data even when that requires compromises to welfare. This tension of serving these sometimes-competing goals may cause moral stress and burnout for people working in animal research (LaFollette et al. 2020; King et al. 2021).

In my experience, veterinarians are more empowered than other laboratory animal care staff and this itself can engender its own suite of moral stressors. Veterinarians vote as ethics committee members, decide how strongly (if at all) to promote the welfare proposals their staff bring to them, and walk a line between being on-site compliance police versus collaborators, even when scientists' animal treatment is less than ideal. In reality, laboratory animal veterinarians have only partial authority and responsibility, as members of oversight committees, for regulatory compliance and for decisions about which projects to approve, and even limited authority over clinical care of animals (Carbone 2004).

## Some Current Issues in Laboratory Animal Ethics

### Rehoming Animals After Use in Research

Animal acquisition has been controversial over the years, including whether shelter and "random source" dogs should be used. Controversial too are questions of what should become of animals if they have completed their role in an experiment and are in good health. Should they be used in another experiment? Culled via euthanasia? Or should they be rehomed, whether for life as a household companion animal or in some sort of retirement sanctuary (Carbone et al. 2003; Fenton 2020; Beagle Freedom Project 2021)?

Legally, rehoming varies widely, with different species receiving different coverage. The US government funds post-research retirement sanctuaries only for chimpanzees (National Institutes of Health 2020). European Union laws encourage rehoming, at least for dogs and cats (Directive 2010/63/EU). At the federal level in the United States, the Guide and the AWA neither encourage nor prohibit rehoming, while several states require efforts to rehome laboratory animals, though usually just dogs and cats (Institute for Laboratory Animal Research 2011; Beagle Freedom Project 2021). Logistically, laboratories planning to find homes for research animals must consider all the health and safety issues that animal shelters consider, as well as ways to assure – possibly by partnering with a local humane shelter – that potential adopters are able to offer the animals a good home.

Is this distinction among species appropriate? Dogs and cats comprise far below 1% of the mammals used in laboratories but they are prioritized in state adoption laws. Mice and rats are much easier to care for, and though they are occasionally adopted, there is little societal demand to find homes for them. What is the ethical basis for distinguishing among individuals within a species? A veterinary college might have teaching use for dog cadavers, for which dogs ending their role in an experiment might be useful. Is it better to purchase new animals for this purpose rather than to use a post-experiment animal who is being considered for adoption? In a strictly consequentialist analysis, the laboratory would simply euthanize the adoption candidate for cadaver use, but for many people, notions of fairness (as well as emotional attachment to animals that staff have come to know) tip the balance toward adoption. Many people consider it unproblematic to kill healthy animals for food or for research if they have lived good lives, but to kill a healthy animal simply because they are no longer needed seems wrong, even if there are costs involved in rehoming (Fenton 2020).

## Genetically Modified (GM) Animals in Research

The invention of technologies to manipulate mouse genes has led to a great increase in the numbers of laboratory mice (Carbone 2021). GM mice have displaced other species in many areas of research.

Animal welfare issues in use of genetic engineering start with the technology itself (BVAAWF/FRAME/RSPCA/UFAW Joint Working Group on Refinement 2003; Ormandy et al. 2011). Many colonies of GM mice are maintained as heterozygous breeders, though only homozygous offspring may be usable for experiments: heterozygous offspring are killed. Animals must be genotyped, usually by amputating some body part (toe, tail tip, ear notch) and typically without anesthesia or analgesia. The technology requires surgery, including vasectomies for males and laparotomy for embryo transplants into foster mothers.

Genetic engineering makes it possible to create animal models of some severe human diseases, such as mice and ferrets with the respiratory disease cystic fibrosis (Leenaars et al. 2020). Beyond physical illness, GM technology can generate mice, monkeys, and other animals born to lives of severe psychiatric problems such as depression or schizophrenia (Jennings et al. 2016; Feng et al. 2020). Thus, genetic modification of laboratory animals presents many animal welfare costs that must be factored into review of any proposed experiments.

Not all GM creates welfare problems. Much of it is welfare neutral and some modifications may even be welfare positive. There is the possibility that animals could be genetically altered to feel less pain, distress, or anxiety: these are not single-gene traits so would need to be further studied to see whether the very modifications that reduce pain somehow increase an animal's propensity to injure itself, or to suffer in some other way.

Genetic modification of laboratory animals also raises ethical concerns apart from the animals' welfare, such as when it blurs lines between human and nonhuman animals. Animals can be "humanized" in various ways. Scientists have injected cells from human fetuses to render them susceptible to the human immunodeficiency virus for experiments, raising ethical concerns about the source of human fetal tissue more than for the welfare or interests of the animals (Legrand et al. 2009). But can animals be too humanized for comfort? As scientists develop the technology, they will make mice whose brains are increasingly human, possibly with expanded cognitive function or more human-like consciousness. Their welfare may be just fine, but as Greely writes, "If we make our models 'too good,' they may themselves deserve some of the kinds of ethical and legal respect that have limited brain research in human beings" (2021).

Finally, there are deontological concerns that extreme genetic modifications can alter an animal's fundamental nature, or telos, in unacceptable ways (Thompson 2010; Rollin 2015). How much and what types of changes should raise these concerns is open for discussion. A rat with green, fluorescent whiskers may yet have its telos largely intact. That same rat engineered to lose the inquisitiveness, playfulness, and sociality so characteristic of that species, or engineered to no longer feel pain or pleasure, may be going too far.

## Animal Husbandry in the Vivarium

In its initial Laboratory Animal Welfare Act (LAWA) of 1966, the US Congress took pains to assure that its coverage of animal acquisition, veterinary care, and housing stopped at the laboratory door (Carbone 2004). The image of science was that animals come to the animal housing facility, or vivarium, and then later leave to enter the laboratory for an experiment from which they never return. That one-way trip sometimes happens, but more often animals are both "on study" and living in the vivarium simultaneously, for days, months, or years. The LAWA's distinction between animal care and housing under veterinarians' jurisdiction, and animal use, under scientists' control, was never entirely realistic, and following exposés of scientists' treatment of laboratory monkeys in the 1980s, the Act was amended to add ethics committee oversight of both care and use of animals, including expanded requirements for exercise for dogs and psychological well-being and environmental enrichment for monkeys (Carbone 2004).

As in farms and zoos, how people house animals has welfare consequences. Are the animals bored? Lonely? Stressed from life with an aggressive cagemate? Cold? Able to hide or to escape bright lights? Acclimated to gentle human touch, or frightened by people? Able to engage in the behaviors they are most motivated to perform? Able to control important parts of their living situation? The ethical requirement to give laboratory animals their best possible lives conflicts with financial and other obstacles that require justification if the quality of the animals' lives is to be compromised.

While a large complex cage does not guarantee good welfare, often laboratory animals do not have large, complex cages to live in. Laboratory animals' enclosures are quite small and quite barren as well (Lahvis 2017; Makowska and Weary 2020). Cost control looms large: a laboratory dog can live far more cheaply in a steel cage or a concrete run than in a home with a yard and a sofa and someone to take them to the beach for a run. Research needs can also result in compromised living situations. Social species may be housed singly to better monitor factors like food consumption. Small cages may allow easier access to manipulate monkeys in physiology experiments. Current rules and regulations contain both engineering standards for animal housing (e.g. that a mouse with litter gets 51 square inches of cage floor area) and performance (animal-based) standards (Institute for Laboratory Animal Research 2011). Given the range of species and housing situations and the range of questions I have outlined, it is not surprising that most current performance standards are broad to the point of vagueness, immeasurable, and difficult to enforce.

The 1985 requirement of the AWA to promote psychological well-being of nonhuman primates became a legal requirement in zoos and laboratories, with "environmental enrichment" a key component. The 2011 Guide broadened this expectation to all laboratory vertebrates, encouraging "enrichment" such as structural additions to enclosures (shelters, nesting material, perches) and manipulable items (foraging devices, toys, chew sticks). While animal welfare science such as preference studies measuring the effort an animal will devote to obtaining these goods can guide practitioners, I offer a note of caution in use of the term "enrichment." The term may imply that meeting animals' physical needs is generally sufficient, and "enrichment" is a little bit extra that we give them out of generosity rather than moral obligation. Laboratory managers and zookeepers might better consider so-called "enrichments" to be the daily standard of care in animal housing, with current unenriched housing situations properly labeled "controlled deprivation" and avoided whenever possible (Burghardt 1996). Scientists sometimes worry that an enriched, complex environment will affect animals' cognitive, physical, and immunological development and, as a result, shift the data outcomes in their experiments (Toth 2015). But if impoverished and enriched environments sometimes result in different experimental data, as they sometimes do, scientists and ethics committees should consider why they think the data from impoverished environments are somehow truer, with an ethical presumption of erring on giving animals the best possible lives (Bayne and Wurbel 2014; Andre et al. 2018).

## Pain Recognition and Management

Pain management for laboratory animals has been an ethical and regulatory imperative for scientists and veterinarians for decades (Carbone 2012a). The 1970 AWA introduced the requirements that adequate veterinary care includes animal pain management and "appropriate use" of anesthetics and analgesics, as determined by the attending veterinarian of the facility, with publicly viewable annual reports of the numbers of animals used and the "pain category" – C, D, or E, as described earlier – of their use. US government principles for laboratory vertebrates similarly require anesthesia and analgesia for procedures that cause more than momentary or slight pain, and euthanasia if pain is untreatable (United States Interagency Research Animal Committee 1985).

Veterinarians have a unique role in managing laboratory animal pain. The AWA requires veterinary consultation when planning potentially painful experiments. The Guide sets what I call a jurisdictional standard: animal pain management is a component of veterinary care, though the ethics committee (on which the institutional veterinarian sits) sets protocol-specific commitments for the research scientist. If animal pain is greater than anticipated, the researcher must contact the veterinarian (Carbone 2012a). Thus, a veterinarian with training in mouse or monkey medicine recommends the combination and doses of pain medications for the animals in their care, and likely, most of the time, the researchers and ethics committees follow the veterinarian's recommendations.

The ethical principle is so clear one might think that there is no ethical challenge here, just the technical challenge of deciding on the right prescription. And it might be, if veterinarians could always identify laboratory animal pain with certainty. Clinical pain diagnosis in the laboratory is a serious challenge. In companion animal practice, a veterinarian works with a client to get a history from someone who spends many hours with their canine companion. The veterinarian's examination includes palpation for painful areas, flexing joints, and watching the animal move. They then work with the client on a therapeutic plan with ongoing client evaluations and adjustments of medication as needed. By contrast, laboratory mice may be observed for just a few seconds a day, with no physical examination or dynamic assessment, and often by researchers without veterinary training, which some veterinarians consider a troubling and unnecessary compromise of animal welfare (Marx et al. 2021).

Welfare scientists are working to validate better pain recognition strategies for mice and other species used in laboratories that would enable veterinarians and researchers to quickly and reliably diagnose and treat animal pain, but so far without substantial success (Mogil et al. 2020). The ethical challenge then is how ethics committees can evaluate protocols if they cannot confidently assess the severity of potential pain or rely on researchers or even veterinarians to have the tools to monitor pain (and, by implication, evaluate the effectiveness of pain medications) during the course of a study. Government guidelines require that, "Unless the contrary is established, investigators should consider that procedures that cause pain or distress in human beings may cause pain or distress in other animals" (United States Office of Science and Technology Policy 1985). Unfortunately, critical anthropomorphism – judiciously applying what we know about humans to other species – does not extend to knowing what drugs at what doses will effectively treat nonhumans' pain (Gross et al. 2003). I am concerned that we laboratory animal practitioners have been underestimating rodent, primate, and other species' pain and bear an ethical responsibility to bring this knowledge to our ethics committees (Carbone 2019a). Ethics committees (and scientists and veterinarians) apply an ethics of uncertainty to these reviews: ethical practice requires acknowledging such factual uncertainties and erring, when possible, on the side of precaution for animals' welfare.

## Unalleviated Pain and Distress

Beauchamp and DeGrazia's principle of no unnecessary harm would suggest that scientists and veterinarians always prevent or treat laboratory animal pain to the best of their ability: they do not (2019). Scientists sometimes see a need to perform experiments that cause pain or distress, and a need to leave the pain untreated out of concern for what drugs might do to the body and to research outcomes. As an example, a scientist might induce painful arthritis in rats in order to test some new pain treatment and will likely have a control or placebo cohort who receive no pain medicines, allowing a clearer comparison between the novel treatment and untreated pain. This sort of situation is covered by the USDA's "Category E" in facilities' annual reports, as described earlier. Every year, some 7–8% of animals are listed as Category E, but as the USDA's AWA enforcement excludes mice and rats, no one is required to use USDA pain categories for these species, therefore no one knows just how many animals in US labs experience unalleviated pain (Marx et al. 2021).

Ethics committee review of "Category E" requires two types of justification (Carbone 2014). *Scientific justification* means that the data truly will be diminished if pain medicines are used, and committees vary in how stringent their standards are. Alongside scientific justification is *ethical justification*, in which "necessary" pain that cannot be alleviated without invalidating the data should only be permissible in studies that address important questions with scientific rigor without reasonable alternatives that are less painful: Beauchamp and DeGrazia's principle of sufficient value to justify harm (2019). Unfortunately, institutional ethics committees may do a thorough review of the scientific justification of a "Category E" study, but much less commonly do a rigorous harm–benefit analysis of whether unalleviated pain should be permissible (Carbone 2019b).

## Summary

With veterinary ethics in clinical practice as the backdrop, I have tried to show how ethics in animal laboratories is similar, but different. In the laboratory, an institution, rather than the veterinarian or the client/owner is legally responsible for animal care and use. In the laboratory, scientists, with veterinary and committee input and oversight, knowingly plan to harm animals, far beyond the temporary harms of surgical neutering or dehorning in companion or farm animal practice. The degree and deliberateness of harming laboratory animals raises important ethical challenges that have been discussed for more than a century. Society accepts this practice, but within limits set by regulations (where they apply). The Three Rs alternatives framework focusing on Replacement, Reduction, and Refinement is a system for identifying and mitigating harms to animals but is mostly silent on what benefits might justify harms. Beauchamp and DeGrazia's six principles of animal research ethics address the harm–benefit calculations that scientists, veterinarians, and ethics committees should perform. Though the daily applied ethics in animal laboratories is largely welfarist, focusing on welfare of sentient animals, it nonetheless treats species of equivalent sentience differently (it is speciesist) and within a species may sometimes treat individuals differently. I have argued here too that serious harm–benefit analyses operate in the face of great uncertainty: uncertainty about the potential benefits to yet-unborn generations (mostly of people, the main beneficiaries targeted in most animal research), but also about how to adequately evaluate and manage the harms to animal species whose welfare remains to be fully studied, using medicines and treatments whose effects on data outcomes are usually not known.

## References

Ainsworth, C. (2006). Scientists share thoughts on animal research. *Nature*. https://doi.org/10.1038/news061211-9.

American Association for Accreditation of Laboratory Animal Care (AAALAC) International (2021a). About: What is AAALAC?. https://www.aaalac.org/about/what-is-aaalac (accessed 20 February 2021).

American Association for Accreditation of Laboratory Animal Care (AAALAC) International (2021b). FAQ: Animals included in the AAALAC International accredited "unit" 2. Invertebrates. https://www.aaalac.org/accreditation-program/faqs/#A2 (accessed 20 February 2021).

American Veterinary Medical Association (AVMA) (2020). AVMA membership 2020. https://www.avma.org/resources-tools/reports-statistics/market-research-statistics-avma-membership (accessed 8 March 2021).

Andre, V., Gau, C., Scheideler, A. et al. (2018). Laboratory mouse housing conditions can be improved using common environmental enrichment without compromising data. *PLoS Biology* 16: e2005019.

Animal Care Panel (1963). *Guide for Laboratory Animal Facilities and Care*. Washington, DC: Public Health Service.

Bailey, M.R. (2018). Love animals? Support animal research. *Lab Animal* 47: 37–38.

Bateson, P. (1986). When to experiment on animals. *New Scientist* 20 February: 30–32.

Bayne, K. and Wurbel, H. (2014). The impact of environmental enrichment on the outcome variability and scientific validity of laboratory animal studies. *Revue Scientifique et Technique (International Office of Epizootics)* 33: 273–280.

Beagle Freedom Project (2021). The Mission. Rescue. Rehab. Repeat. https://bfp.org/mission (accessed 10 May 2021).

Beauchamp, T. and Degrazia, D. (2019). *Principles of Animal Research Ethics*. New York: Oxford University Press.

Bleich, A., Bankstahl, M., Jirkof, P. et al. (2020). Severity assessment in animal based research. *Laboratory Animals* 54: 16.

Burghardt, G.M. (1996). Environmental enrichment or controlled deprivation. *Scientists Center for Animal Welfare Newsletter* 18: 3–10.

BVAAWF/FRAME/RSPCA/UFAW Joint Working Group on Refinement (2003). Refinement and reduction in production of genetically modified mice. *Laboratory Animals* 37 (Suppl. 1): S1–S49.

Carbone, L. (2004). *What Animals Want: Expertise and Advocacy in Laboratory Animal Welfare Policy*. New York: Oxford University Press.

Carbone, L. (2012a). Pain management standards in the eighth edition of the *Guide for the Care and Use of Laboratory Animals*. *Journal of the American Association for Laboratory Animal Science* 51: 1–5.

Carbone, L. (2012b). The utility of basic animal research (in: Animal research ethics: Evolving views and practices, Hastings Center Report). *Hastings Center Report Special Report* 42: S12–S15.

Carbone, L. (2014). Justification for the use of animals. In: *The IACUC Handbook*, 3 e. (eds. J. Silverman, M.A. Suckow, and S. Murthy), 211–237. Boca Raton, FL: CRC Press.

Carbone, L. (2019a). Ethical and IACUC considerations regarding analgesia and pain management in laboratory rodents. *Comparative Medicine* 69: 443–450.

Carbone, L. (2019b). The potential and impacts of practical application of Beauchamp and DeGrazia's six principles. In: *Principles of Animal Research Ethics* (eds. T. Beauchamp and D. Degrazia), 45–61. New York: Oxford University Press.

Carbone, L. (2021). Estimating mouse and rat use in American laboratories by extrapolation from Animal Welfare Act-regulated species. *Scientific Reports* 11: 1–6.

Carbone, L., Guanzini, L., and McDonald, C. (2003). Adoption options for laboratory animals. *Laboratory Animals* 32: 37–41.

De Bruin, W.C., van de Ven, E.M., and Hooijmans, C.R. (2016). Efficacy of soiled bedding transfer for transmission of mouse and rat infections to sentinels: A systematic review. *PLoS ONE* 11: e0158410.

Feng, G., Jensen, F.E., Greely, H.T. et al. (2020). Opportunities and limitations of genetically modified nonhuman primate models for neuroscience research. *Proceedings of the National Academy of Sciences of the United States of America* 117: 24022–24031.

Fenton, A. (2020). Holding animal-based research to our highest ethical standards: Re-seeing two emergent laboratory practices and the ethical significance of research animal dissent. *ILAR Journal* 60: 397–403.

Fernandez-Moure, J.S. (2016). Lost in translation: The gap in scientific advancements and clinical application. *Frontiers in Bioengineering and Biotechnology* 4: 43.

Garner, J.P. (2014). The significance of meaning: Why do over 90% of behavioral neuroscience results fail to translate to humans, and what can we do to fix it? *ILAR Journal/National Research Council, Institute of Laboratory Animal Resources* 55: 438–456.

Greek, J.S. and Greek, C.R. (2004). *What Will We Do if We Don't Experiment on Animals?* Victoria, Canada: Trafford Publishing.

Greely, H.T. (2021). Human brain surrogates research: The onrushing ethical dilemma. *The American Journal of Bioethics* 21: 34–45.

Gross, D.R., Tranquilli, W.J., Greene, S.A. et al. (2003). Critical anthropomorphic evaluation and treatment of postoperative pain in rats and mice. *Journal of the American Veterinary Medical Association* 222: 1505–1510.

Hansen, L.A. and Greek, R. (2013). Evolution and animal models. *JAMA Neurology* 70: 271.

Hay, M., Thomas, D.W., Craighead, J.L. et al. (2014). Clinical development success rates for investigational drugs. *Nature Biotechnology* 32: 40–51.

Hernandez, E., Fawcett, A., Brouwer, E. et al. (2018). Speaking up: Veterinary ethical responsibilities and animal welfare issues in everyday practice. *Animals (Basel)* 8: 15–37.

Institute For Laboratory Animal Research (2011). *Guide for the Care and Use of Laboratory Animals.*, 8 e. Washington, DC: National Academies Press.

Jennings, C.G., Landman, R., Zhou, Y. et al. (2016). Opportunities and challenges in modeling human brain disorders in transgenic primates. *Nature Neuroscience* 19: 1123–1130.

King, M. and Zohny, H. (2021). Animal researchers shoulder a psychological burden that animal ethics committees ought to address. *Journal of Medical Ethics.*. doi:10.1136/medethics-2020-106945.

Kipperman, B., Rollin, B., and Martin, J. (2020). Veterinary student opinions regarding ethical dilemmas encountered by veterinarians and the benefits of ethics instruction. *Journal of Veterinary Medical Education* 48: 330–342.

Kola, I. and Landis, J. (2004). Can the pharmaceutical industry reduce attrition rates? *Nature Reviews. Drug Discovery* 3: 711–715.

LaFollette, H. and Shanks, N. (1996). *Brute Science: Dilemmas of Animal Experimentation.* London: Routledge.

LaFollette, M.R., Riley, M.C., Cloutier, S. et al. (2020). Laboratory animal welfare meets human welfare: A cross-sectional study of professional quality of life, including compassion fatigue in laboratory animal personnel. *Frontiers in Veterinary Science* 7: 114.

Lahvis, G.P. (2017). Unbridle biomedical research from the laboratory cage. *Elife* 6: e27438PG.

Leenaars, C.H., De Vries, R.B., Heming, A. et al. (2020). Animal models for cystic fibrosis: A systematic search and mapping review of the literature – Part 1: Genetic models. *Laboratory Animals* 54: 330–340.

Legrand, N., Ploss, A., Balling, R. et al. (2009). Humanized mice for modeling human infectious disease: Challenges, progress, and outlook. *Cell Host & Microbe* 6: 5–9.

Makowska, I.J. and Weary, D.M. (2020). A good life for laboratory rodents? *ILAR Journal* 60: 373–388.

Marx, J.O., Jacobsen, K.O., Petervary, N.A. et al. (2021). A survey of laboratory animal veterinarians regarding mouse welfare in biomedical research. *Journal of the American Association for Laboratory Animal Science* 60: 139–145.

Mellor, D.J. (2019). Welfare-aligned sentience: Enhanced capacities to experience, interact, anticipate, choose and survive. *Animals (Basel)* 9: 440.

Mogil, J.S. (2019). The translatability of pain across species. *Philosophical Transactions of the Royal Society of London. Series B, Biological Sciences* 374: 20190286.

Mogil, J.S., Pang, D.S.J., Silva Dutra, G.G. et al. (2020). The development and use of facial grimace scales for pain measurement in animals. *Neuroscience and Biobehavioral Reviews* 116: 480–493.

Munoz-Fontela, C., Dowling, W.E., Funnell, S.G.P. et al. (2020). Animal models for COVID-19. *Nature* 586: 509–515.

National Institutes of Health (2020). NIH plan to retire all NIH-owned and -supported chimpanzees. https://www.hhs.gov/guidance/document/nih-chimpanzee-retirement-plan (accessed 10 May 2021).

Niemi, S.M. (2020). Harm-benefit analyses can be harmful. *ILAR Journal* 60: 341–346.

Nuffield Council on Bioethics (2005). *The Ethics of Research Involving Animals*. London: Nuffield Council on Bioethics.

Ormandy, E.H., Dale, J., and Griffin, G. (2011). Genetic engineering of animals: Ethical issues, including welfare concerns. *The Canadian Veterinary Journal. La Revue Veterinaire Canadienne* 52: 544–550.

Ormandy, E.H. and Schuppli, C.A. (2014). Public attitudes toward animal research: A review. *Animals (Basel)* 4: 391–408.

Peterson, N.C., Nunamaker, E.A., and Turner, P.V. (2017). To treat or not to treat: The effects of pain on experimental parameters. *Comparative Medicine* 67: 469–482.

Pew Research Center (2018). Americans are divided over the use of animals in scientific research. https://www.pewresearch.org/fact-tank/2018/08/16/americans-are-divided-over-the-use-of-animals-in-scientific-research (accessed 28 January 2021).

Rollin, B. (2006). *Science and Ethics*. New York: Cambridge University Press.

Rollin, B.E. (2015). Telos, conservation of welfare, and ethical issues in genetic engineering of animals. *Current Topics in Behavioral Neurosciences* 19: 99–116.

Russell, W.M.S. and Burch, R.L. (1959). *The Principles of Humane Experimental Technique*. London: Methuen & Co. Ltd.

Tannenbaum, J. and Bennett, B.T. (2015). Russell and Burch's 3Rs then and now: The need for clarity in definition and purpose. *Journal of the American Association for Laboratory Animal Science* 54: 120–132.

Thompson, P.B. (2010). Why using genetics to address welfare may not be a good idea. *Poultry Science* 89: 814–821.

Toth, L.A. (2015). The influence of the cage environment on rodent physiology and behavior: Implications for reproducibility of pre-clinical rodent research. *Experimental Neurology* 270: 72–77.

United States Department of Agriculture (USDA) (2019). Annual report animal usage by fiscal year. Fiscal year: 2018. https://www.aphis.usda.gov/animal_welfare/annual-reports/Annual-Report-Summaries-State-Pain-FY18.pdf (accessed 22 January 2021).

United States Department Of Agriculture (USDA) Animal Care (2019). Animal Welfare Act and animal welfare regulations. https://www.aphis.usda.gov/animal_welfare/downloads/bluebook-ac-awa.pdf (accessed 27 September 2021).

United States Department Of Agriculture (USDA) (2020). AWA inspection and annual reports. https://www.aphis.usda.gov/aphis/ourfocus/animalwelfare/awa/awa-inspection-and-annual-reports (accessed 15 December 2020).

United States Interagency Research Animal Committee (1985). Principles for the utilization and care of vertebrate animals used in testing, research, and training. *Federal Register* 50.

United States Office of Science And Technology Policy (1985). Laboratory animal welfare; U.S. government principles for the utilization and care of vertebrate animals used in testing, research and training; notice. *Federal Register* 50: 20864–20865.

### Legislation

Animal Welfare Act 1970

Directive 2010/63/EU of the European Parliament and of the Council of 22 September 2010 on the protection of animals used for scientific purposes

Food Security Act 1985, title XVII, subtitle F – Animal Welfare

Health Research Extension Act 1985

Laboratory Animal Welfare Act (LAWA) 1966

# 12

## Food Animals

*Timothy E. Blackwell, Shaw Perrin, and Jennifer Walker*

Ethical issues in all categories of veterinary medicine commonly arise from inherent and unavoidable conflicts of interest (see Chapter 7). According to the American Veterinary Medical Association Principles of Veterinary Medical Ethics #1 (AVMA n.d.a): "A veterinarian shall be influenced only by the welfare of the patient, the needs of the client, the safety of the public, and the need to uphold the public trust vested in the veterinary profession, and shall avoid conflicts of interest or the appearance thereof."

This principle commits veterinarians to at least three stakeholders – the patient, the client, and public safety and trust – but assumes that the interests of these stakeholders are seldom in conflict. This is a false assumption. A fourth important and competing interest pertains to the mental and financial well-being of veterinarians themselves. Conflicts of interest in veterinary medicine are unavoidable. Resolving these conflicts in a professional and ethical manner is the goal.

This leaves us with a landscape of veterinary ethics in which the veterinarian, with little training or guidance, must simultaneously balance the interests of at least four important stakeholders. The landscape becomes more complicated when we consider that the interests of individual animals may conflict with the interests of a group of animals, or the interest of one client, e.g. the seller of livestock, may conflict with the competing interests of other clients, e.g. the buyer of livestock being sold.

This complex ethical setting is common ground for veterinarians regardless of the species they serve. In this sense, food animal veterinary ethics walks the same ground as, for example, companion animal, equine, or laboratory animal ethics. The goal of this chapter is not to portray food animal practice as categorically different than all other practice types, but to highlight specific issues that are more commonly encountered, and uniquely manifested, in food animal practice. Most importantly, we hope to offer guidance on how such conflicts can be managed.

## Ethical Perspectives Regarding Raising Animals for Food

There are those who believe that animal rights and food animal veterinary medicine are incompatible. These people, including some veterinarians, cannot comprehend ensuring the health and welfare of large herds or flocks so that they can be killed for human consumption. A vocal minority of activists and vegan business interests are calling for an end to animal agriculture (Reese 2019). Food animal veterinarians who

*Ethics in Veterinary Practice: Balancing Conflicting Interests*, First Edition. Edited by Barry Kipperman and Bernard E. Rollin.

dedicate their professional lives to ensuring the health and welfare of their patients find these beliefs naive, confused, and culturally contingent. Healthy animals are killed in many veterinary settings, including companion animal shelters and in laboratory and wildlife medicine. Food animal veterinarians are also criticized by some of the public, as well as some of their veterinary colleagues, for supporting and enabling the livestock industry to create ever more intensive animal rearing operations.

It is important for all veterinarians to understand the critical role that food animal veterinarians play in ensuring the health and welfare of animals raised for food. Likewise, it is important for non-food animal veterinarians to have a basic understanding of the importance of livestock production in any sustainable food system. Food animal veterinarians should play a vital role in protecting animal health and welfare on livestock farms. In addition, food animal veterinarians are key in protecting public health by ensuring the appropriate use of pharmaceutical products in livestock production and aiding in the control of food-borne and zoonotic diseases.

For veterinarians and nonveterinarians alike, the concepts of animal rights and animal welfare are not always clearly defined. There are those in the agricultural community who profess to support animal welfare but do not accept the concept of animal rights. Rights are established through laws. Therefore, in most jurisdictions, anticruelty legislation ensures all domestic animals have the right to food, water, shelter, and freedom from unnecessary suffering (Pask 2015). Some animals have these rights enshrined in law and these rights were created to protect their welfare. However, there may not always be a consensus regarding what constitutes adequate shelter or unnecessary suffering, and some animals may be considered exempt from specific protections in some states or municipalities. One cannot be in favor of protecting animal welfare while denying animal rights. Domestic animals have rights specifically to ensure that their welfare is protected.

There is disagreement on what specific rights animals should have. Debating the rights that animals should be given is important and appropriate. Many believe domestic animals have the right to express at least some natural behaviors (Bracke and Hopster 2006). The rights of animals should be debated by the society in which those animals are raised and used. All people are animal rightists if they adhere to the laws of a society that guarantees some basic rights for domestic animals. It is unlikely that people will ever all agree on what rights animals should have but the resulting debates and discussions are important, and veterinarians are well positioned to engage in such debates.

Legitimate animal welfare concerns exist for domestic pet animals, laboratory animals, zoo animals, and domestic animals raised for food. Veterinarians have the experience and education to remedy these animal welfare problems. No one group of veterinarians can claim the moral high ground on animal welfare. All classes of animals that veterinarians deal with have room for improvement when it comes to their welfare and all veterinarians take the same oath to ensure that welfare is appropriate and where it is not, endeavor to improve it.

There will be situations where food animal veterinarians as well as producers are intensively focused on animal profit and productivity at the expense of animal welfare. Developing and enforcing standards to ensure that farm animals are cared for to ensure their welfare in accordance with societal norms is the most effective way to improve the welfare of animals on all farms. Veterinarians, regardless of their personal animal welfare outlook, will remain a valuable resource in ensuring that societal norms are met while maintaining the economic sustainability of an operation.

A common criticism of livestock production is that animals are slaughtered at a young age, long before they have reached their average (or maximum) lifespan (Four Paws International n.d.). This argument is most common among those whose familiarity with animals is based primarily on companion animals. These individuals, veterinarians included, forget that all animal species whether wild or domestic, "overproduce." This is nature's way of attempting to fill a biological niche with the fittest individuals. Without this natural selection, our planet would soon be overpopulated with many more species besides humans. Similar to what occurs naturally, farms resemble stable ecosystems. Although mortality rates are similar between farmed populations and wild populations, domestic animals should not suffer painful deaths from exposure, starvation, predation, etc. as is common in nature.

If a cow–calf operation has a holding capacity of 500 cows producing 450 calves per year with a 30% replacement rate of the cow herd (the number of mature cows that exit the herd due to mortality or poor production), then approximately 300 of the offspring would either have to die or be sold each year to maintain a population within the limit of what the land can support. The difference between the cows and the wildlife that also live on and around the farm is that the farmer, with the assistance of the veterinarian, is responsible for ensuring that all the cattle have food, water, shelter, and freedom from unnecessary suffering. Wildlife do not have these rights or protections and often suffer deaths from starvation, predation, or disease. Farmers ensure that despite a near-identical mortality rate as occurs in stable wildlife ecosystems, death is humane. This enormous responsibility to ensure the health, safety, and welfare of herds and flocks is something that stockpeople and food animal veterinarians take great pride in, and rightly so.

It can be said then that domestic food animals often achieve better states of welfare than their wildlife counterparts. Indeed, those calling for an end to animal agriculture (and thus an end to food animal veterinary practice) have yet to identify a clear alternative plan for repurposing our food-producing animals under better welfare conditions. Calls to stop breeding them are unrealistic and have failed in other species as evidenced by the seemingly intractable feline and canine overpopulation problem. Calls to place these animals on farm "sanctuaries" would require billions of dollars of investment and there would be no guarantee of better animal welfare. While most food animal producers are evaluated and audited for welfare, there is, to our knowledge, no third-party oversight of welfare on farm animal sanctuaries. Mass depopulation of farm animals is theoretically the most effective way to "end" animal agriculture, but this option is likewise unrealistic, problematic from an animal welfare perspective, and is contrary to the very point that animal activists wish to make: that animals have a right not to be killed.

What's left then for those who wish food animal production to end? The market must persuade consumers of animal products not to buy those products. Vegan ideology combined with tech and business interests urge consumers to abandon animal products in favor of diets based only on plants and lab-produced "alternative" proteins. Increasingly, such diets and products are promoted by scapegoating farm animals for causing climate change, thus deflecting attention from fossil fuels while ignoring the carbon sequestration capacities of regenerative agriculture and the importance of livestock manure to plant agriculture (Sims and Maguire 2005; Shober and Maguire 2018). Some veterinarians have joined this chorus for an end to food animal production. However, this approach fails to recognize the harm done to wild animals in plant agriculture (Davis 2003). This approach is also a call for gradual depopulation of food animals – for example, Impossible Food's goal to end cattle production by 2035 (Greenfield 2021). Gradual depopulation of important domestic species is not a serious proposal to improve the welfare of food animals and conflicts with the veterinarian's obligation toward "conservation of animal resources," as specified in the Veterinary Oath (AVMA n.d.c). The broader discussion of food access, food equity, and whether it is even possible to feed the world's population in a sustainable way on a purely plant-based diet is worthy of a chapter in and of itself. Suffice it to say it is our shared perspective that a single solution to global nutrition and sustainability is not tenable.

As veterinarians, we maintain that providing food animals with a good life and a good death is preferable to no life at all. Veterinarians are committed to protecting animal welfare and animal resources. Animal agriculture serves vital public health goals, like providing high-quality protein for human nutrition, just as companion animals serve a legitimate human need for companionship.

## Food Safety and Animal Welfare

All veterinarians have an obligation to public health. For food animal veterinarians, this includes unique responsibilities toward food safety. It is important to make clear the deliberate reference to this section as specific to food animals rather than farm animals. It is critical that all veterinarians recognize and respect the qualification of animals as food. It is also worth noting that the only issues truly unique to food animal practice are the legal and regulatory limitations placed on treatment decisions as they relate to food safety.

The rules in cases of food safety are very clear; all veterinarians, regardless of practice type or patient, are bound to follow the law, specifically the Federal Food, Drug and Cosmetic Act (FD&C Act) (n.d.), established in 1938 to protect the public from pesticide and drug residues in food and water. The use of drugs in food animal medicine has delivered many benefits to the food industry but their use presents potential public health concerns. Historically, the primary concern was the risk of drug residues with the potential to cause human disease or allergic reactions. Today that concern has grown to include the risk of the development of, selection for, and dissemination of antibiotic resistance (Koch et al. 2017). The Food and Drug Administration can limit the use of drugs or an entire class of drugs in any food-producing animal. It is important that all veterinarians accept that any "farm animal" whether considered a "pet" or "production unit" must be treated as if it will end up in the food supply and for this reason every veterinarian should be familiar with or know where to find guidance on making proper treatment recommendations for food animals (Case Study 12.1).

**Case Study 12.1 Food safety vs. animal welfare**

You are a veterinarian in a mixed practice in a semi-rural area. Most of your time is spent in the clinic tending to companion animals, but you share emergency duties with two other veterinarians who serve the mobile practice treating patients on farm. During one of your emergency shifts, you are called to treat Pansy, a three-year-old Nubian female goat. Pansy had been seen earlier in the week by another veterinarian in your practice, diagnosed with pneumonia, placed on Naxcel, a third-generation cephalosporin antibiotic, and the owner was instructed to call if they had not seen improvement in four days.

Upon examination, you confirm that Pansy is bright and alert but has a mild fever and has lung sounds consistent with pneumonia. Although you do not treat a lot of farm animals you remember that there are limitations on what drugs you are allowed to use. You decide a change in course of therapy is warranted and suggest to the owner that treatment be continued but with a different antibiotic. The owner, a cattle rancher, agrees wholeheartedly, telling you that he had suggested to the other doctor to use "this stuff because it works wonders on pneumonia in my cattle." You take the bottle handed to you by the owner and it reads, "Enrofloxacin Antimicrobial Injectable Solution is indicated for the treatment of bovine respiratory disease in beef and non-lactating dairy cattle and for treatment and control of swine respiratory disease." You also note that the label reads "Federal (USA) law prohibits the extra-label use of this drug in food-producing animals."

You are familiar with the drug, having used it often for your dog and cat patients and you agree that it would be your first choice of treatment had this been a pig or beef cow. You also remember that the extra-label use of drugs is allowed under the Animal Medical Drug Use Clarification Act and there are further allowances made under the Minor Use Animal Drug Program, but there are limitations, which often change. To make sure you have the most recent information, you check the Food Animal Residue Avoidance Databank (FARAD n.d.) and find that extra-label use of this class of antibiotics is prohibited. You discover as well that there is no allowance for use of enrofloxacin in minor species. You thank the client for the recommendation but explain that the use of the drug he suggested is prohibited in goats and that you will need either to continue with the present therapy with continued monitoring or switch to a different drug that is allowed for use in goats. The client is insistent that his drug of choice be used and declares that the goat is his son's 4-H pet and is never going to be eaten "so those rules don't apply when it's your favorite goat."

**The conflict:**

You agree the best course of therapy is to change drugs and that enrofloxacin would be the best choice from an efficacy point of view. However, in the eyes of the law, Pansy is a food animal and use of this drug for her treatment is prohibited.

**Considerations:**

The limited availability of treatments for food animals frustrates every food animal veterinarian as does the need to treat every goat, sheep, chicken, cow, rabbit, honeybee, or wildlife as if they will potentially be eaten as food. In this case the conflict is between the veterinarian, client, public safety, public trust, and of course, Pansy, as the stakeholders.

It is reasonable to be persuaded by the owner's plea that Pansy is a pet since he has no intention of using her as food or selling her. It is also tempting to rationalize the use of the enrofloxacin because there are so few drugs available for use in minor species like goats and sheep, and the welfare of these animals should not be compromised simply because a drug manufacturer did not spend the time and money required to earn label approval of the drug for use in this species. It is tempting to make an exception in this case because you trust the client and take him at his word that they would never use this goat as food. Allowing the illegal, extra-label use of enrofloxacin in this case would make your day go a lot smoother: it would make your client happy, and you would avoid the risk of losing a client if he were to get angry or complain to your employer.

There is no way to guarantee that Pansy will never be used as food. Many things can change between now and the eventual end of Pansy's life, all of which are out of your control. As the veterinarian, you can only control what is before you. Once a treatment is initiated under your direction, you are held responsible for any drug residue. On a larger scale, illegal extra-label use of drugs gained a great deal of attention in 2017 when millions of eggs had to be recalled and destroyed across Europe. Over 100 poultry farms in the Netherlands had to be shut down, and the birds destroyed, after it was discovered that a company included fipronil in a "natural remedy" for lice infestation (van der Merwe et al. 2018). Small-scale versions of this issue have been noted in backyard flocks, rendering any eggs from the exposed chickens "contaminated" for an indefinite period.

The rules of extra-label drug use apply to the individual animal regardless of the scale of the operation or the personal and emotional value of the animal. Since the client in this case is a beef producer, he should appreciate your commitment to food safety and protecting the reputation of animal agriculture. This is not always the case, and is rarely the case when it is a client lacking any knowledge of food animal production and regulations. While the law does not make managing this conflict any easier emotionally, it does make the correct course of management clear. When it comes to our professional duty, food safety laws prevail over our personal preferences.

## Individual Animal Care and Welfare in the Practice of Population and Production Medicine

Issues of care and individual medicine within the practice of population medicine are common in practices serving food animals, animal shelters, horse farms, zoos, and wildlife populations.

Animal welfare problems in food animal production can be broadly classified into whole-herd or flock concerns and individual animal problems. Some herd or flock problems result from currently accepted standards of housing and management. Examples of such are gestation stalls for housing pregnant sows or battery cages for laying hens. Although currently accepted by many livestock organizations, these restrictive housing systems are seen as inhumane by the public because of the severe limitations they exert on the expression of normal behavior (Humane Society of the United States 2012). Another category of herd or flock welfare concerns relates to procedures such as castration, dehorning, tail docking, branding, etc. that are commonly performed by stockpeople, may be considered unnecessary, and are often done without the use of effective anesthetics or analgesics.

Individual animal welfare concerns generally involve the suffering of distinct animals within a large production system where appropriate attention to address the suffering of a few animals is not prioritized due to the demands of caring for the remainder of the herd or flock. While this is an important ethical issue for population medicine, it should also be noted that the utilitarian ethics of population medicine – to bring about the greatest good for the greatest number – sometimes results in the sacrifice of some individuals to benefit a larger group of individuals. For example, we may euthanize a dog with rabies, a cow with tuberculosis, or mink with SARS-CoV-2.

Still, food animal veterinarians are sometimes asked how they can work in environments where the welfare of entire herds or flocks as well as of individual animals appears to be of low priority in relation to farm profitability. Case Study 12.2 reflects a scenario where veterinarians may experience conflicts in balancing their professional responsibilities to protect animal welfare.

---

**Case Study 12.2   Providing veterinary service to a sow farm with gestation stall housing**

A new client with a 2400-head farrow-to-wean sow barn asks for assistance to solve a recurring problem with low conception rates. The facility is 10 years old and has been well maintained. Sows are housed in gestation stalls and fed with an automatic drop system once per day. The sows are in good condition with few over- or underconditioned animals. It is a pleasure to work with this client as she is intelligent and pleasant with outstanding pig and people skills. You resolve the infertility issue, and the owner is very pleased. She tells you about her plans to double the herd size. Despite your keen interest in pigs and the swine industry, you are not a proponent of gestation stalls. This is even more the case as group sow housing systems have proven effective from both an economic and animal welfare perspective (Canning et al. 2012; Morgan et al. 2018).

Due to her excellent husbandry skills, the client is producing over 60,000 weaned pigs per year. As a result, the farm generates a healthy return for your practice. Doubling the herd size will result in a proportional increase in income for your clinic. You want this client to succeed but you would prefer that the sows express more of their natural behaviors than the current gestation stalls allow.

Supporting the farmer in her expansion plans can be viewed as part of your professional responsibility. It also means working within a system where animals are held under such restrictive conditions that they have little opportunity to express any natural behaviors. Modern barn construction practices will ensure that a new gestation stall building will remain operational for decades to come.

**The conflict:**

You wish to support this producer in making a major investment in her operation. You are also keenly aware of how this expansion will positively affect the income of your practice. Keeping sows in stalls where they can neither turn around nor fully stretch their limbs has always bothered you and you wish to suggest alternative group sow housing. Your experience as a practitioner has shown you that what one producer can effectively manage, another cannot. The owner is confident in her ability to profitably operate a stall barn and understandably shares her reluctance to invest a large sum of money in an alternative type of facility with which she has no experience. If the owner takes your advice but is unable to operate the new barn to the production level of the current barn, she will suffer significant economic hardship. In addition, the bank may be reluctant to lend a large sum of money to this producer if she decides on a less well-established housing system.

To say that you are in favor of housing sows in groups while most of your clients continue to expand their operations using stall housing seems hypocritical. It is particularly problematic since you profit from every new stall barn in your practice. Friends with no livestock background who have read about the severe restrictions that stall housing places on pregnant sows wonder how you can work with and profit from people who choose to use such restrictive housing practices.

**Considerations:**

Restrictive housing for any animal is generally a compromise between what is best for the owner and for the animal, often in that order of priority. People who are accustomed to seeing a canary in a cage, a snake in an aquarium, a goldfish in a bowl, or a dolphin in a marine park cement pool are often less vocal regarding the very unnatural environment in which these animals exist. For many people, these animal housing arrangements are the only ones with which they are familiar. The same bias exists for swine producers who have known nothing but stalled housing for their entire careers and who have followed the recommendations of university extension agents and agricultural engineers in building and operating such units. An appreciation of this starting point is essential in moving forward toward advocating for less restrictive housing systems for sows.

At the same time, veterinarians must be cautious in promoting less well-documented livestock housing and management systems, particularly where very large capital investments are required. Every housing system is based on specific management practices and expertise and veterinarians are keenly aware of this. Veterinarians have seen all types of housing systems fail when mismanaged. Producers fully appreciate the connection between housing systems and barn management and are cautious about changing to radically different systems without feeling confident that they can manage a new facility. Producers considering new housing arrangements for their livestock seek advice from similar producers who have built and managed the same kinds of systems.

It is the experience of the authors that coercing a client into choosing one housing or management system over another is not advised. A stockperson managing a facility that they were coerced into building often fails to produce satisfactory results. It is too easy to blame problems as they arise on the facility they "knew" would never work. The opposite occurs when the producer makes the decision to change facilities or management techniques themselves. In that case, stockpeople take ownership of problems as they arise and apply their skills and expertise to resolve them. Understanding the importance of peer-to-peer consultations, veterinarians, rather than making recommendations themselves, do well to connect producers with other producers who have experience building and successfully managing housing systems. A peer group of producers who meet in person or virtually to discuss and compare housing, management, and production figures allows more progressive individuals to demonstrate the advantages and disadvantages of innovative alternatives to their peers. Such peer group influence is dramatically more effective in changing the perspective of producers than "expert" advice.

Such an approach has several advantages for the veterinarian. It demonstrates to the client that the veterinarian is engaged in the farmer's expansion efforts and wants the client to make a fully educated decision. It allows the client to compare the full range of options available and to do this through a peer-to-peer format. The veterinarian can still express their personal preference for group housing while allowing the peer-to-peer consultations to exert the major influence.

Some individuals, veterinarians included, question how a colleague who took an oath to protect animal welfare can work with and profit from a farmer who houses their sows in gestation stalls. If a veterinarian would refuse to work with clients using restrictive housing systems on moral grounds, the result is predictable. The producer will find another highly qualified veterinarian to service the herd who has no objections to restrictive housing systems. As a result, little improvement in the welfare of the herd is likely to result.

Working with and gaining the trust and respect of a client provide the opportunity to improve the welfare of all animals on the farm and to communicate your personal welfare ethics through an established relationship. Creating and managing a "consulting cooperative" of food animal clients provides an opportunity for producers to share ideas concerning production, housing, nutrition, and other topics, which can be used to improve the welfare of the animals on the farms.

Refusing to take care of a producer who works diligently to ensure the health and welfare of sows in gestation stalls is no less appropriate than refusing veterinary care for a caged canary or hamster.

## Ensuring Individual Animal Care in a Herd Setting

One difference between practicing individual animal medicine and population medicine involves the care of the individual. In single-patient practice, the totality of care is focused on the individual. In population medicine, by definition, the emphasis is on the herd or flock. Production parameters such as preweaning mortality, culling rate, conception rate, average daily gain, etc. are a major focus of food animal practitioners. These parameters are considered indicative of the combined health and welfare of the individuals in the herd or flock. However, individual animals may be overlooked if the herd or flock is performing up to expectations. This can lead to unintended animal welfare problems.

The problem arises from the fact that a herd or flock may be healthy and thriving while a small percentage of individual animals are suffering from lameness, respiratory disease, diarrhea, or other ailments. Provided these individuals represent a small proportion of the population, they have no noticeable effect on the production values that are closely monitored. Nevertheless, there is real animal suffering that must be attended to but may be overlooked.

There are several reasons why the suffering of individual animals is not adequately attended to in a large-group environment. The very concept of herd health implies a lack of focus on outliers. The greatest returns on time and effort come from managing the group. If feed and water consumption are appropriate, production parameters are hitting preset targets, and the great majority of animals are bright and alert, then "herd health" is good. A much larger effort is required to ensure that every single individual is examined. Unfortunately, when an unfit animal is identified, pens may not be designed for easy separation, examination, and treatment, particularly when only a single caretaker is present. As a result, a wait and see approach is often used hoping that the animal's condition improves on its own. This is seldom in the best interest of the individual animal and can lead to desensitization of the caretaker regarding animal suffering.

In large production settings, the return on treating an individual that is not representative of a larger herd or flock problem is limited. For example, in swine many causes of lameness are challenging to diagnose and even more difficult to treat effectively. It can be equally difficult to identify the reason why an individual animal appears gaunt with no obvious clinical signs, while the remainder of the herd appears healthy and to be eating normally.

Despite these "reasons" for not responding to individual animal ailments within a large herd or flock setting, neither veterinarians nor producers should become complacent regarding the suffering of individuals. It is contrary to the Veterinary Oath and the opposite of what the public expects from veterinarians. Unfortunately, veterinarians focused on food animals receive extensive training in maximizing herd health and productivity but much less practical instruction in addressing individual animal problems within the herd setting. Veterinary curricula should address this deficiency.

Veterinarians should emphasize the importance of maintaining at least one specifically designed hospital pen on every farm. Depending on the size and type of operation, more than one hospital pen may be required. Hospital pens should be designed with the specific needs of animals requiring individual care in mind. They should not be a gated-off corner in the barn or alleyway. Hospital pens should have sound footing, supplemental heat, easy access to appropriate pharmaceuticals, and be placed in a high-traffic area so hospitalized animals are regularly viewed. Provided the reason for using the hospital pen is not a highly infectious disease, most animals will have an increased chance of recovery if not housed alone in a pen. Pen mates often improve the appetite of the sick individual. Care should be taken to ensure the hospital pen mate is not a source of irritation for the compromised individual. Often smaller, more submissive individuals make suitable hospital pen mates for compromised animals.

Veterinarians should ensure that hospital pens do not become hospice pens. Clear, written treatment protocols should be included with every hospital pen. Equally important are stop treatment protocols to ensure that individuals who do not respond to appropriate therapy are euthanized in a timely manner. To ensure that euthanasia is timely and appropriate, veterinarians should train the appropriate stockpeople to recognize suffering, appreciate the importance and responsibility of timely euthanasia, and be competent to perform euthanasia when indicated. This must include ensuring that death has occurred.

## Preventing Individual Animal Welfare Problems

Avoiding individual animal suffering is preferred to treating problems after the fact. Most barns are designed to provide optimal housing for the great majority of animals. However, in any large population there will be a percentage of individuals that are smaller, weaker, or less aggressive and that do not adapt as rapidly to a housing arrangement that is suitable for most of their herd or flock mates. Most of these high-risk individuals are not suffering from a specific disease process. For various reasons, they are not inclined to aggressively compete for the available resources in the pen and this puts them at a significant disadvantage in a large-group situation. Good stockpeople recognize these individuals early but may have limited options to provide the extra attention they require to compete with their herd or flock mates.

It is impractical to design a barn that provides an ideal environment for 100% of the incoming animals when 98% of the animals do not require the extra amenities. However, it is economically sound and welfare appropriate to provide special temporary accommodations for high-risk individuals that need a few days of extra care to adjust to their new environment. Special penning for this group of weaker animals may be similar in design to hospital penning and, on some farms, the same pens can serve both purposes. Specially designed starter penning for weaker individuals should provide less competitive access to feed and water, better footing, additional heat, and more comfortable lying areas. Providing the less competitive animals assistance at the start means less time spent on sick animals later. The weaker cohort in the special needs pen should be able to see and hear the remainder of the herd or flock so that their reintroduction to the large group will be a more seamless transition. These special care pens often have a higher success rate than when they function as hospital pens. Preventing disease in the smaller, weaker cohort is more satisfying and provides greater returns than treating these animals once they succumb to infections.

Understanding the cost effectiveness of both therapeutic and prophylactic pharmaceuticals is critical in ensuring that animal welfare is maximized on modern livestock farms. Veterinarians may struggle to comprehend the reluctance of some producers to use effective vaccinations in their herds. Why would a producer be reluctant to spend $2 on a preventative vaccination program to protect finishing pigs that are worth $190 apiece at market? The reluctance is not as irrational as some may think. If the producer's current cost of production is $180 in a $190 market, adding a $2 vaccination will reduce the farmer's profit on every pig sold by 20%. Few veterinarians would be eager to adopt a strategy that would reduce their income by 20% unless it proved necessary.

Veterinarians as well as producers often misjudge the value of treating individuals. In the above example, if a pig required an additional $40 of care (labor, pharmaceuticals, and feed) to recover from an ailment, some would conclude that adding $40 to the existing $180 cost of production is pointless if the pig is only worth $190. However, if the pig is left untreated and dies, the farmer loses close to $180. If the pig is left untreated but can be sent to a salvage market where they return $90, the farmer may suffer a loss of up to $90. However, if the pig fully responds to the $40 treatment, the farmer loses only $30 ($220 minus $190). It is often cost effective on even the largest production units to build effective hospital pens and to invest appropriate time and resources in helping individuals recover. Ensuring that stockpeople appreciate the importance of individual animal care make them more effective and responsible animal caretakers. Stockpeople feel a sense of pride and accomplishment in identifying ailing individuals and returning them to health and productivity. This increases job satisfaction, often leads to retention of good employees, and improves the bottom line on many farms (Hemsworth and Coleman 2011). Telling a dedicated stockperson that an animal is not worth treating is often both economically and ethically wrong.

Recent technological developments show great promise in helping to quickly identify individual animals in need of medical attention before the onset of overt clinical illness. On dairy farms it is becoming increasingly common to equip animals with wearable bio-monitors able to record resting time, rumination or eating time, body temperature, and other measures important to health and welfare. Additionally, the daily collection of milk from dairy cows allows us to identify milk contents – such as somatic cells – important to cow health. The continued development and implementation of such technology will be of great benefit to producers and veterinarians working to identify individual animals in need of medical care.

## Appropriate Follow-Up Care

An area of ethical concern pertinent to food animal practice is ensuring appropriate follow-up care. Food animal practice has the potential to create these ethical challenges due to the increased demand on a practitioner's time associated with clients who live many miles away. This is less of a problem in practices where the patients come to the clinic. However, when a herd or flock under care is an hour or more away, careful follow-up evaluation of the success or failure of interventions puts an added demand on the practitioner's time. These travel-associated time constraints increase the risk of insufficient follow-up and unnecessary adverse outcomes. Practitioners cannot always expect clients to accurately assess the success of interventions, particularly in cases where they are unfamiliar with disease processes (Sumner et al. 2018). Producers, like veterinarians, have their own daily crises to manage and due to their own time constraints may not critically assess the progress or lack thereof of a veterinary treatment. To avoid moral stress, food animal practitioners should develop a system for monitoring their recommended interventions.

For acutely ill animals, a call or text message the following day emphasizes to the producer that the animal's condition requires close monitoring. In addition, it demonstrates the veterinarian's sincere interest in a positive outcome. For busy practitioners, this next-day check-in can be done by a suitably trained receptionist or technician. For less acute situations, e.g. changing a feeding program for young animals, scheduling a follow-up visit either in person or by phone before you leave the farm has two positive effects. First, it demonstrates your sincere interest in improving the situation on the farm. Second, it provides an incentive for the producer to implement the intervention since they know you will be checking in on their progress at a set date in the future.

Recent developments in telemedicine will be an important tool for case follow-up by food animal practitioners (Patterson n.d.).

## Financial Conflicts of Interest

Financial conflicts of interest are ubiquitous in veterinary medicine. Any practice model where the veterinarian's livelihood is dependent on the income of clients paying for care on behalf of the patient presents the conflict of serving the best interest of the patient while protecting the income stream of the veterinarian. This conflict may be amplified in food animal practice, where it is typical for an individual veterinarian to serve a small number of clients, making the loss of any one client a significant financial risk. Customer dissatisfaction is an ever-present risk to the food animal practitioner's livelihood.

While many companion animal practitioners face similar challenges with the advent of cyberbullying and negative reviews having the potential to negatively impact the business, an important financial conflict in companion animal practice is the profit taken from drug sales. The American Animal Hospital Association (AAHA) Veterinary Fee Reference reports mark-ups ranging from 65 to 113% depending on the type of drug (AAHA 2018). The typical US food animal practitioner may mark up drugs by 2–5%. The reason for the difference is in the volume of drugs a food animal practitioner may sell. Food animal practices that choose to manage distribution of drugs to clients stand to generate significant income if the volume of drug sales is high.

Profit from the sale of drugs therefore represents a clear conflict of interest for all veterinarians. Some food animal practitioners manage this conflict by limiting the sale of drugs on an as-needed basis to those with limited access or use, or by opting to write prescriptions for clients so that they can buy direct from a licensed distributor, effectively limiting any negligible profit to the relatively small number of clients that choose not to buy pharmaceuticals directly. But this does not remove the conflict altogether. Unlike human medicine where, under the Affordable Care Act of 2021 (aka the "Sunshine Act"[1]), the influence of drug companies on treatment decisions has been hampered, veterinarians may accept incentives (hats, jackets, rebates, meals, paid vacations, and other "reimbursements") with impunity. Many veterinarians may not recognize the conflict of interest such "gifts" represent for their practice (Case Study 12.3). The influence of "gifts" on treatment decisions has been well documented. One study suggested that small gifts caused doctors to change their prescription writing behavior (Wood et al. 2017). Still, many veterinarians insist that they are above the sway of fancy dinners and paid fishing trips, and certainly a free pen!

---

**Case Study 12.3   There are no free lunches or kayaking trips**

You have been offered the opportunity for you and your partner to attend a weekend retreat for some needed continuing education (CE) credits, bookended by meals, social events, and "leadership/team building" activities that include whale watching and kayaking. This will be an all-expenses-paid trip courtesy of a pharmaceutical company that manufactures and sells drugs for use in food animals. They have provided the agenda, which includes talks by well-respected academics who will be presenting their latest research. There is also a 30-minute session scheduled to share results of a new prescription drug "X," recently approved for use in cattle.

You accept the generous invitation and inform your clients that you will not be available that weekend to attend this retreat. You earned needed CE, had some fun, got to catch up with some old friends and make new ones. You learned important information regarding disease diagnosis and treatment and about a new product on the market, which is equal in efficacy to other products and easier to administer, but more expensive. A major advantage of this new product is that it requires a single injection under the skin instead of multiple injections in the muscle. A few months later when consulting with a long-time client experiencing a problem with her cows, for which product "X" is labeled, you suggest she begin using this new drug as part of the treatment protocol. Jokingly she responded, "So I'm the one who really gets to pay for your whale watching weekend!"

**The appearance of conflict:**

Accepting any gift has been demonstrated to exert influence on a person's decision-making (Malmendier and Schmidt 2012). Although the decision to recommend product "X" is correct from a medical perspective, as well as from a practical perspective (easier to administer), it is impossible to separate the potential external influence on your treatment recommendation, as the influence is often subconscious. Whether the pharmaceutical company's sponsored trip influenced your decision or not, it nevertheless creates the appearance of having been influenced by gifts from the manufacturer of this new prescription drug.

**Considerations:**

While you believe your client's comment to be in jest, you recognize that she is aware of the potential influence of such business exchanges. You sincerely believe that the recommendation is in her cattle and her best interests. While more expensive, she will only have to give one injection, and it will be much easier and less stressful for the cattle. You have always been concerned that she didn't pull enough cattle for treatment because she dreaded giving repeated shots in the muscle. This is an opportunity to improve welfare with a less painful injection and to ensure more cattle that need treatment receive it. Your clients know you have only their best interest in mind, and they also know that most of the other veterinarians in the area attended the same meeting.

Managing this conflict has proven difficult for the veterinary profession, which has largely resisted following the lead of the human medical professions to curb such influence. In fact, most veterinary conferences continue to be financially supported by pharmaceutical companies, putting in place modest measures to temper influence, requiring presenters acknowledge conflicts of interest and limiting references to product names during plenary or other main sessions while allowing breakfasts, socials, and events to be sponsored along with the ever-present trade-show where pens and other gifts are freely given to veterinarians.

The profession's unwillingness to address this issue can make managing the conflict harder on the individual practitioner, as the acceptance of the practice and denial of the subconscious influence serve to reinforce the false premise that veterinary professionals are somehow above the influence. Some practitioners may choose to take an aggressive approach, accepting nothing of value from any salesperson and choosing not to wear any clothing with a pharmaceutical company name or logo on it, and asking that salespersons or representatives leave product information at the office and schedule appointments to discuss new products or updates during business hours. Others may choose a moderate path, refusing any item of value over a certain dollar amount, allowing for pens, hats, and free lunches but declining invitations to dinners or CE meetings. The fact remains the subconscious pull of reciprocity is powerful, and practitioners should take care to acknowledge the conflict of interest that exists and should certainly be mindful of the appearance of a conflict of interest from the point of view of their client and the public. Still other practitioners choose to manage the appearance of a conflict by simply disclosing it.

By sharing in a public document all gifts (including rebates) received and the valued amount, the practitioner can practice full transparency allowing their clients to then be the judge of whether they were influenced by the pharmaceutical companies. If executed with complete transparency, such disclosure could stand to represent a significant risk to the client–veterinarian relationship as rebates can represent substantial income to the business and be viewed negatively by the client. To take no action to manage the conflict, choosing to believe that one is somehow conscious of their subconscious is to ignore the conflict and the ethical dilemma it presents altogether.

## Emergency Care

Specialty emergency clinics for companion animals are commonplace, especially in urban and suburban settings. This allows many companion animal practitioners the option of referring after-hours emergencies rather than providing that service themselves. In contrast, in the rural setting of food animal practice, the relative paucity of food animal veterinarians and the challenge of transporting large animals are among the reasons why emergency service for food animals falls mostly to private practitioners willing to provide ambulatory service.

The need for emergency services for food animal farms varies greatly by species, location, and size of operation. Some large-scale operations have a veterinarian on staff. Others, particularly many large-scale poultry and swine operations, are often able to handle emergencies following veterinarian-written protocols without needing a veterinary visit. Many producers or their staff can diagnose and treat common diseases, perform euthanasia, or resolve dystocia. The food animal veterinarian's role on such farms has more to do with providing protocols and training to deal with health emergencies rather than to attend personally to each emergency. The rise in interest in telemedicine and teleconsulting will no doubt aid food animal veterinarians who advise and consult in this fashion.

However, in-person veterinary attendance to emergencies remains a much-needed service for smaller farms and for many cattle (both beef and dairy) operations. There is a real demand for these services, but not enough of a demand to allow a market for exclusive emergency services for food animals, as has occurred in many companion animal markets. As part of their commitment to animal welfare and to clients, many food and mixed animal veterinarians provide ambulatory emergency service. But doing so can be taxing on veterinarian quality of life and mental health, particularly in solo or smaller practices and in practices with a large service area. Thus, some food animal veterinarians offer limited or no emergency service, sometimes leaving animals with no veterinary care. Some provide emergency service only to clients, others to both clients and nonclients. This gives rise to an important question: who is a client?

A client can be defined by the requirements of a veterinarian–client–patient relationship (VCPR), including whether, in the past, the veterinarian has seen the animal or group of animals. When that last visit occurred, however, remains poorly defined. Most dairy farms now have a signed VCPR renewed annually. Small-scale or "backyard" producers require service less frequently. In these cases, veterinarians may expand their definition of a current client.

A stable food animal veterinary practice not looking to grow is less likely to provide emergency service to nonclients, while a growing practice may elect to provide expansive emergency services with the goal of growing income, reputation, and acquiring new clients. Given the ambulatory nature of this veterinary care, another important question involves defining a reasonable service area for both clients and nonclients. The drastic and steady reduction in the number of livestock farms means that food animal practitioners are traveling ever longer distances to serve clients and their livestock.

As a profession we must work to ensure that food animals have access to either in-person or veterinary-directed medical care. But many legitimate ethical questions arise as veterinarians weigh the need for emergency service against important personal concerns about quality of life, mental health, burnout, and obligations to clients vs. nonclients (Case Study 12.4).

Principle #7 of the Principles of Veterinary Medical Ethics (AVMA n.d.a) provides specific guidance on veterinary responsibilities for emergency service, but leaves important questions unresolved, especially from the point of view of ambulatory food animal practice:

> In keeping with applicable law, a veterinarian shall, in the provision of appropriate patient care, *except in emergencies*, be free to choose whom to serve, with whom to associate, and the environment in which to provide veterinary medical care.
>
> (italics added)

In general, veterinarians are free "to choose whom to serve" and can establish or cancel a VCPR at any time. The one exception is emergency care. Veterinarians have "an ethical responsibility to provide essential services for animals when necessary to save life or relieve suffering." Such services "may be limited to euthanasia to relieve suffering, or to stabilization of the patient for transport to another source of animal care." Importantly from an ambulatory perspective, veterinarians can choose "the environment in which to provide the veterinary medical care" (AVMA n.d.a).

---

**Case Study 12.4   Offer after-hours service to nonclients?**

You are a mixed animal veterinarian in a rural area where you see a variety of clients with food animals. You and your colleagues offer emergency services for these clients, but debate whether and when to provide such service to nonclients. When on emergency call, you routinely receive requests from nonclients to see their food animals. Some of these owners do not have a veterinarian: others work with a veterinarian who does not provide emergency service or is otherwise unavailable. You sometimes take these calls, sometimes not, and recognize that you don't have a consistent way of deciding which calls to take and which to refuse. There are a handful of solo and mixed animal practitioners in your area who see food animals, but the nearest 24-hour university referral clinic is over 300 miles from your rural clinic. You call a meeting to discuss with your colleagues how best to approach nonclient emergencies.

**The conflict:**

Providing emergency service is in accord both with the Principles of Veterinary Medical Ethics and a valid VCPR, which requires that the veterinarian "is readily available for follow-up evaluation or has arranged for the following: veterinary emergency coverage, and continuing care and treatment" (AVMA n.d.b). Providing such emergency coverage is easier for multi-doctor practices. For this reason, we recommend that practitioners, when not available to provide emergency service for their clients, seek arrangements with other local veterinarians to provide that coverage.

  Should this clinic also serve nonclients in emergencies? The Principles of Veterinary Medical Ethics certainly imply that we have "an ethical responsibility" to serve these clients when "essential services" such as euthanasia or the life of the animal are at stake. When we are not available to provide such services, we should be able to provide referral. But in this case, it is not realistic to refer, say, a down cow to a specialty university clinic 300 miles away. Many food animal cases require ambulatory veterinary care.

**Considerations:**

We suggest that providing emergency service to nonclients should be left to the discretion of veterinarians. We also suggest that a practice establish guidelines to help owners, associates, and staff make these decisions. While it may ultimately be left up to the individual on call, it is helpful at a minimum to have guidelines for the defined service area and limits therein. Food animal veterinarians have a responsibility to their clients but some question whether that responsibility extends to every owner of a food animal in their service area. Responding to every emergency call from nonclients can lead to overwork, stress, and poor quality of life. Recent efforts by many in the veterinary community to improve the mental health and quality of life for veterinarians are laudable. The decision whether to serve a nonclient can legitimately depend on several factors, such as distance to the client, current physical and mental state of the veterinarian, and whether the veterinarian or practice is looking to gain new clients.

Those who are able and willing to serve nonclients in emergencies provide essential services to many food animals in immediate need of medical care and may then choose to price those services accordingly. This may be seen by some clients as being taken advantage of, or simply an attempt to dissuade emergency service requests.

The moral stress and demands of providing emergency service to food animal clients are real for veterinarians, affecting their mental and physical health. The formation of peer-to-peer groups designed to facilitate discussion about these issues is one way veterinarians can help each other reduce moral stress and improve quality of life.

## Conclusion

Like all veterinarians, food animal practitioners meet "ethical dilemmas on a day-to-day basis" (Tannenbaum 1995). Many of these dilemmas are identical to, or variations on, dilemmas faced routinely by veterinarians working on non-food animal species, such as financial conflicts of interest or conflicts between obligations to clients and patients. There is a need for more active discussion and research on food animal veterinary ethics and the inclusion of food animal ethics in veterinary curricula and in policy and training developed by organizations such as the American Association of Bovine Practitioners, American Association of Swine Practitioners, AVMA, and the Society for Veterinary Medical Ethics.

## Note

1 The Physician Payments Sunshine Act – also known as section 6002 of the Affordable Care Act of 2010 – requires medical product manufacturers to disclose to the Centers for Medicare and Medicaid Services any payments or other transfers of value made to physicians or teaching hospitals including meals and reimbursements for attending continuing education events. It also requires certain manufacturers and group purchasing organizations to disclose any physician ownership or investment interests held in those companies.

## References

American Animal Hospital Association (AAHA) (2018). *The Veterinary Fee Reference: Vital Statistics for Your Veterinary Practice*. Lakewood, CO: AAHA.

American Veterinary Medical Association (AVMA) (n.d.a). Principles of veterinary medical ethics. https://www.avma.org/resources-tools/avma-policies/principles-veterinary-medical-ethics-avma (accessed 10 October 2020).

American Veterinary Medical Association (AVMA) (n.d.b). The veterinary-client-patient relationship. https://www.avma.org/resources-tools/pet-owners/petcare/veterinarian-client-patient-relationship-vcpr (accessed 10 October 2020).

American Veterinary Medical Association (AVMA) (n.d.c). Veterinarian's Oath. https://www.avma.org/KB/Policies/Pages/veterinarians-oath.aspx (accessed 10 October 2020).

Bracke, M.B.M. and Hopster, H. (2006). Assessing the importance of natural behavior for animal welfare. *Journal of Agricultural and Environmental Ethics* 19: 77–89.

Canning, P., Zurbrigg, K., and Blackwell, T. (2012). Comparing feed efficiency and reproductive performance of gestating sows housed in conventional and group gestation. *Proceedings of the Annual Meeting of the American Association of Swine Veterinarians*, 305–306. Perry, IA: AASV.

Davis, S.L. (2003). The least harm principle may require that humans consume a diet containing large herbivores, not a vegan diet. *Journal of Agricultural and Environmental Ethics* 16: 387–394. https://doi.org/10.1023/A:1025638030686

Federal Food, Drug and Cosmetic Act (FD&C Act) (n.d.). Federal Food, Drug and Cosmetic Act (FD&C Act). https://www.fda.gov/regulatory-information/laws-enforced-fda/federal-food-drug-and-cosmetic-act-fdc-act (accessed 3 July 2021).

Food Animal Residue Avoidance Databank (FARAD) (n.d.). Prohibited and restricted drugs in food animals. http://www.farad.org/prohibited-and-restricted-drugs.html (accessed 3 July 2021).

Four Paws International (n.d.). The life expectancy of farm animals. https://www.four-paws.us/campaigns-topics/topics/farm-animals/life-expectancy (accessed 21 December 2021).

Greenfield, P. (2021). 'Let's get rid of friggin' cows' says creator of plant-based 'bleeding burger'. Guardian. https://www.theguardian.com/environment/2021/jan/08/lets-get-rid-of-friggin-cows-why-one-food-ceo-says-its-game-over-for-meat-aoe (7 January 2021).

Hemsworth, P.H. and Coleman, G.J. (2011). *Human–Livestock Interactions: The Stockperson and the Productivity and Welfare of Intensively Farmed Animals*.Wallingford: CAB International.

Humane Society of the United States. (2012). An HSUS report: The welfare of intensively confined animals in battery cages, gestation crates, and veal crates. https://www.humanesociety.org/sites/default/files/docs/hsus-report-animal-welfare-of-intensively-confined-animals.pdf (21 December 2021).

Koch, B.J., Hungate, B.A., and Price, L.B. (2017). Food-animal production and the spread of antibiotic resistance: The role of ecology. *Frontiers in Ecology and the Environment* 15 (6): 309–318.

Malmendier, U. and Schmidt, K. (2012). You owe me. National Bureau of Economic Research https://www.nber.org/system/files/working_papers/w18543/w18543.pdf (21 December 2021).

Morgan, L., Klement, E., Novak, S. et al. (2018). Effects of group housing on reproductive performance, lameness, injuries and saliva cortisol in gestating sows. *Preventive Veterinary Medicine* 160: 10–17.

Pask, J. (2015). Overview of Canada's anti-cruelty laws. Michigan State University College of Law. https://www.animallaw.info/article/overview-canadas-anti-cruelty-laws (21 December 2021).

Patterson, G. (n.d.). Productionvet NOW: The leading virtual care platform for veterinarians. https://vetnow.com/production-animal-veterinarian (21 December 2021).

Reese, J. (2019). *The End of Animal Farming*. Boston, MA: Beacon Press.

Shober, A.L. and Maguire, R.O. (2018). Manure management. In: *Reference Module in Earth Systems and Environmental Sciences* (ed. S.Elias). Amsterdam: Elsevier https://doi.org/10.1016/B978-0-12-409548-9.09115-6.

Sims, J.T. and Maguire, R.O. (2005). Manure management. In: *Encyclopedia of Soils in the Environment* (ed. D. Hillel), 402–410. Amsterdam: Elsevier. https://doi.org/10.1016/B0-12-348530-4/00515-4.

Sumner, C.L., Von Keyserlingk, M.A.G., and Weary, D.M. (2018). Perspectives of farmers and veterinarians concerning dairy cattle welfare. *Animal Frontiers* 8 (1): 8–13. doi:10.1093/af/vfx006.

Tannenbaum, J. (1995). *Veterinary Ethics: Animal Welfare, Client Relations, Competition and Collegiality*. St. Louis, Mosby.

van der Merwe, D., Jordaan, A., van den Berg, M. et al. (2018). Case report: Fipronil contamination of chickens in the Netherlands and surrounding countries. *ECVPH Food Safety Assurance* 7: 567–584. https://doi.org/10.3920/978-90-8686-877-3_23.

Wood, S.F., Podrasky, J., McMonagle, M.A. et al. (2017). Influence of pharmaceutical marketing on Medicare prescriptions in the District of Columbia. *PLoS ONE* 12 (10): e0186060. https://doi.org/10.1371/journal.pone.0186060

# 13

## Equines

*David W. Ramey*

## Introduction – What is Ethics?

Ethics is a very old field of philosophy that involves systematizing, defending, and recommending concepts of right and wrong conduct. Etymologically, the term ethics originates with horses, coming from the Greek word *ethos*, meaning "accustomed place" (as in "the habitat of horses," *Iliad* 6.511, 15.268).[1] One of the earliest examples of a code of professional ethics is the Hippocratic Oath, sometimes summarized as, "Above all, do no harm." Ethical concepts are commonsense, but they can be very difficult to apply, especially in some areas of equine practice. A more detailed explanation of the principles of ethics is found in Chapter 4.

One of the easiest ways to offend someone is to call them unethical. Furthermore, a suggestion of even marginally unethical behavior often leads to a defense along the lines of, "Everyone has their own ethics." The inherent assertion is undoubtedly true; one person's moral and ethical judgments may clearly differ from another's. As a result, even if individuals share some of the same ethical beliefs, they may disagree about how to behave in certain moral or ethical situations. But while people may have their own sense of ethics – that is, their own sense of right and wrong – some practices are clearly better (and therefore more ethical) than others. Practices that are kinder, fairer, in the interest of the horse's long-term health, supported by sound scientific evidence, and more honest are generally more ethical than practices that are mean-spirited, unfair, destructive to the horse's health, not supported by science, or untruthful. While everyone involved in the care of horses should strive to be ethical, this goal applies especially to veterinarians, who claim to be experts in horse health and welfare, and who expect people to trust them based on that assertion.

## Why Are Ethics Important in Equine Practice?

People who are perceived as being more ethical – kinder, fairer, etc. – are generally thought of more highly than people who are considered less ethical. In surveys of professions, nurses generally get high marks because (i) they are thought of as honest, and (ii) they do so much for other people (Gallup 2020). On the bottom end of the scale tend to be professions such as lawyers, used car salesmen, and members of the United States Congress: these individuals may have the reputation of being in their job mostly

*Ethics in Veterinary Practice: Balancing Conflicting Interests*, First Edition. Edited by Barry Kipperman and Bernard E. Rollin.
© 2022 John Wiley & Sons, Inc. Published 2022 by John Wiley & Sons, Inc.

for their own benefit. Veterinarians tend to rate up near the top of professional surveys in ethical behavior, even higher than physicians (Kedrowicz and Royal 2020).

In equine clinical practice, many people claim to have expertise: some of these individuals work in areas that are legally considered the practice of veterinary medicine. These people, many of whom do not have veterinary degrees, may claim special knowledge, or even a level of skill higher than veterinarians, including "dentists," "chiropractors," "massage therapists," "laser therapists," etc. As a result, it is important that veterinarians distinguish themselves from other, self-proclaimed experts in horse health. Veterinarians can be distinguished from other individuals who claim to be experts in animal health in three primary areas: ethics, scientific research, and because of their education, in medical and welfare concerns of all animals (a sort of special knowledge).

Thus, ethical practice offers veterinarians a unique opportunity to distinguish themselves as trusted providers of equine care. On the other hand, unethical conduct threatens to undermine the special status given to veterinarians. If veterinarians are perceived as acting unethically (i.e. not acting in the best interest of horses), society may be (and has been) motivated to act. In fact, people do not have to use veterinarians. Ethical conduct is one good reason why people might be inclined to use veterinary services; thus, ethical conduct is not only an ideal it is also good business.

Perhaps most importantly, ethical conduct builds trust. A strong veterinarian–client relationship, which is essential to building and maintaining a successful clinical practice, relies on trust. While it can be hard to gain and maintain, trust can be easily lost, particularly if a veterinarian is perceived as being dishonest or unethical.

## What Behaviors Characterize Ethical Professional Conduct?

Ethical standards and behavior provide confidence to the public about the reliability and actions they can expect when using the services of a professional. Professional organizations break down their ethical codes of conduct into discrete components (American Veterinary Medical Association [AVMA] n.d.). These components include:

- Honesty: Truthfulness and straightforwardness along with the absence of lying, cheating, or theft. This would include honesty about the potential effectiveness of treatments being offered, or honesty about the results of diagnostic tests.[2]
- Integrity: An adherence to moral principles.
- Transparency: Operating in such a way that it is easy for others to see what actions are being performed.
- Accountability: Answerability, blameworthiness, liability, and the expectation of assumption of responsibility for one's actions.
- Confidentiality: The expectation that the veterinarian will hold secret all information relating to a patient unless there is consent permitting disclosure from the client.
- Objectivity: Fairness, having no personal stake, factuality, and nonpartisanship (i.e. not acting in one's own self-interest).
- Respectfulness: Courteous regard for people's feelings.
- Obedience to the law: If there are laws relevant to the practice of veterinary medicine, obviously, it is unethical not to follow them.

## What Is a Horse?

The horse as a biological system has been studied for centuries. That study has resulted in a great deal of special knowledge that is not easy for lay people to understand or apply. Veterinarians are generally qualified to provide veterinary care based on their special knowledge; that is, veterinarians know how to anticipate what will happen to a horse after various pharmaco-medical interventions. However, there is no clear social consensus when it comes to how horses should be considered and treated.

Part of the difficulty with discussing ethics in equine practice is that there are at least two very disparate opinions as to the status of horses in society. There are also different opinions about what constitutes appropriate care. One view would be that horses are akin to companion animals (e.g. dogs and cats). Under such a view, horses are animals to be kept and cared for, essentially in perpetuity. These horses are essentially considered to be part of an extended human family and may be treated accordingly with little consideration of pecuniary measures of value.

Another perspective would be that horses are valued primarily for their ability to perform, either in various types of work, or in various competitions for money and/or prizes. As such, these horses may be viewed more like commodities.[3] That is, their inherent value may not be so much as an individual animal as it is a means to make a living and/or to bring acclaim to the humans that use them. Any number of "performance" horses may fall under this heading: racehorses, jumping horses, cutting horses, etc. There are various types of working equids as well.

Working and performance horses may be well attended while they are active, but such attention may not always be in the best interest of their long-term health (e.g. stress from prolonged stall confinement, inability to move freely, a variety of medications given to enhance performance or being fed high amounts of grain concentrates). In addition, horses that may be somewhat unhealthy, e.g. a horse with an osteoarthritic joint, may be treated in hopes of prolonging their performance lives without consideration of the long-term aspects of such treatment. For some of these horses, once their performance days are finished, their usefulness may be finished as well.

## What Makes Ethical Discussions in Equine Practice so Difficult?

Ethical equine veterinary practice would be much easier if veterinarians could always simply do what is in the best long-term health interests of the horse and not charge for doing so. However, the fact is, veterinary medicine is a business. While horse owners typically don't begrudge veterinarians the right to make a living, and while veterinarians have an ethical obligation to take care of themselves and their families, ethical lines can become blurry if the primary focus in taking care of or using horses is to make money.

In an ideal world, the best ethical conduct benefits everyone involved in the clinical interaction. However, in equine practice there are often many interested parties involved in therapeutic decisions regarding horses: owners, trainers, and riders, as well as independent entities, such as those who manufacture products. These individuals may have different interests. Unfortunately, due to various pressures from interested parties, the individual who may receive the least consideration – at least in the long term – is the horse.

## The Stakeholders in Ethical Discussions About Horses

If it is reasonable to assert that veterinarians should act ethically, and if ethical practice improves the public's perception of professions, one might reasonably wonder why it is necessary to have discussions on ethics at all, and why ethical practice may sometimes seem to be such an elusive goal. To answer these questions, it is necessary to look at the participants in clinical transactions in equine practice and then examine the obstacles to ethical behavior.

### Veterinarians

The veterinarian's ethical responsibility to him- or herself, as well as to the horse, should ideally come before the demands of the client. Otherwise stated, a veterinarian shouldn't do what he or she doesn't feel is right. Unfortunately, clients can put a good deal of pressure on veterinarians to provide treatments, not only to enhance performance, but also in end-of-life situations, where clients may push to prolong a horse's life even at the cost of its suffering. While doing what the client wants may increase client satisfaction, at least short term, in human medicine working to make the client happy is associated with *worse* outcomes and *greater* costs (Fenton et al. 2012). In veterinary medicine, client satisfaction has been inversely associated with the mental health of the veterinarian (Perret et al. 2020).

In addition to an intellectual and emotional undertaking, equine practice is also a business by which veterinarians support themselves and their families. As such, the veterinarian's obligation to him- or herself may be used as justification for putting the veterinarian's needs above ethical obligations to the horse, the horse owner, or society. However, ethics that is overly self-directed tends to foster irresponsible and dishonest conduct. Ultimately, conduct that considers only the veterinarian undermines the integrity of both the individual and the veterinary profession.

### Clients, Owners, and Trainers

Veterinary medicine differs from most of human medicine in that the client and the patient are not the same individual (or species). The human medical model most closely aligned with veterinary medicine is pediatric medicine. In pediatric practice, patient decisions are made without the input of the patient: someone else makes treatment decisions and pays the bills.

Although many clients want only what is best for their animals, others – particularly in performance horse disciplines – may have competing interests. For example, the goal of getting to the next show, the next race, or the next event may be more important to a client or trainer than the long-term health of the horse. Some clients may even be willing to risk injury to the animal in the pursuit of short-term gain.

In addition, clients can sometimes stand in the way of effective treatment, often demanding treatment – or lack of treatment – because of their "love" for their horse(s). A veterinarian is not ethically obliged to simply accede to a client's demands. The veterinarian's ethical responsibility to self and to the horse supersedes such demands. Veterinarians who act at the whim of a client also put themselves in a vulnerable position should a procedure go wrong: the defense, "I was just doing what the client wanted," is not tenable should an adverse reaction occur, and the procedure is not justifiable medically. The law generally assumes that the veterinarian's primary duty is to the animal and not to the client (McEachern and Weedon 2004).

Still, in the eyes of the law, owners have virtually complete autonomy regarding their animals, except for laws prohibiting overt cruelty and neglect. Owners may choose not to treat a sick horse, not to euthanize a suffering horse, or may demand therapy that may not be in accordance with the best interests of the horse, or that is even allowed by law. This situation can create a major problem for veterinarians who want to act only in the interest of the horse. The veterinary clinician does not often have the power of law behind them to force the owner to take (or prevent) action. Thus, although some veterinarians may see their role as analogous to pediatricians, society (i.e. the legal system) has not yet caught up with the ethics underlying that view, even though many members of society would probably agree with it.

The veterinarian's most powerful tool for getting clients to act in the best interest of the horse is their Aesculapian authority. This is the traditional "godlike" place of honor given to physicians in society, referring to Aesculapius, the Greek and Roman god of medicine and healing (Rollin 2002). However, this authority can easily fail if veterinarians do not fulfill their ethical responsibilities. For example, a veterinarian could advocate for an unproven therapy without disclosing this, causing the client to waste time and money, with no benefit for the animal. This action would be clearly unethical, lacking both honesty and transparency. If such actions were discovered, this would reflect poorly on the veterinarian as well as the veterinary profession.

Clients have few ethical responsibilities to their veterinarians. For example, one would hope that clients might be ethically obliged to pay their bills, to tell the truth about their horse(s), as well as to share information with the veterinarian about their concerns and expectations. However, in equine practice, one quickly realizes that in some cases, these hopes are futile. In fact, horse owners have neither the ethical responsibility nor legal obligation to employ veterinarians. In veterinarian–client relations, ethical obligations can be something of a one-way street. Thus, it is in the self-interest of veterinarians to seek out clients who act responsibly and who also have the best health interests of their horses in mind.

## Organizations

When members of the public lack training and expertise, they can be easily exploited. Thus, to prevent exploitation of the public and to preserve their own integrity, most professions have internally enforced ethical codes of practice to which members of the profession are expected to adhere. These codes allow a profession to define a standard of conduct. Ethical standards also help maintain the public's trust in a profession, encouraging the public to continue seeking their services.

### Breed Associations and Competition Bodies

The equine world is filled with various breed organizations and competition bodies that have their own rules and standards pertaining to the care and treatment of horses. For example, tail blocking is prohibited by law in several states and is against the rules of most show and breed organizations (Hepworth-Warren 2017). Ethical conduct on the part of veterinarians would mandate that they follow those rules (American Association of Equine Practitioners [AAEP] 2010).

### Veterinary Professional Organizations

Veterinary organizations have their own codes of ethics and have the authority to enforce those codes, usually by not allowing or rescinding membership. Self-policing allows a profession to maintain control over the standards to which they are held. Stringent self-policing serves as one way to handle internal problems within a profession and is an alternative to public relations campaigns to repair the damage that can occur when such internal problems are exposed. Unfortunately, self-policing attempts often fail because of the inherent conflicts of interest that occur. For example, whereas the legal profession has a model ethical code and more than 400,000 members, its members are not held in high esteem: in fact, the legal profession is routinely the brunt of jokes about its lack of ethics.

An organization may be loath to criticize the unethical practices of its members because of fears of bad publicity or loss of revenue. Consequently, in cases in which professional bodies are expected to regulate their own ethics, there are opportunities for such bodies to become self-serving. If professional bodies fail to regulate their own ethics, it can cast an entire profession into disrepute and lead to onerous external regulation. In the world of equestrian sport, this has happened and is happening. For example, the Horseracing Safety and Integrity Act was signed into law at the end of 2020, in part to address society's ethical concerns about horse racing (United States Congress 2020).

It would follow that veterinarians should also be active in self-policing their colleagues to maintain a high standard of practice. However, individuals may also be reluctant to criticize colleagues because of fear of being ostracized or of reprisal. Even the vernacular used to describe individuals who point out unethical practice is couched in pejorative terms (e.g. "ratting out," "snitching," "squealing"). Regardless, outside agencies are more than happy to make sure that veterinarians practice ethically and responsibly; veterinary malpractice law is rapidly evolving in the United States. Thus, it is as important for professional organizations to act ethically and responsibly as it is for its individual members.

## Manufacturers

Advertising and sponsorship are everywhere in equestrian events: manufacturers even serve as sponsors for many breed and professional organizations. This is ethically problematic since it may make unsuspecting horse owners more likely to purchase products that may not be effective treatments for their horses. From an ethical point of view, advertising should always be truthful and not make false or misleading claims: however, this is often not the case. The primary goal of manufacturers is to sell products. As a result, advertisers may fail to provide information about the risks of treatment or may not disclose that a product has not been shown to be effective. This is particularly problematic in the supplement industry, which, because of federal legislation is loosely regulated to the point that products do not have to meet scientific standards for efficacy, purity, quality, or content, provided they do not make direct therapeutic claims (United States Congress 1994). It follows that those veterinarians who recommend – or worse, sell and profit from – such products are acting in an ethically questionable manner.

## Society

Social responsibility is the concept that an individual has a responsibility to society: these responsibilities are beyond the individual's immediate self-interest (profit, professional success, etc.). Ethically speaking, "success" should be measured not only by how much money is made or how many horses are seen, but also by how many horses and people are helped. As such, "Equitarian" endeavors, or providing volunteer assistance at rescue facilities, pony clubs, or other organizations, are good examples of veterinarians fulfilling their ethical responsibilities to society. Such actions benefit the veterinary profession as well as the individuals who participate in such endeavors by generating goodwill and positive press.

Society largely allows veterinarians to regulate themselves based on two perceptions: (i) that veterinary medicine is a profession with "special knowledge"; and (ii) that veterinary medicine fulfills its obligations (including ethical ones) to the horse, horse owners, and society. Even so, society does not necessarily grant veterinarians a free pass pertaining to special knowledge. Indeed, laws pertaining to the regulation of veterinarians are mutable and have been amended to allow the practice of various modalities by non-veterinarians in individual states.

The mere holding of a veterinary license does not guarantee that the practice of veterinary medicine will retain its protected status. To help retain that status, veterinarians should consider it their ethical responsibility to society to advance knowledge of the practice of veterinary medicine. Veterinarians should use their knowledge to come up with better approaches for diagnosis and treatment, to confirm the utility of existing treatments, and to discard ineffective treatments.

Perceptions of how the veterinary profession is fulfilling its obligations to society are also important. It has been said that "Perception is reality"; the way others perceive veterinarians is "reality" for the veterinarian. For example, if veterinarians are perceived as "in it for the money" or as acting in ways deemed merely to protect their own turf – as opposed to acting in the best interest of the horse – society may choose to ignore the veterinarian's voice when discussing its concerns about horses, and it has frequently done so.

Whereas veterinarians may have ethical obligations to society, society has essentially no ethical obligations to veterinarians, or even to horse owners. Since most of society does not own horses, societal concerns are directed to the perceived welfare of horses, often without the benefit of direct experience or knowledge. In addition, societal concern for equine welfare appears to be increasing.

For example, society regulates how owners can keep horses; there are laws pertaining to horse welfare and abuse. Owners who fail to care for their horses in accordance with societal standards can have their horses taken away from them; individuals who treat their animals in a particular fashion can be fined or jailed. There are numerous examples of society's interest in the ethical treatment of horses. For example, the failure of the Tennessee Walking Horse industry to protect horse welfare led to federal legislation banning the practice of "soring." Soring is the practice of inflicting pain on the legs and hooves of horses with caustic chemicals, chains, and other objects to artificially create the high-stepping gait known as the "Big Lick" (United States Department of Agriculture/Animal and Plant Health Inspection Service [USDA/APHIS] 2020). Numerous other examples of societal regulations in the horse world – made with or despite advice from the veterinary community – include:

1) Federal legislation banning horse slaughter has been proposed and introduced in the US Congress several times, most recently in 2021 (American Society for the Prevention of Cruelty to Animals [ASPCA] 2021). Such proposed laws have been introduced over the objections of both the AAEP and the AVMA. It is inarguable that they were introduced because of societal concerns.
2) The Pregnant Mare Urine (PMU) Industry. The PMU Industry[4] was the subject of intense societal scrutiny in the late twentieth and early twenty-first centuries. As a result of that pressure, improved regulations were put in place concerning care of the mares and foals. Although criticism still exists, published ethical standards and regulations might have helped prevent some of the furor that was directed at that industry.
3) The carriage horse industry. Although many feel that horse-drawn carriage rides are picturesque and romantic ways to see major metropolitan areas, others feel that it is a form of equine abuse, and carriage horses have been banned in some cities (Newswire 2020). Ultimately, the fate of the carriage horse industry will result from a tug of war between those two interests. Those interested in maintaining a viable carriage horse industry would do well to ensure that their horses are treated ethically and humanely and do so vocally and transparently: for example, by publishing guidelines and schedules for examinations and treatment, to allay concerns from those who feel that carriage horses should be banned from city streets (ASPCA n.d.).

## Horses

The ethical responsibilities of horse ownership, societal interests in horse welfare, and veterinary medical treatment should dovetail, all working together for the best interest of the horse's health. The veterinarian's ethical duty is to the horse: consequently, veterinarians must avoid orders or requests from a third party that are not in the best interest of the patient. Unfortunately, client demands – for example, for "better" performance – may not be in the best long-term health interest of the horse. This fact sometimes makes the veterinarian's goal of ethical practice in the best interest of the horse's health difficult.

In addition, societal concerns – even if they are well-meaning – may not be expressed in ways that are beneficial for the horse. For example, while the goal of allowing horses to run free on the range in the American West may be laudable, it may not be in the best interest of the horses if there is not sufficient range to sustain them or there is a lack of sufficient predators to control their herds (Bureau of Land Management [BLM] 2020). Nevertheless, by virtue of their special knowledge about horses, ethical veterinarians are in the best position to advocate for the welfare of the horse, and it is to the ultimate advantage of both the horse and the veterinary profession that they do so.

## Relevant Ethical Issues

### Selling, Promoting, and Prescribing Products

The fact that veterinarians profit from what they sell is full of ethical landmines. For ethical reasons, physicians cede the prescription of, and payment for, medications to pharmacists so that they will not be perceived as having a conflict of interest. While veterinarians can ethically both sell and prescribe prescription medications, and while horse owners usually don't mind paying for something that was prescribed for a horse, the inherent conflict of interest is apparent. Keeping the horse's and owner's best interests at the forefront of treatment decisions may help alleviate ethical concerns.

There are several advantages when clients purchase their medications from veterinarians, all of which are consistent with good medicine and ethical practice:

- Veterinarians have medications in stock and can dispense medications immediately.
- Veterinarians can answer questions, provide instructions for use, and demonstrate how to give medications.
- Medications prescribed by veterinarians have been handled properly and have been controlled from the point of manufacture through distribution and dispensing, providing clients quality assurance.

There are many businesses that show little concern for any of these ethical issues associated with selling prescription medications. However, "fighting fire with fire" by offering drugs on demand, or as an agent of a pharmaceutical company not directly involved in clinical care of the horse, is unethical. Furthermore, in most states it is unlawful for a veterinarian to write a prescription or dispense a drug outside a veterinarian–client–patient relationship (AVMA n.d.). On the other hand, in most states, when a client requests a prescription from a veterinarian for a horse that is under the veterinarian's care instead of purchasing the medication directly from the veterinarian, the veterinarian is generally obliged to provide it.

The fact that veterinarians may ethically sell products does not mean that all products are sold or recommended ethically. When horses require treatment for disease or injury, it is in their best interest, and an ethical imperative, that they receive the treatments that are most likely to be effective and that they are not given treatments which have no measurable effects. Furthermore, if a treatment has not been shown to be effective, ethical principles of informed consent demand that clients be told about its potential limitations (see Chapter 5). A person selecting a therapy for a horse must fully understand:

- The nature of the treatment.
- Reasonable alternatives to the proposed intervention.
- The relevant risks, benefits, costs, and uncertainties related to each treatment.

The failure to provide necessary information so that the client fully understands what is known about the potential risks and benefits of a treatment is an ethical failure on the part of the person providing treatment.

Furthermore, from an ethical perspective, therapies should neither be promoted nor prescribed based on criteria that are not relevant to the likelihood of a successful outcome for the horse. Promoting or prescribing a therapy using terminology such as, "new," "natural," "holistic," "not 'Western' medicine," "cutting edge," or "ancient" is ethically questionable. None of these adjectives – even if accurate – has anything to do with whether the treatment helps the horse. Instead, it is an effort to promote a therapy to people of a certain mindset. Any term has ethical implications if it implies a level of expertise that other veterinarians do not have. Except for veterinary specialists certified by the AVMA, descriptive titles may only reflect the personal philosophy of the veterinarian, or the circumstances under which they have chosen to practice. Such titles can be ethically troublesome if they are used primarily for public relations purposes.

## Experimental Treatments

It is an unfortunate fact that not all conditions of the horse have cures. Furthermore, some treatments available for horses result in healing that may be less than ideal (e.g. treatment for injuries to the digital flexor tendons). As a result, all parties in equine medical transactions are eager for better alternatives for many conditions.

Experimental treatments are an ethical dilemma in equine practice. There is a high degree of uncertainty with many treatments currently being advocated. Under such circumstances, it is impossible for an owner to give truly informed consent. Influenced by the promotion of and desire for newer and more effective treatments, veterinarians may have to choose between using a treatment of proven effectiveness and one with medical "promise." In equine medicine, treatments are usually released well in advance of a significant body of research, and such research as may be conducted is usually based on small sample sizes. Long-term follow-up is generally lacking. Furthermore, conflicts of interest can arise when the veterinarian owns (and must pay for) the product or service that the veterinarian is also recommending.

Unfortunately, the search for newer, "cutting-edge" treatments can be an ethical trap. Misleading and/or unclear information can skew owners' expectations of experimental treatments (Marks and Hahn 2020). Marketing for such treatments usually reaches the horse-owning public well in advance of any evidence for their effectiveness. Horse owners may be willing to try to do anything for their horse, even without knowing if the proposed treatment is safe or effective, and even if such treatments are expensive. However, ethical veterinary practice requires balancing the hopes of clients against ensuring that clients are properly informed and that the horse is not put at risk of harm. Such treatments may simply increase the cost of care with no measurable benefit to the horse. Veterinarians should act in the best interest of the horse and the client, and not in their own self-interest.

If a therapy offers only promise and the effects haven't been scientifically proven, the correct term for the treatment is "experimental." There is nothing wrong with an experimental treatment, of course. Experimental therapies such as stem cells, gene therapy, and platelet-rich plasma (PRP) are currently employed in the treatment of conditions such as osteoarthritis or injuries of tendons and ligaments (to name a few). One benefit of such treatments is that they are individualized: that is, they are made from the horse's own cells. However, the marketing of such products is often ethically questionable. Implying that a therapy is "new," "promising," or "advanced," or that it is "regenerative" (implying that the treatment replaces the lost or injured tissue with new tissue that is the same as the lost tissue, or at least improves the speed or quality of healing) might inappropriately influence an owner's expectation of success and lead them to choose such therapies, even when there is no advantage compared with conventional treatments.

It is certainly possible to provide such products or services ethically. However, providing treatments of unknown benefit to the horse carries many ethical responsibilities. It is important that clients have access to impartial and accurate information and are made aware of uncertainties about possible outcomes when deciding about trying an experimental treatment. Clients should be advised that:

1) The therapy that is being proposed may not be approved by the US Food and Drug Administration (FDA) (or other governmental oversight body).
2) Their horse is not part of a clinical trial. That is, the client is being asked to pay for a treatment where the benefit is unknown, the cost is certain, and the treatment results are not being compiled.
3) If such information is available, clients should be informed regarding other horses that have been treated, comparing how treated horses did in comparison to non-treated horses. However, it may be impossible for a client to give informed consent unless a therapy is honestly represented.
4) Clients should be informed of what to do about adverse reactions.

Many conditions of the horse require better treatments. But it is one thing to have a person agree to participate in an experiment with their horse: it is quite another to sell that person on the "promise" of an attractively named therapy and not bother to keep track of the results. Due to such concerns, in 2019, the FDA issued a warning to consumers about stem cell therapies (USFDA 2019).

From an ethical point of view, the level of evidence for an experimental therapy must be communicated to the client. Ethical veterinarians should operate according to their best assessment of the current data, considering the relative risks and benefits of different strategies and the evidence for them. Healthcare decisions made for the horse should be made with the horse's best interests in mind and should not be influenced by extraneous factors such as the veterinarian's self-esteem.

## Performance Horses

If one believes that it is acceptable for horses to be used in sporting activities for the enjoyment of people (a hotly contested topic), then it seems inarguable that those animals should be as healthy as possible when they perform. As such, treatments to restore health and welfare where disease previously existed – antibiotics to treat respiratory infections, surgeries to correct repairable fractures, etc. – are certainly not only ethical, but part of the veterinarian's responsibility to the horse, themselves, and society.

However, returning a horse to normal so that they can perform to their capabilities is not necessarily the goal of treating horses in competitions. For example, some clients may want "increased performance" so that they can get a ribbon, belt buckle, money, or some other prize. Other horses have demonstrable musculoskeletal problems and may be expected to perform despite those problems if competition circumstances demand. Veterinarians may get in an ethical bind by attempting to provide treatments to enhance performance, or to provide treatments to allow a horse to perform despite ongoing injury.

Unfortunately, care of performance horses may result in inherent conflicts of interest. While the primary duty of the equine veterinarian is to the horse, the goal of long-term good for the horse's health and having it compete may conflict. Since the veterinarian may be employed by individuals whose primary interest is short-term gain, the professional success of a veterinarian working under such circumstances may rely on keeping the horse in competition, which may also mean advocating for short-term success at the risk of long-term detriment. If this conflict influences the veterinarian's actions, the veterinarian can ultimately be held accountable.

Similarly, the veterinarian may be involved when a horse is returning to competition after injury. In most cases, owners and trainers want to return the horse to competition as soon as possible. Rest and rehabilitation might be best for the horse's long-term health: however, rest might mean the horse misses an important competition. If the horse wins, it's value may increase: if it competes, it risks reinjury. Under such circumstances, the veterinarian can find themselves in a difficult dilemma, risking criticism if advising that the horse is held out of competition, but also if the horse is returned to work too early and sustains additional injury. Awareness of these conflicts is the first step to acting ethically.

Horses have no knowledge of the nature of performance and competition. A horse who finishes last in a race is not concerned by their "failure" to win; a horse who doesn't switch their leads behind is clearly not hampered by the "problem." Horses who fail to perform to expectations, although otherwise healthy, are a clear target for those who claim to be able to affect performance by some intervention, be it a veterinary treatment, a supplement, or some form of "alternative" therapy (see Case Study 13.1). Without evidence that a problem really exists, and that the treatment might be effective, promoting such a therapy would likely waste time and the owner's money, and subject the horse to risk (of treatment) without expected benefit. Those circumstances may seem unethical, but they form the focus of a good deal of product and service promotion, and, unfortunately, occur in every segment of the equine industry.

In human medicine, where issues concerning ethics and competitive sports are regularly discussed, there is no universally accepted code of ethics. However, the International Federation of Sports Medicine declares, "It is the responsibility of the sports medicine physician to determine whether the injured athletes should continue training or participating in competition" (International Federation of Sports Medicine n.d.). From a legal liability standpoint, veterinarians should be mindful of the risks they take when they treat horses to get them to perform while injured.

Rules regarding the use of performance-enhancing drugs are explicitly stated by some equestrian sport organizations (United States Equestrian Federation 2021) but are conspicuously absent in others. It's unethical to use a prohibited substance; however, just because a medication is not a prohibited substance does not also mean that it is ethically appropriate to use it. For example, while a sedative medication may be prohibited in competition, an herbal sedative preparation is not an acceptable alternative: the intent of the rules is that horses are not sedated. Efforts to limit drug use in performance horses are undermined when a substance is used because, "It doesn't test" (i.e. the substance is not detectable). Of course, the veterinarian should not use any drug that is likely to adversely affect the horse's health.

In the heat of competition, with money, reputations, and prizes at stake, an equine veterinarian can be placed in a difficult spot. Unless a horse performs to expectations, the owner/trainer will have concerns that the considerable investment made in maintaining the horse is being wasted. For some owners, that investment is the primary consideration and horses are expected to "earn their keep." Not doing what the client wants risks losing the client. Alternatively, doing what the client wants may not be in the best interest of the horse. Some clients may choose to retain equine veterinarians not because they are ethical, but because they are not. In some environments, ethical concerns for the welfare of the horse are not viewed as a virtue, and veterinarians who refuse to practice according to client expectations of "increasing" or "improving" performance may not be retained.

However, even in performance situations, there are usually clear ethical lines. For example, it would be obviously unethical to inject a local anesthetic into a horse's osteoarthritic joint prior to performance, not only because there are regulations against such practice, but because such an action would put the life of both horse and rider at risk. Similarly, one could not ethically support giving a horse a nonsteroidal anti-inflammatory drug to mask a viral respiratory disease-induced fever: such an action would put not only the health of the treated horse at risk, but also the health of other horses.

To be clear, not all medication that is administered to performance horses is given unethically. In fact, in some cases, ethical lines may be quite blurry. For example, in racing horses, Furosemide has been shown to both increase performance and decrease the incidence of exercise-induced pulmonary hemorrhage (Knych et al. 2018). One can easily argue either side of the question of whether Furosemide should be used prerace: on the one hand, it enhances performance (and possibly the risk of injury), and on the other since it decreases bleeding from the lungs, it is beneficial for the horse's health. As another example, administering a nonsteroidal anti-inflammatory drug may improve the health and welfare of the horse if given postrace to relieve soreness, but may be entirely unethical prerace if given to mask limb soreness, due to both applicable regulations as well as to increased risk of injury to horse and rider.

To a certain extent – and partially due to a lack of concern for ethical obligations to society – decisions about treatments to "improve" equine performance are being taken out of the hands of the veterinary profession, horse owners, and trainers. Society has clearly expressed its distaste for the use of performance-enhancing medications in all human sporting endeavors. Further, society is expressing increasing interest in equine welfare, and is frowning on what it perceives (rightly or wrongly) as an indiscriminate use of performance-enhancing treatments. Because of societal concerns, many performance horse endeavors are coming under increasing scrutiny, and society is stepping in to regulate such endeavors based on its concern for the health and welfare of the horses: witness US legislation pertaining to "soring" of Tennessee Walking Horses (Cota 2021), horse slaughter (ASPCA 2021), and newly proposed federal legislation for oversight of the thoroughbred racing industry (US Congress 2020).

**Case Study 13.1    A performance horse for which "hock injections" have been requested**

A horse trainer employs you to attend to most of the horses in his stable. He presents a 12-year-old Warmblood gelding for hock injections because the horse is not jumping to expectations. He states that he has known the horse for two years and that the horse periodically requires "maintenance" to jump properly. He requests that you inject the horse's hocks, without giving additional detail (e.g. which of the joints of the tarsus, which medication should be used, etc.) You watch the horse move and do not detect lameness, and the horse willingly goes over jumps.

**What should you do?**

Ethical analysis:
The relevant interests in this ethical dilemma include the horse, the trainer, the horse's owner, the veterinarian, and the veterinary profession. You suspect that there is nothing wrong with the horse: however, the trainer is making demands consistent with his experience and expectations for horses that are in jumping training.

Choices include:

1.  Inject the horse's hocks, per the trainer's request.
2.  Persuade the trainer that you would like to do a lameness examination prior to considering treating the horse.
3.  Contact the owner and discuss the situation prior to examining or treating the horse.
4.  Suggest another mode of treatment.
5.  Treat the horse and suggest that other horses in the barn may need the same "routine" treatment.
6.  Refuse to treat the horse.

Owner or trainer requests for specific treatment are common in settings where horses are used for performance. Many owners and trainers have been "educated" that performance horses may require occasional therapeutic injections due to inflammation caused by performance, for chronic joint problems such as osteoarthritis, or even for joint "maintenance," where horses may be believed to need periodic interventions due to the putative wear and tear on joints from competition. Therapy driven by owner or trainer demands is an unfortunate part of performance horse practice, because they may ascribe "failures" of performance to an underlying physical cause instead of behavioral causes, rider effects, or other possibilities.

The expedient approach might be to inject the horse's hocks and fulfill the trainer's expectations. This also economically benefits you. Furthermore, the ritual of injecting the hock might induce a perceived benefit via the placebo effect and reinforce the perception that you have a special skill needed for the horse to perform (Arnold et al. 2020). Assuming that there is nothing wrong with the horse, performing the procedure requested would subject the horse to some risk without expected benefit (Steel et al. 2013). If the risk outweighs the potential benefit, there is neither a scientific nor ethical rationale for the procedure.

In addition, such an approach also may cause moral stress. Under such circumstances, the veterinarian is no longer working as a health professional: rather, he or she is working as a technician-on-demand. One could attempt to rationalize such a decision to treat based on the premise that it may prevent a future problem, but under that rationale, one could argue for injecting dozens of joints, or performing numerous unnecessary procedures. Further, performing services on demand may reflect poorly on the veterinary profession. Instead of being viewed as diagnosticians and advocates for equine health, veterinarians who inject joints under such circumstances may be viewed as solely acting in their own interest, or as acting to pursue revenue, but certainly not as acting in the best interests of the horse.

Attempting to persuade the trainer or owner to allow for an examination prior to proceeding with any procedure would certainly advocate for the horse's interest. However, suggesting an examination may be considered by some trainers as an affront to their authority. Thus, the veterinarian should be careful to acknowledge the expertise of the trainer while at the same time asserting their concern that the best care be delivered to the horse.

Contacting the owner of the horse prior to engaging in the procedure also runs the risk of alienating the trainer/agent. While your ultimate obligation is to the horse and horse owner (who pays the bills), direct communication with the horse owner can occasionally cause conflict, especially if there is a misunderstanding or misinterpretation. Thus, it is in the veterinarian's interest to make sure that all parties are properly informed and that communication channels are clear.

Suggesting another, less invasive mode of treatment would mediate the potential risk of direct harm from an intra-articular injection and may be considered as a "lesser evil."

Treating the horse and suggesting that other horses that have not been examined might benefit from the same treatment would be clearly unethical.

Refusing to treat the horse, while an ethically tenable position, would almost certainly result in the loss of the client. However, refusing to simply treat on demand would help avoid long-term consequences, such as moral stress (see Chapter 22) from abrogating your responsibility to the animal. Unfortunately, in many cases, economics plays a large role in the decision-making process.

Ideally, discussing a horse's condition and the best treatment options (including no treatment) with the owner, trainer, agent, and/or other caretakers (e.g. farriers) is the most likely means for finding a solution for the horse that achieves the greatest benefit for everyone involved. Furthermore, alternative solutions may be discovered. On the other hand, if the owners or trainers insist on a course of action despite the veterinarian's attempts to act in the horse's best interest, the veterinarian may be forced to realize that the ethics of the owner and/or trainer/agent may not be congruent with theirs and may be faced with difficult decisions.

## Inevitability and the Illusion of Futility

"If I don't do it, somebody else will." This is a well-known and time-honored rationalization, suggesting that no matter what action is taken by an individual, a particular outcome is inevitable (Glover and Scott-Taggart 1975; Fisher and Ravizza 1991). The rationale is clear enough. An action, for example, administering a forbidden substance to a horse, is objectionable. The concern is that if the veterinarian who is present does not undertake the action, someone else will, and the substance will be administered regardless: a single person's act of omission is therefore insignificant. Consequently, the veterinarian may conclude that there is no point in not giving the substance, because it will not prevent the action, and business will be lost. The presumption is that ethical refusal to do the right thing will only hurt the ethical person without preventing the unethical action. Under such circumstances, actions become Darwinian, in which the goal becomes survival.

Such Darwinian behavior was captured by Joseph Heller in his 1961 novel, *Catch-22* (Heller 1961).

"From now on I'm thinking only of me."

Major Danby replied indulgently with a superior smile, "But, Yossarian, suppose everyone felt that way?"

"Then," said Yossarian, "I'd certainly be a damned fool to feel any other way, wouldn't I?"

Of course, this rationale is faulty, self-serving, and absurd. If a group of young people were to come across a solitary old person, and one of the group decided that the old person should be robbed, the rest of the group would not be blameless if they decided to participate in the robbery because it was going to happen anyway. In that same vein, it could be argued that it is more humane for an unethical procedure (i.e. tail blocking or cutting a tail) to be performed by a veterinarian, with the use of aseptic technique, adequate sedation, and postprocedure analgesia, than it is to subject the animal to the risk of such procedures performed by an untrained individual. When considered in a vacuum, that is undoubtedly the case; invasive procedures should be performed by trained individuals with the use of adequate postoperative analgesia. However, the assertion that an action is inevitable overlooks the fact that it would still be unethical, and its performance by veterinarians would only serve to perpetuate the unethical practice. Thus, it could not be condoned. In fact, the inevitability rationale is only invoked when someone has something to lose (i.e. business) by not doing the dubious action, or something to gain (i.e. money) by doing it. In fact, there are times when someone else will *not* perform the unethical action.

Furthermore, the impact of refusal to act unethically can also lead to a good result, even when the action happens. The individual's determination to do right is always desirable. Clearly, invoking inevitability is merely an excuse for not acting in the best interest of the horse.

## Protecting the Veterinary Turf

In equine practice, many individuals who are *not* veterinarians assert that they provide care that is critical for the health of horses. Veterinarians may be concerned about loss of revenue to such individuals. Such concerns have led veterinarians to co-opt terms from other professions to try to buttress their own authority or to distinguish themselves from their colleagues (e.g. "chiropractor" or "podiatrist"). This linguistic legerdemain is ethically questionable: imagine the outcry from the veterinary profession if a Doctor of Chiropractic (DC) were to identify as a "veterinarian." However, such vernacular also gives horse owners very little ability to distinguish veterinarians from other providers of equine health services. It takes no small amount of hubris to assert that a veterinarian is doing "chiropractic" on horses better or worse than a licensed DC who went to school to do chiropractic (merits of the associated procedures notwithstanding). Similarly, veterinarians who provide special products or supplements may have a difficult time distinguishing themselves from other purveyors of such products.

Veterinarians who perform necessary services, supported by good science, knowledge, and ethics are in the best position to build client trust. Other attempts to maintain professional hegemony over the horse's care are likely to be derided as "turf protection" or as being "in it for the money" by those with competing interests. The veterinary turf is best protected when the welfare of the horse is the primary consideration.

## When Treatment Goals Collide

Other difficult ethical dilemmas may occur when a client's ideology differs from that of the veterinarian. Consider a horse suffering from chronic laminitis, in which there are no realistic options except euthanasia. Despite many veterinarians' opinions that euthanasia decisions should be left up to the client, there are cases in which the client refuses to let go, and the horse suffers. In such cases, a veterinarian should consider doing whatever it takes to end the animal's suffering and pull out all stops to persuade the owner to euthanize, if, in the veterinarian's judgment, the animal has no positive quality of life left.

Therapies given to "do everything possible" or that lack evidentiary foundation can prolong animal suffering and waste client resources. Giving such therapies is not irrational, as it provides hope and a sense of control over the horse's disease. However, veterinarians are not ethically obligated to provide, or even to discuss, therapies that the veterinarian deems to be futile (see Chapter 10). Clinical decisions in such circumstances must follow both clinical judgments about the therapy's chance of success as well as consideration of the client's goals (Lantos et al. 1989). If a client demands an essentially harmless but probably worthless therapy, perhaps the best a veterinarian can do is articulate their reasons for rejecting the therapy in question and attempt to continue to advocate for the horse.

Even when treatment goals collide, ethical veterinarians should consider continuing to work with their clients, in part to help ensure that unscrupulous practitioners or the cost of new treatments do not cause financial hardship or burden, and in part to keep the client focused on objective milestones that signify efficacy or lack thereof.

## Conclusions

If it were easy to be ethical, there would be no need for discussions on ethics. While doing the right thing and acting fairly and ethically is at the foundation of building a professional reputation, there are times when telling the truth or refusing to perform a procedure may result in loss of the client and may not be in a veterinarian's immediate self-interest. There are times when acting ethically carries a cost. Ultimately, the acid test of one's character and commitment to ethics is whether they will do the right thing even if it is not necessarily in their immediate best interest to do so.

To a certain extent, ethical conduct constrains a practitioner's ability to do what they – or even the client – wants. While some may chafe at such constraints, the legal system stands ready to provide a reminder that there are limits to the veterinarian's autonomy. The fact is that veterinary professionals cannot simply do whatever they want. On the other hand, pressures applied by owners, trainers, and riders may mean that ethical conduct, with the horse's best health interests as the primary goal, may not be valued. Nevertheless, if ethical practice is perceived as the standard by which veterinarians should operate, ethical veterinarians and the organizations they represent should lead the fight against unethical practices. If not, societal concerns about unethical practices open the door to the legal profession and legislators to redress ethical complaints.

Although ethical practice can be a challenge for equine veterinarians, strict attention to ethical practice provides an opportunity for veterinarians to separate themselves from other providers of products and services to horse owners. Ethics is a powerful driver of clients' perceptions of trust, honesty, and professionalism. If veterinarians are perceived as practicing for the benefit of the horse, their opinions and expertise are likely to be solicited: on the other hand, if they are perceived as being in it for themselves, they may be heavily criticized (Bogdanich et al. 2012). Professional organizations representing veterinarians should advocate strongly for the ethical treatment of horses and especially before public pressure requires that they do so. Leaders can strongly influence unethical behavior in the workplace. Vocal advocacy for the welfare of the horse and ethical conduct only serves to benefit equine veterinarians, as well as the veterinary profession.

## Notes

1 Late Latin borrowed the Greek word as *ethicus*, the feminine of which *ethica*, for "moral philosophy," is the origin of the modern English word "ethics".
2 In 2019, a lawsuit was filed alleging falsification of radiographic records of Thoroughbred sales yearlings. https://horseplayusa.com/lawsuit-against-hagyard-equine-medical-reveals-misdating-of-auction-x-rays. The Kentucky State Board of Veterinary Medicine investigated the claims and settled with eight veterinarians, ordering them to make "administrative payments" to offset the costs of the investigations (Voss 2019).

3  The two positions are not mutually exclusive.
4  The PMU industry collects urine from pregnant mares as a source of an estrogen conjugate sometimes used in hormone replacement for postmenopausal women to relieve the symptoms of menopause.

## References

American Association of Equine Practitioners (AAEP) (2010). Ethical and professional guidelines. https://aaep.org/guidelines/aaep-ethical-and-professional-guidelines (accessed 20 June 2021).

American Society for the Prevention of Cruelty to Animals (ASPCA) (n.d.). Policies and positions: Carriage horses. https://www.aspca.org/about-us/aspca-policy-and-position-statements/carriage-horses (accessed 19 June 2021).

American Society for the Prevention of Cruelty to Animals (ASPCA) (2021). Animal welfare groups commend federal lawmakers for reintroducing bill to ban horse slaughter. https://www.prnewswire.com/news-releases/animal-welfare-groups-commend-federal-lawmakers-for-reintroducing-bill-to-ban-horse-slaughter-301295437.html (accessed 19 June 2021).

American Veterinary Medical Association (AVMA) (n.d.). Principles of veterinary medical ethics of the AVMA. https://www.avma.org/resources-tools/avma-policies/principles-veterinary-medical-ethics-avma (accessed 19 June 2021).

Arnold, M.H., Komesaroff, P., and Kerridge, I. (2020). Understanding the ethical implications of the rituals of medicine. *Ethics in Medicine* 50 (9): 1123–1131.

Bogdanich, W., Drape, J., and Ruiz, R. (2012). Racing economics collide with the veterinarian's oath. *New York Times* http://www.nytimes.com/2012/09/22/us/at-the-track-racing-economics-collide-with-veterinariansoath.html (accessed 20 June 2021).

Bureau of Land Management (BLM) (2020). BLM begins new fertility control trial as overpopulation of wild horses and burros on public lands reaches new heights. https://www.blm.gov/press-release/blm-begins-new-fertility-control-trial-overpopulation-wild-horses-and-burros-public (accessed 19 June 2021).

Cota, J. (2021). Why are U.S. lawmakers taking an unusual step to fight horse soring? *American Farrier's Journal*. https://www.americanfarriers.com/blogs/1-from-the-desk-of-afj/post/12665-why-are-us-lawmakers-taking-an-unusual-step-to-fight-horse-soring (accessed 20 June 2021).

Fenton, J.J., Jerant, A.F., Bertakis, K.D. et al. (2012). The cost of satisfaction: A national study of patient satisfaction, health care utilization, expenditures, and mortality. *Archives of Internal Medicine* 172: 405–411.

Fisher, J.M. and Ravizza, M. (1991). Responsibility and inevitability. *Ethics* 101 (2): 258–278.

Gallup (2020). Honesty/ethics in professions. https://news.gallup.com/poll/1654/honesty-ethics-professions.aspx (accessed 19 June 2021).

Glover, J. and Scott-Taggart, M. (1975). It makes no difference whether I do it or not. *Proceedings of the Aristotelian Society* 49: 171–209. Supplementary Volumes.

Heller, J. (1961). *Catch-22*. New York: Simon and Schuster.

Hepworth-Warren, K. (2017). The truth about tail blocks. *Equus* 476 https:// equusmagazine.com/horse-world/tail-blocks-truth (accessed 20 June 2021).

International Federation of Sports Medicine (n.d.). Code of ethics. https://www.fims.org/ about/code-ethics (accessed 20 June 2021).

Kedrowicz, A.A. and Royal, K.D. (2020). A comparison of public perceptions of physicians and veterinarians in the United States. *Veterinary Sciences* 7: 50.

Knych, H., Wilson, W.D., Vale, A. et al. (2018). Effectiveness of furosemide in attenuating exercise-induced pulmonary haemorrhage in horses when administered at 4- and 24-h prior to high-speed training. *Equine Veterinary Journal* 50 (3): 350–355.

Lantos, J.D., Singer, P.A., Walker, R.M. et al. (1989). The illusion of futility in medical practice. *The American Journal of Medicine* 87 (1): 81–84.

Marks, P.W. and Hahn, S. (2020). Identifying the risks of unproven regenerative medicine. *Journal of the American Medical Association* 324 (3): 241–242.

McEachern, M.M. and Weedon, G.R. (2004). Modern trends in veterinary malpractice: How our evolving attitudes toward nonhuman animals will change veterinarian medicine. *Animal Law* 10 (125): 125–161.

Newswire (2020). Horse carriage ban: Chicago's 2020 "feel good story". https://apnews. com/article/health-coronavirus-pandemic-animal-welfare-lung-disease-diseases-and-conditions-a7bdd31bffb2c182a07e54a0a29a4279 (accessed 19 June 2021).

Perret, J., Best, C., Coe, J. et al. (2020). The complex relationship between veterinarian mental health and client satisfaction. *Frontiers in Veterinary Science* 7: 92.

Rollin, B.E. (2002). The use and abuse of Aesculapian authority in veterinary medicine. *Journal of the American Veterinary Medical Association* 220 (8): 1144–1149.

Steel, C.M., Pannirselvam, R.R., and Anderson, G.A. (2013). Risk of septic arthritis after intra-articular medication: A study of 16,624 injections in thoroughbred racehorses. *Australian Veterinary Journal* 91 (7): 268–273.

United States Congress (1994). Dietary Supplement Health and Education Act of 1994. https://ods.od.nih.gov/About/DSHEA_Wording.aspx (accessed 20 June 2021).

United States Congress (2020). Horseracing Integrity and Safety Act of 2020. https://www. congress.gov/bill/116th-congress/house-bill/1754/text (accessed 20 June 2021).

United States Department of Agriculture/Animal and Plant Health Inspection Service (USDA/APHIS) (2020). Horse Protection Act. https://www.aphis.usda.gov/aphis/ ourfocus/animalwelfare/SA_HPA (accessed 22 December 2021).

United States Equestrian Federation (2021). Drugs and medications. https://www.usef. org/compete/resources-forms/rules-regulations/drugs-medications (accessed 4 August 2021).

United States Food and Drug Administration (USFDA) (2019). FDA warns about stem cell therapies. https://www.fda.gov/consumers/consumer-updates/fda-warns-about-stem-cell-therapies (accessed 19 June 2021).

Voss, N. (2019). Hagyard settles lawsuit with veterinarians over contract dispute. Paulick Report. https://www.paulickreport.com/news/the-biz/hagyard-settles-lawsuit-with-veterinarians-over-contract-dispute (accessed 19 June 2021).

## 14

# Animals in Zoos, Aquaria, and Free-Ranging Wildlife

*Sathya K. Chinnadurai, Barbara de Mori, and Jackie Gai*

## Introduction

The fundamental ethical concern in veterinary practice – whether veterinarians should prioritize animal or client/owner interests – becomes quite difficult to address when dealing with wild animals, both free-ranging and in human care. Clients can be individual owners, but also zoos, sanctuaries, rescue centers, game reserves, and so on, and conflicts arise not only between the animal and client, but also between the interests of the individual animal and those of the species or population it belongs to. Approaches to addressing these conflicts are influenced by our beliefs regarding the duties humans have to wild animals: do humans regard wild animals as belonging to nature or as being dependent on humans? Alternatively, should we treat them as pests when they conflict with our interests, or as ambassadors for their species when we keep them in zoos and sanctuaries? Depending on the different values we place on wild animals in these different scenarios, veterinarians working with them can be challenged by ethical concerns that may be a source of moral distress (see Chapter 22).

There are myriad moral concerns and ethical dilemmas veterinarians encounter when devoting their professional expertise to wild animals, starting with the large number of species they must deal with. Medical knowledge of a single species can be very limited, so very often veterinarians must base treatment or anesthetic protocols on those of similar species. Being advocates and "speaking up" for the interests of wild animals can be very challenging and may be perceived as contentious or confrontational. Most of the challenges are similar to those encountered in other sectors of veterinary practice and are dependent on the differing moral status attributed to the animals. For example, if an individual wild animal belongs to a private owner, veterinarians will probably treat them as a pet or companion, with the additional challenge of dealing with a wild animal. In another example, if an individual animal is perceived as surplus in a population management scenario under human care, veterinarians may be required to euthanize a healthy animal, as occurs for domestic animals raised for food or research purposes.

When it comes to conserving biodiversity, whether the individual animal belongs to an endangered species or a common one may make a difference in the quality of veterinary care we can provide. When dealing with free-ranging wildlife, additional challenges arise: do we let nature take its course or do we intervene to care for an injured animal in the wild? What about rescuing an injured animal for the purpose of being released if that animal is conceived of as belonging to an invasive species that instead

*Ethics in Veterinary Practice: Balancing Conflicting Interests*, First Edition. Edited by Barry Kipperman and Bernard E. Rollin.
© 2022 John Wiley & Sons, Inc. Published 2022 by John Wiley & Sons, Inc.

should be subjected to a culling intervention? All these challenges are in addition to the more common ethical problems (see Chapter 7) veterinarians face when dealing with their responsibilities to animal patients.

## Wild Animals in Human Care: Zoos and Aquaria

Over the past two centuries, zoological parks have changed their core missions from being focused solely on the exhibition of wild and exotic animals for the purpose of visitor entertainment to being advocates for the conservation of wild animals and their habitats. While these objectives have evolved, the fundamental business of exhibiting animals to the public to advance the mission has remained the same, with advancements made in the science of animal care, nutrition, welfare, and veterinary medicine. Veterinarians often find themselves at the interface of advancing the institution's goals and assuring individual animal welfare. At times, the business of operating a zoo and the needs of the individual animal may not align and a veterinarian may have to navigate competing interests.

An essential challenge arises with the desire to exhibit a wild animal in an environment other than its natural habitat. The animals kept in zoos are a subset of their species in the wild, a species that may be threatened with extinction. Conway summarizes the moral dilemma central to wild animals in captivity: "it is a paradox that so many human beings agonize over the well-being of an individual animal yet ignore the millions daily brutalized by the destruction of their environments" (1995). The central ethical challenges for a professional working with wild animals in a zoo or aquarium include: (i) Is it ethical to maintain a wild animal in captivity at all? If (i) is justified, then (ii) are there specific uses that are justified (breeding, conservation, education, research) and uses that are not justified? (iii) Do the uses of an individual animal for the conservation of its species ever supersede the needs of that individual animal? Lastly, (iv) for the veterinarian, are medical interventions performed solely for the purpose of managing a species in captivity that are of no benefit to the individual animal (i.e. artificial insemination, avian deflighting, surgical sterilization) justified as a means of advancing the mission of the zoo?

### Definitions

A zoo or zoological garden has been defined as "an establishment where wild animals are kept for exhibition (other than a circus or pet shop) to which members of the public have access, with or without charge for admission" (UK Government 1981). While this technical definition may apply to any number of institutions exhibiting wild animals, each of the multitudes of "zoos" has different management practices, falls under different regulatory oversight, and applies a wide range of standards. Thus, each institution may be very different in practice. The American Association of Zoos and Aquariums defines a zoological park or aquarium as:

> a permanent institution which owns and maintains wildlife, under the direction of a professional staff, provides its animals with appropriate care and exhibits them in an aesthetic manner to the public on a regularly scheduled,

predictable basis. The institution ... shall further be defined as having as a core mission the exhibition, conservation, and preservation of the earth's fauna in an educational and scientific manner.

*(AZA 2022)*

Similarly, the European Association of Zoos and Aquaria requires that zoos in the European Union participate in conservation research and training and promote public awareness on conservation (EAZA 2013). The goals of promoting conservation, education, and animal care unite modern zoos. Some smaller, privately owned facilities, which best fall under the description of "menagerie," also characterize themselves as zoos, even with a limited focus on education and conservation. Other institutions that maintain captive wildlife include sanctuaries, which may keep retired or unwanted exotic animals from zoos, circuses, or private individuals.

## Stakeholders

As with any animal industry, there are competing interests in the operation of zoological institutions or aquaria. In companion animal practice, the veterinarian serves both the client and the animal: in the zoo industry there is the added layer of meeting the organization's missions, the broader needs of the populations, and the needs of species conservation. In some cases, care may be prioritized for animals that are more genetically valuable or for individuals that have higher reproductive potential. Each of the stakeholders (except the animals) has input into the management and care of an individual animal.

### Internal Stakeholders

Zoo and aquarium professionals fall into a few distinct categories, each with a different role to play in the care of the animals of the collection.

#### Animal Caretakers

The animal care staff in a zoo may consist of animal keepers, managers, curators, and veterinarians. Each of these individuals may have different goals for the animals in their care within the scope of the zoo's mission. Animal keepers have a wide range of experience and backgrounds, work closely with the animals, and are likely to form a strong human–animal bond (Hosey and Melfi 2012). This relationship of keeper staff with the animals may result in personal attachment as strong as a person with their pet, which may affect their objective assessment of the animal's quality of life and decisions on management and euthanasia (Hosey and Melfi 2012). Curators are charged with the comprehensive management of the animal collection and must balance the needs of an individual animal with the needs of the species population and the desire to have exhibit-quality animals in adequate quantities to meet public expectations. Medical, management and euthanasia decisions are typically made by veterinarians in conjunction with the curator, but both must consider the emotional attachment of the keeper staff to an animal whom they have formed a relationship with since birth. Seemingly clear logistical decisions based on prognosis, quality of life, and resources may be clouded by the personal desires of the care staff, and the managers and veterinary staff have a responsibility to both the animals and the keepers who care for them.

### Administration

As a business, even if it is nonprofit, the administration of a zoo has to consider not only the animals and employees, but also the financial solvency of the organization. This includes budgeting of veterinary care, food choices, and facility modifications. There is also an ongoing need to maintain positive public and donor perceptions. So, care of the animals must be transparent, but also easily explained and understandable to the public and funding agencies.

### Animals

The animals themselves are critical stakeholders. Each individual animal's care and welfare should be monitored and managed to the greatest extent possible. Every animal is unaware of its place in the greater mission of the institution or conservation and consideration of its individual needs must be made and assessed constantly.

## External Stakeholders

### Regulators, Local Agencies, and Accrediting Groups

Zoos, aquaria, and sanctuaries are governed by several national, international, and local regulations. Many of these regulations establish a safety net of minimum standards, and institutions should strive to exceed many of these standards.

Welfare guidelines pertaining to wildlife in human care have been set forth by a multitude of organizations, including the World Organisation for Animal Health (OIE 2021), and extrapolation to wild animals can be made from similar information in the American Veterinary Medical Association (AVMA) Animal Welfare Principles (AVMA n.d.). The US Department of Agriculture (USDA) sets minimum standards of care for exhibited species and oversees enforcement of the Animal Welfare Act (AWA) (USDA 2021). The AWA requires all facilities that exhibit animals regulated under the Act (primarily mammals) to ensure veterinary oversight of their programs by retaining an attending veterinarian to provide care and husbandry advice. The veterinarian must have training and experience in the care and management of the species being attended. The USDA also conducts both announced and surprise inspections to licensed premises to assess many aspects of animal care and use, including the provision of veterinary care.

The US Fish and Wildlife Service, National Marine Fisheries Service, and state and local wildlife agencies are all charged with the protection of some threatened and endangered species and may provide direction on the management of certain taxa. Many zoos are funded and under the jurisdiction of city or county agencies. In rare cases, the direct care and management of a species may be dictated by a local government, in some cases by officials with no animal experience. Public pressure may dictate legislation with direct impact on the institution, managers, or veterinarians making decisions for the animals in their care.

Several nongovernmental organizations provide an additional level of inspection and quality control above the minimum standards set by governmental agencies. Accreditation by the Association of Zoos and Aquariums (AZA) (United States), European Association of Zoos and Aquariums (EAZA), the World Association of Zoos and Aquariums (WAZA), The Global Federation of Animal Sanctuaries (GFAS), and others have established additional standards and an inspection and accreditation process for zoos, aquaria, and sanctuaries. Other non-zoo-based groups offer certifications for zoos and aquaria in humane care of animals.

In the United States, the primary accreditation body is the AZA. The AZA provides external assessment and certification of zoos and aquaria and operates programs for global population management with taxon-specific animal care guidelines. The AZA has a recently established animal welfare standard, in accordance with the WAZA's animal welfare strategy (WAZA 2015), which states that:

> The institution must follow a written process for assessing animal welfare and wellness... This process should be both proactive and reactive, transparent to stakeholders, and include staff or consultants knowledgeable in assessing animal welfare, and quality of life for animals showing signs of physical or mental distress or decline. Animal welfare/wellness refers to an animal's collective physical and psychological states over a period of time and is measured on a continuum from good to poor.
>
> *(AZA 2022)*

### Public and Zoo Guests

Because the core business model of zoos involves exhibiting animals to the public, zoos must provide a valued experience for the guests that are their primary customer. In some cases, this involves exhibiting relatively common species (some large carnivores, pinnipeds, giraffes) that may be popular attractions, but have a lower conservation value than other more threatened, less charismatic species. Similarly, public desire to see certain species may result in animals being held and displayed in unsuitable climates. For example, giraffes are a very common and popular species, but are not adapted to the cold temperatures found in many northern zoos. The conservation and research arms of most zoos are supported, in part or whole, by the income generated by public guests. This requires a constant maintenance of visitor-pleasing attractions, including the nonanimal business operations of food service, games, rides, and other attractions, and those operations must work in concert with the animal operations to complete the guest experience.

At a public display institution, visitors have expectations to see animals throughout the business day. This limits the ability to remove animals from exhibit for medical care and hospitalization. Some basic aspects of medical care, including shaving and bandaging, may alter the guests' experience and temporarily render an animal as being of lower exhibit quality. Consistent messaging and transparency is essential to maintaining public trust and interest.

### Animal Rights Advocates

Sometimes the veterinarian may need to balance the ideal medical care or management of an animal with public perception. This may include preemptive messaging to address likely concerns from organizations opposed to animals in zoos and aquaria.

## Ethical Considerations for Keeping Animals in Zoos

Zoos are focused on conservation, education, sustainability, and entertainment. The broader question is whether these reasons justify captivity of wild animals. Before discussing *how* zoos should best care for their animals, the question should be asked *if* zoos should have them in the first place. This discussion is expanded when we consider the differing needs of certain species. Taylor contends that "if significant benefits can be shown, then captivity for at least some animals might be defensible, [but] it would appear that the burden of proof rests most heavily on the zoo to demonstrate that the benefits of captivity to the continued preservation of the species outweigh the costs incurred to the freedom of the individuals" (2014).

Zoos often balance the interests of multiple stakeholders with animal welfare (Hosey et al. 2013). Animals in a zoo collection are typically considered to serve a specific purpose, such as exhibit, breeding, conservation, or education. Animals that no longer serve these purposes may include animals that are off public display for health reasons or collection plans resulting in surplus animals maintained in off-exhibit holding areas in perpetuity. The ethics of caring for these animals in the numbers needed is a balance between maintaining a viable genetic pool of animals and the space, staffing, and husbandry resources needed to provide for those animals. An ongoing ethical concern is whether zoos should be responsible for the lifelong care of animals that were previously useful but now no longer serve the zoo's mission. If such animals are to be removed from the zoo, who is responsible for identifying an ethical means of disposition, and how?

## Animal Welfare Considerations for Keeping Wild Animals in Captivity

While it may be possible to ethically keep certain species in manmade enclosures, it may be challenging or impossible to house other species in an exhibit that meets the animals' physical and psychological needs. Fraser (2009) argues that focus should be placed on meeting the needs of basic health and function, natural living, and affective behaviors.

### Basic Health and Function

This is the primary purview of the zoo veterinarian, in conjunction with animal managers, caretakers, and nutritionists. A comprehensive veterinary program considers species-specific needs with a focus on individual animal care. The approach to animal care in a zoo is an extension of the individual animal and herd management practices taught in veterinary school, with less immediate focus on the global conservation status of the species.

### Natural Living

Some aspects of natural living are lost in a captive setting. It is obvious that a bird may not be able to exhibit its full repertoire of flight in an aviary. An anteater may not have unlimited access to native insects to forage on throughout the day. There are also potentially negative aspects of natural living that are removed in the captive setting. Some animals will compete for mates and sometimes fight a conspecific to the point of maiming or death. This is typically managed in a zoo with either physical separation or behavioral modification (gonadectomy, pharmacotherapeutics) and while this might support the goal of improving health and function, it eliminates an aspect of natural living. In some situations, the medically prudent decision to separate an animal for surgery and treatment of a wound might be a significant stressor for a social species forced to live alone.

### Affective Behaviors

Animal emotions and motivations for animal behaviors are receiving greater scrutiny and study in zoos and aquariums. This field of study typically falls to a growing body of welfare scientists with input from veterinary behaviorists and animal care professionals.

## Prioritization of Care and Conservation

Zoos and aquaria face the challenges of limited resources when advancing their missions. Finite cost concerns, space, staffing, and time necessarily dictate which species and which individuals can be kept, displayed, cared for, and conserved. Powell et al. (2019) argue that certain species need to be prioritized for ex situ conservation based not only on their proximity to extinction, but also on the likelihood of maintaining a healthy sustainable population. Some species may be so far depleted that extraordinary measures to save the last one or two individuals may do nothing for saving the species. Conversely, some species that are threatened, but not yet in dire straits, may benefit most from focused conservation efforts to prevent further decline. In a zoo, this may affect allocation of resources to certain species and even certain individuals, and can directly affect the ability of a veterinarian to care for a patient. A fractured leg in a common species may entail a different outcome than one in a high-priority conservation species. While attention to individual welfare is consistent between the cases with provision of analgesia, the more common animal may be euthanized while more extensive measures are taken for the endangered animal. This is similar to working with a private owner who determines the financial extent of care that their animal receives: a zoo might have to do the same based on the assigned value of the individual.

These limitations are not only financial, but also affect space allocation. With a limited amount of space and housing available, a zoo must determine how much is allocated to exhibit animals and to off-exhibit captive propagation, including so-called assurance colonies. The off-exhibit holding and breeding spaces do not generate revenue for the zoo but are essential to maintaining a genetic store house. With these limitations on exhibit, holding, and breeding spaces, nonreproductive animals, especially some male animals, have been subjected to population management euthanasia (culling) (Powell and Ardaiolo 2016; Powell et al. 2018).

## Ethical Considerations for the Veterinarian

As with any animal industry, a zoo veterinarian faces the daily challenge of making decisions in the best interest of an individual animal's welfare while balancing the desires of the keepers who maintain a close personal attachment to the animal and the mission of the institution. Similar to private practice, there are financial limitations placed by the fixed resources of nonprofit institutions and the need to balance the cost of care for thousands of animals.

The competing interests of species conservation, individual animal welfare, public perception and enjoyment, and financial solvency raise multiple ethical challenges for the zoo or aquarium veterinarian. In some cases, especially when the veterinarian is part of an outside contract service, the veterinarian may not be party to the management decision-making process and instead may only be included after critical decisions have been enacted. For example, a veterinarian may not be included in the decision-making process on sourcing new animals from the wild. This is still a fairly common practice, especially with reptiles, amphibians, and fishes, and a decision may be made either to improve genetic diversity or to acquire a species that is not available from captive propagation. While not involved with the decision to source the animals from the wild, the veterinarian is charged with treating medical conditions that result from that decision. In some cases, wild-caught animals may carry foreign parasites, may not be acclimated to the captive diet causing gastrointestinal symptoms, and may have prolonged periods of maladjustment to captivity resulting in stereotypical behaviors such as pacing, head-bobbing, or feather destruction. These are repetitive behaviors with no obvious goal and function that are assumed to be associated with poor welfare.

Collection of animals from the wild can create other ethical challenges for the veterinarian and the institution. In addition to the medical and husbandry challenges and the acclimation stress of bringing a wild animal into captivity, there are ethical questions associated with the potential stress and trauma of removing animals from the wild and the potential damage to fragile wild populations and ecosystems. Loss of genetic diversity inherent with captive breeding from a small founder population can cause inbreeding depression and reduce individual animal fitness. This genetic limitation is self-perpetuating with increasing infertility and reproductive abnormalities in inbred populations. Wild collection and importation of new founder animals allows for diversification of the genetic pool but can be a stressor on both the individual animal and the source population. Aquaria still rely heavily on wild collection of fishes and there is little information about the sustainability of these practices. This places the veterinarian in the challenging situation of treating both hereditary diseases made worse by inbreeding and conditions associated with the transition to captivity.

Similarly, a veterinarian may not have input into the design of a habitat but be expected to treat medical conditions that arise from exposure to inappropriate temperatures, humidity, or ambient light. Exhibiting animals with extensive housing and husbandry needs is challenging, as "natural" conditions may be impossible to replicate in a zoo or aquarium resulting in poor welfare. Many "captivity-related" medical conditions are the result of housing animals in an environment that is very different from what centuries of evolution have prepared them for. A North American zoo will have a different temperature, humidity, and diversity of available natural forage materials than an animal's range habitat in sub-Saharan Africa. While accommodations are made to replicate the native environment, a veterinarian must be prepared to treat conditions related to inappropriate or inadequate husbandry. They should be comfortable raising ethical concerns related to captive husbandry and be appropriately positioned in the institutional hierarchy to have those concerns addressed.

Some social species (naked mole rats, African painted dogs, some primates, many fishes, and invertebrates) naturally live in groups with intense competition with conspecific injury, aggression, and even death being commonplace. In a captive setting there is the simultaneous desire to prevent injury and death while still providing for natural living. In many cases these may be mutually exclusive. Natural living as a multifaceted concept includes both positive and negative impacts on an individual animal's health and welfare. Humans working with captive wildlife must make the decision about which natural behaviors to allow and which to restrict. The veterinarian, in conjunction with animal managers, must make decisions on the extent of medical intervention and the effect that will have on an animal's social standing. As stated by Learmonth (2019), "Not all natural behaviors, nor natural environments, are to the benefit of animals in a captive setting, and practical application of the natural living concept has flaws. Expression of natural behaviors does not necessarily indicate positive well-being of an animal." As a veterinarian, the option for intervention might include observation only and allowing "nature to take its course," allowing a degree of conspecific aggression and mortality in a colony of animals. In other situations, an individual may be temporarily or permanently removed from a social grouping for its own safety, but then is forced to live alone or in a small group.

Many elective procedures performed by veterinarians on a nondomestic animal may be performed solely for the purpose of making an animal more suitable to a zoo, similar to declawing of domestic cats (see Chapter 10). Some commonly performed examples include deflighting procedures on birds, which can range from noninvasive flight-feather trimming to surgical distal wing amputation in hatchlings (pinion). Less common techniques such as tooth reduction and declawing of large felids (*Panthera* spp.) are typically not performed in accredited zoos and are discouraged by the AVMA. Declawing of large felids performed for any reason other than medical necessity is prohibited by the USDA for all regulated animal facilities (USDA 2006).

For many government-owned or operated zoological institutions in the United States, medical records for all animals are freely accessible by the public through the Freedom of Information Act. As such, it is exceedingly easy for any individual to obtain copies of a complete medical record and choose to distribute it to the media or public. While this unfettered access is a boon for accountability and transparency, it is possible to selectively excerpt any portion of the medical record to promote an agenda with verbiage taken out of context. As such, a veterinarian must remain vigilant to write records that are not only complete and accurate but can withstand scrutiny from the public. This can be challenging in cases of illness or injury that is partially the result of substandard husbandry conditions or human error. Conditions such as pododermatitis can occur commonly in captive birds and can be ameliorated with improving husbandry, but discussion of the etiology and the treatment in a medical record requires some admission of guilt for the poor husbandry. The veterinarian must balance the expectations of accuracy, transparency, and patient advocacy in a way that is complete and honest with a focus on improving care without laying blame.

There are many privately owned and operated exotic animal display facilities that frequently operate without the oversight of accreditation bodies. As animal exhibitors, they fall under the regulatory arm of the USDA Animal Care, but often operate with limited staff and rarely have a staff veterinarian. The veterinarian providing care for such facilities, or for private owners of wild animals, faces an ethical dilemma: by providing care to animals with compromised welfare, is the veterinarian enabling ownership and exhibit of animals in a manner the veterinarian finds substandard? While each animal may require the care of a veterinarian, the provision of that care in some cases may not remedy the suffering of animals in these facilities. Does providing immediate care for an animal that is being kept in a deficient situation enable that owner to continue "business as usual"? Does providing medical care to animals in dangerous and inhumane situations, knowing that they will continue to be kept in those settings, implicitly support the operations? These circumstances have further come to light with popular reality television programs focused on exotic animal ownership and exhibition.

Some of the most challenging ethical quandaries for a zoo veterinarian surround captive population management (Asa et al. 2014; Penfold et al. 2014). Limited space and resources require constant population control, which is often paradoxical because many zoo-housed animals are there for the purpose of reproduction, but that reproduction must be controlled in a way that allows appropriate housing, care, and disposition of animals. The goal of managing population numbers can be met by several methods, each with physiological consequences for the animal and ethical implications for the clinician. In many species, years spent not breeding, either due to contraception or being held without a mate, are associated with reproductive pathology and infertility. Multiple zoo-based reviews confirm that reproductive cycling without pregnancy negatively impacts future fertility (Hermes et al. 2004; Asa et al. 2014; Penfold et al. 2014). The clinician, the zoo, and population managers are left with the quandary of needing to keep a young animal from reproducing due to inadequate space for offspring, while knowing that the longer that the animal remains sterile, the less likely it is to conceive, essentially taking it out of the reproductive pools. Contraception and reproductive management are a huge ethical concern for zoos. In most cases, to promote conservation, responsible breeding and propagation of species are paramount, but with successful propagation, there is concern for available space and housing of nonreproductive animals. In the past few decades, the success of contraceptives has helped curb this population overgrowth, but at the same time leaves some animals reproductively inert.

Euthanasia of healthy "surplus" animals is one of the most contentious ethical dilemmas for zoo veterinarians. Regardless of the reasoning for euthanasia, culling, or humane killing, the task usually falls to the zoo veterinarian to carry out. For a clinician who is trained to treat, heal, and cure, it is antithetical to be asked to kill a healthy animal for the needs of population management. Sometimes the distaste for population management euthanasia limits discussion of the topic and may leave a veterinarian unprepared for the emotional toll of the task. Because of the effects of medical contraception on future fertility, some institutions may choose to allow animals to reproduce, knowing that there is not enough space to accommodate their offspring. In the wild, large litter sizes are often a means of countering high neonatal mortality, but with medical care in captivity those pressures do not exist, resulting in so-called surplus animals.

If surplus animals cannot be placed at other zoos, the choice may be made to cull them. Some argue that this process is the most akin to natural living. It allows a female animal to experience the natural activities of pregnancy and rearing young and allows the juvenile a short, but healthy life. If the method of euthanasia is humane, is the killing of a young healthy animal any less ethically sound than killing an old, healthy animal? Does killing negatively affect its welfare, and is this more problematic for younger animals (see Chapter 21)? Is it more ethical to house surplus animals in overpopulated enclosures or send them to institutions with lower animal welfare standards just to allow them to live, even if that longer life means added suffering? These very challenging questions get to the heart of each of the ethical dilemmas discussed earlier for the zoo veterinarian. Is the welfare and sustainability of the species population paramount, or does the final ethical judgment rest with the individual animal (Case Study 14.1)?

**Case Study 14.1 Options for population management in African painted dogs**

Background: African painted dogs (*Lycaon pictus*) are an endangered species kept in zoos in the United States and Europe. This species has many physical similarities to the domestic dog and as such is regarded by the public as having similar appeal. Despite the physical similarities, differences in demeanor and social structure makes medical management challenging. With any endangered species, maintaining female reproductive potential is critical to the survival of the species. With painted dogs, females reach sexual maturity at approximately 12–18 months. Litter sizes can vary considerably, from 2 to 20 pups with an inter-birth interval of 12 months. Contraception and multiple nonpregnant cycles lead to reproductive pathology and future infertility. Complications from extended nonpregnant periods include pyometra (uterine infection) and cystic endometrial hyperplasia (Asa et al. 2014; Langan and Jankowski 2019).

Scenario: As part of the zoo's management plan, breeding-age African painted dogs will be exhibited, but there is not room to house more than five or six animals. At this time there is no option for external placement of puppies at other zoos, but there likely will be in the future. The zoo director is asking for veterinary guidance on the best strategy for housing reproductive-age animals together without exceeding the housing capacity of the exhibit.

Ethical analysis:

Conflicting interests in this situation include: the species population (in terms of maintaining the future reproductive potential of breeding age females); the individual breeding dogs themselves; any potential puppies; zoo management, which is exhibiting the animals; the public who are paying to see animals on exhibit; the animal caretakers; and the veterinarian who is tasked with carrying out any medical intervention or culling.

Choices include:

1. Allow the animals to breed naturally and either:
   - Accept some natural pup mortality and attempt to find placement for the pups once they mature.
   - Induce medical abortion during pregnancy.
   - Cull surviving puppies.
2. Temporarily contracept the females by hormone implant and accept the risk of uterine pathology and loss of future reproductive potential.
3. Permanent sterility (ovariohysterectomy) assuring no future conception or uterine pathology but subjecting some animals to a surgical procedure and loss of future reproductive potential.
4. Separate the animals by sex, which is contradictory to their normal social structure and may cause stress to animals due to social separation from conspecifics and limited space for each single-sex group. Also, accepting the risk of uterine pathology and loss of future reproductive potential.

In species with large litter sizes, there are often more offspring produced than will survive to adulthood. With painted dogs, there are often more puppies than there is space for, and choices must be made about how to house and maintain those surplus animals. Culling surplus puppies is routine practice in many parts of the world, thereby "mimicking" normal neonatal mortality rates. The veterinarian, as the advocate for the animals, is tasked with maintaining the welfare, fertility, and health of the female dogs and their puppies. Zoo management must balance the need to display animals for public enjoyment and education with the conservation of genetically diverse captive populations.

If the zoo and the veterinarian choose the most "hands-off" approach of displaying sexually intact males and females together, inevitable breeding will result in puppies that need housing once they mature. There is benefit to the adults as they can maintain more normal social dynamics between sexes and between adults and young. This aspect of "natural living" allows for the closest replication of wild dynamics, but comes with consequences. In this species, it is common for a conspecific animal to perform infanticide or injure a pup, resulting in the need for medical intervention. The choice is then between letting nature take its course and allowing an animal to die, or separating it to allow medical care, which might make it difficult to reintegrate that individual into the pack. Those pups that survive to adulthood may need to be placed in another zoo at maturity. If there is not space available, a zoo may be forced to house the surplus animals in a smaller habitat or off-display holding area.

Should the veterinarian suggest temporary contraception or separation by sex, there are well-documented effects of repeated nonreproductive cycles on uterine health (Asa et al. 2014; Penfold et al. 2014) including causing a life-threatening pyometra or endometrial hyperplasia, which may render an animal infertile (Lamglait et al. 2015). These choices, while ideal and convenient in the short term, carry lifelong consequences for the individual and the population. Rendering female dogs infertile reduces the population size, thereby reducing genetic diversity. This loss of genetic diversity in painted dogs can contribute to inbreeding and associated inherited defects such as heart disease (Langan and Jankowski 2019).

Medical abortions and permanent sterility are medical and surgical options, respectively, to minimize surplus offspring. Both procedures are medically invasive and carry no benefit to the dam herself. If a medical or surgical intervention is chosen to limit litter size, the cost is paid by the dam, but saves the need for culling of puppies. These procedures have the potential for pain, infection, or other complications. A dilemma then arises about the relative impact on the adult female versus the unborn puppies.

Lastly, culling of surplus puppies allows the adults to live the most natural life and limits the incidence of uterine pathology and surplus animal numbers. In this scenario, puppies would be born naturally, reared by the dam until maturity, and at the time of natural weaning or separation would be culled. The choice to cull healthy animals has an immense personal toll on the staff and veterinarians and is not widely practiced in the United States. There is the added challenge of messaging for a public that may not see any benefit to the killing of healthy animals, as seen with the global public outcry over the euthanasia of Marius the giraffe at the Copenhagen Zoo in 2014. The benefit of this choice is the maintenance of reproductive potential and the ability for the pack to experience natural birth and rearing.

## Free-ranging Wildlife

### Veterinary Practice in Wildlife Management Agencies

Agencies such as federal, state, and Tribal Fish and Wildlife Services employ veterinarians to assist in protecting endangered and threatened species through field conservation efforts, reestablishing animals in historic ranges via captive breeding programs, and providing technical advice and expertise to develop regulations pertaining to hunting, population management, and conservation of species and their habitats. Veterinarians may perform hands-on medical procedures such as chemical immobilization for translocation of animals, placement of radio tracking collars, and investigation of disease outbreaks. Advanced degrees or postgraduate coursework in epidemiology, wildlife ecology, and related fields are helpful and may be required for careers working with free-ranging wildlife (Florida Fish and Wildlife Conservation Commission n.d.).

The focus of the wildlife veterinarian employed by these agencies is more often animal health at the population and ecosystem level, rather than on the treatment of individual animals. While veterinary care may be provided to individual wild animals, the veterinarian in this type of practice is also mindful of that individual's role as a member of a population or group of animals. Because of this Respect for Nature ethical perspective (see Chapter 4), medical intervention may not be provided to sick or injured animals in favor of "letting nature take its course." Witnessing, but not acting upon, the perceived suffering of a wild animal may be distressing to both the wildlife veterinarian and members of the public.

Management of population size, herd health, and ecosystem health often involves allowing, or even encouraging, licensed members of the public to hunt and fish. A substantial source of revenue for the operation of fish and game or fish and wildlife agencies is derived from the sale of hunting and fishing licenses. Veterinarians employed by these agencies may very rarely be directly involved with hunting and fishing activities, but these activities are a large part of the "culture" of the agency and the ethical dichotomy of killing wild animals to protect them (i.e. killing deer to prevent their overpopulation and starvation due to limited prey/resources) is ever present.

When wild animals are captured for purposes such as relocation, placement of tracking devices, or biological data collection, some may be harmed or killed in the process. Capturing ungulates such as deer, elk, and bighorn sheep may involve pursuing animals with a helicopter to a desired location, shooting them with darts containing anesthetic drugs, restraining them with nets, and other invasive handling techniques. Tracking devices such as collars around the neck or surgically implanted radio transmitters may cause harm to animals (Arnemo et al. 2018). While the purpose of such operations is to benefit the animals, injury or death may be caused in the process as a result of hyperthermia, capture myopathy (exertional rhabdomyolysis), and trauma. The goal is to keep the percentage of animals harmed or killed low, but there are certain levels of expected and *acceptable losses* in such operations (Schemnitz et al. 2009). The wildlife veterinarian must accept that even with expert skill and planning, their actions may directly harm or kill otherwise healthy wild animals.

Animals that are relocated into areas different from where they were found may displace or outcompete resident animals in the new area, so careful consideration must be given to potential harm to the wild population. For example, introducing an apex predator such as a mountain lion to an area where resident mountain lions have established territories and there is a finite source of prey could have a negative impact on the welfare of those established lions. The wildlife veterinarian must not only consider the welfare of the animal being relocated but also the welfare of the other animals already living in the relocation area, which may be affected by the introduction of a new animal.

## Wildlife Rehabilitation

Wildlife rehabilitation is dedicated to treating individual animals that have been orphaned or injured, with the goal of returning them to the wild once healed. Veterinarians working in wildlife rehabilitation centers grapple with ethical considerations on almost a daily basis. Animals that enter the care of a rehabilitation center typically undergo a triage process by a trained individual upon admission. The primary question asked during this process is: is it likely that medical care will restore this animal to full function so it can be returned to the wild? If the animal has sustained an injury that renders it permanently unable to cope in the wild, it is usually humanely euthanized. As an example, an eagle with a badly damaged eye has lost its binocular vision, and therefore cannot focus on prey well enough to capture and kill it, so is likely to die of starvation if released.

Wild animals may be *physically* able to survive in the wild, but if they become habituated to people while under human care, they cannot be released. Great care must be taken to prevent wild animals from being attached to, and dependent upon humans during the rehabilitation process to maximize the animal's chances of survival once returned to the wild. Animals deemed nonreleasable due to physical or behavioral conditions are sometimes kept in captivity to be displayed as education specimens or "ambassadors" for their wild conspecifics. Nonreleasable animals may also be euthanized even though great time and effort has been put into healing them if they are ultimately deemed behaviorally unsuitable for caged life or if there is no available cage space for that animal in the captive world. The decision to either euthanize a nonreleasable animal or to keep it permanently captive often falls on the veterinarian's shoulders, who should take into consideration the animal's unique temperament and perceived adaptability to a captive environment.

One should also consider the potential effects on genetic fitness of the wild population when returning orphaned, sick, or injured animals to the wild after rehabilitation. What were the reasons that brought them into human care in the first place? If humans had not intervened, these individual animals likely would have died, and would have never bred and contributed their genes to their population. Are wildlife rehabilitators interrupting "nature's way" by interfering with natural selection? Or are they doing a net good for nature by repairing damage to wild animals that was caused by humans?

Veterinarians in small or mixed animal private practice may occasionally be presented with an injured or orphaned wild animal by a Good Samaritan. While the veterinarian may render emergency care to stabilize the patient, they should be transferred to the care of a licensed rehabilitator in the area. When transfer is not immediately possible or there is no licensed facility nearby, the veterinarian should be aware of local, state, and federal laws governing wildlife to avoid legal trouble. There are rules describing how long it is legal to possess a wild animal, how and where it can be legally released, and what types of injuries are incompatible with life in the wild. There are many differences in handling and treatment protocols for wild animals compared with domestic animals, and veterinarians interested in rendering aid to wild animals should seek additional training in wildlife care to best serve these patients.

## Disease Transmission Between Humans and Wild Animals

Wild animals may harbor pathogens that are harmful to humans, representing a significant reservoir for emerging zoonotic diseases (Jones et al. 2008). Viral diseases such as rabies, severe acute respiratory syndrome (SARS-CoV-2 [Covid-19]), Middle East respiratory syndrome (MERS), hantavirus, monkeypox, and avian influenza are a few examples of zoonotic diseases that may be transmitted from animals to humans. Measures such as culling healthy animals may be taken to control a perceived threat of zoonotic disease, directly impacting the welfare of those animals (van Herten and Bovenkerk 2021).

*Reverse* zoonotic disease transmission occurs when humans infect an animal with a disease that may become harmful to the population or species once that infected animal is released. A key example of a potentially harmful reverse zoonotic disease is the transmission of SARS-CoV-2 (Covid-19) and pandemic H1N1 influenza from humans to vulnerable species (Sooksawasdi Na Ayudhya and Kuiken 2021). The introduction of a potentially harmful or lethal disease into a vulnerable wild population (and its ecosystem) could be catastrophic to an endangered species. Even if a human pathogen doesn't harm wild animals, those animals could serve as a reservoir of disease that could be transmitted back to humans in a more pathogenic form due to genetic mutations creating new and more deadly variants. Often on the frontline of human–animal interaction, wildlife veterinarians must carefully consider planned work involving wildlife, balancing the need to protect public health, while mitigating risk of doing harm to their animal patients.

## Invasive Species

Wildlife veterinarians may be involved with situations where the life of one species must be prioritized over that of another species (Case Studies 14.2 and 14.3). "Invasive species" are animals that are not native to an area and are having a negative impact on historically resident native species. Invasive species may have been artificially introduced to an area by humans or they may have moved into a new area on their own. If the invasive species is affecting the survival of a threatened or endangered species, it may be subject to an eradication program where members of the invasive species are killed to protect the native species and its ecosystem. Veterinarians may be directly involved in eradication programs, capturing and euthanizing animals deemed invasive as part of an organization's mission to protect native wildlife.

## Wild Animals as "Nuisances"

Wild animals, *even in their own native habitat*, may be deemed as nuisances or pests when they are perceived as a threat to humans or human interests. Wildlife veterinarians may be involved when a wild animal has become a "nuisance" to humans and therefore intervention is deemed necessary (Case Studies 14.4 and 14.5).

**Case Study 14.2**

Barred owls, native to the east coast of the United States, have gradually moved west in recent years and are now displacing native and endangered spotted owls that live in the Pacific Northwest by outcompeting them for food and shelter. To protect the spotted owl, barred owls are being shot or caught and euthanized.

**Case Study 14.3**

A Good Samaritan brings an injured Red-Eared Slider turtle to a wildlife rehabilitation center. It was found on a busy street with a cracked shell, presumably hit by a car. It is alert, active, and seems healthy other than the injury, which can be repaired. These turtles are popular in the pet trade, and people have illegally released pet turtles to the wild, where they have become invasive species in many states, displacing native turtles from habitat and food sources. Because the Red-Eared Slider is considered an invasive species in several states, it is illegal to rehabilitate and release to the wild. Bound by state regulations, the veterinarian must either euthanize the turtle, or refuse to accept it for care.

   Wildlife rehabilitators face the issue of invasive species daily when orphaned or injured animals are presented for care, as only animals that are native to their area may be legally released to the wild. Those that are deemed invasive must either be euthanized or kept in captivity.

**Case Study 14.4**

A bear cub is approaching people at a public park and vocalizing. The cub is too young to survive on his own in the wild, so it is assumed that he has been separated from his mother. It will be difficult to raise him in captivity to an age where he can survive on his own without reinforcing his dependence on humans in the process. Releasing an animal that has no fear of humans and sees them as a food source creates a dangerous situation. Humane euthanasia may be an appropriate option for the cub; however, publicity surrounding this case places public pressure on wildlife agencies to "rescue" him, even though rescue means that he will likely spend the rest of his life in a cage and never experience life as a wild bear.

**Case Study 14.5**

Coyotes occupy both wildlands and cities throughout North America, and as highly intelligent omnivores they are extremely adaptable to living near people. In some areas, coyotes kill and eat domestic cats and other small pets that may be roaming unsupervised outdoors. When coyotes find such easy prey, their close proximity to people may pose a threat to small children. The task of euthanasia may fall to the wildlife veterinarian when public safety takes priority over the welfare of the coyotes.

### Conflict with Animal Agriculture and Fisheries

Wildlife veterinarians often become involved when disease transmission may occur between wildlife and domestic livestock. To mitigate risk of disease spread, the veterinarian must consider the interests of livestock producers (largely driven by economics), as well as the health and welfare of both livestock and wildlife (Case Study 14.6). Wild animals may compete with people for the same resource and when this happens, the wildlife veterinarian may be expected to intervene (Case Study 14.7).

---

**Case Study 14.6**

Tule elk roamed much of California until they were hunted to near-extinction in the 1800s. A small herd discovered in 1874 was protected, and their offspring were re-established in areas they once occupied, including a herd in a coastal National Park. This growing population of elk is simultaneously a conservation success story and a problem to the ranches surrounding the park (Watt 2015). Livestock producers are concerned about the potential transmission of Johne's disease (a disease of economic significance) from the elk to their cattle, and want the elk herd to be moved, killed, or reduced in size by allowing hunting. A large segment of the public is opposed to hunting, and wants the elk protected. Fences keep the elk confined and away from cattle, but also limit access to food and water sources, with detrimental effects on the elk. Wildlife veterinarians may be involved on both sides of the dispute – monitoring elk for disease and signs of starvation or dehydration, and at the same time advising ranchers on keeping their livestock safe, therefore protecting their economic interests.

---

**Case Study 14.7**

A popular source of food and recreation for people, some populations of salmon and steelhead trout in the Pacific Northwest are threatened or endangered. Wild sea lions rely on these fish as a primary food source, and so they are perceived as both competition to human interests and a threat to the fish population. Wildlife veterinarians working for government agencies may be asked to assist in trapping and euthanasia of sea lions, whose interests take lower precedence than those of humans and fish.

---

## Conclusion

Working with wild animals, whether in human care or in the wild, presents unique ethical challenges for the practicing veterinarian. First and foremost, wild animals' interests are not represented by one "owner," and multiple stakeholders may have legal and ethical interests in their welfare. Veterinary care and possession of wild animals are usually regulated by multiple governmental agencies. Wildlife veterinarians must also be knowledgeable regarding applicable laws and regulations. In many cases, wild animals are considered the property of the public, so public opinion may influence the degree and methods of veterinary interventions that may be employed. Wildlife practitioners must also balance the welfare of the individual animal with the interests of its group or species and human interests. Navigating these often-competing viewpoints requires the willingness to advocate for animal welfare and the capacity to recognize and address ethical conflicts.

# References

American Veterinary Medical Association (AVMA) (n.d.). AVMA Animal welfare principles. https://www.avma.org/resources-tools/avma-policies/avma-animal-welfare-principles (accessed 28 November 2021).

Arnemo, J.M., Ytrehus, B., Madslien, K. et al. (2018). Long-term safety of intraperitoneal radio transmitter implants in brown bears (*Ursus arctos*). *Frontiers in Veterinary Science* 5: 252.

Asa, C.S., Bauman, K.L., Devery, S. et al. (2014). Factors associated with uterine endometrial hyperplasia and pyometra in wild canids: Implications for fertility. *Zoo Biology* 33 (1): 8–19.

Association of Zoos and Aquaria (2022). The accreditation standards & related policies. https://assets.speakcdn.com/assets/2332/aza-accreditation-standards.pdf (accessed 28 November 2021).

Conway, W. (1995). Zoo conservation and ethical paradoxes. In: *Ethics on the Ark: Zoos, Animal Welfare and Wildlife Conservation* (eds. B.G. Norton, M. Hutchins, E.F. Stevens, and T. Maple), 1–12. Washington, DC: Smithsonian Institution Press.

European Association of Zoos and Aquaria (2013). The modern zoo: Foundations for management and development. https://www.eaza.net/assets/Uploads/images/Membership-docs-and-images/Zoo-Management-Manual-compressed.pdf (accessed 8 February 2021)

Florida Fish and Wildlife Conservation Commission (n.d.). Becoming a conservation veterinarian. https://myfwc.com/research/wildlife/health/conservation-veterinarian (accessed 28 November 2021).

Fraser, D. (2009). Assessing animal welfare: Different philosophies, different scientific approaches. *Zoo Biology* 28 (6): 507–518.

Hermes, R., Hildebrandt, T.B., and Göritz, F. (2004). Reproductive problems directly attributable to long-term captivity – Asymmetric reproductive aging. *Animal Reproduction Science* 82: 49–60.

Hosey, G. and Melfi, V. (2012). Human–animal bonds between zoo professionals and the animals in their care. *Zoo Biology* 31 (1): 13–26.

Hosey, G., Melfi, V., and Pankhurst, S. (2013). *Zoo Animals: Behaviour, Management, and Welfare*. Oxford, UK: Oxford University Press.

Jones, K.E., Patel, N.G., Levy, M.A. et al. (2008). Global trends in emerging infectious diseases. *Nature* 451 (7181): 990–993.

Lamglait, B., Trunet, E., and Leclerc, A. (2015). Retrospective study of mortality of captive African wild dogs (*Lycaon pictus*) in a French zoo (1974–2013). *Journal of Zoo and Aquarium Research* 3: 47 51.

Langan, J.N. and Jankowski, G. (2019). Overview of African wild dog medicine. In: *Fowler's Zoo and Wild Animal Medicine Current Therapy*, Vol. 9 (eds. R.E. Miller, N. Lamberski, and P. Calle), 539–547. Saint Louis, MO: Elsevier Saunders.

Learmonth, M.J. (2019). Dilemmas for natural living concepts of zoo animal welfare. *Animals* 9 (6): 318.

OIE (World Organisation for Animal Health) (2021). Terrestrial Animal Health Code. https://www.oie.int/en/what-we-do/standards/codes-and-manuals/terrestrial-code-online-access (accessed 28 December 2021)

Penfold, L.M., Powell, D., Traylor-Holzer, K. et al. (2014). "Use it or lose it": Characterization, implications, and mitigation of female infertility in captive wildlife. *Zoo Biology* 33 (1): 20–28.

Powell, D.M. and Ardaiolo, M. (2016). Survey of US zoo and aquarium animal care staff attitudes regarding humane euthanasia for population management. *Zoo Biology* 35 (3): 187–200.

Powell, D.M., Lan, J., and Eng, C. (2018). Survey of US-based zoo veterinarians' attitudes on population management euthanasia. *Zoo Biology* 37 (6): 478–487.

Powell, D.M., Dorsey, C.L., and Faust, L.J. (2019). Advancing the science behind animal program sustainability: An overview of the special issue. *Zoo Biology* 38 (1): 5–11.

Schemnitz, S.D., Batcheller, G.R., Lovallo, M.J. et al. (2009). Capturing and handling wild animals. In: *The Wildlife Techniques Manual* (ed. N.J. Silvy), 232–269. Baltimore, MD: Johns Hopkins University Press.

Sooksawasdi Na Ayudhya, S. and Kuiken, T. (2021). Reverse zoonosis of COVID-19: Lessons from the 2009 influenza pandemic. *Veterinary Pathology* 58 (2): 234–242.

Taylor, M.A. (2014). Zootopia – Animal welfare, species preservation and the ethics of captivity. *Poultry, Fisheries & Wildlife Sciences* November 12: 1–4.

UK Government (1981). UK Zoo Licensing Act. https://www.legislation.gov.uk/ukpga/1981/37 (accessed 30 November 2021).

United States Department of Agriculture (2006). Information sheet on declawing and tooth removal. https://www.aphis.usda.gov/animal_welfare/downloads/big_cat/declaw_tooth.pdf (accessed 30 December 2021).

United States Department of Agriculture (2021). Animal welfare inspection guide. https://www.aphis.usda.gov/animal_welfare/downloads/Animal-Care-Inspection-Guide.pdf (accessed 30 November 2021).

van Herten, J. and Bovenkerk, B. (2021). The precautionary principle in zoonotic disease control. *Public Health Ethics* 14 (2): 180–190.

Watt, L.A. (2015). The continuously managed wild: Tule Elk at Point Reyes National Seashore. *Journal of International Wildlife Law & Policy* 18 (4): 289–308.

World Association of Zoos and Aquariums (2015). Caring for wildlife: The world zoo and aquarium animal welfare strategy. https://www.waza.org/priorities/animal-welfare/animal-welfare-strategies(accessed 14 January 2022).

# 15

# Exotic Pets

*Michael Dutton*

## Contemporary Exotic Pet Information

A growing area of pet ownership currently includes what are termed exotic pets. The American Veterinary Medical Association (AVMA) categorizes these as specialty and exotic pets (AVMA 2018). Table 15.1 shows ownership of exotic pets and trends from 1996 to 2016. As a comparison, almost 70 million dogs and 74 million cats in the United States were owned in 2016 (AVMA 2018).

Exotic pets are popular for several reasons. They are unique pets and for their owners that uniqueness is desirable. Exotic pets may be the only choice in certain situations. If an owner has a fur allergy, owning a bird or reptile may be the only viable option. In some cases, the smaller exotic companion mammals (ECMs) such as hamsters or gerbils are viewed as "starter" pets for young children given their small size and minimal housing requirements. Certain exotic pets undergo a period of being trendy or a fad. This can be seen in Table 15.1 for ferrets, who were very popular in the early 2000s but now number half of what they did in 2006.

**Table 15.1** Exotic pet ownership and trends (AVMA 2018).

| | Percentage of US households who owned specialty or exotic pets | | | | |
|---|---|---|---|---|---|
| | 1996 | 2001 | 2006 | 2011 | 2016 |
| Fish | 6.3% | 6.1% | 7.8% | 6.5% | 8.3% |
| Rabbits | 1.9% | 1.7% | 1.6% | 1.2% | 1.2% |
| Ferrets | 0.4% | 0.5% | 0.4% | 0.3% | 0.3% |
| Reptiles | 1.5% | 1.6% | 2.0% | 2.5% | 2.9% |
| Pet livestock | 0.5% | 0.4% | 0.6% | 0.6% | 0.4% |
| Pet poultry | 0.3% | 0.3% | 0.4% | 0.9% | 1.1% |
| | Specialty and exotic pet populations on 31 December | | | | |
| Fish | 55,554,000 | 49,251,000 | 75,898,000 | 57,750,000 | 76,323,222 |
| Rabbits | 4,940,000 | 4,813,000 | 6,171,000 | 3,210,000 | 2,243,609 |
| Ferrets | 791,000 | 991,000 | 1,060,000 | 748,000 | 500,801 |
| Reptiles | 3,479,000 | 2,875,000 | 3,854,000 | 5,298,000 | 6,032,066 |
| Pet livestock | 6,083,000 | 2,936,000 | 10,995,000 | 5,045,000 | 1,785,618 |
| Pet poultry | 4,423,000 | 2,894,000 | 4,966,000 | 12,591,000 | 15,367,327 |

*Ethics in Veterinary Practice: Balancing Conflicting Interests*, First Edition. Edited by Barry Kipperman and Bernard E. Rollin.
© 2022 John Wiley & Sons, Inc. Published 2022 by John Wiley & Sons, Inc.

The suitability of having exotic animals as pets can be determined by considering two questions. The first question is how domesticated is the exotic animal? That is, pets that are bred, kept by humans, and are tame. The common ECMs, along with chickens, probably meet the definition of domestication the best. The other suitability question is the ability to keep the exotic pet in an environment that closely mimics its natural state. This pertains to housing, diet, and environmental enrichment. The capacity to meet these requirements often depends on the owner's resources and finances. Whereas the housing requirement for a rabbit is minimal, appropriate housing for a reptile taking heat and humidity requirements into account can be costly.

Often, notably for the avian or reptile and amphibian groups, the cost of purchasing the pet is only a small component of the overall cost of ownership. Providing appropriate husbandry, especially the housing component, can be a significant initial and ongoing cost. In some cases, the owner is reluctant to maintain appropriate husbandry due to the costs. Not having appropriate housing can severely impact the health of an exotic animal, so it is paramount that all costs are considered before obtaining an exotic pet. Chapter 8 discusses the cost of ownership of pets in more detail.

Resources for owners include the Internet, experienced exotic pet owners, local enthusiast clubs, pet store personnel, and veterinary staff.

## The Veterinarian Skill Set

Veterinary specialists in exotic pet medicine exist worldwide, but they are a small minority of veterinarians. Of the approximately 105,000 veterinarians in the United States, approximately 13% are specialists (AVMA n.d.). In the United States, the American Board of Veterinary Practitioners certifies specialist veterinarians in avian practice, ECM practice, and reptile and amphibian practice: about 120 are avian specialists, about 25 are ECM specialists, and about 20 are reptile and amphibian specialists (AVMA n.d.). Requirements to obtain veterinary specialist status are numerous and rigorous including years of experience and training, peer-reviewed publications, extensive continual education, and successfully passing a comprehensive examination. In the United States, specialists must also complete ongoing requirements to maintain their certification.

Exotic pet owners expect to obtain veterinary care at a level commensurate with the care of dogs and cats (Rosenthal 2006), therefore the veterinary profession should provide similar services and levels of care for these exotic pets as they would a traditional pet. It is estimated that of the 15% of US veterinary practices that see exotic pets, most of these offer minimal services beyond examinations and vaccinations (Kohles 2010). So, there is a significant disparity between what veterinarians should provide, what the public expects, and what is occurring in reality. As training in veterinary school is quite limited (Rosenthal 2006), the primary means of obtaining proficiency with exotic animals is via continuing education and training of the current staff or to hire exotic pet-competent veterinarians and staff (Doneley 2005).

Although most canine and feline practice equipment and medications can be easily used for exotic pets, the ethical question is whether a minimally competent or exotic pet-incompetent veterinary staff should be performing veterinary services on these unique animals that have special needs and complex enrichment requirements. An analogy is whether you should offer equine services if you are primarily a canine and feline practitioner. Most small animal veterinary graduates have taken equine classes and had hands-on training but decline to treat horses once in practice due to a lack of experience, expertise, and confidence. It is incumbent on the minimally skilled veterinarian to either improve their competency or seek a referral option for their exotic patients for the health and well-being of the exotic pet. A minimally capable or inexperienced veterinarian should not be treating these complex patients. Veterinarians may argue that suboptimal veterinary care is better than no care. That position is no longer justifiable given the myriad ways veterinarians and their staff can improve their skill set.

For the veterinarian who wants to be proficient in exotic pet medicine, these are means of achieving this:

1. Hire and train veterinary staff with expertise. Having one to three veterinary staff members who are well versed in exotic pets relieves pressure from the veterinarian to do all the history taking and handling routine exotic pet telephone calls.
2. Have protocols for annual examination, annual recommended diagnostic testing, and, in the case of ferrets, vaccinations.
3. The veterinarian, and ideally, the exotic pet-knowledgeable veterinary staff must receive annual continuing education. The past 10 to 15 years have seen significant increases in medical knowledge and techniques available for exotic pets. The way to become competent is through continuing education, internships, and/or residencies. Unless the veterinarian is planning for the majority of their caseload to be exotic pets, continuing education is the most common route to gain exotic pet knowledge. Subscriptions to exotic pet journals are necessary. Most major continuing education organizations offer wet labs, which are invaluable to learn new skills. Membership in the Association of Exotic Mammal Veterinarians (www.aemv.org), the Association of Avian Veterinarians (www.aav.org), and the Association of Reptile and Amphibian Veterinarians (www.arav.org) is highly recommended. In addition to these organizations' journals, they offer excellent continuing education. In the United States, they have consolidated their continuing education offerings in a multiple-day seminar called ExoticsCon (www.exoticscon.org).
4. Develop an after-hours emergency venue for exotic pets. Many states require that veterinarians offer clients emergency services either on site or at a convenient emergency facility. If a local ER offers exotic pet services, then this is a nonissue. If they do not, then consider asking if you can help train the local ER staff in basic exotic pet triage to satisfy any state requirements.
5. Lastly, proficiency comes with experience. The more the veterinary staff does and experiences, the better they will become in handling exotic pets.

To be competent in exotic pet medicine requires time, money, and resources on the part of the veterinary staff. If the veterinarian and staff are unwilling to invest in improving their skills, then one must consider whether this is an appropriate veterinary service to offer.

## Overview of Treating Exotic Pets

Although there is discussion within the veterinary community whether exotic animals are appropriate to have as pets (Hess et al. 2011), exotic pets comprise approximately 22% of the veterinary companion animal market (Kohles 2010). If the veterinary staff feels that having exotic pets or a particular set of exotic pets is not appropriate, then that facility should not see those species. Veterinary teams that commit to treat exotic pets should do so fully and completely, realizing that owners can be as committed to their gerbil as to a dog (Brown and Nye 2006). In the author's experience, the human–exotic pet bond is as strong as that seen with dogs, cats, and horses. As with other species receiving veterinary care, the veterinarian's role can be defined as providing the client with four pieces of information: the diagnosis, the treatment, the prognosis, and the cost. All decisions made after this information has been provided are for the client, and the client alone, to make. If veterinarians do not make value judgments regarding an animal's worth, it is often surprising what an exotic pet owner will pursue (Doneley 2005).

From a business aspect, ancillary services such as vaccinations, preventive medications (such as heartworm and flea/tick preventives), and dietary products play minimal if any role in income generation. In the author's practice, the average transaction fee (ATF) for exotic pets is 30% less than for dogs and cats. Possible ways to increase this ATF include delegating select services to staff such as beak trims, freeing up the veterinarian's schedule for more in-depth exotic pet services. Increasing your competency through training and addition of specialized equipment (such as a ventilator for anesthesia) can increase the ATF. For the veterinarian willing to commit to full-service and advanced exotic pet care, the overall gross revenue from exotic pets can be equal to a similar dog and/or cat practice.

Treating exotic pets presents challenges for the veterinary staff and practice. One important consideration is the high number of emergencies and fatalities that occur since exotic pets are usually presented late in the course of their disease. Many of these diseases are due to inadequate husbandry on the part of the owner. The poor prognoses associated with these circumstances can add to the emotional toll on the veterinary staff, who may justifiably wonder what the outcome would have been "If only we were able to see the pet sooner." Regularly seeing animals succumb to preventable problems can be emotionally draining and lead to compassion fatigue.

Another concern is public health and safety of the pet, owner, and veterinary staff. In this category are zoonoses and pet biosecurity. Many exotic pets have zoonotic potential to humans. As an example, Salmonella is a known pathogen in turtles. Biosecurity relates to the owner's ability to maintain an appropriate hygienic environment and precautions to minimize spread of pathogens between pets or from pet to owner. Professionals should directly address the biosecurity of the pet's veterinary care.

As in other species, the Five Freedoms should be the guiding principles for assessing the welfare of an exotic pet (Webster 2016). Briefly these are:

1. **Freedom from hunger and thirst** – by ready access to fresh water and a diet to maintain full health and vigor.

2. **Freedom from discomfort** – by providing an appropriate environment including shelter and a comfortable resting area.
3. **Freedom from pain, injury or disease** – by prevention or rapid diagnosis and treatment.
4. **Freedom to express normal behavior** – by providing sufficient space, proper facilities and company of the animal's own kind.
5. **Freedom from fear and distress** – by ensuring conditions and treatment which avoid mental suffering.

For exotic pets, all five need to be addressed in the context of their species-unique needs. Examples include the following:

1. Diets for particular species can be unique and may be difficult to obtain.
2. Creating an appropriate environment can be expensive.
3. Many exotic pets hide pain and illness until disease is advanced.
4. Expressing normal flight or foraging behavior may be difficult to achieve in the confines of a room or house.
5. Recognizing fear and distress can be difficult in some exotic pets.

EMODE is a concept that combines the Five Freedoms along with public health and safety concerns to determine the ease of maintaining an animal that maximizes its wellness (Warwick et al. 2014; Webster 2016). Table 15.2 presents a comparison of exotic pets to dog and cat ownership to illustrate that exotic pets are more difficult to manage on the part of owners and veterinary staff.

**Table 15.2** EMODE includes considerations regarding both the care of the animal with respect to its biological needs as well as human health and safety concerns (Warwick et al. 2014).

| Easy | Moderate | Difficult | Extreme |
|------|----------|-----------|---------|
| | | Invertebrates | |
| | | Fishes | |
| | | Amphibians | |
| | | Reptiles | |
| | | Birds | |
| | | Mammals (unusual) | |
| | | Mammal – primates | |
| | Domesticated animals | | |
| | Dogs and cats | | |

## Exotic Pet Groups

Veterinarians typically see one or more of three large groups of exotic pets. These include avian pets, ECMs, and reptiles and amphibians. Under the avian grouping, a significant subset includes backyard or small flock poultry patients. ECMs include species such as rabbits, ferrets, and rodents. Fish are the most common exotic pet, but the vast majority do not receive veterinary care due to the low perceived value of fish compared with the cost of veterinary care and the limited knowledge about the availability of veterinary services for aquatic animals (Loh et al. 2020). These two deficient areas should be addressed by the veterinary community to improve veterinary care for fish. For the purposes of this chapter, fish and less common and illegal exotic pets will not be covered.

## Avian – Nonpoultry

Properly owning and maintaining a bird entails a number of requirements common to owning any exotic pet. These include proper diet, housing, environmental enrichment items, and easily cleaned food and water bowls. Purchase prices can range up to several thousands of dollars. Usually, the size of the bird and the abundance or scarcity of a particular bird species determine the price when purchased through a pet store or breeder. Prices can be discounted when purchased through rescues or the Internet. These latter venues are common sources since many birds parrot size and larger have more than one owner through their lifetime.

The main reasons for relinquishment are noisy, messy, and potentially destructive behaviors (Hoppes and Gray 2010). Birds may be relinquished to a new owner who may not be any better suited to handle these problems by providing the appropriate husbandry and resources to ameliorate any behavioral or medical concerns. Improving owner retention is a multifaceted problem that has no clear answer. Remedies such as fines or restricted laws have not been effective (Perdomo et al. 2021).

One area that veterinarians can significantly impact is owner education on the behavioral and husbandry needs of birds before and after purchase. The Internet can play a vital role here through the use of species-specific websites (www.theparrotforum.com as one example), although some sites are not well curated. Reaching out to the public by attending pet expos, giving lectures at hobbyist clubs, and engaging with pet stores is beneficial for all stakeholders. Many locales mandate a "veterinarian of record" where the veterinarian is required to assist the store in managing their exotic pets. In these instances, reviewing client education materials and discussing issues you commonly see with new owners is advised. From a business perspective, leaving a professionally designed brochure for the veterinarian's services to be provided with each sold exotic pet can gain a new client for the practice.

Probably the most common ethical issue for veterinarians caring for these birds is improper husbandry, especially diet. Therefore, a thorough investigation of the bird's environment, diet, lighting schedule, and enrichment is paramount as part of the veterinary visit. If it is a recently acquired bird, the new owner may not have any knowledge of these items from the prior owner. As a veterinarian consulting on a new bird with an unknown history, it is prudent to assume the worst: an all-seed diet, limited cage space, poor lighting, and poor enrichment as a baseline. Having a thorough discussion about these potential shortcomings with owners can help determine what areas to prioritize. This history taking can occur by avian-knowledgeable staff or online surveys in addition to time spent in the exam room with the veterinarian. The veterinarian must also gauge how much information or education is too much at one time for the owner. If the goal is to have an educated client who can better care for their pet, then splitting up large amounts of information may be best. In the author's experience, most owners are very appreciative of any information the staff can provide. We are seen as the experts by the client.

Avian pets are the most likely species to show signs of maladaptive behaviors because of poor husbandry. The most visually evident maladaptive behavior is feather destructive behavior (FDB). It is beyond the scope of this chapter to explore the pathophysiology and possible treatments for FDB. Briefly, the lack of appropriate environmental enrichment along with possible poor dietary choices lead birds to excessively pluck their feathers. FDB is a coping mechanism based on a stereotypical behavior (Rubenstein and Lightfoot 2014). It does not occur in birds in the wild, leading one to assume there is some deficiency in the captive environment. Therapies include appropriate diet, adequate sleep, lighting, and environmental enrichment to replace normal flock behaviors (Stelow 2021). Many times, FDB cannot be resolved completely, and the pets live with this abnormality through their life. FDB has been estimated to occur in 15% of captive birds (Chitty 2003).

### Avian – Poultry

Poultry, through years of breeding and human interaction, are considered domesticated. Treating poultry typically falls into two categories. The first category is where the veterinarian is expected to serve the common good of the small flock intended to produce meat or eggs with the understanding that poor performing (e.g. no longer producing eggs) individuals may be culled and others euthanized to determine an etiology to benefit the remaining flock members and the owner's financial interest. Ethically, this can be termed the "greater good" theory or utilitarianism and is practiced in most production animal endeavors. Husbandry concerns include appropriate housing, protection from predators, diet, and environmental enrichment. Most small flock poultry are housed outside in protected coops that can be easily accessed in inclement weather, fed prepackaged diet from the local feed store, and can forage in the yard. As with any pet, the owner has an ethical obligation to meet the Five Freedoms. In my experience, these poultry generally have these basic needs met.

The second category is the chicken who is considered a personal pet and thought of as akin to a dog or cat with the concurrent human–animal bond. Many times, this pet chicken is one who started as a flock member but due to personality or uniqueness evolved to "pet" status during its lifetime. Most of these chickens are past their prime egg laying years and are laying few, if any, eggs. Most chickens live no longer than five years. Medical and ethical concerns for these pets are the same as for "flock" chickens in terms of husbandry, diet, and environmental enrichment. Because of the bond between owners and pet chickens, in the author's experience, many pet chicken owners are willing to pursue veterinary services. A common medical issue is due to reproductive disease requiring a salpingohysterectomy (removal of the oviduct, but not the ovary), which is an extensive and expensive surgery. Treating obvious reproductive diseases such as egg peritonitis with only medical therapy can be unrewarding and prolongs potential suffering of the pet chicken. Many times, the humane action is to euthanize the pet chicken in these cases.

## Birds in the Pet Trade

Although international conservation treaties (Convention on International Trade in Endangered Species of Wild Fauna and Flora [CITES] n.d.), national law (Fish and Wildlife Service [FWS] n.d.), and local municipality rules exist to prevent this, it is estimated that two to five million birds are illegally traded per year (Bergman 2009). The global illegal pet trade is estimated to be worth US$10 billion per year (Harris et al. 2015). This trade is causing depletion of a number of wild bird populations (Peng and Broom 2021). Approximately one-third (>400) of all globally threatened bird species are thought to be affected by overexploitation for food or the cage bird trade (BirdLife 2008). Veterinarians should ideally promote the purchase of captive-bred birds, but most owners do not consult with their veterinarian prior to the purchase of a pet bird. Corporate pet stores are regulated by most states, leaving expos, Internet searches, and flea markets as likely sources for the purchase of a wild-caught bird. Many times, captive-bred birds are free of various diseases wild-caught birds may carry.

It is imperative for the veterinary staff to inquire about the origin of the pet bird, although the actual origin does not lessen the veterinarian's responsibility to treat the pet and serve as an educational resource for the owner. Most US state laws do not require the veterinarian to report wild-caught birds to the authorities. However, some states do prohibit ownership of certain species of birds due to the fact they may be considered an invasive species if the pet escapes. It is up to state regulations whether these illegally owned birds need to be reported to the authorities. In the author's experience, owners of illegal pets do not seek veterinary care to avoid any legal repercussions.

By discussing the issues with wild-caught animals (e.g. depletion of wild populations, animals not adapted for human ownership, a high number of animals die during capture and transport, and zoonotic disease potential) with veterinary clients, some pressure may be exerted on the illegal pet trade. It appears that regulations regarding the illegal pet trade can have some effect, as evidenced by a 90% drop in the illegal bird trade in the European Union since a 2005 ban (ScienceDaily 2017)

## ECMs

Unlike pet birds, many common ECM species are thought to be domesticated. Almost all ECMs are captive-bred from hobbyists or companies dedicated to breeding them. The major welfare concern of ECM's is the provision of appropriate husbandry and diet. Appropriate diets are readily available at several locations such as pet stores.

## Rabbits

Because rabbits are social animals, they should be raised in groups of at least two with adequate space to hop and run around for several hours a day and have toys or objects to manipulate (Crowell-Davis 2007). The cost of ownership for a rabbit is low. Diets are inexpensive and easily located. Housing needs are minimal since many roam throughout the house. They can be litter box trained, which removes a hygienic concern for the owner. Many rabbits live 8–10 years.

Frequently seen medical issues are related to substandard husbandry. Education of the owner is paramount to improve the rabbit's quality of life. Two physiological characteristics predispose rabbits to common medical issues. The first is they are hind-gut fermenters where fermentation of high-fiber, low-energy food takes place in the cecum of the gastrointestinal tract. Rabbits also exhibit cecotrophy, which is the ingestion of cecotrophs (e.g. night stools) for nutrient extraction. When the normal movement of food is impaired because of insufficient fiber, abnormal gas and a slowing down of digestion can occur. This is called gastrointestinal stasis, which can be fatal.

Rabbits also continually grow their teeth (elodont), requiring a constant wearing down by chewing fiber in the diet. When the diet is deficient in fiber, dental overgrowth occurs, impairing ingestion of food, which can result in starvation. From the rabbit's perspective, chewing fiber and roughage provides enrichment (Baumans 2005).

Rabbits can be very easily stressed, and ethically it is incumbent on the owner and veterinarian to minimize stress. Situations that can be stressful to a rabbit include (Australia Agriculture n.d.):

- Novelty (new environments, transport, strangers)
- Sudden or loud noises
- Inability to express natural behaviors (inadequate exercise, lack of environmental enrichment, can't escape stressful events)
- Pain, discomfort, or illness
- Boredom
- Insufficient space
- No access to food or water
- Social stress through lack of or loss of companionship or too many individuals in a confined space
- Insufficient temperature control or ventilation.

The goal is to minimize stress by providing enrichment (such as chewing roughage), areas for the rabbit to retreat to if needed, areas to roam and explore at the rabbit's pace, along with fresh food and water. Veterinarians should consider offering house call visits to minimize stressors. During the veterinary visit, discussion of how to mitigate other stressors can be completed. There are a number of useful rabbit care sites available on the Internet that both the veterinary staff and owner can review to help (https://rabbit.org/frequently-asked-questions).

## Ferrets

Ferrets are a common ECM due to their extroverted nature. Their small size (usually less than 1 kg) makes them an ideal exotic pet for small living quarters. Many localities have banned ferret ownership due to cases of biting children and an unsubstantiated assumption that they are a natural reservoir of rabies, and prospective owners should check local laws. Some localities also ban veterinarians from caring for ferrets and it is up to the veterinarian to determine how local laws pertain to their practice. Ferrets have a life span of eight years and commonly develop diseases such as hyperadrenocorticism (70% of ferrets affected) (Simone-Freilicher 2008), insulinoma (25%) (Chen 2008), lymphoma (11%) (Antinoff and Hahn 2004), and dilated cardiomyopathy. These diseases typically are not curable and there may be considerable expense in managing them. Ferrets as pets are less common now than 10–15 years ago possibly due to the emotional and financial burden of these conditions on owners.

Most ferret illnesses are slow to develop, are usually visibly evident, and are chronic in nature. This gives owners time to research the illness, make financial arrangements for treatment, and deal with quality-of-life concerns at a more measured pace. Ill ferrets typically decline slowly, and the owner may not be sure if this is due to "old age" or progression of the disease. Therefore, it can be difficult for owners to determine when euthanasia is appropriate. This is where the veterinary staff can be invaluable in providing criteria about the pet's quality of life. For the diseases listed in the previous paragraph, the veterinary conversation starts when the diagnosis is made. For these diseases, well-developed medical algorithms with expected outcomes, prognosis, and life expectancy are established. By being candid at the initial veterinary visit, both the client and veterinary staff can discuss options for treatment and when an appropriate time is for euthanasia. For example, the development of recurring hypoglycemic seizures while the ferret is being treated for insulinoma is usually a sign that euthanasia should be considered.

As with other exotic pets, ferrets may transmit zoonotic diseases. One current concern is the potential for ferrets to carry severe acute respiratory syndrome–coronavirus 2 (SARS-CoV-2) virus. Fortunately, the Covid-19 virus is poorly transmitted from ferrets and they do not seem to be a reservoir for human infection (Shi et al. 2020).

## Rodents

This group includes the hystricognath rodents (guinea pigs and chinchillas) and myomorph rodents (rats, mice, gerbils, and hamsters). Guinea pigs live an average of 4–8 years, chinchillas average 8–10 years, while the myomorph rodents typically live no more than 2.5 years. Cost of ownership for rodents is low. Appropriate caging and diet are readily available. There are few special requirements (such as dust baths for chinchillas). The larger-sized rodents can roam free in the house while the smaller rodents are typically housed in species-appropriate habitats. Possibly due to their short lifespan, many of the myomorph rodents are treated symptomatically when they become ill, while the hystricognath rodents are more likely to receive extensive veterinary care for their ailments.

Like rabbits, guinea pigs and chinchillas have elodont teeth where the incisors and cheek teeth continually grow. They are also hind-gut fermenters. The common medical problems that occur are the same as for rabbits, namely dental issues and gastrointestinal stasis. These disorders can be expensive to treat and often occur acutely, which can leave the owner emotionally or financially challenged to make medical decisions. In the author's experience, recurring dental and gastrointestinal issues typically are treated by clients since the prognosis for full recovery is good.

In rats, neoplasia is common, and is often mammary related. It can occur at a young age and the tumors can grow quite large becoming painful and impinging on the rat's mobility. Preventive treatment is via ovariohysterectomy between three to four months of age (Hotchkiss 1995). Client education by the veterinary staff is the key to promote rat spaying. Spaying a rat costs approximately the same as spaying a dog, which typically lives five to seven times longer, and that cost can be a deterrent. Exotic pet surgery has a number of technical concerns such as the small size of the pet, tissues being more friable, and anatomic issues that are unique relative to dogs or cats. Additionally, most veterinarians have limited exotic pet surgery experience from veterinary college training.

A common ethical issue for hamsters and gerbils is they are typically purchased as "starter" pets for young children. Studies have shown that companion animals help child/adolescent development in the areas of self-esteem, loneliness, intellectual development, and increased social competence (Purewal et al. 2017). It appears that these benefits are stronger with owning a dog or cat as opposed to other types of pets (Vizek-Vidović et al. 1999). While owning a pet can be a predictor for young adults to be more empathic, more prone to helping professions, and more oriented to social values (Vizek-Vidović et al. 2001), it can be argued that leaving the primary responsibility of pet ownership to a child increases the possibility of poor husbandry that is potentially harmful to the animal. When these animals are ill, veterinarians, for the most part, will take the child's concerns into account but leave the final decision to the parent.

### Reptiles and Amphibians

Reptiles and amphibians are collectively called "herps" since the branch of biology dedicated to these two classes is herpetology. The cost of ownership varies by species and should be researched prior to purchase. Herps require extremely specific husbandry and often the cost of animal purchase is lower than the cost of appropriate caging, mechanical systems for heat and humidity, monitoring equipment, and maintaining an appropriate diet. The lifespan of herps varies greatly with some species living just a few years and others such as some tortoise species living 60–80 years or more. As with other long-lived pets, a transition plan is necessary, especially for the older owner.

Most herps tend to be solitary and do not need large areas to roam. As such, their actual cage can be smaller than for a similar sized ECM or bird. One thing to consider is the eventual adult size of the herp. Most amphibians do not grow extensively, whereas reptiles can become quite large as they mature. Some snakes such as boas range from 3 to 13 feet in length at adulthood. All aspects of husbandry need to be increased as the reptile grows, so more or larger heat sources, more equipment to regulate humidity, etc. Unless husbandry is modified appropriately, overcrowding, nonhygienic environment, and lack of adequate nutrition can occur.

Most illness (including death) is related to the owner's failure to provide adequate husbandry. For the veterinarian, it can be challenging to find a proper balance between educating the owner and being sensitive to their emotional state associated with imparting bad news. Because husbandry is so important, a thorough review of the reptile or amphibian's habitat and diet is of utmost importance. There are several informative websites that provide lists of particular species needs in terms of diet along with environmental optimal temperature zones for both day and night, humidity, and length of daily ultraviolet radiation or UVB exposure.[1] The veterinary history should include when equipment was purchased, as many UVB lamps lose their potency approximately nine months after beginning use. The UVB frequency is not visible to the human eye. UVB meters can be purchased but may be costly. An alternative is to purchase a new bulb every six months.

A common lizard disease is nutritional secondary hyperparathyroidism or metabolic bone disease due to inadequate calcium in the diet. Other lizard diseases include infectious stomatitis, dermatitis due to poor shedding, and gastrointestinal impaction caused by pica from eating the cage substrate. All of these are preventable diseases with proper husbandry. Unfortunately, frequently the first veterinary visit is due to illness. Ideally, the first visit would be a healthy pet exam and include a thorough discussion of husbandry. Promoting the veterinary skills of your facility to pet stores, online, and by hobbyist club visits can be one way to discuss the importance of that first well pet visit.

Herps are a potential zoonotic hazard, and this should be discussed with their owners during the veterinary visit. One of the more common concerns is salmonellosis. The US Centers for Disease Control and Prevention (CDC) recommends that children under the age of five years not have herps as pets for this reason (CDC n.d.). The CDC also recommends owners over the age of 65 not have herps as pets since they are at higher risk for infection. The veterinarian should also be aware of any state or local restrictions as many states prohibit the private ownership of venomous snakes due to concerns of them acting as invasive species.

## Husbandry and Role of the Veterinary Team

Good husbandry is paramount to having a healthy and enriched exotic pet. Exotic pets present unique and specialized husbandry needs that both the owner and the veterinarian need to know. Each species in the group has its own unique husbandry requirements. For avian and herp pets, a common veterinary rule of thumb is that over 90% of medical issues are caused by improper husbandry. In a clinical setting, this results in much more focus on history taking including diet, size of enclosure, heat, humidity, and environmental enrichments. The proactive veterinary staff member sees this as a significant opportunity for client education.

An experienced veterinary staff member can greatly supplement information obtained on the Internet for almost all clients, especially first-time owners of exotic pets. The staff should have at their disposal good client educational materials and a willingness to take the time to listen to the client and appropriately answer their concerns. For client educational materials, directing owners to specific websites is useful. Veterinary professional sites such as Veterinary Information Network (www.vin.com) have downloadable client education sheets that can also be used. Having client education handouts for common problems while discussing the issues with the owner is a time saver in a busy practice.

Appropriate owner education starts from the first telephone call. In many cases, what triggers the call from the owner is some type of abnormal behavior or sign of illness. A physical exam appointment should be made at the earliest possible time. A rule of thumb in dealing with exotic pets is that by the time the owner recognizes illness, you must consider it already at a moderate to advanced stage. It is an extremely knowledgeable and attentive owner who notes early and minor illness.

Once the appointment is made, a pet's history form should be completed, and it should be detailed and very specific. Ideally, clients can complete these forms at home, or it can be more of a checklist that the veterinary staff member goes over with the client. Having clients write down what they are feeding or obtaining a picture of the food label is invaluable. For herps, knowing what equipment clients have and when they obtained it can be vital in determining if equipment failure may be an etiology for an illness.

The examination process should be appropriate to the species. It should be conducted in a quiet setting and start with a visual assessment of the pet. Depending on that assessment, parts of the examination along with diagnostics may need to be staged to minimize life-threatening complications due to stress. Respiratory distress or recumbency should be treated with a grave prognosis and the owner should be informed of such. Fear Free LLC has a webinar that outlines many steps to make the exam process stress-free for birds.[2] Similar concepts can be used for ECMs and herps. Most ECMs and herps travel without any overt signs of stress. Birds may be better handled via a veterinary house call visit. Alternatively, for an established patient, telemedicine may be useful. The veterinarian needs to be cognizant of the rules governing telemedicine consultations in their area.

## Environmental Enrichment

Exotic pets are complex animals with species-specific needs. The mortality rates of captive exotics are high, quality of life is often compromised, and lifespans are often not reached (Free-Miles 2019). One estimate has the death rate of reptiles kept in captivity during their first year of acquisition at 75% (Toland et al. 2012)! Ethically, it can be difficult to justify keeping exotic pets in artificial environments, so it is necessary for the owner to maximize environmental enrichment. The concept of environmental enrichment is to provide pets a stimulating and appropriate environment to maximize their well-being (Rupley 2015). When done correctly, the exotic pet should thrive. Given the wide scope of exotic pet species, environmental enrichment for a particular species should be researched before purchasing the pet. If this cannot be provided, then the owner should be discouraged from owning an exotic pet. This is where the veterinary staff plays a key role in the health of the exotic pet. Of the three exotic groups, birds need the greatest amount of environmental enrichment while ECMs and herps are easier to provide appropriate enrichment for. If an owner cannot afford a suitable environment for an exotic pet, then a veterinary discussion on another, better suited, exotic pet should occur.

Operant learning using positive reinforcement (rewards) to shape desirable behaviors and eliminate undesirable ones (Langlois 2021) is a great way to challenge these highly intelligent animals to learn new things while also developing a strong social bond with their owners.

## Where to Rehome an Exotic Pet

Exotic pets sometimes need to be rehomed. The reasons for rehoming are comparable with those for other traditional species and include moving, death of an owner, allergies, and inability to maintain a good quality of life for the exotic pet (Grant et al. 2017). In the case of larger birds, their loud vocalization, especially in the morning and night, is a common reason for surrender. Since some exotic pets are long lived, such as larger birds and tortoises, conversations with owners about plans for rehoming these animals in case of death should be approached during one of the veterinary visits. The goal is to prevent an exotic pet from being placed into a rehoming situation where the new owners are not capable of properly caring for the animal.

Unlike dogs, cats, and horses, rehoming an exotic pet can be more difficult due to a paucity of available rescues and shelters. Having a list of local rescue shelters and a list of reputable clients who would take on an exotic pet is necessary for the veterinary staff. Also, one must be cognizant of what species is being rehomed where. Rehoming a macaw to a client who has never had a bird before would be discouraged since this species of bird requires more owner resources in terms of equipment, food, and time. For example, a macaw, if not properly approached and handled, can cause serious human injury from their bites. Again, the veterinary staff can do much of the research and client communication to make a rehoming situation successful.

## Case Studies

A common theme with Case Studies 15.1–15.4 is that many illnesses in exotic pets are largely prevented by proper nutrition, habitat, environmental enrichment, and an appropriate human-pet bond. Consequently, the veterinary staff must summon the courage to have difficult conversations that diplomatically discuss the failure to manage their exotic pet correctly. The author has found that actively listening to the client's concerns, answering questions, and discussing ways to improve husbandry go a long way in improving the welfare of exotic pets.

> ### Case Study 15.1  Owner reluctance to do testing in older parrot with weight loss
>
> Ms. Simmons presents a 20-year-old male eclectus parrot, Polynesia, who is lethargic and losing weight. She would like to discuss quality-of-life issues. She has had Polynesia his entire life. The other bird in the house (African grey) has no apparent illness. Ms. Simmons wants to "do right" by Polynesia and he is a dear companion. In the past, she has declined recommended baseline bloodwork and radiographs as part of annual visits since the bird has not shown any signs of illness. Testing was advised, but the owner requested a therapeutic trial instead. After further discussion, testing was approved.
>
>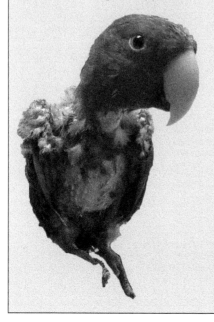

| Pertinent topic | Answer |
| --- | --- |
| Diet | Mostly seed with human food and vegetables. |
| Prior history | Has had feather destructive behavior (FDB) for 12+ years. FDB lesions have been stable for that time. |
| Exam findings | Distended coelom. Mild tachycardia. FDB lesions. Weight loss of 15% over past six months. |

| Question | Answer |
| --- | --- |
| Who are the relevant interests? | Given the exam findings, Polynesia most likely has a serious disease. The owner has a strong emotional attachment to Polynesia but was reluctant to pursue diagnostics. The veterinarian has a duty to relieve animal suffering. |
| What are the strengths of each interest? | Polynesia has a strong interest since his health/life is at stake. He is healthy enough to obtain blood samples and radiographs without compromising his well-being. |
| How do these interests conflict? | The major conflict is that the bird's life is dependent on the owner's decisions. Her reluctance to do testing to determine what is wrong with Polynesia may be monetary in nature or she may be afraid that the tests will reveal significant or life-threatening disease. After initial declination of testing, the veterinarian advocated for how testing may benefit Polynesia. |
| What are the available choices and their potential consequences for each interest? | Choices include: 1. Do testing now. Modern point-of-service equipment and staff trained to do an avian complete blood count (CBC) mean we would have information within 30 minutes. Ethically, obtaining a diagnosis (if possible) to start therapy sooner or to make a quality-of-life decision would be the preferred action for the bird. 2. Monitor Polynesia, recheck in one week, and obtain a new weight. This may delay any possible treatment, prolong suffering, and potentially worsen prognosis. |
| Are there any relevant laws or codes of conduct to consider? | Since Polynesia is not in any visible distress, any laws related to animal cruelty or abuse are not relevant at this time. |
| Choose a course of action or inaction Have I advocated for my patient/s to the best of my ability? | Testing revealed severe liver enlargement, coelom fluid, and elevated liver enzymes. Neoplasia is considered the likely cause as opposed to fatty liver syndrome. Further diagnostics including ultrasound and fine needle aspirate of the liver were offered but were declined. Euthanasia was recommended but was declined. The owner elected for a conservative approach and wanted to try "something" to see if it would help. A course of milk thistle was dispensed as a liver protectant, but the veterinarian discussed that this would be unlikely to improve his condition. Polynesia stopped eating 10 days later. On recheck, he had lost more weight and had worse coelom distension. Euthanasia was elected. This case exemplifies the challenges faced by veterinarians when advocating for patients conflicts with owner desires due to financial or emotional concerns. Therapeutic trials are often requested as they allow time for owners to cope with a terminal diagnosis, provide a sense of hope, and are perceived to be benign. Although these seldom cause harm, they can prolong suffering while the owner awaits a beneficial response that may not occur. Frequent follow-up is pivotal in ensuring such trials are of limited duration. |

**Case Study 15.2   The appeal of the exotic pet has worn off**

Ms. Childers' son has gone to college and left managing his pet water dragon, Draco, to his mother. Ms. Childers knows nothing about caring for the pet and her son left little direction for her. Today's visit is to understand more about Draco and how to care for this animal. During the exam, she mentions that she feels the pet's appeal has worn off for her son and she is concerned she will be stuck caring for the pet for the next few years.

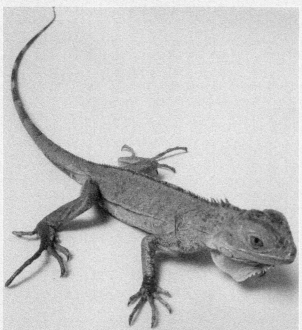

| Pertinent topic | Answer |
| --- | --- |
| Diet | Appropriate for this species. |
| Husbandry | Review of the heat, humidity, and terrarium structures was appropriate. |
| Exam findings | A little thin with discoloration of some toes. It was felt that this was more a humidity issue. |

| Question | Answer |
| --- | --- |
| Who are the relevant interests? | Draco is stable and has adequate husbandry. Draco is completely dependent on the collaboration between the mother and son as caretakers. |
| | The mother is the present caretaker of the pet. |
| | The son also has an interest since he originally owned Draco and provided most of the care until now. |
| What are the strengths of each interest? | Draco has an interest but since he is currently being well cared for, the stronger interest is who will be his long-term caretaker. In this aspect, the mother and son have stronger interests that could be considered equal (at some time the son will come home from college). |

| How do these interests conflict? | The mother is not happy to care for a pet she has no emotional bond with. Instead, her emotional bond is with her son. Fortunately, Draco is well maintained and is not in danger at this time due to this conflict. This is subject to change. |
| --- | --- |
| What are the available choices and their potential consequences for each interest? | 1. For Draco, none.<br>2. For the mother, either maintain Draco or consider rehoming. This should be done in agreement with the son.<br>3. For the son, have a discussion with his mother about what is best for Draco. The veterinarian can help facilitate that conversation. |
| Are there any relevant laws or codes of conduct to consider? | Since the pet is fine and appears to be well maintained, no laws or codes come into play. |
| Choose a course of action or inaction<br><br>Have I advocated for my patient/s to the best of my ability? | The mother chose to maintain care of the pet. It is anticipated when Draco can move to college with the son, Draco will do so. As long as the same level of care for Draco can occur at college, the veterinarian is satisfied with this decision.<br><br>This case illustrates that circumstances can change, and the exotic animal's care may be transferred to another person who has minimal knowledge of their unique requirements, potentially endangering their health and welfare. In this case, change in care was known in advance and steps should have been taken to smooth the transition from the son to the mother. |

### Case Study 15.3  Gecko with inadequate husbandry

Mr. Desmond presents Rango, a male gecko. He has been listless for the past one to two weeks. Today, Rango is not eating or moving.

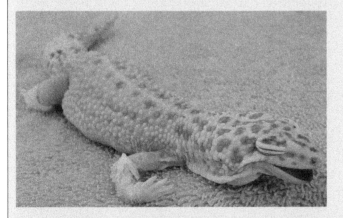

| Pertinent topic | Answer |
| --- | --- |
| Diet | Crickets were the mainstay of the diet. No supplemental calcium is provided. |
| Husbandry | Review of the heat, humidity, and terrarium structures shows it is appropriate. |

| Exam findings | Pathologic fractures of both antebrachia. Retained shed of skin from molting. Flexible mandible ("rubber jaw"). Listless. Based on the exam findings, a tentative diagnosis of secondary nutritional hyperparathyroidism (metabolic bone disease or MBD) was made. |
| --- | --- |

| Question | Answer |
| --- | --- |
| Who are the relevant interests? | Rango is experiencing poor quality of life and pain. |
| | The owner has shown some initiative by bringing Rango in for an exam. The veterinarian has an interest in ending the suffering of the animal. |
| What are the strengths of each interest? | Rango has the strongest interest since he has a life-threatening disease. |
| How do these interests conflict? | Rango is in a situation where medical intervention may not be enough to save him. For the owner, this would mean incurring veterinary costs and performing nursing care at home. MBD is a chronic disease that may take weeks to months to resolve. It is the duty of the veterinary staff to inform the owner that this could have been prevented by providing appropriate husbandry and to offer an accurate prognosis. |
| What are the available choices and their potential consequences for each interest? | 1. Perform tests to confirm the diagnosis. Since the exam findings are classic for MBD, this step probably can be skipped. |
| | 2. Treat in-hospital for one to three days to stabilize the pet and manage pain. |
| | 3. Treat as an outpatient with calcium injection, subcutaneous warmed saline, and removal of retained shed. Send home with oral calcium, force-feeding formula, and analgesic for pain. Demonstrate to the owner how to administer so mandibular fracture will not occur. Ensure they understand that any fractures will be permanent and may hinder mobility. |
| | 4. Euthanasia. |
| Are there any relevant laws or codes of conduct to consider? | This may legally fit the definition of cruelty. Unfortunately, in exotic pet medicine, this is a common occurrence. Veterinarians are mandated to report suspected cruelty in certain states in the United States (Wisch 2020). It is up to the veterinary staff to determine who to report cruelty cases to. Often, the scope of the local authority's jurisdiction is limited to dogs, cats, livestock, and horses (Animal Law 2003). Depending on the local animal cruelty reporting rules, local authorities may not pursue the complaint. |
| Choose a course of action or inaction<br><br>Have I advocated for my patient/s to the best of my ability? | Due to costs, the owner elected for outpatient therapy (no. 3). Follow-up calls at 1 day, 7 days, and 14 days showed the pet was doing well in terms of mobility and attitude but was not eating on his own yet. He was still being fed by the owner. |
| | As many exotic pets are presented to the veterinarian when they are already exhibiting moderate to severe illness, many nutritional and husbandry-based diseases do not resolve quickly. For MBD, it can be months if not a year before a full recovery. Prevention is the key, and the onus of appropriate husbandry is on the owner. The veterinary staff is there to educate and support the owner in their management of the exotic pet. |

**Case Study 15.4   Bird that is overly bonded to owner bites the spouse**

Mr. Evans has a nine-year-old female cockatoo, Tequi, who adores him. But in the past six months, when his wife has approached Tequi, she has become aggressive and bitten her.

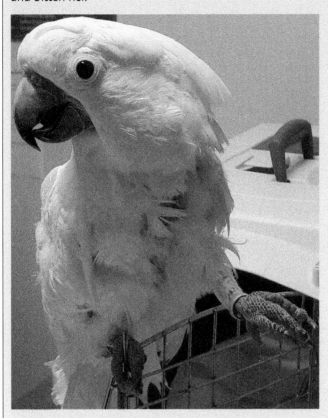

| Pertinent topic | Answer |
|---|---|
| Diet | 50% pellets with the other 50% being seeds, nuts, and people food. Mr. Evans allows the pet to eat from his plate. |
| Husbandry | Cage size and number and types of toys are appropriate. Things to improve are the use of captive foraging (i.e. prolonging time for bird to find its food and eat it), more variety in toys, and sufficient sleep for Tequi. |
| Exam findings | Mild feather loss on the keel. The rest seems appropriate. |

| Question | Answer |
|---|---|
| Who are the relevant interests? | The bird is exhibiting mate-related aggression, a maladaptive behavior due to inappropriate social bonding and close interaction between Mr. Evans and Tequi. This behavior is a manifestation of stress. |
| | Mr. Evans does not see a big concern because he enjoys the attention of the pet. |
| | Mrs. Evans is the recipient of Tequi's inappropriate behavior. The behavior can be hazardous since Mrs. Evans has been bitten previously. |

| | |
|---|---|
| What are the strengths of each interest? | Mrs. Evans has the strongest interest since she is the recipient of the aggression. |
| | Tequi's undesirable behavior is a product of the poor social husbandry by Mr. Evans. |
| How do these interests conflict? | If the social dynamics can be changed, Mr. Evans will lose his desired interactions with the pet, but Mrs. Evans will have a better dynamic between her and the pet. |
| What are the available choices and their potential consequences for each interest? | 1. Do nothing. The aggressive behavior may put the bird at risk of relinquishment or euthanasia. |
| | 2. Change to a more appropriate diet along with captive foraging and more complexity and variety of toys. |
| | 3. Initiate the recommendations outlined in no. 2 and work on changing the social interactions of the three parties. This involves time and labor for the family. |
| | In the author's experience, most owners opt for option no. 3 since it is a winning solution for all: Tequi is happier, Mrs. Evans is happier, and Mr. Evans has removed a source of stress. |
| | It is then up to the veterinary staff to outline a plan to address all aspects of option no. 3. |
| Are there any relevant laws or codes of conduct to consider? | Since the pet is fine and appears to be well maintained, no laws or codes come into play. |
| Choose a course of action or inaction<br><br>Have I advocated for my patient/s to the best of my ability? | The owners were counseled on changing the social dynamics and modifying the diet. Follow-up visits have shown a better social dynamic with Tequi being more tolerant of Mrs. Evans. |
| | Birds have specific and varied social interactions with other birds, animals, and humans. Overbonding is a common issue and a discussion with an avian-experienced veterinarian could have prevented this conflict. |

## Notes

1. https://zoomed.com/search-by-animal-caresheets is one site for UVB information.
2. Veterinary Certification Program – Avian | Fear Free Pets.

## References

American Veterinary Medical Association (AVMA) (n.d.). AVMA American Board of Veterinary Specialties. https://www.avma.org/education/specialties (accessed 12 February 2021).

American Veterinary Medical Association (AVMA) (2018). *2017–2018 Edition AVMA Pet Ownership And Demographics Sourcebook*. Schaumburg, IL: AVMA.

Animal Law (2003). State and municipal regulation of dogs. https://www.animallaw.info/article/state-and-municipal-regulation-dogs (accessed 22 March 2021).

Antinoff, N. and Hahn, K. (2004). Ferret oncology: Diseases, diagnostics, and therapeutics. *Veterinary Clinics: Exotic Animal Practice* 7 (3): 579–625.

Australia Agriculture (n.d.). Guidelines for keeping pet rabbits. https://agriculture.vic.gov. au/livestock-and-animals/animal-welfare-victoria/other-pets/rabbits/guidelines-for-keeping-pet-rabbits (accessed 8 February 2021).

Baumans, V. (2005). Environmental enrichment for laboratory rodents and rabbits: Requirements of rodents, rabbits, and research. *Institute for Laboratory Animal Research* 46 (2): 162–170.

Bergman, C. (2009). Wildlife trafficking: A reporter follows the lucrative, illicit and heartrending trade in wild animals deep into Ecuador's rain forest *Smithsonian Magazine* 16: 34.

BirdLife (2008). Nearly half of all bird species are used directly by people. http://www. birdlife.org/datazone/sowb/casestudy/98 (accessed 7 February 2021).

Brown, S. and Nye, R. (2006). Essentials of the exotic pet practice. *Journal of Exotic Pet Medicine* 15 (3): 225–233.

Chen, S. (2008). Pancreatic endocrinopathies in ferrets. *Veterinary Clinics: Exotic Animal Practice* 11 (1): 107–123.

Chitty, J. (2003). Feather plucking in psittacine birds 1. Presentation and medical investigation. *Practice* 25 (8): 484–493.

Convention on International Trade in Endangered Species of Wild Fauna and Flora (CITES) (n.d.). CITES homepage. www.cites.org (accessed 1 February 2021).

Crowell-Davis, S. (2007). Behavior problems in pet rabbits. *Journal of Exotic Pet Medicine* 16 (1): 38–44.

Doneley, R. (2005). Ten things I wish I'd learned at university. *Veterinary Clinics: Exotic Animal Practice* 8 (3): 393–404.

Fish and Wildlife Service (FWS) (n.d.). Wild Bird Conservation Act. https://www.fws.gov/ international/laws-treaties-agreements/us-conservation-laws/wild-bird-conservation-act.html (accessed 10 February 2021).

Free-Miles, S. (2019). Exotic pet welfare and ethics. In: *British Small Animal Veterinary Association Congress Proceedings*, 270–271. Quidgely, UK: BSAVA.

Grant, R., Montrose, V., and Wills, A. (2017). ExNOTic: Should we be keeping exotic pets? *Animals* 7 (6): 47.

Harris, J.B.C., Green, J., Prawiradilaga, D.M. et al. (2015). Using market data and expert opinion to identify overexploited species in the wild bird trade. *Biological Conservation* 187: 51–60.

Hess, L. (2011). Exotic animals: Appropriately owned pets or inappropriately kept problems? *Journal of Avian Medicine and Surgery* 25 (1): 50–56.

Hoppes, S. and Gray, P. (2010). Parrot rescue organizations and sanctuaries: A growing presence in 2010. *Journal of Exotic Pet Medicine* 19 (2): 133–139.

Hotchkiss, C. (1995). Effect of surgical removal of subcutaneous tumors on survival of rats. *Journal of the American Veterinary Medical Association* 206: 1575–1579.

Kohles, M. (2010). *Marketing and Growing an Exotic Pet Practice*. Australia: Association Avian Veterinarians Australasian Committee – UEP.

Langlois, I. (2021). Medical causes of feather damaging behavior. *Veterinary Clinics: Exotic Animal Practice* 24 (1): 119–152.

Loh, R., Vukcevic, J., and Gomes, G. (2020). Current status of aquatic veterinary services for ornamental fish in Australasia. *New Zealand Veterinary Journal* 68 (3): 145–149.

Peng, S. and Broom, D. (2021). The sustainability of keeping birds as pets: Should any be kept? *Animals* 11: 582.

Perdomo, E., Araña Padilla, J., and Dewitte, S. (2021). Amelioration of pet overpopulation and abandonment using control of breeding and sale, and compulsory owner liability insurance. *Animals* 11 (2): 524.

Purewal, R., Christley, R., Kordas, K. et al. (2017). Companion animals and child/adolescent development: a systematic review of the evidence. *International Journal of Environmental Research and Public Health* 14 (3): 234.

Rosenthal, K. (2006). Future directions in training of veterinarians for small exotic mammal medicine: Expectations, potential, opportunities, and mandates. *Journal of Veterinary Medical Education* 33 (3): 382–385.

Rubenstein, J. and Lightfoot, T. (2014). Feather loss and feather destructive behavior in pet birds. *Veterinary Clinics: Exotic Animal Practice* 17 (1): 77–101.

Rupley, A. (2015). Wellness management and environmental enrichment of exotic pets. *Veterinary Clinics: Exotic Animal Practice* 18 (2): ix–x.

ScienceDaily (2017). EU trade ban brings down global trade in wild birds by 90 percent. https://www.sciencedaily.com/releases/2017/11/171122151048.htm (accessed 1 March 2021).

Shi, J., Wen, Z., Zhong, G. et al. (2020). Susceptibility of ferrets, cats, dogs, and other domesticated animals to SARS–coronavirus 2. *Science* 368 (6494): 1016–1020.

Simone-Freilicher, E. (2008). Adrenal gland disease in ferrets. *Veterinary Clinics: Exotic Animal Practice* 11 (1): 125–137.

Stelow, E. (2021). Avian behavior consultation for exotic pet practitioners. *Veterinary Clinics: Exotic Animal Practice* 24 (1): 104.

Toland, E., Warwick, C., and Arena, P. (2012). The exotic pet trade: Pet hate: Exotic pet-keeping is on the rise despite decades of initiatives aimed at reducing the trade of exotic and rare animals. Three experts argue that urgent action is needed to protect both animals and ecosystems. *Biologist* 59: 14–18.

United States Centers for Disease Control and Prevention (CDC) (n.d.). Safe handling of pet reptiles & amphibians. https://www.cdc.gov/healthypets/pets/reptiles/safe-handling.html (accessed 13 February 2021).

Vizek-Vidović, V., Štetić, V., and Bratko, D. (1999). Pet ownership, type of pet and socio-emotional development of school children. *Anthrozoös* 12 (4): 211–217.

Vizek-Vidović, V., Arambasic, L., Kerestes, G. et al. (2001). Pet ownership in childhood and socio-emotional characteristics, work values and professional choices in early adulthood. *Anthrozoös* 14 (4): 224–231.

Warwick, C., Steedman, C., Jessop, M. et al. (2014). Assigning degrees of ease or difficulty for pet animal maintenance: The EMODE system concept. *Journal of Agricultural and Environmental Ethics* 27: 87–101.

Webster, J. (2016). Animal welfare: freedoms, dominions and "A life worth living". *Animals* 6 (6): 35.

Wisch, R. (2020). Table of veterinary reporting requirement and immunity laws. https://www.animallaw.info/topic/table-veterinary-reporting-requirement-and-immunity-laws (accessed 26 March 2021).

# 16

## Integrative Medicine

*Narda G. Robinson*

## Introduction

Integrative veterinary medicine (IVM), a field also known as "complementary and alternative veterinary medicine," "holistic medicine," "unconventional," and "natural medicine," first began in the 1970s in North America and has expanded ever since. IVM "describes the combination of complementary and alternative therapies with conventional care and is guided by the best available evidence. Veterinarians frequently encounter questions about complementary and alternative veterinary medicine (CAVM) in practice, and the public has demonstrated increased interest in these areas for both human and animal health" (Memon et al. 2016).

IVM presents a gamut of opportunities and difficulties when it comes to ethical practice. Even the title that one employs to describe it carries a considerable amount of nuance and implications as to its relationship with the "other," "conventional," "allopathic," or "mainstream" methodologies. The cumbersome nomenclature reflects the difficulty in separating diverse types of practices, each with their own origins from human medicine, scientific and unscientific foundations, proponents, and critics. Both "sides" should eschew the term "traditional" medicine as it introduces confusion. That is, is the speaker referring to "traditional" in the modern sense, talking about contemporary treatment with pharmaceuticals and surgery, or are they commenting on indigenous folk-medicine approaches that predate the scientific era?

Most veterinarians who incorporate techniques outside of those typically taught in veterinary curricula prefer the term "integrative." This sidesteps the awkwardness of "CAVM" as well as excludes the name "alternative," which implies treatments *other than* mainstream methodologies. "Holistic," which is missing its "w" ("wholistic"), suggests that its practitioners consider the entire patient. However, this invites a backlash from "conventional" veterinarians, who also insist that they view patients in their entirety. "Natural" medicine may have sufficed decades ago, but highly technical approaches such as photomedicine, pulsed electromagnetic field therapy, and electroacupuncture are not found in nature. So, in keeping with the prevailing opinions as to the ideal terminology, this chapter will use the term IVM when provided by veterinarians, and IM (minus the "V") for those situations in which a nonveterinarian or individuals with unknown credentials deliver this type of care. It contains an overview of the field, the pros and cons of each modality, and a case study that illustrates the ethical opportunities and pitfalls that IVM treatments present. The ethics of IVM impact the patient, the client, the profession, veterinary education, and scope of practice.

*Ethics in Veterinary Practice: Balancing Conflicting Interests*, First Edition. Edited by Barry Kipperman and Bernard E. Rollin.
© 2022 John Wiley & Sons, Inc. Published 2022 by John Wiley & Sons, Inc.

## Expanding Acceptance of IVM

As scientific support for IVM grows, its legitimacy and acceptance are similarly expanding. In fact, the convergence of science-based integrative medicine, fear-free veterinary care, integrative rehabilitation, and bond-centered practice is producing a new vision of what constitutes "typical" veterinary practice. Furthermore, veterinarians are encountering a burgeoning level of enthusiasm among clients for IVM for a wide range of problems in their animals. A survey of 423 horse owners found that 96% had used integrative medicine approaches (whether provided by a veterinarian or not) on their horse (Thirkell and Hyland 2017). The most popular therapies included massage (71%), chiropractic manipulation (59%), and magnet therapy (54%). Most (81%) expressed openness to instituting new treatments without consulting their veterinarian. This is concerning as it can result in potential harm to the treated horse and/or riders. Notably, only half of those surveyed stated that they were "very satisfied" with their "regular" veterinarian. A recent study of 204 horse owners found that 52% contacted an IM therapist before a veterinarian for back pain (Gilberg et al. 2021). Only 10–15% did not use any IM method for prevention or after injury.

Most veterinary teaching hospitals provide IVM services (Memon et al. 2021). Shmalberg et al. (2019a) analyzed the nature of canine and feline patients referred for acupuncture and herbal therapy to an academic veterinary teaching hospital. This two-year retrospective study found dogs (92%) far more frequently referred for treatment than cats (8%) and the most common problems noted were musculoskeletal (27%), neurologic (17%), oncologic (15%), and dermatologic (11%) in nature. Acupuncture in its various forms (dry needling (95%), electroacupuncture (26%), and pharmacopuncture (the injection of vitamins into points) (24%) was the most common therapy provided, followed by herbal supplements (76%). It should be noted, however, that one of the authors is also a manufacturer of Chinese herbal mixtures in addition to working as a professor at the same institution. The same authors published a three-year retrospective analysis of equine patients referred for acupuncture and herbal medicine (Shmalberg et al. 2019b). The three most common problems for which horses presented included musculoskeletal issues (62%), gastrointestinal dysfunction (9.5%), and anhidrosis (6%). Once again, acupuncture constituted the most common treatment (90%). A report of IM therapists treating dogs in Sweden found that the most frequently used methods were massage, stretching, and acupressure (Sohlberg et al. 2021).

Veterinary students who receive exposure to IVM during school or earlier may decide to pursue this type of work upon graduation. Some even report that this was the driving force for their pursuing a career in veterinary medicine (personal communication). More seasoned veterinarians may transition to IVM after they have grown weary with corporate pressures (see Chapter 17) and the limited and sometimes stressful treatment options that may cause the patient to fear the practitioner. Many welcome the opportunity to learn new ways to help their patients heal that provide comfort, restore functional homeostasis, and have a rational basis with evidence of effectiveness. On the other hand, some veterinarians pursue treatment methods that fail to meet requirements for a scientific basis and supportive evidence, whether IVM or "conventional."

## Choosing "Conventional" vs. IVM Approaches

Scientific evidence of effectiveness cannot be the only criterion of what constitutes "good care." Other relevant factors include risks of treatment, potential complications, pain, and debility that may arise, costs, recovery time, and client's informed consent. Ethically, clients should receive a complete picture based on evidence of the range of options available. However, surgeons, for example, may not have studied the effectiveness of nonsurgical options, including IVM techniques such as medical acupuncture, massage, movement therapy, and photomedicine. Moreover, veterinary orthopedic surgeries can earn practitioners thousands of dollars for each procedure, with the tibial plateau-leveling osteotomy (TPLO) costing $5000 or more. Could this also constitute a conflict of interest between what is best for the patient and best for the practice's "bottom line"?

How do results compare between the TPLO and a nonsurgical approach with IVM and rehabilitation for patients with injured cranial cruciate ligaments? To date, no research exists that directly compares a multimodal IVM protocol with the TPLO. Furthermore, IVM methodologies offered by one practitioner may vary in number and type from those of another, in addition to tailoring treatment selections for each patient's individual needs. A study comparing the TPLO with something as simple as a custom-made stifle joint orthotic indicated "high owner satisfaction rates for both interventions" (Hart et al. 2016). In this case, if a brace that costs under $1000 could allow patients to avoid the risk of severe and costly complications, even without the addition of IVM, why are veterinarians not learning more about nonsurgical options? Could this stem, at least in part, from the limited to nil exposure to IVM that most veterinary schools offer students? Only 30% of veterinary colleges reported offering a formal course in IVM and only 77% offered "some level" of instruction in IVM, with acupuncture and rehabilitation as the most popular modalities covered in the curriculum (Memon et al. 2021). Could a conflict of interest on the part of a teaching institution that nets high profits from TPLOs dissuade faculty from promoting nonsurgical options, especially given the heavy reliance that academia has developed on corporate funding? Where are the ethical discussions on this?

In addition to the pain and invasiveness of the TPLO, the procedure may lead to numerous complications, some severe, painful, and debilitating in an unacceptably (to this author) high percentage of patients. As stated by Bergh and Peirone, "Ten to 34% of TPLO surgical procedures are reported to experience a complication and approximately two to four percent require revision surgery to address a complication" (2012). Soft tissue complications include laceration of regional blood vessels, ligaments, and tendons. Severe blood loss may result from damage to local arteries. Measures instituted to reduce the risk of soft tissue damage, such as the introduction of gauze sponges to decrease iatrogenic tissue trauma, may deposit debris into the wound and lead to tissue reactions, infections, and the formation of a draining tract. Intraoperative complications range from tibial and/or fibular fracture to broken hardware, i.e. bits of screws, pins, drill bits, etc. The authors list over 20 postoperative complications, ranging from meniscal tear to patellar tendonitis, pivot shift, delayed union, internal tibial torsion, implant failure, and more. In contrast, medical acupuncture, photomedicine, massage, and movement therapy all have extremely low rates of injury and complications.

An IVM approach for cranial cruciate ligament injury offers a multimodal, relatively pain-free treatment series that addresses the plural causalities of ligamentous deterioration and its consequences *instead of* altering the limb's configuration. As we apply critical scrutiny to *all* practices, we should also weigh the ethical pros and cons of the physiologic considerations, pain and stress, financial impacts, and long-term risks of each approach. An exhaustive comparison of conventional and IVM procedures for common problems in veterinary practice would be a worthy undertaking but is beyond the scope of this chapter.

## Types of IVM Care

For all IVM therapies, the first step in treating animals safely and effectively involves an accurate assessment and delineation of the patient's problems. Human practitioners who apply their techniques to animals have neither the requisite veterinary education nor the experience in the field that veterinarians do. Clients who take their animal to a human acupuncturist, chiropractor, or massage therapist often fail to recognize the vast differences and the risks involved. These issues reinforce the need for all IM and IVM providers to maintain a science-based, evidence-informed perspective and to eschew archaic methodologies.

### Acupuncture

The scientific approach to acupuncture often called "medical acupuncture," evolved from ancient Asian methods during the 1980s with the development of the American Academy of Medical Acupuncture and other physician acupuncturist groups in Europe. A British group defines "Western" medical acupuncture as "a therapeutic modality involving the insertion of fine needles; it is an adaptation of Chinese acupuncture using current knowledge of anatomy, physiology, and pathology, and the principles of evidence-based medicine" (White 2009).

#### Mechanism of Action

Acupuncture involves inserting thin, sterile, solid needles into specific sites on the body called "acupuncture points." Acupuncture points, arranged in lines called "channels" (or "meridians"), typically follow neurovascular routes or myofascial cleavage planes. The anatomic structures within the needle's vicinity activate a cascade of autoregulatory and physiologic responses within the central, peripheral, and autonomic nervous systems. The nature of the effects engendered corresponds to the "job" of the structure activated. That is, needling an acupuncture point on the face alters the resting tone of the trigeminal and facial nerves. Most often, the outcomes of needle stimulation include analgesia, reversal of central or peripheral sensitization, and normalization of myofascial tone and function. This phenomenon is called neuromodulation. Electroacupuncture (EA) amplifies the neurophysiologic changes engendered by needling: an electrical lead attaches to the shaft of the acupuncture needle, which then functions as an electrode which delivers a stimulus of varying frequencies that modulate neuronal activity.

These modern, biologically based mechanisms replace the metaphorical concepts of chi (Qi), i.e. what Traditional Chinese Medicine (TCM) practitioners call "energy," which they claim circulates throughout the body through invisible "meridians." TCM providers allude to prescientific-era metaphorical causes of disease such as wind, heat, cold, dampness, and dryness. Furthermore, TCM practitioners utilize primitive, folkloric assessments such as tongue diagnosis and pulse diagnosis to determine their acupuncture and herbal prescriptions, despite the lack of validation of these methods for all species. This amounts to prescribing treatments based on faith or empirical observations, leading to less-than-ideal results. Whereas a scientifically trained medical acupuncturist selects points in a systematic manner, seeking to restore proper function in central, peripheral, and autonomic nervous system pathways, a TCM practitioner relies either on point "formulae" that are general in nature or a set of bizarre, exotic ideations and rituals of examination, such as Yamamoto Scalp Acupuncture, Korean Hand Acupuncture, Five Elements, etc.

Fortunately, the effects of needling provide sufficiently strong homeostatic influences that even if a TCM-based practitioner believes they are working through quasi-religious processes, the effects on the body may nevertheless be helpful. That said, a more precisely designed needling protocol assembled by a medical acupuncturist would more directly and profoundly address patients' specific problems.

### Indications

Research on acupuncture to treat naturally occurring disease most commonly includes dogs with intervertebral disc disease (IVDD) and horses with back pain or laminitis. For thoracolumbar (TL) IVDD in dogs, EA combined with conventional medical treatment led to a shorter time to recover both ambulation and deep pain sensation than did conventional care alone (Hayashi et al. 2007). Other studies indicate that EA for dogs with TL IVDD decreased pain, reduced incidence of relapse, and facilitated return to function (Laim et al. 2009; Han et al. 2010). Researchers typically evaluate EA rather than dry needling alone, finding that EA yields superior results for this condition (Dragomir et al. 2021).

Equine research has revealed similar outcomes, as EA outperformed phenylbutazone for the alleviation of TL back pain (Xie et al. 2005). Treatment with dry needling, hemoacupuncture (bleeding of points with a lancet), or aquapuncture (or "pharmacopuncture," if involving the injection of medication or vitamins into points) resulted in a significant reduction in the severity of lameness (Faramarzi et al. 2017).

Additional indications for acupuncture, as shown for humans, include chronic pain (Yuan et al. 2016; Vickers et al. 2018), neurologic injury or disease (Fan et al. 2018), immune dysfunction (Kim and Bae 2010), digestive disorders (Li et al. 2015), reproductive disturbances (Zhu et al. 2018), cancer-related pain (Chiu et al. 2017), and more.

### Contraindications

Acupuncture has a strong safety record, and few contraindications exist including pregnancy, tumor or infection in sites chosen for needling, bleeding disorders, and conditions wherein introducing a sharp object into the body could be injurious, such as in aggressive or extremely fearful patients.

### Adverse Effects

When performed by a scientifically based, anatomically aware practitioner, acupuncture has a low rate of complications in my experience. The scientific background and knowledge of anatomy should inform the acupuncturist about safe depths of needling: this helps to avoid severe complications such as organ puncture and injury to large vessels (Peuker et al. 1999).

## Manual Therapies

Manual therapies refer to interventions involving the hands. Two common examples in veterinary medicine include massage (Gilberg et al. 2021) and chiropractic. While applications of manual therapies frequently relate to musculoskeletal discomfort and/ or dysfunction, other indications include lymphedema, immune dysregulation, nerve compression, and visceral dysfunction.

### Massage

Massage techniques vary widely ranging from light to heavy pressure and from slow to invigorating techniques and styles. A common approach called Swedish massage incorporates several maneuvers such as effleurage (stroking and gliding), tapotement (percussion), petrissage (kneading), and friction massage (vigorous rubbing in a targeted zone requiring special attention).

#### Mechanism of Action

Massage focuses on soft tissue elements – muscles, fascia, tendons, nerves, and other intervening soft tissues. The neuromodulatory and homeostatic effects of massage regulate the autonomic nervous system and confer analgesia: many of the mechanisms overlap with those described for acupuncture. Furthermore, mechanical influences of massage can alleviate tissue swelling and lymphatic congestion.

#### Indications

Benefits of massage include pain and stress reduction, improved gastrointestinal motility, immune regulation, and mood elevation. Numerous applications thus arise in intensive and palliative care, oncology, pain medicine, rehabilitation, and sports medicine (Formenton et al. 2017). An uncontrolled, retrospective study on the effects of massage therapy on pain and quality of life in dogs concluded that treatment reduced the severity of myofascial and musculoskeletal pain (Riley et al. 2021).

#### Contraindications

Certain conditions and types of patients may preclude the safe and effective delivery of massage therapy to small animals, compelling the provider to either avoid a problematic area or select a different modality. Patients who are especially fragile or ill need to receive briefer and gentler treatments with less digital pressure and compression. One should avoid massage directly to neoplastic lesions, recent surgical sites, highly inflamed tissue, and infected areas. Animals that are aggressive, febrile, or in shock are typically considered unsuitable for massage.

#### Adverse Effects

As with acupuncture, thorough and science-based education in massage would make injury from the intervention unlikely. Those who provide massage should tailor treatment for certain conditions and types of patients. A massage therapist with insufficient awareness of nonhuman anatomy and tolerance for pressure could injure an animal with excessive force, especially if that patient has medical issues such as disk disease, spinal instability, or cancer (Miwa et al. 2019). For these reasons and more, jurisdictions that allow human massage therapists to work with animals need to ensure that the practitioners work closely with veterinarians. This may translate to a requirement for supervision, whether direct or indirect.

## Chiropractic

The terms "animal chiropractic," "veterinary manual therapy," and "animal adjusting" typically refer to a procedure called high velocity low amplitude thrusting. Those that provide the service may claim that this technique improves a wide variety of problems but, when pressed, fail to be able to explain how it works or show any evidence of efficacy or safety.

### Mechanism of Action

Chiropractors claim to treat "subluxations," which in this parlance describes minor misalignments of the vertebrae or ribs, in contrast to the standard medical definition of a partial dislocation. However, the idea that one is "putting back into place" a rib or a vertebra has amassed criticism. More likely, the sudden forces applied to a joint incite a volley of mechanoreceptor firing and create conditions that may restore joint motion, safely or unsafely. No one chiropractic technique has been shown to be superior to another, and as aforementioned, little to no chiropractic research is available on animals, so safety and effectiveness remain in question.

### Indications

Limited data exist for chiropractic in dogs, cats, or horses. This has not stopped animal chiropractors and their veterinary proponents from promoting chiropractic for a gamut of problems including idiopathic lameness, intervertebral disc disease, wobbler syndrome/cervical vertebral insufficiency, spondylosis, cauda equina syndrome, urinary incontinence, neuropathies, postsurgical rehabilitation, trauma, and organ pathology (Taylor and Romano 1999; American Veterinary Chiropractic Association 2021). However, many of these conditions may constitute contraindications.

### Contraindications

Contraindications for chiropractic include conditions that weaken bone or other structural elements such that applying a rapid thrust to a vulnerable spine or limb could lead to serious injury. Examples include deossifying or destabilizing conditions such as hyperadrenocorticism, neoplasia, secondary renal hyperparathyroidism, degenerative joint disease, and disc disease.

### Adverse Effects

The way that an "animal chiropractor" or "animal adjuster" performs the therapy on an animal varies widely. They may only use their hands or rely on a mechanical device. Force may be minimal or much greater, as when a chiropractor "adjusts" a horse with a mallet and a block of wood. Excessive pressure from forceful thrusts of chiropractic has the potential to injure organs, vessels, neural tissue, and/or bones (Swait and Finch 2017).

Injuries from chiropractic usually result from trauma to the spinal cord or brain that arise from blood vessels, discs, or nervous tissue that have been damaged with the thrust (Boucher and Robidoux 2014). Human neurological and neurosurgical reports have revealed an association between stroke and upper cervical manipulation (Turner et al. 2018). The mechanism of injury often involves arterial dissection or spasm (Gomez-Rojas et al. 2020). The author has been informed about anecdotal incidents involving horses being injured and expiring following cervical spinal adjustments.

### Controversies

In addition to the risk of injury, the lack of a clear mechanism of action, and unknown effectiveness, controversy arises from the fact that manual therapies may be delivered by nonveterinarians. While scope of practice challenges apply to every other treatment mentioned in this chapter, the damage that chiropractic can do to an animal supersedes most other IM care.

Furthermore, nonveterinarians' lack of familiarity with animal behavior, with veterinary medicine and zoonotic diseases, and proper restraint techniques can pose risks to therapists, bystanders, and patients. Lay chiropractors, specifically, may not have suitable liability insurance coverage for such incidents, exposing the veterinarian supervising their work to unexpected malpractice claims. Finally, one must consider, as with Traditional Chinese Veterinary Medicine (TCVM), whether veterinary schools should teach IVM methods that lack evidence of safety and effectiveness. This includes chiropractic.

## Photomedicine

Photomedicine involves the application of light to the body to support healing and lessen pain. Photomedicine devices may deliver the light as a laser beam ("laser therapy") or light-emitting diodes (LEDs). As with acupuncture and massage, laser therapy provides analgesia, myofascial relaxation, and circulatory support. In contrast to the physical stimulation of needling and hands-on therapy, photomedicine accomplishes its healing influences through photons that act on cells. Therefore, treatment effectiveness and the types of responses seen depend heavily on if and how light enters living tissue.

### Mechanism of Action

For tissue to absorb light and alter its physiology, a photochemical or photobiologic event must take place. A "photoacceptor" molecule, also known as a "chromophore," responds to light by initiating a series of physiologic responses. When a chromophore (such as cytochrome c oxidase in the mitochondrial respiratory chain) absorbs a photon, a series of reactions takes place that influence oxidative states, tissue growth, circulation, and various signaling pathways related to phenomena such as the modulation of immunologic and inflammatory responses (Chung et al. 2012; Mokmeli and Vetrici 2020). The term "photobiomodulation" describes these events, incorporating in its name the impact of *photons* on the individual's *biology*, with the outcome of *modulating*, or normalizing, physiologic states.

### Indications

Photomedicine, whether with laser therapy or LEDs, has shown effectiveness for the following conditions in humans and experimental animals:

- Musculoskeletal pain (postsurgical, sports injury, fracture, etc.) (Gendron and Hamblin 2019);
- Inflammation and edema (e.g. mastitis, otitis, soft tissue trauma, etc.) (Hamblin 2017);
- Joint disease (cranial cruciate ligament disease or injury, arthritis, elbow dysfunction, etc.) (Al Rashoud et al. 2014);
- Wound healing, especially when delayed (Tatnatsu-Rocha et al. 2016);
- Alopecia (Avci et al. 2014);
- Central nervous system injury and degeneration (Hashmi et al. 2010);
- Peripheral nerve injury (Sasso et al. 2020);
- Internal organ dysfunction (Liebert et al. 2017);
- Oral mucositis in cancer patients (Zadik et al. 2019).

### Contraindications

One should avoid applying laser therapy to a neoplastic or malignant tumor, a hyperactive thyroid gland, areas of active hemorrhage, the eye, and the pregnant uterus. Laser is also contraindicated in cases of lymphoma and for patients on immunosuppressive medications as laser therapy has immunostimulatory effects. In immature patients, higher-powered laser therapy devices may stimulate premature closure of epiphyses. This caution is warranted over long bones in animals less than one year old. For patients on photosensitizing pharmaceuticals or botanicals, treatment intensity should be lowered. For example, photosensitizing agents such as hypericin in Saint John's wort may augment the dermatologic impact of laser light (Cotterill 2009).

### Adverse Effects

The main risks of laser therapy pertain to eye damage and thermal burns. Laser light can damage the retina and other components of the eye. Laser goggles, too frequently omitted for those in the vicinity, protect against indirect exposure but not direct. Tattoos, when lasered, can become extremely painful due to the absorption of light and the generation of heat at the tattoo site. Questions remain about the ability of laser therapy to stimulate neoplastic growth and if so at what wavelengths and powers.

### Controversies

Questions remain about proper "dosing" of light in nonhuman species, as well as the long-term safety of high-powered treatment such as that delivered by Class IV units in veterinary medicine. Too few users (veterinarians and veterinary technicians) understand the scientific basis of photobiomodulation and the different tissue responses to a spectrum of wavelengths, pulsing regimens, and other treatment parameters. They default to a "point and shoot" approach, aware of little more than how to turn on the machine and where to aim the applicator. This does a disservice to animals, who may experience thermal burn or vision loss from an improperly applied beam (Ma et al. 2019).

### Botanical Medicine

Herbal (botanical) medicine refers to the practice of prescribing plant products for the treatment of disease. Herbal medicine is one of the oldest forms of treatment; even animals self-medicate with plants. Some researchers have suggested exploring how and why animals self-medicate to elucidate ways that humans might also derive benefits and discover novel treatments for problems such as cancer (Dominguez-Martin et al. 2020).

The indications, contraindications, and adverse effects of botanical medicine would directly correspond to their pharmacologic actions, dose administered, herb–drug interactions, manufacturing quality or lack thereof, patient health or illness, and more.

Evidential support concerning use of plant products in veterinary patients remains scarce (Shmalberg et al. 2019b). Consequently, for veterinarians who seek a science-based rationale for their botanical recommendations, one tends to make inferences from human studies, realizing the risks and limitations of doing so. However, one area of veterinary herbal research, i.e. cannabis-derived hemp extracts, is expanding rapidly (Cital et al. 2021). Indications including pain management, mechanisms of action, guidelines for quality control verification, and doses are becoming available. In fact, laws are beginning to change to allow veterinarians to discuss and/or prescribe products such as cannabidiol (CBD) (Nolen 2021).

On the other hand, while practitioners apparently feel quite comfortable recommending a Chinese herb called *Yunnan Paiyao* to prevent hemorrhage, little rigorous research exists to support this practice (Robinson 2016). Nonetheless, one can earn a certification in Traditional Chinese Veterinary Herbal Medicine (TCVHM) wherein one can make diagnoses and select remedies based heavily on folkloric assessments such as tongue and pulse diagnosis. Both methods lack validation and reliability across all species, including human.

### Additional Controversies with TCVHM

Chinese herbal mixtures may contain endangered flora or fauna (Cheung et al. 2020) as well as insects, worms, heavy metals, undisclosed pharmaceuticals (St-Onge et al. 2015), and a host of other undesirable ingredients (Bi et al. 2020). Some TCVHM remedies contain undisclosed quantities of herbal strychnine (a potent neurotoxin) or aconite (both cardiotoxic and neurotoxic). The identity and/or amount of each constituent in a product may be kept secret by the manufacturer. Proprietary compounds put patients and practitioners at risk because the veterinarian has no knowledge of the full list or amount of ingredients in a product. This violates the American Veterinary Medical Association (AVMA) Principles of Veterinary Medical Ethics (PVME), which advise against recommending or prescribing products with secret ingredients: "Veterinarians shall not promote, sell, prescribe, dispense, or use secret remedies or any other product for which they do not know the ingredients" (AVMA n.d).

When manufacturers keep their recipes secret, this raises the possibility of liability and injury if the patient or a human in the household (toddler, etc.) ingests tablets with an unknown quantity of highly toxic ingredients. This becomes even more problematic when the label lists strychnine and aconite by their *Pinyin*, rather than English, names, thereby disguising the nature of the bottle's contents.

Chinese "herbal" medicine is actually a misnomer, as Chinese "herbs" may not be derived from plants at all. Animal-based ingredients such as testis, penis, placenta, and horn found in Chinese herbal medicines harbor potential for zoonotic disease transmission. In addition to health concerns, products from animals in Chinese so-called "herbs" contribute significantly to animal mistreatment and the endangerment of species such as the tiger and rhinoceros. The benefits of these illegally derived compounds are unproven and typically folkloric, exacerbating the misery caused by wildlife poaching and trafficking in Asia and Africa.

### Homeopathy

Homeopathy is a practice initiated in the late eighteenth century by the German physician Samuel Hahnemann. Hahnemann based homeopathy on the notion that "like cures like" (National Center for Complementary and Integrative Health 2021). He posited that a small amount of a substance could cure the symptoms a patient was showing that that very same substance would *produce*, if provided in larger amounts.

#### Mechanism of Action

No known, or even credible mechanisms of action exist by which extremely dilute homeopathic preparations might have a therapeutic effect. Indeed, researchers struggle to convincingly demonstrate clinical differences between homeopathic remedies and placebo in rigorously designed studies (Doehring and Sundrum 2016; Cukaci et al. 2020). As a result, most authorities consider that any clinical outcomes obtained from homeopathic remedies are based on a placebo effect.

#### Indications and Contraindications

Although largely unsupported by research, homeopaths contend that their remedies can benefit patients with almost any condition, including cancer, despite having little to no rigorous research to support their claims. We should not be asking what homeopathy should or shouldn't be used for: instead, we should ask why anyone is using this in animals at all (AVMA 2013, 2017).

#### Adverse Effects

The most likely adverse effect of homeopathy would be delay of proper diagnosis and treatment, as those who practice "classical" homeopathy advise against mixing the "subtle healing energies" of the remedy-coated sugar pills with pharmaceuticals or other healing interventions. This type of mindset lands homeopathy in the *alternative* medicine camp rather than IVM, in that it dissuades combining techniques to give the animal the best chance of recovery.

#### Controversies

Ethical questions arise when practitioners prescribe unapproved and untested homeopathic remedies for animals who are ill, infectious, and/or painful. It is unethical and misleading to offer an ineffective treatment to patients and their caregivers. The unscientific premise of homeopathy calls into question its legitimacy.

## Regulatory and Legal Concerns

Each year, states and provinces across the United States and Canada, respectively, face pressure to allow nonveterinarian healthcare providers direct access to animals. These practitioners range from chiropractors and acupuncturists to massage therapists and physical therapists. Too often, laws change to grant these rights before veterinary medical associations can organize an effort to stop the process. In 2019, the AVMA updated an overview of scope of practice laws regarding CAVM and other practice act exemptions (AVMA 2021). Keep in mind that rarely does a practice act become *more* restrictive. Instead, the ingress of human practitioners into companion animal and equine practice steadily grows.

Sometimes, this arrangement represents a compromise between the human profession (in this case, chiropractic) and the veterinary profession's representatives in the state in which the change in law is up for debate. Some veterinarians would prefer not to relax laws and allow nonveterinarians to work on animals without direct supervision, citing issues of potential problems such as misdiagnosis and maltreatment. Others welcome more providers to treat animals: they may feel that animals are underserved (a claim that chiropractors have been known to make) and that clients should have the "right" to seek whatever types of treatments and practitioners they want to treat their animals (another contention made by chiropractors to state regulatory authorities).

Chiropractors will also cite "restraint of trade" when pushing to gain entry to animal work – the same argument they lodged successfully against the American Medical Association in the mid-twentieth century. However, several differences exist between treating humans as a human-trained healthcare provider and demanding access to nonhumans. Obviously, the human biped's form and function differ from the horse, dog, and cat. Moreover, nonhumans experience a wide range of diseases and injuries that veterinarians learn how to diagnose and treat, but chiropractors do not. With practically no studies on the safety and effectiveness of chiropractic manipulation in nonhumans, how can one argue that animals will benefit and not be injured? (And how can veterinary schools allow faculty to practice and promote chiropractic when they are precisely the ones who should be performing research to *test* these approaches before instituting them in a *veterinary* teaching hospital?)

In some instances, as with chiropractic, for example, states may require a special "certification" that requires a human chiropractor to have satisfied requirements from a self-proclaimed certifying body. They may have to attend a specific number of hours of coursework, complete testing by an "approved" course, and agree to practice in accordance with the guidelines set forth by the certifying body and the state board of chiropractic. So, what is "certification"? Essentially, anyone can "certify" anyone in anything. On the one hand, dedicating 50–150 hours to learning a rational, evidence-informed technique such as medical acupuncture has a science-based foundation as strong as many other practices taught to veterinarians during their professional school years. On the other hand, one can spend five minutes on the internet and obtain certification as a Reiki (energy healing) master. In their work, they may claim to connect with an animal's "spirit" guides. This involves "interspecies telepathic communication" as the Reiki master "listens" to what the patient communicates to them. If the animal "dislikes" taking antiepileptic medication every day, for example, the practitioner may relay this to the client, who then has a quandary. Do they listen to what the animal "wants" or rely on their primary care veterinarian's recommendations?

Thus, while a veterinarian's license to practice veterinary medicine usually allows them to include IVM, more nonveterinarians are gaining access to treating animals by applying continual pressure to state regulatory authorities. Legislators may possess little background in science and animal healthcare, so arguments made by veterinarians about the need to protect the health and safety of veterinary patients may make little impact. Even state veterinary boards may seem ineffectual to resist the ongoing onslaught of human healthcare providers in this regard. Their "customer" is the consumer, and veterinarians that volunteer their time to serve on the state board have limited capacity to resist organized assaults on the state's practice act, at least over time. This explains why, in jurisdiction after jurisdiction, more nonveterinarians are advertising their nonhuman work. They may make unjustified claims and try to convince the public that *they* are the true experts in each modality. Veterinarians who seek training or "certification" from courses taught by these human healthcare providers (such as chiropractors) who are seeking more rights to work with animals lend credence to these practices.

Changing laws to ease access to animals by nonveterinarians may invite a host of unintended consequences. With chiropractic, for example, beyond the wide array of manipulative approaches they may apply to an animal, they may make nutritional recommendations, sell clients supplements for the animal, discourage vaccines, and perform their own kind of "diagnosis," which they disguise by using a term, "functional neurology." Functional neurology represents a means by which they employ a surrogate (often the client) to touch the animal. With the client touching the animal, the chiropractor tests the strength of the client's deltoid muscle of the other outstretched arm. This supposedly indicates the vitality of an "energy circuit" going through the animal to the client. The chiropractor may ask the client to hold a vial that has a supplement (nutraceutical) or vitamin. If the client can resist the chiropractor's downward pressure on the outstretched arm, that reflects strengthened "energy" and the chiropractor will recommend that the client purchase that supplement. While this scenario sounds outlandish, this method of selling supplements has existed for decades within the chiropractic profession.

So, what if problems arise related to IM, whether one holds a veterinary license or not? What if a client makes a complaint to the state veterinary board or pursues other legal recourse? As stated by Pugliese et al. (2019), "In veterinary malpractice litigation, standards of care expressed in guideline statements could influence the civil and penal courts in the decision-making process." However, they also indicate, "Despite their popularity, clinical practice guidelines (CPGs) are not used often in clinical practice and their use remains controversial." Furthermore, "The majority of CPGs are based on trials considering homogenous populations." In veterinary medicine this is a limiting factor in their application, because in clinical practice, patients are rarely homogenous (i.e. species, breed, body weight, etc.). This author would also add that those who develop CPGs may, like many veterinary healthcare professionals, lack an adequate understanding of what IVM is, the pitfalls of unscientific practices, and how a rational IVM approach to a clinical condition may provide superior results, even if the evidence is only now emerging. As such, an implicit bias *against* IVM practice may exist based on lack of knowledge about the discipline's complexity and those modalities that *do* meet scientific muster.

In a commentary, "A new look at standard of care," Block (2018) exposes the fluidity and confusion surrounding what standard of care (SOC) constitutes. He cites a definition from 1837, one of the oldest legal references available, as what "an individual under a duty of care must have proceeded with such reasonable caution as a prudent man would have exercised under such circumstances" (*Vaughan vs. Menlove*, cited in Block 2018). By 1966, in veterinary case law, Block recounts the SOC definition as "the standard of care required of and practiced by the average reasonably prudent, competent veterinarian in the community" (*Dyess vs. Caraway*, cited in Block 2018). He notes that one court emphasized that SOC fails to outline clear, practical, clinically relevant recommendations and instead alludes to what the *average* practitioner would do – not the best or the most well-informed. As such, SOC does not constitute "best practices," the "gold standard," or "ideal care." Instead, SOC compares a veterinarian's action to prevailing community standards. In other words, SOC can vary according to geography, and not on scientific or evidential reasoning. Focusing too much attention on SOC, rather than *quality* of care, could put animal health and welfare in jeopardy. In this case, "majority rule," as opposed to factual analysis, may exert a downward pressure on practice standards and keep outdated, unnecessarily invasive procedures in place when equally or more effective IVM approaches warrant broader introduction into first-line care.

Consequently, veterinarians navigating the multimodal field of IVM face a steep challenge when designing documents on informed consent (see Chapter 5). Listing every potential benefit and adverse effect for each modality offered, for the specific condition(s) an animal has, may quickly become insurmountable. That said, it is unlikely that many/any veterinarians also list all the potential complications of the TPLO, or present the comparative, evidence-based outcomes of a surgical vs. nonsurgical approach to presumed cranial cruciate ligament injury.

## Ethical Aspects

While veterinarians have responsibilities to meet standards of accountability to their patients, clients, society, public health, and the profession, do human healthcare professionals who push to legally work with animals? And who writes these standards, publishes them, with what biases, industry connections and conflicts of interest, and based on what evidence? In fact, the term "evidence-based medicine" is glaringly absent from the AVMA PVME (AVMA n.d.).

"Allopathic" practitioners often press veterinary IVM providers for more research proof. However, does the veterinary profession expect the same degree of evidence from them, for their "conventional" treatments involving drugs and surgery? A recent commentary notes a lack of such standards for many common invasive procedures (Vigano et al. 2019):

> What's the strongest evidence in surgery? The lack of evidences [*sic*] to guide practice. Several justifications have been advanced, including difficulty randomizing patients for surgical interventions, large benefits from innovative procedures that do not need confirmation, and peculiarities of surgical patients that preclude applicability of any fixed rule. In this scientific anomaly, surgical education became studded with myths that inappropriately gained the rank of evidences [*sic*].

The veterinary profession has little evidence to support many of its routine practices. Rarely do surgeons select techniques based on double-blind, controlled studies. Furthermore, how forthcoming are veterinary school faculty members about the funding they receive from pharmaceutical or surgical supply companies, and how do these affiliations impact what they teach?

### Potential for "Opportunism"

Some critics have suggested that IVM practitioners may be opportunistic when offering clients treatments that support comfort, quality of life, and mobility near the end of life. This represents a narrow and uninformed view of what IVM care offers and what motivates IVM practitioners. The evidence for IM benefits (Kogan et al. 2017) throughout the life cycle and especially in a hospice setting underscores the value of having these methods available for clients to improve their animal's welfare in the last months of life and aid owners in preparing for end-of-life decisions. In many areas of the country, IVM has become so popular and sought after that veterinarians find their practices overbooked: they are not seeking to add "hopeless" cases to their rosters.

Instead, though, we might ask what constitutes a "hopeless" case. Is this a patient for whom medications and surgery were tried and didn't work? If so, could other healing methods have produced better outcomes? Why weren't they offered earlier? If we are to provide a balanced view of the ethics of IVM, then the notion that drugs and surgery are "legitimate" whenever offered and that promoting IVM is "opportunistic" and "baseless" needs to shift and is doing so.

To wit: more clients are seeking nonsurgical approaches for their animals with IVDD and cranial cruciate ligament degeneration. While "doing nothing" is an option for both approaches, and some animals recover spontaneously, most suffer from ongoing pain and debility that IVM could successfully address in several ways. For both conditions, IVM eliminates the risk of surgical complications and euthanasia from failed surgery. And yet, in many settings, clients are not even informed about IVM options (Case Study 16.1).

---

**Case Study 16.1 A client seeks IVM care without referral from their veterinarian**

Gonzo is an 11-year-old neutered male Labrador retriever with multiple orthopedic and neurologic problems including back pain, neck pain, and gait abnormalities. He previously had bilateral TPLO stifle surgeries, after which he exhibited persistent and progressive pain and lameness. An MRI of his spine indicated protruding intervertebral disks at multiple sites in his neck. Gonzo's primary care veterinarian, Dr. X, prescribed gabapentin, meloxicam, and strict cage confinement for six to eight weeks, with Gonzo only allowed out of his kennel for "bathroom breaks." He discussed two other options: euthanasia or surgery.

After four weeks, Gonzo weakened further and was reported to be "depressed." Marie, his human mom, found out about your IVM practice from a friend who'd had good results for her own dog after TPLO surgery. She is seeking a second opinion. She hesitantly asks what options are available, admitting that when she inquired about IVM options, Dr. X dismissed them, insisting that acupuncture is "just a placebo" and would provide no benefits. She cannot bear to see Gonzo continue this way and is considering euthanasia, as she cannot afford surgery and would prefer not to put him through any more surgeries.

Physical examination confirms widespread myofascial dysfunction, upper motor neuron injury of the cervical spinal cord, an asynchronous gait indicative of caudal cervical compressive myelopathy, and significant tenderness to palpation in and around both stifles.

**What should you do?**

Ethical analysis:

Relevant interests in this ethical dilemma include Gonzo, the client, Dr. X, the veterinary profession, and you. You are concerned that Dr. X did not refer Gonzo and wish to gain the confidence of both Marie and Dr. X to give Gonzo the best chance for improved quality of life.

Choices include:

1. Discuss the impact of unaddressed myofascial pain syndrome on Gonzo's quality of life with Marie. Describe the pros and cons of a spectrum of integrative medical options and how they may benefit Gonzo, including his prognosis with each. Suggest a month or two of medical acupuncture and related techniques and modifying his pain medications, along with a careful rehabilitation program to improve his mobility via a series of supportive movement therapies. Offer to meet in person or by telemedicine to monitor Gonzo's mobility and pain issues. Reassure Marie that she is welcome to continue with Dr. X as her primary veterinarian and to seek a surgical consult if she'd like at some later date.

2. Offer to speak with Dr. X to inform him about the scientific justification for medical acupuncture and related techniques, along with supportive rehabilitation measures, and hope that he supports these considerations for Gonzo, which may facilitate owner approval and compliance. One might mention that research on human patients with spinal cord injury has shown that many prefer and benefit from integrative rehabilitation approaches such as acupuncture, magnet therapy, cannabis, physiotherapy, and therapeutic exercise (Heutink et al. 2011; Kizhakkeveettil et al. 2014) and share your experience treating patients like Gonzo. Send Dr. X records of your IVM treatment so that he is apprised of the approaches instituted and of Gonzo's response.

3. If Marie prefers that Dr. X not be informed, a dilemma is created. Veterinarians have a fiduciary duty to serve the client because the client is paying them. Because a client engages a practitioner with the assumption that the doctor is serving their interests, the client expects loyalty to them. But what about your professional obligation to Dr. X? According to the AVMA PVME, "When a client seeks professional services or opinions from a different veterinarian without a referral... With the client's consent, the new attending veterinarian should contact the former veterinarian ... before proceeding with a new treatment plan" (AVMA n.d.). Ideally, you would try to persuade Marie that keeping Dr. X informed is best for Gonzo, but this may then jeopardize your newly established relationship with Marie.

4. Recommend euthanasia because medications haven't helped, kennel confinement has substantially reduced Gonzo's quality of life, and Dr. X does not appear to support IVM therapies.

> Intervertebral disc disease, a common canine affliction, can cause pain, weakness, muscle tension, inflammation, circulatory compromise, neurologic impairment, and paralysis. Clients facing the expense, fear, and psychological impact of having their dogs undergo surgery should be educated on the risks and benefits of surgical versus nonsurgical approaches. Marie has already expressed reluctance to pursue surgery, and the measures that Dr. X has recommended are not benefiting Gonzo and, in fact, have led to a decline in his physical and emotional state.
>
> In a recent report, more than half of equine veterinarians in Sweden did not offer IVM, and 55% referred patients for IVM or IM services (Gilberg et al. 2021). A study of Swedish small animal practitioners found that 39% did not use IVM (Sohlberg et al. 2021). Integrative medicine and rehabilitation practitioners may suffer moral distress (see Chapter 22) if they feel compelled to euthanize patients based on the assumption that all effective nonsurgical treatments have been tried and failed or because owners are emotionally exhausted from seeing their pet suffer.
>
> Many veterinarians who practice medical acupuncture, photomedicine, and rehabilitation have experienced success and joy when seeing patients improve that others had given up on (Frank and Roynard 2018). Clients and practitioners who pursue IVM may benefit from knowing that they explored all reasonable, rational, and justifiable means of providing comfort and supportive care in the final stages of an animal's life, instead of regretting a premature euthanasia decision or a highly invasive and traumatic procedure.

## The Future of IVM

In their commentary on informed consent, Fettman and Rollin (2002) encourage veterinary clinicians to acquire sufficient knowledge to educate their clients about the pros and cons of IVM:

> Complementary and alternative veterinary medical (CAVM) practices should be held to the same ethical and evidential standards as conventional medicine. Even if a veterinarian is disinclined to recommend CAVM approaches, the owner may request information regarding the comparative risks and benefits of CAVM compared with conventional management. It will likely become more common for clients to request some combination of complementary and conventional medical practices (integrative medicine) in the management of animals, or to seek alternative approaches alone when traditional management has failed to induce a satisfactory result.

IVM is changing veterinary medicine, not only by introducing new methodologies, but also by calling into question long-held assumptions about "gold standard" approaches to common conditions. The growth in substantiation for IVM practices should cause practitioners to ask, "Is surgery really the treatment of choice for intervertebral disc disease, when medical acupuncture and related techniques such as photomedicine have such strong scientific support for spinal cord injury?" Also, "Why am I expected to refer my patients with suspected cranial cruciate ligament injury to an orthopedic surgeon when there are so many other less invasive modalities that may be equally effective?"

At the same time, all veterinarians should question the ethics of teaching unscientific approaches such as TCVM to students at an AVMA-accredited veterinary college and offering formal internships in the Chinese medicine approach (Xie and Wedemeyer 2012). Moreover, as noted previously, conflicts of interest abound that may influence what is promoted or taught at veterinary schools.

Clearly, the time has arrived to take IVM seriously, regarding both the benefits it can offer when scientifically supported and the harms that can result from unscrutinized and untested assumptions and practices.

## References

Al Rashoud, A.S., Abboud, R.J., Wang, W. et al. (2014). Efficacy of low-level laser therapy applied at acupuncture points in knee osteoarthritis: A randomized double-blind comparative trial. *Physiotherapy* 100 (3): 242–248.

American Veterinary Chiropractic Association (2021). Why animal chiropractic/ indications for care. https://www.animalchiropractic.org/find-a-doctor (accessed 16 September 2021).

American Veterinary Medical Association (AVMA). (n.d.). Principles of veterinary medical ethics of the AVMA. https://www.avma.org/resources-tools/avma-policies/ principles-veterinary-medical-ethics-avma (accessed 16 September 2021).

American Veterinary Medical Association (AVMA) (2013). A debate on homeopathy. https:// www.avma.org/javma-news/2013-03-01/debate-homeopathy (accessed 16 September 2021).

American Veterinary Medical Association (AVMA) (2017). A closer look at veterinary homeopathy. https://www.avma.org/javma-news/2017-05-01/closer-look-veterinary-homeopathy (accessed 16 September 2021).

American Veterinary Medical Association (AVMA) (2021). 2019 Model Veterinary Practice Act (Section 15 updated January 2021). https://www.avma.org/sites/default/ files/2021-01/model-veterinary-practice-act.pdf (accessed 29 December 2021).

Avci, P., Gupta, G.K., Clark, J. et al. (2014). Low-level laser (light) therapy (LLLT) for treatment of hair loss. *Lasers in Surgery and Medicine* 46 (2): 144–151.

Bergh, M.S. and Peirone, B. (2012). Complications of tibial plateau levelling osteotomy in dogs. *Veterinary and Comparative Orthopaedics and Traumatology* 25: 349–358.

Bi, Y., Bao, H., Zhang, C. et al. (2020). Quality control of Radix Astragali (the root of *Astragalus membranaceus* var. *mongholicus*) along its value chains. *Frontiers in Pharmacology* 11: 562376.

Block, G. (2018). A new look at standard of care. *Journal of the American Veterinary Medical Association* 252 (11): 1343–1344.

Boucher, P. and Robidoux, S. (2014). Lumbar disc herniation and cauda equina syndrome following spinal manipulative therapy: A review of six court decisions in Canada. *Journal of Forensic and Legal Medicine* 22: 159–169.

Cheung, H., Doughty, H., Hinsley, A. et al. (2020). Understanding Traditional Chinese Medicine to strengthen conservation outcomes. *People and Nature* 3: 115–128. doi:10.1002/pan3.10166.

Chiu, H.Y., Hsieh, Y.J., and Tsai, P.S. (2017). Systematic review and meta-analysis of acupuncture to reduce cancer-related pain. *European Journal of Cancer Care* 26 (2): 1–17. doi:10.1111/ecc.12457.

Chung, H., Dai, T., Sharma, S.K. et al. (2012). The nuts and bolts of low-level laser (light) therapy. *Annals of Biomedical Engineering* 40 (2): 516–533.

Cital, S., Kramer, K., Hughston, L. et al. (2021). *Cannabis Therapy in Veterinary Medicine. A Complete Guide*. Cham, Switzerland: Springer.

Cotterill, J.A. (2009). Severe phototoxic reaction to laser treatment in a patient taking St John's wort. *Journal of Cutaneous Laser Therapy* 3 (3): 159–160. doi:10.1080/147641701753414988.

Cukaci, C., Freissmuth, M., Mann, C. et al. (2020). Against all odds-the persistent popularity of homeopathy. *Wiener Klinische Wochenschrift* 132 (9–10): 232–242.

Doehring, C. and Sundrum, A. (2016). Efficacy of homeopathy in livestock according to peer-reviewed publications from 1981 to 2014. *Veterinary Record* 179 (24): 628.

Dominguez-Martin, E.M., Tavares, J., Rijo, P. et al. (2020). Zoopharmacology: A way to discover new cancer treatments. *Biomolecules* 10: 817.

Dragomir, M.F., Pestean, C.P., Melega, I. et al. (2021). Current aspects regarding the clinical relevance of electroacupuncture in dogs with spinal cord injury: A literature review. *Animals* 11: 219.

Fan, Q., Cavus, O., Xiong, L. et al. (2018). Spinal cord injury: How could acupuncture help? *Journal of Acupuncture and Meridian Studies* 11 (4): 124–132.

Faramarzi, B., Lee, D., May, K. et al. (2017). Response to acupuncture treatment in horses with chronic laminitis. *Canadian Veterinary Journal* 58 (9): 823–827.

Fettman, M.J. and Rollin, B. (2002). Modern elements of informed consent for general veterinary practitioners. *Journal of the American Veterinary Medical Association* 221 (10): 1386–1393.

Formenton, M.R., Pereira, M.A.A., and Fantoni, D.T. (2017). Small animal massage therapy: A brief review and relevant observations. *Topics in Companion Animal Medicine* 32 (4): 139–145.

Frank, L.R. and Roynard, P.F.P. (2018). Veterinary neurologic rehabilitation: The rationale for a comprehensive approach. *Topics in Companion Animal Medicine* 33 (2): 49–57.

Gendron, D.J. and Hamblin, M.R. (2019). Applications of photobiomodulation therapy to musculoskeletal disorders and osteoarthritis with particular relevance to Canada. *Photobiomodulation, Photomedicine and Laser Surgery* 37 (7): 408–420.

Gilberg, K., Bergh, A., and Sternberg-Lewerin, S. (2021). A questionnaire study on the use of complementary and alternative veterinary medicine for horses in Sweden. *Animals* 11: 3113.

Gomez-Rojas, O., Hafeez, A., Gandhi, N. et al. (2020). Bilateral vertebral artery dissection: A case report with literature review. *Case Reports in Medicine* 2020: 8180926.

Hamblin, M.R. (2017). Mechanisms and applications of the anti-inflammatory effects of photobiomodulation. *AIMS Biophysics* 4 (3): 337–361.

Han, H.-J., Yoon, H.-Y., Kim, J.-Y. et al. (2010). Clinical effect of additional electroacupuncture on thoracolumbar intervertebral disc herniation in 80 paraplegic dogs. *The American Journal of Chinese Medicine* 38 (6): 1015–1025.

Hart, J.L., May, K.D., Kieves, N.R. et al. (2016). Comparison of owner satisfaction between stifle joint orthoses and tibial plateau leveling osteotomy for the management of cranial cruciate ligament disease in dogs. *Journal of the American Veterinary Medical Association* 249 (4): 391–398.

Hashmi, J.T., Huang, Y.Y., Osmani, B.Z. et al. (2010). Role of low-level laser therapy in neurorehabilitation. *Physical Medicine and Rehabilitation* 2 (12, Suppl. 2): S292–S305.

Hayashi, A.M., Matera, J.M., and Pinto, A. C.B. de C.F. (2007). Evaluation of electroacupuncture treatment for thoracolumbar intervertebral disk disease in dogs. *Journal of the American Veterinary Medical Association* 231 (6): 913–918.

Heutink, M., Post, M.W., Wollaars, M.M. et al. (2011). Chronic spinal cord injury pain: Pharmacological and non-pharmacological treatments and treatment effectiveness. *Disability and Rehabilitation* 33 (5): 433–440.

Kim, S.K. and Bae, H. (2010). Acupuncture and immune modulation. *Autonomic Neuroscience: Basic & Clinical* 157 (1–2): 38–41.

Kizhakkeveettil, A., Rose, K., and Kadar, G.E. (2014). Integrative therapies for low back pain that include complementary and alternative medicine care: A systematic review. *Global Advances in Health and Medicine* 3 (5): 49–64.

Kogan, M., Cheng, S., Rao, S. et al. (2017). Integrative medicine for geriatric and palliative care. *The Medical Clinics of North America* 101 (5): 1005–1029.

Laim, A., Jaggy, A., Forterre, F. et al. (2009). Effects of adjunct electroacupuncture on severity of postoperative pain in dogs undergoing hemilaminectomy of acute thoracolumbar intervertebral disk disease. *Journal of the American Veterinary Medical Association* 234 (9): 1141–1146.

Li, H., He, T., Xu, Q. et al. (2015). Acupuncture and regulation of gastrointestinal function. *World Journal of Gastroenterology* 21 (27): 8304–8313.

Liebert, A., Krause, A., Goonetilleke, N. et al. (2017). A role for photobiomodulation in the prevention of myocardial ischemic reperfusion injury: A systematic review and potential molecular mechanisms. *Scientific Reports* 7: 42386.

Ma, J., Yang, X., Sun, Y. et al. (2019). Thermal damage in three-dimensional vivo bio-tissues induced by moving heat sources in laser therapy. *Scientific Reports* 9: 10987.

Memon, M.A., Shmalberg, J., Adair, H.S., III et al. (2016). Integrative veterinary medical education and consensus guidelines for an integrative veterinary medicine curriculum within veterinary colleges. *Open Veterinary Journal* 6 (1): 44–56.

Memon, M.A., Shmalberg, J.W., and Xie, H. (2021). Survey of integrative veterinary medicine training in AVMA-accredited veterinary colleges. *Journal of Veterinary Medical Education* 48 (3): 289–294.

Miwa, S., Kamei, M., Yoshida, S. et al. (2019). Local dissemination of osteosarcoma observed after massage therapy: A case report. *BMC Cancer* 19: 993.

Mokmeli, S. and Vetrici, M. (2020). Low level laser therapy as a modality to attenuate cytokine storm at multiple levels, enhance recovery, and reduce the use of ventilators in COVID-19. *Canadian Journal of Respiratory Therapy* 56: 25–31.

National Center for Complementary and Integrative Health (2021). Homeopathy: What you need to know. https://www.nccih.nih.gov/health/homeopathy (accessed 17 October 2021).

Nolen, R.S. (2021). Nevada veterinarians can treat patients with certain cannabis products. https://www.avma.org/javma-news/2021-10-01/nevada-veterinarians-can-treat-patients-certain-cannabis-products (accessed 21 November 2021).

Peuker, E.T., White, A., Ernst, E. et al. (1999). Traumatic complications of acupuncture. Therapists need to know human anatomy. *Archives of Family Medicine* 8 (6): 553–558.

Pugliese, M., Voslarova, E., Biondi, V. et al. (2019). Clinical practice guidelines: An opinion of the legal implication to veterinary medicine. *Animals (Basel)* 9 (8): 577.

Riley, L.M., Satchell, L., Stilwell, L.M. et al. (2021). Effect of massage therapy on pain and quality of life in dogs: A cross sectional study. *Veterinary Record* 189 (11): e586.

Robinson, N.G. (2016). Yunnan Baiyao: Facts and myths. https://www.cliniciansbrief.com/article/yunnan-baiyao-facts-myths (accessed 18 October 2021).

Sasso, L.L., de Souza, L.G., Girasol, C.E. et al. (2020). Photobiomodulation in sciatic nerve crush injuries in rodents: A systematic review of the literature and perspectives for clinical treatment. *Journal of Lasers in Medical Sciences* 11 (3): 332–344.

Shmalberg, J., Xie, H., and Memon, M.A. (2019a). Canine and feline patients referred exclusively for acupuncture and herbs: A two-year retrospective analysis. *Journal of Acupuncture and Meridian Studies* 12 (5): 160–165.

Shmalberg, J., Xie, H., and Memon, M.A. (2019b). Horses referred to a teaching hospital exclusively for acupuncture and herbs: A three-year retrospective analysis. *Journal of Acupuncture and Meridian Studies* 12 (5): 145–150.

Sohlberg, L., Bergh, A., and Sternberg-Lewerin, S. (2021). A questionnaire study on the use of complementary and alternative veterinary medicine for dogs in Sweden. *Veterinary Sciences* 8: 331. https://doi.org/10.3390/vetsci8120331.

St-Onge, M., Vandenberghe, H., and Thompson, M. (2015). Thyroid storm caused by Chinese herb contaminated with thyroid hormones. *American Journal of Case Reports* 16: 57–59.

Swait, G. and Finch, R. (2017). What are the risks of manual treatment of the spine? A scoping review for clinicians. *Chiropractic & Manual Therapies* 25: 37.

Tatnatsu-Rocha, J.C., Ferraresi, C., Hamblin, M.R. et al. (2016). Low-level laser therapy (940nm) can increase collagen and reduce oxidative and nitrosative stress in diabetic wounded mouse skin. *Journal of Photochemistry and Photobiology B* 164: 96–102.

Taylor, L.L. and Romano, L. (1999). Veterinary chiropractic. *Canadian Veterinary Journal* 40: 732–735.

Thirkell, J. and Hyland, R. (2017). A survey examining attitudes towards equine complementary therapies for the treatment of musculoskeletal injuries. *Journal of Equine Veterinary Science* 59: 82–87.

Turner, R.C., Lucke-Wold, B.P., Boo, S. et al. (2018). The potential dangers of neck manipulation and risk for dissection and devastating stroke: An illustrative case and review of the literature. *Biomedical Research and Reviews* 2 (1). doi:10.15761/BRR.1000110.

Vickers, A.J., Vertosick, E.A., Lewith, G. et al. (2018). Acupuncture for chronic pain: Update of an individual patient data meta-analysis. *The Journal of Pain* 19 (5): 455–474.

Vigano, L., Giuliani, A., and Calise, F. (2019). The dilemma of surgical research between evidences and experience, impact factor and innovation. *Updates in Surgery* 71 (3–5).

White, A. (2009). Western medical acupuncture: A definition. *Acupuncture in Medicine* 27 (1): 33–35.

Xie, H., Colahan, P., and Ott, E.A. (2005). Evaluation of electroacupuncture treatment of horses with signs of chronic thoracolumbar pain. *Journal of the American Veterinary Medical Association* 227 (2): 281–286.

Xie, H. and Wedemeyer, L. (2012). The validity of acupuncture in veterinary medicine. *American Journal of Traditional Chinese Veterinary Medicine* 7 (1): 35–43.

Yuan, Q.-L., Wang, P., Liu, L. et al. (2016). Acupuncture for musculoskeletal pain: A meta-analysis and meta-regression of sham-controlled randomized clinical trials. *Scientific Reports* 6: 30675.

Zadik, Y., Praveen, R.A., Fregnani, E.R. et al. (2019). Systematic review of photobiomodulation for the management of oral mucositis in cancer patients and clinical practice guidelines. *Supportive Care in Cancer* 27 (10): 3969–3983.

Zhu, J., Arsovska, B., and Kozovska, K. (2018). Acupuncture treatment for fertility. *Open Access Macedonian Journal of Medical Sciences* 6 (9): 1685–1687.

## 17

## Corporate Veterinary Medicine

*Thomas Edling*

## Introduction

As we discuss corporate veterinary medicine, I will define a corporation as a large company or group of companies that is controlled together as a single organization (Cambridge Dictionary n.d.). This definition conveys what most people refer to when corporate veterinary medicine is considered. In fact, most veterinary businesses are legally structured as corporations to provide the owner legal protection but are not thought of as corporate veterinary medicine.

The history of veterinary corporations is relatively short, beginning in 1987 when VCA (Veterinary Centers of America Inc.) purchased its first independently owned veterinary clinic. Shortly after that Banfield/Medical Management International, Inc. began its corporate climb and in 1994 PetSmart teamed up with Banfield to open veterinary clinics in their stores. Mars, Inc. stepped into the veterinary clinic business in 1994 when it became a part owner of Banfield Pet Hospital. Since that time Mars became the sole owner of Banfield and, in 2015, Mars bought BluePearl. Then, in 2017, Mars purchased VCA Inc. and, in 2018, Mars crossed the ocean to Europe with the purchase of Linnaeus, followed by AniCura. Veterinary Specialty Hospital, the first specialty referral and emergency practice in Hong Kong, was purchased by Mars in 2020 along with Veterinary Emergency & Specialty Hospital in Singapore (Mars Veterinary n.d.).

What is happening in veterinary medicine is simply the common business practice of "roll up." This is a successful strategy in which a large company purchases successful smaller companies and folds them together into a larger corporation. Private equity firms are eager to offer funding for these ventures as they recognize the relatively safe investment and good returns veterinary companion animal practices provide. Currently, it is estimated that veterinary corporations own over 10% of general companion animal practices and close to 50% of specialty referral practices (Tanella 2020). Small private practices with one or two practitioners are not generally the target of veterinary corporations simply because the economics do not work in the favor of larger corporations. Veterinary corporations are here to stay and there is no reason to believe this trend will slow or stop soon.

From a business viewpoint, veterinary corporations provide advantages over small private clinics such as economy of scale when purchasing medications, equipment, and supplies. Corporations will also be well versed in successful business aspects and will have employees skilled in these practices. They may also offer a more standard work schedule for employees. Some corporate practices may also provide standards of

*Ethics in Veterinary Practice: Balancing Conflicting Interests*, First Edition. Edited by Barry Kipperman and Bernard E. Rollin.

care for the veterinarians working in their clinics. These can be very helpful documents that elevate the care for pets but may also be too prescriptive and restrict a veterinarian's clinical judgment.

In contrast to working for veterinary corporations, the advantages of owning small private practices are considerable. Owners have autonomy over their workplace regulations, settings, and practice without oversight other than their state veterinary licensing board. Private practice ownership comes with many perks as well as the numerous headaches of managing any small business.

When most veterinarians graduate from veterinary school, they take the oath of the American Veterinary Medical Association (AVMA), which outlines societal expectations of veterinarians (AVMA n.d.a). Additionally, veterinarians working in the United States are expected to adhere to the ethical code of conduct described by the AVMA, the Principles of Veterinary Medical Ethics (PVME) (AVMA n.d.b). Veterinarians should study these guiding documents to help them better understand their professional obligations as these ethical guidelines should be followed by veterinarians under all work conditions.

Many of the concerns expressed about corporate veterinary practices arise from corporate goals not aligning with the Veterinary Oath or PVME. This chapter will address potential conflicts that can arise between corporate business management goals and the individual veterinarian's professional ethics.

## Corporate Owned Clinical Veterinary Practices

### Frontline Clinical Veterinarians

Frontline veterinarians are the first to see an animal when they come into the clinic and are the professionals interfacing between the client/pet and the corporation. There can be several ethical challenges for veterinarians in this position as they attempt to apply the overarching guidance from the corporation in situations they encounter. At times, the corporate guidance may not be specific enough, or the corporate guidance may be overly restrictive. These circumstances may lead to concerns and possibly direct conflict with the veterinarian's personal and professional ethics.

Take for example a situation where a veterinarian sees an animal owned by a person who does not have the economic means to pay for the care necessary to help the pet. The veterinarian may attempt to offer multiple levels of care with differing costs for the client and patient to no avail. In some instances, the client simply cannot afford the needed care. The veterinary corporate policy may be very clear that discounts will not be given to clients that do not fit into categories such as military, first responders, elderly, guide dog, etc. The veterinarian has an ethical dilemma. They would very much like to help the client and pet but are not allowed to do so. What should they do? Should they attempt to "massage" the charges by coding incorrectly in the computer management software? Is it ethical to falsify the computer records? Does falsifying the computer records also falsify the medical records? Is it ethical to lower costs when the lost money will be absorbed by the corporation? Is this fair to the corporation? They can reach out to their supervisor but know in the past that has resulted in a denial of permission to discount services. These situations are common (see Chapter 8), and a veterinarian should anticipate this occurring in order to have the ability to develop viable solutions. What is the ethical stand to take?

Consider a similar situation in which an owner requests that cosmetic surgery be performed on their pet (see Chapter 10), which is allowed by the corporation but is ethically untenable to the veterinarian. The corporation is clear that those types of surgeries will be performed and actively advertises the procedures to the public. What should the veterinarian do? The clinician may attempt to discuss the medical and ethical concerns with the client to dissuade them from having the surgery performed on the pet. In an ear cropping example, many people do not understand the trauma and pain involved in cutting off much of the pinna and, once explained, will elect not to proceed. But this may result in lost revenue for the corporation and the veterinarian. Another solution would be for the veterinarian to transfer the case to a colleague in the practice who is willing to perform the procedure. It would be advisable to have these conversations with a supervisor prior to them happening so a logical and reasonable solution can be determined. Situations that are fully supported and encouraged by the corporation but are not acceptable to the veterinarian are a common occurrence. What else could the veterinarian do in this circumstance?

It is a common practice in corporate veterinary clinics to have well-defined financial production goals for veterinarians. In most cases, these production goals are tied to the veterinarian's pay and, if not met, they may be used to downgrade the veterinarian's compensation. From the corporation's viewpoint, production goals integrated with compensation may motivate veterinarians to work hard and consider the business aspects of the practice. Production-based pay may also discourage veterinarians from discounting and giving away services. From many veterinarians' perspectives, production-based pay encourages them to focus more on money than on practicing the best medicine. This system encourages veterinarians to pursue the maximum fees during every visit instead of providing the best animal and customer care. Should the veterinarian recommend the most expensive diagnostic work-up to pad the bill? Those tests may help the veterinarian understand the patient's medical condition, but are they necessary? In some of these situations the veterinarian must choose between practicing good medicine and a good paycheck. What should the veterinarian do?

It can be difficult to counsel clients and diagnose a complicated medical issue in the approximately 15 minutes allotted for consultations. Should the veterinarian take the time needed to help the patient or keep on schedule? If the veterinarian elects to stay longer with the client and put themselves behind schedule, should they make up for the extra time by advising clients to purchase unnecessary supplements or products such as shampoos? Another common tactic encouraged by some corporations is to "upsell" medications when less expensive medications would work equally well. I have witnessed corporations that post running totals of each veterinarian's statistics, such as per-client charges and total income, in the break room to encourage competition. All these situations can induce ethical turmoil for veterinarians as the push for profit can be a driving factor in lieu of proper care.

Referring a patient in need of care or expertise (see Chapter 10) that is not available at a veterinary clinic can cause stress when corporate guidelines, written or implied, discourage referral outside the corporation. Keeping a patient "in-house" when it should be referred is also a violation of the PVME. In times of financial hardship, should practices continue treating an animal unsuccessfully simply to increase the clinic's financial gain? This is a significant ethical problem as most veterinarians find it difficult to justify keeping the patient when they know the animal would be better served elsewhere. Another ethical question is should a clinic encourage their veterinarians to perform all available diagnostic tests on a patient prior to referring them to a specialist? This helps meet the financial criteria required by the corporate guidelines. Yet, this may reduce client resources needed to permit the specialist to help the patient. Justifying actions based on financial and not medical reasoning is an ethical dilemma faced by many veterinarians. What is the answer?

Another related aspect of this theme is when veterinarians are treating terminally ill patients. The ethical practice would be to have a frank discussion with the owner about long-term outcome, quality of life, and costs. Some corporations encourage veterinarians to continue to treat the patient right up to the last minute when that might not be the best option for the client and patient. Some owners will continue to the very end without regard for costs. Other clients may elect humane euthanasia when all aspects of the situation have been discussed. Is it unethical for clients to be encouraged to continue futile treatments primarily to raise more revenue for the clinic?

One concern that can be a significant cause of stress is continuing a relationship with a client who consistently acts or speaks improperly or abuses the veterinary staff because they provide considerable income to the clinic. These clients may have multiple animals and never ask about the expenses associated with caring for their pets. Written and unwritten corporate guidelines can make it difficult to "fire" this type of client because there would be perceived financial loss. These clients can lower the morale of the clinical team and be the cause of absenteeism, elevated levels of anxiety, and employees quitting. When an abusive client is allowed to remain, the ethical quandaries that occur generally become much worse for the clinic than the financial loss of firing the client. What is an ethical method for handling these clients?

One of the positive financial aspects of a corporation owning several clinics is the purchasing power acquired due to economy of scale. The more a corporation purchases, the better price it can obtain from the supplier. This can also bring about ethical issues as decisions can be made to purchase a medication that might not be the best choice but was offered at the most economical price or margin. In some corporations, purchasing decisions are made by nonveterinarians without veterinary oversight. This can lead to frontline clinicians being forced to use medications that are not the best option for their patients. This ethical quandary can be considerable as the veterinarian will not see the response to treatment they would expect if the appropriate medication were available. In some circumstances nonveterinarians in upper management may pressure clinicians to use medications with a higher profit margin. This situation may occur because the manager does not have the medical background to be able to understand the differences between the medications but does understand the costs and profit margins involved. I have seen this circumstance be the cause of a veterinarian quitting their job. How should veterinarians manage these situations? Will they lose standing in their job if they request availability of medications with lower profit margins?

Another situation that may be exacerbated by corporate guidelines is convenience euthanasia (see Chapter 21). This topic presents the veterinarian with a complex moral issue to navigate. This end-of-life quandary can be further complicated by a corporate policy that requires or strongly encourages the veterinarian to perform this service.

What should the veterinarian do when faced with a euthanasia request based on client convenience? What are their options? What if the owner tells the veterinarian they are going to initiate legal proceedings against the corporation if they do not euthanize their pet?

A corollary to convenience euthanasia is the situation where an animal is insured, and the insurance company has authorized euthanasia with a payout going to the owner. The animal has a condition that can be treated with a good chance for a positive outcome. The veterinarian discusses treatment options with the owner, but the owner elects for euthanasia to collect the insurance money. This situation can become more convoluted if the corporation has a business relationship with the insurance company, which may influence the veterinarian's decision. What options does the veterinarian have in this case?

## Frontline Veterinary Managers in Clinical Settings – Single and Multiple Facility Management

In several corporations, veterinarians who have proven themselves to be worthy of advancement will be promoted to a frontline veterinary manager with direct supervision over other veterinarians. They may supervise veterinarians at a single facility or at multiple clinics. In all cases, the role of the supervisor is to be available, pay close attention to situations as they arise, and use teachable moments to help their veterinary team deal with medical, ethical, and business concerns. This supervision is especially important for veterinarians in their first few years out of school.

In many practices this is a proven, successful model for advancement and a desired role. In other situations, the supervisory role may not be welcome but become a burden that the veterinarian is not ready to undertake. Should the veterinarian accept the new role even though they do not want the added burden? Does not accepting the promotion hurt the veterinarian's chances for promotion in the future or job security?

Supervision of veterinarians brings all the issues and concerns of the frontline veterinarian along with the added stress of corporate managerial expectations. Supervisors can learn the system and be the "protector" who allows their employee practitioners to function relatively free from corporate stress. Conversely, they may not only pass on the stressors due to corporate oversight but compound concerns.

Supervision also generates an entirely new set of ethical issues, especially when the person is supervising veterinarians in their own cohort. When an individual from a cohort is singled out and elevated to a managerial position, it is common for some individuals in the cohort to have resentment toward the supervisor. The resentment can be worsened if the new supervisor was not seen as a competent clinician. It can also be taxing if supervisory roles reverse, and the veterinarian finds that a previous employee is now their supervisor.

Supervising under a corporate umbrella can be both an effective means to advancement and disadvantageous. If the corporation has a well-run business management system and a well-structured and implemented training program, the ethical dilemmas can be substantially reduced. If the business is poorly managed or there is no training program and corporate support, supervision can be career ending. The management expectations and parameters established by the corporation will be essential in allowing for success. Time and training are crucial as most veterinarians do not have any formal training in how to supervise. Being a very good veterinarian does not translate into being a competent supervisor. Veterinarians elevated to supervisory roles need to be trained and provided the opportunity to learn managerial skills including time off from their normal clinical duties to be an effective supervisor. Some corporations expect veterinarians placed in managerial positions to continue to see their normal case load while managing a team. This added work can cause ethical concerns due to limited time and conflicting interests as a dual manager/clinician. With limited time, managers may schedule themselves the best shifts for financial gains or start practicing in a way that will lead to poor ethical choices for the patient. How do veterinary managers resolve the ethical dilemma created by serving both their clients and patients as a veterinarian and the corporation as a manager when the goals of each role conflict?

Managers may also be held accountable for the financial goals of the team as opposed to only being responsible for the quality of their medical care. If they are responsible for both financial goals and quality of care, there can easily develop conflicting interests that will cause ethical problems for the supervisor and clinicians. This can be a significant cause for concern if the goals are unrealistic or if the manager is new, poorly trained, or has an underperforming team.

When determining who to promote to supervisor, some corporations will promote the veterinarian who produces the highest average client transaction fees. If production is the only criterion for promotion, it is possible that the veterinarian being elevated to supervisor is not the most qualified supervisor or the most competent veterinarian. If this is the case, the veterinarians supervised by this person can have ethical issues due to the supervisor's below-average clinical skills or poor management style. The ethics of the supervisor may also be brought into question. Ethical issues due to poor supervision can range from a supervisor scheduling a veterinarian to undesirable shifts, offering favoritism, promoting poor clinical ethics that are more profitable, and scheduling preferred individuals to shifts that historically provide a higher per-client income stream. What can veterinarians in this situation do to abide by their personal ethics?

Supervision generally carries performance appraisals of colleagues as part of the job requirement. Performance appraisals will be based on the values of the corporation and may lean heavily toward income production. Early in a veterinarian's career the veterinarian will not have the experience to recognize, diagnose, and treat patients as competently and quickly as they will after several years of practice. This can lead to ethical concerns if the newer veterinarian is evaluated by the same parameters as a seasoned professional. Newer veterinarians caught in this web may start to try and gain economic ground by hurrying their appointments, ordering unnecessary diagnostic tests, and using medications with a higher profit margin in the hopes of obtaining a better corporate assessment. Competent supervisors will be able to recognize this pattern and coach the newer veterinarian not to take these short cuts if the corporation allows new veterinarians to have an adequate learning curve for growth. If the corporation does not allow the supervisor to adjust for new veterinarians in their appraisals, ethical issues will arise for both the supervisor and the veterinarian. In addition, the new veterinarian may develop habits that conflict with their personal ethics. What can the supervisor do in this situation? What can the inexperienced veterinarian do when facing these ethical challenges?

Managing clinicians in a single facility is difficult and managing veterinarians in multiple facilities is an even greater challenge. The task of overseeing multiple facilities is often more than double the supervision of a single clinic. The more employees a supervisor manages, the fewer hours in the day are available for clinical work. It is not uncommon for a veterinarian to become overwhelmed by this type of supervisory role. Many anxieties and ethical conflicts arise from corporate decisions that can place an unhealthy burden on a veterinarian in a supervisory role. The ethical concerns evolving from these situations can arise from the supervisor and the supervisor's employees. It can be difficult for a manager who is being overworked to communicate the need for help to their supervisor, which leads to significant problems for all involved. These multi-facility supervisory roles are the direct result of corporate control over multiple locations. This is the business model and is not concerning unless the supervisor does not have the training or aptitude, which may not be determined until situations causing ethical problems are well established. What can the managing veterinarian do in these situations?

Hiring effectively is a critical aspect of any veterinary organization and one of the most difficult tasks. Many aspects of the business and attributes of the candidates must be assessed before deciding to hire someone. In a corporation that provides proper guidance and oversight, the process can be successful. Many candidates look good on their curriculum vitae (CV) and are good practitioners, but not all will fit well with the team. Everyone has a different way of communicating, practice style, personality, sense of humor, and work ethic. A veterinarian trained in spay and neuter surgeries by a humane/shelter organization is professionally qualified for that work environment but might not fit into a clinic that is principally focused on high-end medical care and customer service. They may also be the best clinician ever hired at that location. Personal interactions are critical and the importance of hiring the correct fit cannot be overemphasized. To achieve the best outcome, the direct supervisor of the new hire should be involved in the hiring process. When people are hired by a remote office and simply plugged into open spots without significant input from the supervisor of the team, the opportunity for problems to develop is significant. After the hire, a set protocol should be followed to assess new hires in a timely fashion so problems can be caught and addressed early. What methods can supervisory veterinarians use to help new team members fit into their existing organization?

## Veterinarians in Upper Management with Corporate Oversight

In corporations, it is common to select veterinarians who have shown aptitude in supervisory roles for positions of upper management such as a regional director or similar position. These jobs require a significantly different skillset as the work no longer requires day-to-day oversight of clinical veterinarians but understanding the business aspects of veterinary clinics. This transition can be challenging as the veterinarian may want to continue hands-on clinical work. Again, training is important along with a clear understanding of roles and responsibilities. These positions often require the veterinarian to make decisions that are more business based than clinically based. Common ethically challenging situations arise such as how to balance the ledger book with the cost of clinical excellence, selecting pay rates for veterinarians and staff, and personality and communication conflicts between upper management and employees. These are all areas that are unique to veterinarians working in corporations and are points where ethics can come into play. Veterinarians in these positions must straddle the fence between thinking like the trusted veterinary professional seeking the best solution for a client and their animal and following the corporate directives that may conflict with what is best for the animal.

## Retail Pet Stores and Independent Veterinarians

Major retail pet store chains contract with independent veterinarians to provide care for the animals in their stores. Most pet stores in the United States do not sell dogs and cats but sell nontraditional companion animals. These animals include common pet rodent species such as hamsters, guinea pigs, and mice; some reptile species such as bearded dragons, leopard geckos, and corn snakes; and bird species such as budgerigars, cockatiels, and conures. If the stores offer grooming, boarding, or daycare/training services, the corporation will also contract with veterinarians to provide services, on an emergency basis, in the event a dog/cat is injured during grooming, or an animal becomes ill during training or boarding. The larger corporate stores will have the veterinarian under contract including payment and pricing details to provide services. In some states, there is a requirement for an independent veterinarian, licensed in that state, to develop and oversee a program of adequate veterinary care for pet stores.

When there is need for a veterinarian, a store employee will contact the veterinary clinic with information about an illness, injury, or need for vaccinations. The veterinarian is permitted to offer advice or care instructions via phone or other electronic means in accordance with the state's veterinarian–client–patient relationship (VCPR) guidelines. The veterinarian will generally determine designated times each week to visit the store or have a store employee bring the ill or injured animal to the veterinary hospital for treatment. Depending on the severity of the illness or injury and the retail pet store's ability to provide appropriate housing and treatment, the animal will either stay at the veterinary clinic or return to the store. Business relationships between retail pet stores and veterinarians can be beneficial for the animals, veterinarian, and pet store. There can also be instances where the relationship deteriorates. In some instances, the store may attempt to persuade the veterinarian to provide services that conflict with the state VCPR guidelines, such as treating an animal who has not been seen by the veterinarian with remaining medication from a previous patient. Ethical concerns may arise if the store pressures the veterinarian and/or threatens to end the contract with the veterinarian. What should the veterinarian do in the case of a store animal who needs urgent care but cannot be seen immediately? Should they let the store treat the pet with left-over medications that might help even if the veterinarian has not personally seen the pet?

The animal care staff of large pet store chains that employ independent veterinarians are instructed to follow the policies and procedures developed by corporate veterinarians. These regulations cover animal husbandry (substrate, temperature, light, food, water, etc.), when to seek veterinary care, receiving animals from animal suppliers, cleaning and disinfecting habitats, as well as many other aspects of animal care. Occasionally, a store employee may intentionally or unintentionally alter the care instructions for an animal or group of animals housed in the store. This can result in husbandry mistakes, which lead to medical problems for the animal(s) involved. The contracted veterinarian working with the store may question the reasoning behind the animal's care and be told by an employee that the store was following corporate policy. If the veterinarian questions the policy, the employee may insist there is nothing that can be done, which places the veterinarian in a difficult position. In some cases, the veterinarian may know the store did not follow policy but does not want to confront the store. The veterinarian may try to contact the corporate veterinary offices to obtain clarification and choose not to let the corporation know the store is not following protocol so they do not damage the relationship with the store employees. These circumstances can place the veterinarian in a position where the ethics of caring for an animal treated in a manner that caused disease come into question. Should the veterinarian do what they think is best for the animal with the understanding that moving in that direction will cause a significant rift between the veterinarian and the local store employees? What are the options for the veterinarian in this situation?

Most nontraditional or exotic companion animals (see Chapter 15) that retail pet stores sell to the public in North America come from breeders, mostly in the United States. The breeders either sell the animals directly to the stores or sell the animals to distributors that provide the animals to the pet stores. The large retail chains receive animal shipments on a weekly basis or more often depending on the animal species, holding capacity, and public demand for the animal. In most cases the animals bred and distributed to the stores are healthy when delivered and are provided good care in the stores. In some circumstances a problem will occur with a breeder or distributor and an animal will be ill or injured upon arrival at the pet store. If the animals from a specific supply company are consistently ill or injured, it can become ethically challenging for the independent veterinarian to continue to work with the pet store if they do not believe the store is attempting to work with the supplier to solve the problem.

The veterinarian's ethical dilemma when facing continual medical problems in pet store animals is compounded by the pet store employees' desire to help the animals. The pet store employees may look to the veterinarian to help their animals if they have been unable to get a satisfactory solution from their corporation. Chronic animal health issues make the veterinarian's job exceedingly difficult when animals continue to suffer and there does not appear to be any movement from the corporation to resolve the issues. The veterinarian is caught between the corporation, the store employees, and their own ethical concerns over animal suffering. What should the veterinarian do in this circumstance? Should they continue to work toward a solution that helps the animals in the store? What recourse might they have?

There are numerous circumstances where ethical concerns arise in these relationships due to the business decisions of the corporation. Some retail pet stores sell animals that have health concerns due to the genetics involved in breeding color morphs or hairless varieties. An example is the ball python spider morph, which is a coloration/pattern of the ball python. This snake has a genetic defect leading to a neurological disorder, the "wobble syndrome." Some corporate pet stores continue to sell this color morph even though they know about the associated problems. Other issues may arise due to ethical concerns about animals that are collected from the wild or that might be difficult for a hobbyist to maintain well in their home. Most species of freshwater fish are bred in captivity in Asia or the United States, while most species of marine fish are collected from the wild. The wild collection of fish is controlled and regulated but continues to be controversial. Groups such as Rising Tide are improving the breeding of marine aquatic life, but there will always be some species of fish that will be collected from the wild.

Veterinarians who work with corporate pet stores should learn about their corporate business practices and decide whether they can reconcile possible ethical concerns with their own ethics. Should veterinarians work on wild collected animals from pet stores? Should veterinarians work with pet stores that sell animals with known genetic problems? If the veterinarian decides not to work with the store, who will be there for the animals?

Veterinarians working for corporate pet stores should review and understand their euthanasia practices prior to starting work. The pet store will have euthanasia guidelines that will involve the contracted veterinarian. Corporate pet stores typically follow the AVMA guidelines for euthanasia (AVMA 2020) and expect the contracted veterinarian to follow their corporate guidance. In some corporate stores, only veterinarians are allowed to euthanize an animal other than aquatic life, but in other stores employees may euthanize small rodents and reptiles. The store veterinarian may be called upon to train employees on how to correctly perform euthanasia. An example is in states where pet store employees are allowed to euthanize healthy mice and rats that are going to be fed to a customer's reptile. The store veterinarian may be asked to demonstrate and train how to euthanize the rodents. The veterinarian should think through this situation before it arises. Should the veterinarian supervise or condone euthanasia of healthy animals slated for reptile food?

In a different situation, a store may have a nontraditional companion animal who is terminally ill and more than likely is going to die within the next 24 hours. The store might not allow the veterinarian to euthanize the animal due to the costs of the veterinary visit. It is clear the animal is suffering and the ethical thing to do would be to euthanize the animal, but because the store manager is trying to save money, the store might not allow the veterinarian to perform the ethical treatment. In some cases the veterinarian will not know this situation has occurred, and in others the veterinarian will be called and asked their opinion but not be allowed to provide the service. The veterinarian may find out during a subsequent visit or phone conversation that the animal suffered and died without intervention. Should the veterinarian have a frank discussion with the store manager about the ethics of the situation? Should the veterinarian continue to work with the store? It can be easy for veterinarians to criticize pet stores for substandard care. It is more challenging to try and help the store understand animal pain and suffering and work with them to establish boundaries and practical guidelines for when to help end suffering via humane euthanasia. These ethical actions by the veterinarian could also help improve corporate practices.

## Veterinarians Working for Corporate Pet Stores as Advisors

Another role for veterinarians working for corporations includes work that is not in a clinical position but as a full-time corporate advisor. These veterinarians are expected to be the voice of the animals that the corporation sells. This can be a very challenging endeavor as the work performed by veterinarians in these corporate positions covers a wide gamut of potentially difficult issues.

Corporate advisor veterinarians are generally employed as a director or vice president and are involved with developing the policies and procedures the retail store employees use to provide care for the animals in their stores. These include all aspects of animal care from habitat design, food, treats, supplements, water, substrate/bedding, lighting, temperature, humidity, and cage accessories such as hide boxes and climbing vines. Other areas of policy development encompass protocols for caring for animals that are ill or injured, quarantine, biosecurity, veterinary care protocols, cleaning and disinfecting policies and procedures, and euthanasia guidelines. Veterinarians in this capacity will also be the subject matter expert helping to develop training materials for the store employees to assist them in following the animal care policies and procedures. Additional aspects of these veterinary jobs involve working with store buyers to locate and purchase the products used by the store to help care for the animals. These include all the consumable products such as food, supplements, bedding/substrate, as well as the store habitats and personal protective equipment used by store employees to clean and disinfect the habitats.

In all these areas of veterinary involvement ethical questions can arise. For example, in meetings with animal food manufacturers, a veterinarian might be asked to help decide which food is best for a specific animal sold by the store. The veterinarian may make a recommendation to the buyer on which food to purchase based on the nutrition, palatability, ease of storage, and other factors relevant to the animals' welfare. The buyer may hear the veterinarian's recommendation and reasoning then return to the veterinarian with a counterproposal supporting a different food that is less expensive. The less expensive food may be nutritionally acceptable but is not as palatable or is more difficult to feed. It is not the best choice but is it good enough? Where does the veterinarian draw the line and how far should they go to support their choice? Variables are abundant in these situations, and it can be easy to be influenced by forces not necessarily in line with the best choice for the animal. Supervisors may pressure the veterinarian to support the less desirable food choice because the supervisor plays golf with the owner of the food manufacturing company. The food manufacturer may be a major supporter of a charity organization the corporation supports and expects a quid pro quo for their donations. The veterinarian can be caught in the middle. On one side the less desirable food may be acceptable in the short term while the animal is in the store, so the ethical concern may not be significant. The veterinarian should recognize that if they do not support the less desirable food, they may no longer be included in future food buying discussions and may lose their influence over animal nutrition for the store animals.

Corporate advisor veterinarians will also be involved in developing standards for the companies that supply animals to the stores. There is a large pet industry associated with breeding and distributing small nontraditional companion animals including rodents, rabbits, ferrets, reptiles, fish, birds, and other animals such as hedgehogs. The larger pet corporations develop standards for these breeders and distributors and perform audits to help ensure the animals are being bred, cared for, and distributed in a safe and healthy fashion. On occasion, an audit might bring to light an area where a breeder or distributor has not met the animal care standards required by the pet store. The infraction may be small and easily alleviated with basic instructions. In this case the infractions are resolved, and the companies continue to work together. On the other hand, the violation may be so egregious that the business relationship should be terminated with the breeder/distributor.

If the company terminates the relationship immediately, what happens to the animals at the breeder/distributor facility? Should the pet store continue to buy the animals from the breeder/distributor facility until all animals designated for them have been purchased knowing that some of the animals are ill or injured and will require veterinary care? Some of the illness issues may not reveal themselves until the animals have been distributed to multiple stores and the stores will be required to take care of the animals. This not only puts a financial burden on the stores but also initiates significant concerns associated with the store employees being forced to care for ill animals. Most store employees go out of their way to take exceptional care of the animals in their charge. It takes an emotional toll on store employees to work with sick and injured animals. The corporate veterinarian will be involved with these decisions and must understand the ethical dilemmas involved. What is the correct ethical decision?

## Marketing, Education, and Other Ethical Concerns for Corporate Veterinary Advisors

Marketing is one area of the corporate world in which veterinarians may also be involved. Marketing campaigns strive to entice people to purchase products by making encouraging claims about the product. In some instances, the marketing claims espoused by the product manufacturer are not supported by evidence-based science. The veterinarian may be brought in to decide what can be stated and how far the manufacturers' claims may be stretched before they are blatantly false. There may be a significant gray area between known facts and marketing claims. There can also be a considerable ethical predicament when company executives support inaccurate manufacturing claims that would possibly allow the product to sell better. Does the veterinarian support manufacturer claims that are less than truthful or insist upon evidence-based statements only? There are consequences for both actions. On the ethical side, the veterinarian is morally correct and has the satisfaction of knowing the ethical decision was made not to support the inaccurate claims. On the other side, the veterinarian may now be seen as a person who is not a team player and may not be asked for their advice next time. If the veterinarian goes along with the marketing scheme, does that give them leverage during the next marketing meeting to make changes to messaging and bring some science to the ad campaign? If the veterinarian does not support the campaign, will they be ostracized and not get the next promotion or pay raise? What is the correct ethical decision?

The corporate world is a much different environment than the clinical veterinary world. In the clinical world, most veterinarians have the same basic knowledge level and speak the vocabulary of veterinary medicine. Veterinarians have similar understandings of disease processes, medications, surgical procedures, and basic nutrition. In the corporate world, there will be no one else with the same grasp of veterinary knowledge except other veterinarians working for the corporation. There will be people who have a particularly good understanding of animals and their care, but their veterinary knowledge will be limited. Most people in the company will be playing on a somewhat level field, while the veterinarian will be the outsider.

This distinction is made to demonstrate that nobody in the corporation will be able to understand how a veterinarian views the ethical and health issues pertaining to the animals.

Consequently, educating nonveterinarians in a corporation can be challenging. It can be difficult for a veterinarian to convince others that concepts the employees have learned from lay sources are incorrect. For example, dog food manufacturers know that human marketing concepts are very influential. Grain-free and gluten-free marketing are prime examples. These marketing concepts are used because pet owners believe grain-free and gluten-free are better for them and they want their pets to have similar benefits. It can be challenging to convince company executives that grain-free and gluten-free are human nutritional concepts and are not science-based veterinary concepts. Attempting to explain science-based information to people without a background in science is difficult. It can turn into an ethical concern because the veterinarian may be asked to help support the marketing and educational campaigns for these products. When a retail corporation supports a major marketing claim they invest a significant amount of time and effort into store employee education. The educational program is designed to teach the store employees how to sell the product. If the veterinarian is asked to be a subject matter expert and help design the educational materials, it can be tricky when there is no science to support the marketing claim. Is it ethical to support a program teaching that grain-free is best for dogs when science does not support this? How does the veterinarian keep their moral compass when the marketing program is moving forward and they are expected to contribute?

Pet retail corporations have animal buyers who are tasked with bringing in new species of animals that will sell and make good pets. This can be challenging because there is not an abundance of new small animals, birds, reptiles, or fish that fit this bill. Corporate advisor veterinarians work closely with the animal buyers to help decide which of these new animals meet the requirements for a healthy pet. Most "new" animals in the pet world are color or hair morphs of known species. Some of these animals have been developed by years of specific breeding and are healthy. Others have genetic defects that render them potentially less healthy.

For example, a few years ago breeders started producing "skinny pigs," which are guinea pigs with little or no hair. These animals have a genetic defect that does not allow their hair to develop normally, resulting in predominantly hairless animals. Having no hair is abnormal and can cause health concerns associated with thermoregulation, skin problems such as excessive dryness, and possible immune system complications. These animals are being sold through most retail pet stores as well as on the internet. What is the ethical stance of the corporate veterinarian? Do they refuse to allow the animal to be sold by the corporation? Will their refusal make any difference? Do they work to develop standards for providing care for the animal inside the store as well as educational materials for prospective owners to use to properly care for their new pet at home? Corporate veterinarians are commonly faced with these issues.

Corporate advisor veterinarians are also asked to decide how much care store employees should provide to ill and injured animals in their stores. State and local laws concerning veterinary care and pet store animals vary greatly. The Animal Welfare Act and most state laws define veterinary care that must be provided for dogs and cats in pet stores but do not provide direction for nontraditional companion animals. A few states and localities provide some direction on veterinary care for non-traditional companion animals. Animal care teams supported or led by corporate veterinarians are tasked with developing protocols on when and how a store employee should intervene when an animal is sick or injured. The protocols also determine when veterinary care should be sought. Corporate policies generally provide direction to all employees in all states. Should there be different levels of care for animals in states or localities that do not require animals to receive veterinary care? Should there be a single medical directive for all stores? When should veterinary intervention be sought? Should it be sought for all species, even a $2 mouse? The office visit will be substantially more than the cost of many animals sold in stores. Should animals under a certain price be denied veterinary care and only expensive animals receive care? Where is the ethical line in the sand drawn for an animal that needs veterinary care in a pet store? In a person's home, small rodents generally do not receive veterinary care. If the animal that became sick in the store did not get sick until it was purchased and home with the new owner, it probably would not receive medical care. Is there an ethical difference? Should store employees be allowed to use products sold in the stores to treat the animals without veterinary supervision? These are ethical questions that surround the day-to-day decisions of corporate veterinarians.

In the first few years of this millennium most major retail pet store chains sold antibiotics and other "treatments" over the counter (OTC) to the public. These medications were developed by companies to "treat" problems such as diarrhea in rodents, eye problems in reptiles, and fin rot in fish, just to name a few. Few if any of these "medications" are manufactured with the quality control standards mandated by law for human and animal pharmaceutical companies. In addition, few if any of these "medications" have been tested for efficacy in any of the animals listed on their labels. Many of these antibiotics are similar to human medications and are known to be purchased and given to humans as treatments. There are intriguing "loopholes" in the Federal Drug Administration (FDA) laws pertaining to OTC products designated for animals. In addition, the FDA has more pressing issues to deal with and not enough staff to provide substantial time to this issue. Although the products might not be technically legal to sell, all pet stores were selling them, and the FDA did not intervene. People with no training in diagnosing or treating pets are purchasing these products and "treating" their pet and in some instances, their children and themselves.

In the best-case scenarios, these products do no harm, but then the pet may not receive needed medical care from a veterinarian. In the worst cases the product could cause a worsening of the pet's disease, and the pet dies. Since most people do not take their small nontraditional pets to a veterinarian for treatment, what is the problem with providing the pet owner a possible cure for their animal? Aquatic life antibiotics are a large component of the OTC products, and there are very few veterinarians qualified to treat fish. It is also uncommon for a person to seek veterinary advice for their fish. Should the fish owner have the same flip of the coin chance to help their animal with an OTC product? In addition, the OTC antibiotic products account for several million dollars in sales for the large retail pet stores. With OTC antibiotic products there is also another major concern about creating antimicrobial resistance. In 2009 one major pet chain stopped selling all OTC antibiotics while others continue to sell them today. What should the ethical position be for the corporate veterinarian? Should they take a stance? Should the veterinarian work to convince the corporate leaders that the "right thing to do," the ethical position, is to stop selling these products, which will reduce the corporation's income? Is this an issue that a veterinarian should address? Is there someone in the company who has better training to address the issue? Is there a right answer?

Another aspect of corporate veterinary oversight in the retail pet industry revolves around nonconsumable products sold by the company. Veterinarians in these positions are tasked with developing a review process to determine if products should be sold. These products can range from dog collars and cat food bowls to bird cages and chew toys. The products originate in numerous countries around the world and, in most cases, there are no industry standards. Should the veterinarian establish new standards for the welfare of the animals, even if the new standards would be disruptive to manufacturers, or keep the status quo? For example, what if the standard bird cage found on retail shelves for a budgerigar (*Melopsittacus undulatus*), commonly known as a budgie, which is approximately $12'' \times 9'' \times 12''$, is too small to meet the budgie's physical and behavioral needs?

To develop new standards for cage sizes that better fit the needs of the bird would force manufacturers to retool their manufacturing facilities and make new forms for the plastic cage base. These costs would be substantial for the manufacturer. The increased manufacturer costs would be passed on to all retailers as the cage price would increase and retail stores would be forced to change their store shelf layouts to accommodate larger cages. Concurrently, new shipping boxes would have to be developed along with all the marketing information and pictures needed to adorn the outside of the shipping box. Overall, millions of dollars would be spent and countless hours invested just to create a better bird cage. In addition, the major manufacturers that did not conform to the new standard would lose their contract with the large retailer. Is there an ethical imperative for the veterinarian to make the changes to meet the needs of the bird? What is the "cost" to the veterinarian inside the corporation for being disruptive? What is the ethical "cost" for not making such a decision when there is a clear need? Is it the veterinarian's responsibility to try to improve the lives of all animals within their circle of influence?

Everywhere a veterinarian works, if animals are involved, zoonotic diseases transmissible to humans are a concern. In the corporate retail pet industry, most pets have the capacity to carry and spread zoonotic diseases. Fortunately, most of the zoonotic diseases are common and do not cause significant illness when animals are handled properly. Developing educational materials that help owners keep their pets at home in a safe fashion is part of a corporate veterinarian's purview. Veterinarians in these positions are also called upon to develop the biosecurity standards that help protect store employees during their daily tasks.

Should developing new protocols for lowering the incidence of zoonotic diseases in pet store animals be a corporate veterinarian's concern? Is there an ethical position that allows a veterinarian to ignore working toward improving the lives of people and animals? For example, if there are methods that can be used to help breeders reduce the burden of *Salmonella* in reptiles, should a corporate veterinarian pursue that goal? What if the corporation discourages the veterinarian from following that goal due to the concern that the new methods might temporarily reduce the number of animals available for sale? Or due to concern that it will raise the cost of the reptile species and put the company at a competitive disadvantage? What are the veterinarian's ethical choices under these circumstances?

## Closing Thoughts

Corporate veterinary practices will continue to increase in number and employ more veterinarians. Corporations are discovering that the education veterinarians receive can be harnessed to help in advisory and other roles. This trend will continue and veterinarians who choose to work within the corporate structure should educate themselves on the intricacies of the corporate environment so they can be ready for the challenges they will face.

In this chapter I have raised some of the ethical concerns facing veterinarians working for corporations. We have looked at veterinarians working in clinical positions as well as veterinarians employed in more of an advisory role to corporations. Both situations continually place the veterinarian in positions of ethical conflict. Veterinarians in clinical practice must attempt to adhere to their oath to be the beloved and trusted veterinary professional and use their hard-earned skills to help their clients and animals. At the same time the veterinarian must exist within a corporate framework that in some instances is in direct conflict with their Veterinary Oath and ethical principles. The veterinarian in the corporate advisory role works in an environment where they may be the only professional voice for the animals in their corporation. They are guided by the same veterinary principles and must find ways to uphold that oath while managing the ethical situations surrounding them by reconciling the concerns specific to corporations.

In all these circumstances, it is helpful to refer to the Veterinary Oath (AVMA n.d.a) and PVME (AVME n.d.b) of the AVMA to help guide the decision-making process. The Veterinary Oath clearly states that veterinarians are required to use their "scientific knowledge and skills for the benefit of society, through the protection of animal health and welfare, the prevention and relief of animal suffering, the conservation of animal resources, the promotion of public health and the advancement of medical knowledge." The first AVMA veterinary ethics principle states, "A veterinarian shall be influenced only by the welfare of the patient, the needs of the client, the safety of the public, and the need to uphold the public trust vested in the veterinary profession and shall avoid conflicts of interest or the appearance thereof." It will also be beneficial to read Chapters 4, 7, and 23 of this text, which provide ethical frameworks to help readers address ethical problems.

The ethical identity of veterinarians develops before entering veterinary school. It is based on the numerous interactions, learning experiences, and observations of mentors and other influential people in the veterinarian's life. It is formed by interactions with animals that our society recognizes as pets, production animals, and wildlife. The process is shaped by social and religious beliefs. When an influential veterinary professor, clinician, or employer makes an ethical decision, it undoubtedly is noticed, whether it is discussed or not (this is known as the hidden curriculum). At some point, veterinarians read the Veterinary Oath and AVMA principles and decide where they fit into their professional identity and hopefully discus ethical concerns in veterinary school classes or informally with classmates.

All veterinarians are faced with ethical dilemmas (see Chapter 7) and must make decisions whether they are ready to make them or not. The aftermath of those decisions continuously shapes the veterinarian's identity. The best advice I can offer to veterinary students is to take this seriously and attempt to think through as many scenarios and circumstances and the related ethical decisions as possible before graduating and facing unanticipated ethical decisions. Practice making ethical decisions to help define what you believe is right.

Veterinarians working in privately owned and corporate owned clinics, as employees, practice owners or supervisors, as corporate advisors, in laboratories, food and fiber production, pharmaceutical representatives, etc. all have a circle of influence. It is my belief that it is our duty as veterinarians to continually do our best to better the lives of animals under our influence. This is a marathon not a sprint. Sometimes working within a corporation involves acquiescing to a partial compromise so in the future you can make far-reaching changes that will improve the lives of animals. It can be a fine line to walk, and success will not always be achieved. Learn from the experiences and continue to press ethical issues that are best for the animals. Continue to think through ethical situations and discuss ethics with your colleagues. Discuss ethics with your supervisors and those making decisions for your corporation. Corporations may appear to be large autonomous organizations that make decisions by committee. In fact, corporations are very prone to outside influence and there is an individual behind every decision. Most individuals in pet-related corporations do care about animals and wish to do what is right for the animals in their charge. Sometimes they simply need a gentle reminder.

As a veterinarian working within the pet industry, I was surprised at how often colleagues directly attacked my integrity for working within a pet store corporation. I am certain they did not understand or see the entire picture and were clouded by the standard misperceptions surrounding the pet industry. It is far easier to criticize something you do not understand than to become involved and help. One of the best ways to change a system that needs assistance is from within. When you see a problem, address it within the system and continue to press it until you have resolution. Find like-minded people and move forward. Stay the ethical course and continue the fight as the animals may not have any other advocates. Continue to follow your ethical guidepost to pave the way for positive change for animals, veterinarians, and society. You and your ethic are intertwined. Dealing with difficult ethical situations and fighting to improve the lives of the animals within your circle of influence will remind you of who you are and why you became a veterinarian.

The worst sin towards our fellow creatures is not to hate them, but to be indifferent to them: that's the essence of inhumanity.

George Bernard Shaw

## References

American Veterinary Medical Association (AVMA) (n.d.a). Veterinarian's Oath. https://www.avma.org/resources-tools/avma-policies/veterinarians-oath (accessed 9 November 2021).

American Veterinary Medical Association (AVMA) (n.d.b). Principles of Veterinary Medical Ethics. https://www.avma.org/resources-tools/avma-policies/principles-veterinary-medical-ethics-avma (accessed 9 November 2021).

American Veterinary Medical Association (AVMA) (2020). Guidelines for the euthanasia of animals. https://www.avma.org/resources-tools/avma-policies/avma-guidelines-euthanasia-animals (accessed 9 November 2021).

*Cambridge Dictionary* (n.d.). Corporation. https://dictionary.cambridge.org/us/dictionary/english/corporation (accessed 9 November 2021).

Mars Veterinary Health (n.d.). Stronger together: Introducing our family of veterinary practices and labs. https://www.marsveterinary.com/who-we-are/our-companies (accessed 9 November 2021).

Tanella, P.H. (2020). The corporatization of veterinary practices in America – Will you be a part of it? https://www.veterinarypracticenews.com/myvpnplus/the-corporatization-of-veterinary-practices-in-america-will-you-be-a-part-of-it (accessed 9 November 2021).

# Section 4

# Emerging Ethical Concerns

**18**

# Animal Use in Veterinary Education

*Andrew Knight and Miriam A. Zemanova*

## Historical Perspective

Historically, and still contemporaneously in many veterinary schools, terminal use of animals to teach surgical, and less often, clinical procedures such as resuscitation, is commonplace. Terminal use means that the animals are killed at the completion of the educational task (or tasks in the case of multiple survival procedures). By the mid-1980s however, there was growing societal appreciation of animals as beings with moral status and interests worthy of protection (Lairmore and Ilkiw 2015). A survey of veterinary schools across the United States and Canada indicated considerable change in the traditional reliance on terminal laboratories to teach veterinary surgery, with increasing use of cadavers and inanimate models (Bauer 1993). Nevertheless, 27% of veterinary schools were still killing animals before recovery from anesthesia, with 69% using terminal exercises in small animals, and 20% using them in large animals.

Within the United States, although invasive procedures and terminal surgeries continued in most schools, the majority were offering alternatives by 2004 (Anon. 2004). In recent years, the replacement of terminal animal use within veterinary surgical training has been gaining pace. Veterinary schools that have eliminated such animal use include the School of Veterinary Medicine at Tufts University (the first veterinary school in the United States to eliminate all terminal procedures in all species), the University of Pennsylvania, Michigan State University, The Ohio State University, the University of California, Davis, and, in 2020, Tuskegee University. In 2021, the College of Veterinary Medicine at Colorado State University has begun developing a roadmap "to move the school away from the use of terminal procedures for teaching and replacing that component with activities of equal or greater educational value by using models, cadavers, virtual reality, and supervised surgical experiences on live animals in real-life settings, such as in spay-neuter clinics" (McReynolds 2021). Established in 1998, the Western University College of Veterinary Medicine is one of the most recent US veterinary schools. It promises students "An opportunity to learn how to heal animals without harming them for educational purposes. This is our guiding reverence for life philosophy" (Western University of Health Sciences 2020). However, most US and international veterinary schools still harm and kill animals for teaching purposes.

## Animal Impacts

Large numbers of animals are used for educational purposes. Global laboratory animal use for all purposes was estimated at 192 million in 2015 (Taylor and Alvarez 2019). It has been estimated that in any country, animal use in education and training amounts to 1–10% of the total number of reported animals (Akbarsha et al. 2013). This means an estimated 2–19 million animals are used for educational purposes worldwide, each year. Within the 27 European Union (EU) Member States, approximately half a million animals in total were used for the purposes of education and training from 2015 to 2017 (European Commission 2020) – an average of 165,000 animals annually. It is important to note that only animals protected by the EU Directive 2010/63 (i.e. vertebrates and cephalopods) are included in the national statistical reports. Animals who are bred (potentially for other purposes), killed, and their cadavers then used in educational procedures – as is common within anatomy courses, for example – are not included in these statistical reports. The actual number of animals used in education and training is therefore likely to be higher than these estimates.

Many of the animals used in demonstration experiments or terminal procedures suffer significant harms to their welfare, including initial sourcing and transportation, the involuntary disruption of their social networks, confinement, fear, and pain (Knight 2011). Veterinary laboratories teaching clinical skills may be stressful for animals. For instance, transrectal palpation training increases cortisol hormone levels in cows (Giese et al. 2018) and horses (van Vollenhoven et al. 2017), which is indicative of acutely stressful conditions. Finally, the animals do not directly benefit from participation, and many are killed when the educational task is completed.

With respect to terminal animal use, it has often been asserted that when humanely inflicted, such as under anesthesia after a surgical procedure, death is not harmful to an animal (Webster 1994). As we've noted elsewhere (Zemanova et al. 2021) however, "Modern conceptualizations of animal welfare … understand that good welfare requires not just the avoidance of negative states, but the experience of positive states. Death permanently prevents such positive states, and indeed, the achievement of any other interests animals could seek to fulfill during the remainder of their lives" (Yeates 2010; Jensen 2017). Accordingly, death is in fact one of the most profound harms that can be inflicted, barring exceptional cases such as genuine euthanasia of those faced with severe, ongoing suffering, with a poor prognosis for recovery.

## Human Impacts

The impacts on animals used for educational purposes are well documented. Potential adverse effects on participating students and staff are less commonly recognized.

Live animal use incurs risks of injuries such as bites, scratches, and kicks from large animals, as well as allergic reactions – a common occupational hazard for animal workers. Additionally, anatomy specimens are normally preserved using chemicals of high toxicity – sufficient to prevent colonization by all bacteria, molds, and other organisms. These can create health hazards through direct exposure or aerosolization (Bhat et al. 2019). This creates potential for legal liability should exposure-related adverse effects result. In the experience of one of us (AK) and colleagues from leading veterinary schools internationally, compliance with personal protective equipment such as gloves, gowns, and masks is sometimes lacking (Knight 2007a).

Other impacts are educational and psychological. The invasive nature of animal use within demonstration experiments and surgical training, and the killing of animals for cadaver sourcing, naturally incur high potential for stress within students drawn to the veterinary profession by a desire to care for animals (Capaldo 2004) (see Chapter 22 for a more thorough discussion of moral stress). A recent report of US veterinary students found that helping animals was the most common choice selected as an important reason for becoming a veterinarian (Kipperman et al. 2020). Moral stress can create multiple, adverse impacts. First, such mental turmoil has considerable potential to interfere with the cognitive processes involved with learning and memory, decreasing educational effectiveness. Surveys of veterinary students participating in invasive animal laboratories have identified that they are often distracted from relevant scientific concepts by the plight of their animals, and the necessity of maintaining life and appropriate anesthetic management, which is made considerably more challenging by their lack of experience and supervision (Knight 2011).

Some students find such experiences so upsetting that they may be considered to have suffered psychological trauma (Capaldo 2004). More subtle, but arguably more profound effects appear common. Cognitive dissonance is a discordance between behavior and beliefs (Engel et al. 2020). In this case, the behavior is harmful educational animal use, and the belief is that animals are sentient and should not be harmed. People normally resolve cognitive dissonance by either altering behavior or beliefs. Some students resolve this conflict by leaving or not participating in the exercise or declining to apply for admission – an alteration of behavior. For example, while in veterinary school in the 1980s, one of the editors (BK) boycotted a laboratory in which beagles were to be injected with an intravenous overdose of digoxin while connected to an electrocardiogram (EKG) monitor until death was confirmed. This drug's effects of causing cardiac conduction blockade followed by cardiac arrest and death were well documented (Atkins and Ames 2018). Hence, widespread continuation of harmful animal use within veterinary schools systematically discriminates against empathic students opposed to harming animals in the absence of overwhelming necessity, making it less likely such students will become veterinarians.

Unfortunately, most students appear to resolve this mental conflict by changing their beliefs, rather than their behavior. Arluke and Hafferty (1996) showed that learning experiences perceived as morally wrong initially lead to ethical uneasiness, but then often progress to desensitization, through the use of rationalizations to justify the behavior concerned. Many veterinary students may therefore start to believe that animals are less deserving of moral consideration. The decreasing awareness among veterinary students of animal sentience (specifically, hunger, pain, fear, and boredom in dogs, cats, and cows) throughout their veterinary courses (Paul and Podberscek 2000), the decreased likelihood of fourth-year students providing analgesia when compared with second- or third-year students (Hellyer et al. 1999), and the inhibition of normal development of moral reasoning ability during the four years of veterinary school (Self et al. 1991) have all been documented within veterinary student cohorts.

This may also represent "compassion fatigue" – a diminished ability to empathize, or feel compassion for others (Pereira et al. 2017). Numerous studies indicate declining empathy for animals as veterinary students progress through training programs (Colombo et al. 2016).

These are all desensitization-related phenomena. They are psychological adaptations to the cognitive dissonance created by curricular requirements to harm and kill sentient creatures when such measures do not appear to be clearly justified.

The pressure on such students is immense. Students know that refusal to participate could threaten careers they have put enormous effort into achieving and leave them with university debts that can reach several hundred thousand dollars, without the professional ability to repay them. Acting in accordance with one's convictions in such circumstances requires considerable courage, and a willingness to risk incurring very serious consequences. Consequently, it is unsurprising that most alter their beliefs, rather than their behavior.

Ultimately, those few students who do not alter their beliefs may not graduate, and those who remain often appear to alter their beliefs, becoming veterinarians with a diminished appreciation of animal interests, and of their capacity for suffering. These outcomes constitute profound harms to the students in either group. Veterinary patients are also potentially at risk when veterinarians are subsequently less likely to consider animals as sentient, or to warrant appropriate analgesia. Some evidence also suggests the veterinary profession at large is less progressive on animal welfare and advocacy issues than society reasonably expects (Knight 2008; Kipperman et al. 2018).

## Humane Alternatives

Many humane alternatives have been developed for laboratories in which animals are harmed or killed, and successfully implemented within veterinary curricula internationally. These include computer simulations and videos of professionally performed dissections (prosections) and experiments, noninvasive self-experimentation, ethically sourced cadavers, preserved anatomical specimens, models, mannequins and surgical simulators, and supervised clinical experiences (Knight 2011).

### Computer Simulations and Videos

The first computer simulations had simplistic user interfaces. Modern simulations include video clips of animal experiments, showing resultant effects (Figure 18.1), and virtual equipment and body parts, such as nerves and muscles (Figure 18.2). Dissection simulations may offer virtual dissecting kits, from which students must select appropriate tools (Figure 18.3). Correct choices may be rewarded by still images and videos of professionally performed dissections. These prosections successfully preserve and display structures that may be destroyed during student dissections (Figure 18.4). Histological (microscopic) anatomy of tissues and organs may be displayed alongside the gross (macroscopic) anatomy (Figure 18.5).

Some simulations are freely available via the Internet, such as those at www.humanelearning.info. Others are available for a fee, such as the "Virtual Canine Anatomy" program from the Colorado State University College of Veterinary Medicine and Biomedical Sciences (http://www.cvmbs.colostate.edu/vetneuro). The latter provides key information about many anatomical structures (Figure 18.6). Other simulations such as Pro-dissector's "Face" (Figure 18.7) allow students to click on certain muscles, which then contract, displaying the effects on the visible tissues. Simulations may also provide functional diagrams of working organs (Figure 18.8).

They may illustrate surface anatomy (Figure 18.9) and allow rotation to obtain different views (Figure 18.10). They may even provide information about the natural history of the species in question.

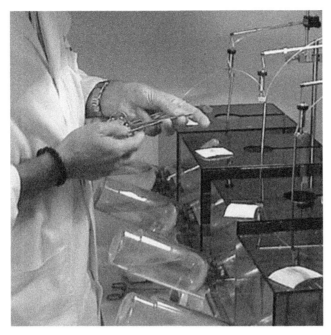

**Figure 18.1** Modern simulations may include video clips of animal experiments (*Source*: Knight 2012, figure 02, p. 2, with permission of ALTEX Proceedings).

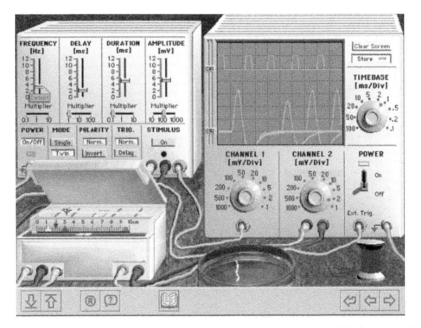

**Figure 18.2** Modern simulations may include virtual equipment and body parts such as nerves and muscles (*Source*: Knight 2012, figure 04, p. 2, with permission of ALTEX Proceedings).

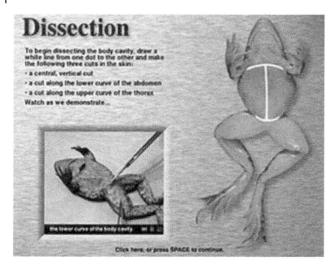

**Figure 18.3** Dissection simulations may require students to use virtual tools appropriately (*Source*: Knight 2012, figure 05, p. 2, with permission of ALTEX Proceedings).

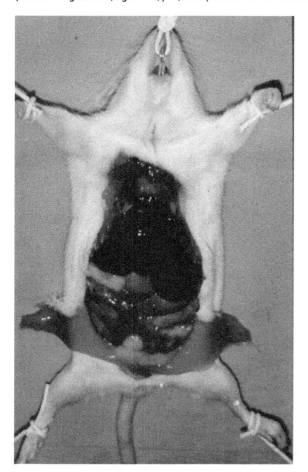

**Figure 18.4** Professionally performed dissections ("prosections") preserve and display structures sometimes destroyed during student dissections (*Source*: Knight 2012, figure 06, p. 3, with permission of ALTEX Proceedings).

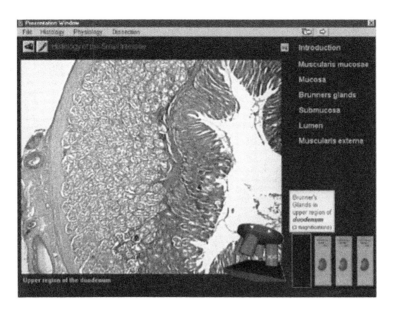

**Figure 18.5** Histological anatomy may be displayed alongside gross anatomy (*Source*: Knight 2012, figure 07, p. 3, with permission of ALTEX Proceedings).

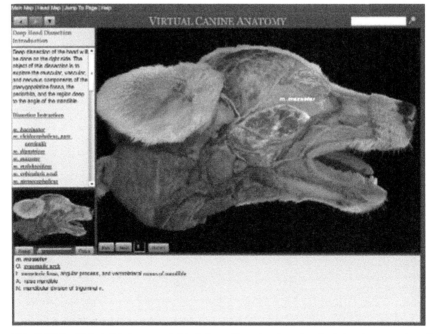

**Figure 18.6** Simulations may provide information about anatomical structures, such as the points of origin and insertion of muscles, their innervation and function (*Source*: Knight 2012, figure 08, p. 3, with permission of ALTEX Proceedings).

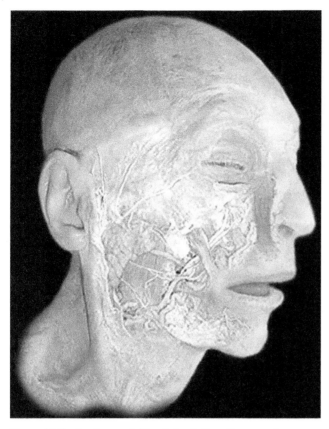

**Figure 18.7** Prodissector's "Face" simulation allows students to contract selected muscles to observe their effects (*Source*: Knight 2012, figure 09, p. 3, with permission of ALTEX Proceedings).

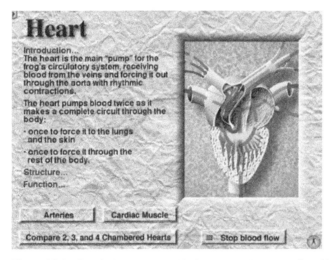

**Figure 18.8** Simulations may provide functional diagrams of working organs (*Source*: Knight 2012, figure 10, p. 4, with permission of ALTEX Proceedings).

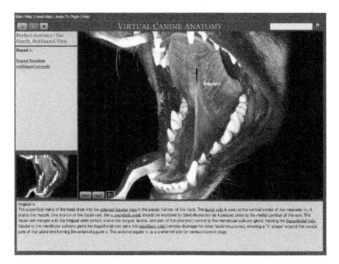

**Figure 18.9** Simulations may illustrate surface anatomy (*Source*: Knight 2012, figure 12, p. 4, with permission of ALTEX Proceedings).

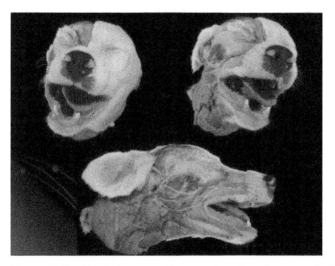

**Figure 18.10** Simulations may allow rotation of specimens to obtain different views (*Source*: Knight 2012, figure 13, p. 4, with permission of ALTEX Proceedings).

### Noninvasive Self-experimentation

Noninvasive experiments conducted on oneself or classmates may be used to investigate and demonstrate physiological principles, such as responses of heart rate or blood pressure to exercise, lung capacity, the effects on visual fields of phenomena such as blind spots or after-imaging, and many others (Lutterschmidt and Lutterschmidt 2008).

### Ethically Sourced Cadavers

Ethically sourced cadavers are obtained from animals who have been euthanized for medical reasons, for severe and intractable behavioral reasons, or who have died naturally, or in accidents. In contrast, killing animals for other reasons is ethically controversial, and such cadavers cannot be legitimately classified as ethically sourced, although they are sometimes misrepresented as such. This includes killing animals specifically for teaching purposes, or in slaughterhouses or animal shelters due to pet overpopulation, or when surplus to the needs of animal industries, such as greyhound racing or biomedical research.

Client donation programs within veterinary teaching hospitals provide most ethically sourced cadavers, and others may be sourced from partner veterinary clinics. These may be used for learning anatomy, clinical skills, and surgery. In contrast to the anatomical uniformity supplied by the greyhound cadavers often used in anatomy laboratories, ethically sourced cadavers may demonstrate normal biological variation, e.g. between dog breeds. They may be accompanied by clinical histories, and may allow comparison of normal and pathological tissues, increasing their educational efficacy for veterinary students. A significant number of US and international veterinary schools have established client donation programs for ethical cadaver sourcing (Kumar et al. 2001; Knight 2011).

## Preserved Specimens

Whether ethically sourced or not, animal specimens may be preserved in several ways. This can allow their reuse for years. Potted specimens are preserved using powerful chemicals designed to prevent tissue dissolution and bacterial putrefaction along with color preservatives (Figure 18.11). Colored casts of blood vessels and airways may be made after perfusion of these vessels with colored dyes (Figures 18.12 and 18.13). The surrounding tissues are dissolved by weak acids over prolonged periods. Plastination involves several chemical steps, as well as evacuation. The water and lipids within tissues are replaced by polymers, yielding a plastic texture, and removing most of the odor. Very large animals have been successfully plastinated (Figure 18.14).

## Models, Mannequins, and Surgical Simulators

Many models and mannequins have been designed to illustrate anatomy. Others have been created for clinical skills training for veterinary or medical students, or laboratory technicians. Such skills may include venipuncture (blood sampling using faux blood solutions), endotracheal intubation, thoracocentesis, bandaging, splinting, resuscitation, arterial pulse palpation, and auscultation of heart and breath sounds via a stethoscope (Figures 18.15 and 18.16).

There has been an increasing interest in the use of simulation training within veterinary education. Surgical simulators include soft tissue and orthopedic models and mannequins (Figures 18.17 and 18.18). Systems such as the Pulsating Organ Perfusion Trainer (Figures 18.19 and 18.20) use real organs sourced from slaughterhouses or elsewhere. The major blood vessels are perfused with faux blood solution using a closed circulatory system. This system includes a pulsatile pump that simulates a beating heart. This creates bleeding when vessels are deliberately or inadvertently cut, allowing practice of *hemostatic* (to control hemorrhage) surgical techniques. Surgery may be practiced via both conventional approaches and endoscopic incisions and equipment.

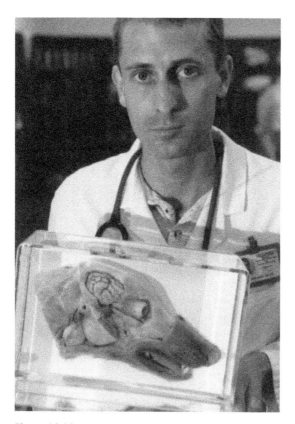

**Figure 18.11** Author Andrew Knight as a veterinary student, with a potted, prosected canine head (*Source*: Knight 2012, figure 16, p. 5, with permission of ALTEX Proceedings).

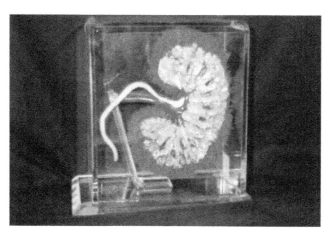

**Figure 18.12** Cast of the vasculature of the bovine kidney (*Source*: Knight 2012, figure 17, p. 6, with permission of ALTEX Proceedings).

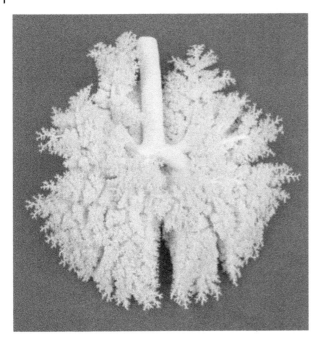

**Figure 18.13**   Cast of the airways of the canine tracheobronchial system (*Source*: Knight 2012, figure 18, p. 6, with permission of ALTEX Proceedings).

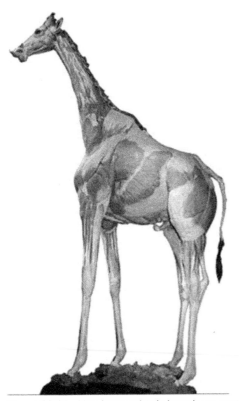

**Figure 18.14**   Very large animals have been successfully plastinated (*Source*: Knight 2012, figure 19, p. 6, with permission of ALTEX Proceedings).

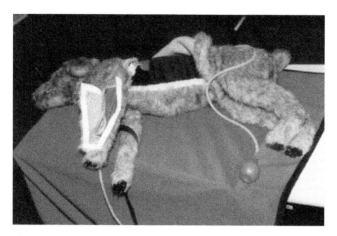

**Figure 18.15** Mannequins such as Rescue Critters' Critical Care Jerry allow veterinary students to practice numerous procedures and auscultation. A wide range of normal and pathological heart and breath sounds may be auscultated. (*Source*: Knight 2012, figure 20, p. 7, with permission of ALTEX Proceedings).

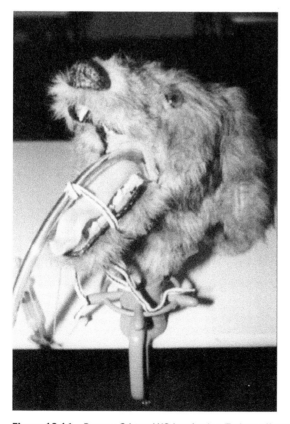

**Figure 18.16** Rescue Critters' K9 Intubation Trainer allows veterinary students to practice endotracheal intubation (*Source*: Knight 2012, figure 21, p. 7, with permission of ALTEX Proceedings).

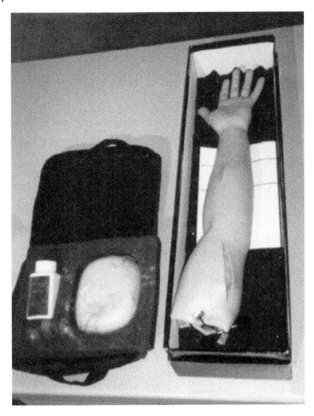

**Figure 18.17** Surgical simulators include soft tissue models and mannequins (*Source*: Knight 2012, figure 22, p. 7, with permission of ALTEX Proceedings).

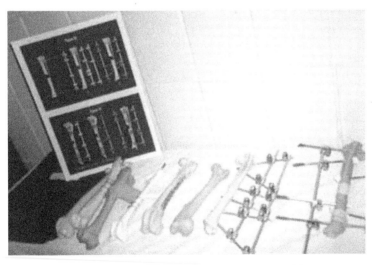

**Figure 18.18** Simulated bones can be used for practicing orthopedic procedures (*Source*: Knight 2012, figure 23, p. 7, with permission of ALTEX Proceedings).

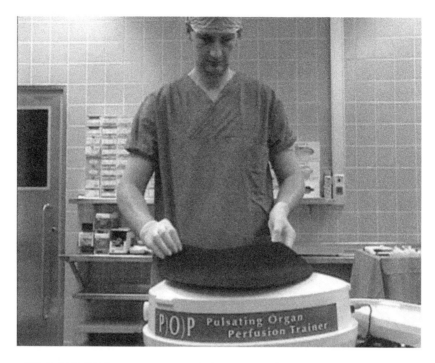

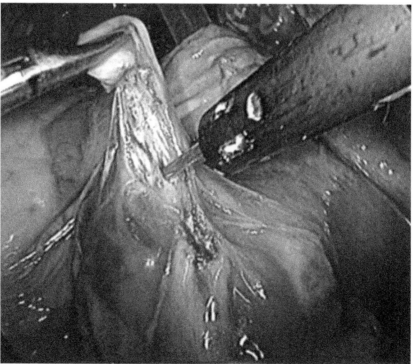

**Figures 18.19 and 18.20** The Pulsating Organ Perfusion Trainer (*Source*: Knight 2012, figures 24 and 25, p. 8, with permission of ALTEX Proceedings).

It has also been recognized that skills developed during video gaming correlate with increased laparoscopic surgical skills, and training curricula have been proposed that would include video games (Levi et al. 2019). Haptic simulators are even more advanced. These provide tactile feedback to students' instruments and fingers that is anatomically appropriate depending on their locations within simulations, such as a virtual bovine rectum (Figure 18.21). Haptic simulators are also used in endoscopic surgical training. The designer of the haptic bovine rectal palpation simulator-Professor Sarah Baillie, has also created equine colic and feline abdominal palpation simulators.

### Supervised Clinical Experience

In most countries, veterinary surgery has traditionally been learned through practicing surgical procedures on healthy animals, which are then killed at the end of these "terminal" procedures. However, many veterinary schools have now introduced humane alternatives. These ideally comprise three main stages. First, students practice basic manual skills such as instrument handling and suturing using knot-tying boards, plastic organs, and other models. Second, they participate in simulated surgery using ethically sourced cadavers. Third, students observe, assist with, and then perform beneficial surgery under close supervision on real patients, similarly to the training of human surgeons (Knight 2011). Animal shelter neutering programs are a very popular example of the latter, within humane veterinary surgical courses (Howe and Slater 1997).

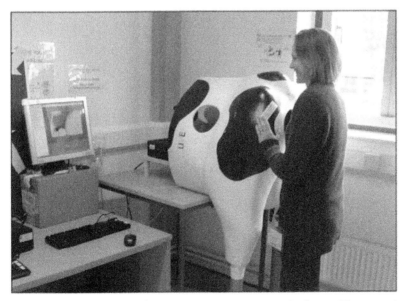

**Figure 18.21** University of Queensland veterinary student Dr. Bryony Dixon practices pregnancy diagnosis using a haptic bovine rectal palpation simulator at England's Royal Veterinary College in 2008. In 2011 Dr. Dixon became one of the first University of Queensland students to graduate without participating in harmful animal use (*Source*: Knight 2012, figure 26, p. 8, with permission of ALTEX Proceedings).

## Educational Efficacy

Veterinary education has been evolving to keep up with scientific advances and novel approaches in clinical practice, while continuing to comply with the public expectation of training competent clinicians (Dilly et al. 2017). However, one of the biggest obstacles to embracing humane teaching methods appears to be uncertainty about their efficacy in achieving desired learning outcomes (Zemanova et al. 2021). We recently analyzed publicly available nontechnical summaries of projects using animals for the primary purpose of education and training within the EU (Zemanova et al. 2021). This analysis indicated two main reasons provided by educators and researchers for continued animal use: (i) belief in the necessity of using a living animal for "proper" learning; and (ii) the perceived lack of an adequate alternative. Our recent systematic review identified 50 relevant peer-reviewed studies published since 1968, of which 13 focused on veterinary education (Zemanova and Knight 2021). Twelve of the 13 veterinary studies showed equivalent or superior teaching efficacy of humane teaching methods (Table 18.1).

Studies have compared learning outcomes for surgical skills in students trained using dog cadavers with those of students trained using live dogs. They found no significant difference in speed and performance of the surgical task (Carpenter et al. 1991), or overall skills (Pavletic et al. 1994). Five studies compared surgical training outcomes using live dogs and models. The assessment of the learning outcome of the humane method was predominantly either equivalent (Greenfield et al. 1994, 1995a) or superior (Olsen et al. 1996; Griffon et al. 2000). Only one study reported inferior learning outcomes. Smeak et al. (1994) created a hollow organ model, which proved to be inappropriate for training of the surgical task during the course of the study. The model had increased fragility, with suture pull-through occurring despite appropriate placement and tension. This study highlighted the need for an appropriate model design to ensure teaching efficacy.

Apart from models, some techniques can be successfully taught through videos or simulations. McCool et al. (2020) showed that human virtual reality endoscopy trainers could be successfully used to teach endoscopy skills to veterinary medicine students. Abutarbush et al. (2006) evaluated two teaching modalities providing instruction in equine nasogastric intubation. Students taught through a self-learning computer module performed better than students exposed to a live demonstration, not only during knowledge assessment but also in task performance. Two other studies focused on tasks performed on horse models or simulators: injecting the jugular vein (Eichel et al. 2013); and transrectal palpation and ultrasonography (Nagel et al. 2015). The fact that students were able to train repeatedly on a simulator led to significantly better performance and confidence in comparison with students in a control group, who could learn only through a live demonstration (Eichel et al. 2013), or train on a live horse for a limited amount of time (Nagel et al. 2015). Finally, Winder et al. (2018) demonstrated that even online learning can be just as effective in learning specific procedures.

Numerous studies have evaluated the performance of humane teaching methods in veterinary education, without any direct comparison with harmful animal use. For instance, in a study by Langebæk et al. (2015), students reported increased levels of

**Table 18.1** Studies in veterinary education and training, comparing the learning outcome of a humane teaching method in comparison with harmful animal use (data from Zemanova and Knight 2021)

| Study | Country | Species | Humane method | Student numbers: humane method (total students) | Assessment of learning outcome | Learning outcome of humane method |
|---|---|---|---|---|---|---|
| Carpenter et al. 1991 | United States | Dog | Ethically sourced cadaver | 12 (24) | Task performance | Equivalent |
| Greenfield et al. 1994 | United States | Dog | Model | 36 (36) | Task performance | Equivalent |
| Pavletic et al. 1994 | United States | Dog | Ethically sourced cadaver | 12 (48) | Skills assessment by employers | Equivalent |
| Smeak et al. 1994 | United States | Dog | Model | 20 (40) | Task performance | Inferior |
| Greenfield et al. 1995a | United States | Dog | Model | 18 (36) | Task performance | Equivalent |
| Olsen et al. 1996 | United States | Dog | Model | 20 (40) | Task performance | Superior |
| Griffon et al. 2000 | UK | Dog | Model | 20 (40) | Task performance | Superior |
| Abutarbush et al. 2006 | Canada | Horse | Computer simulation | 27 (52) | Exam; task performance | Superior |
| Eichel et al. 2013 | Germany | Horse | Model | 12 (24) | Task performance | Superior |
| Nagel et al. 2015 | Austria | Horse | Simulator | 8 (25) | Task performance | Superior |
| Winder et al. 2018 | Canada | Cow | Online learning | 23 (43) | Task performance | Equivalent |
| Davy et al. 2019 | United States | Dog | Video | 19 (38) | Task performance | Equivalent |
| McCool et al. 2020 | United States | Dog | Virtual reality simulation | 6 (12) | Task performance | Equivalent |

competence, confidence, and anatomic knowledge after having used a low-cost model for canine ovariohysterectomy training. Similar results were reported by Annandale et al. (2020): training on an ovariohysterectomy model significantly decreased surgical time when later performing a live animal ovariohysterectomy. In another study, veterinary students who participated in anesthesia-focused simulations before a live animal anesthesia exercise showed significant improvements in their operational performance (Jones et al. 2019).

Simulators and mechanical models can be used to practice a task repeatedly, in a standardized environment, at the student's own speed, without any potential risk to patients (French et al. 2021; Silva et al. 2021). Even low-cost, low-tech simulators can be useful for practice. For example, Williamson et al. (2019) compared two canine celiotomy closure models: low-fidelity and high-fidelity. Both of them helped improve surgical skills among veterinary students. Participants in a study (Hage et al. 2016) rated a low-cost, self-developed model of ultrasound-guided pericardiocentesis as useful and realistic. Andrade et al. (2020) constructed a model of the cardiovascular system with simple materials such as plastic bottles, transparent tubing, and rubber balloons. Most students in the study found the model to be a more efficient and satisfactory learning method than a traditional lecture.

## Other Benefits of Humane Alternatives

Logistical considerations are important to educators, particularly the cost and time required to use various teaching modalities. Economic considerations have been one of the major drivers of humane teaching methods internationally, because these methods are often cheaper than methods that rely on harmful animal use. Educational animal use incurs costs associated with animal purchase, transportation, housing, feeding, veterinary care when necessary, experimental anesthesia, euthanasia, and disposal. When these costs occur every year, for considerable numbers of animals, such costs can become substantial.

Many alternatives, however, are reusable, and can be used largely cost-free, for years, once the initial purchase has been made. Initial costs are often comparatively affordable. Most computer simulations, for example, are available for a few hundred dollars or less, and some clinical or surgical skills trainers can be even cheaper. The financial advantages of alternatives have been demonstrated in several studies (e.g. Dewhurst et al. 1994; Craven and Goh 2018), and are likely to become increasingly important as economic pressures on universities continue to rise in many countries.

Time savings may also be considerable. In his description of nerve physiology experiments, Clarke (1987) provides insights as to why this is beneficial:

> Previously, ..., considerable time would be taken dissecting a viable sciatic nerve preparation..., at which point there would be a distinct possibility that the nerve was no longer viable. It is often a tired and irritable student who finally comes to the point in the experiment of measuring changes in response. Such a student is not in the optimum frame of mind to either perform the experiment with the due care and attention required or to think about the neurophysiological concepts involved. With the simulation, such problems are eliminated. Not only is much more time devoted to the experiment, but time is available to explore the subject in greater depth.

One of us (AK) can personally attest to the accuracy of this description, as this exact experiment was part of his veterinary physiology course when he was a student at Australia's Murdoch University. A study demonstrated that computer simulations can save teaching time, as well as money, and can be effective and enjoyable for biomedical student learning (Dewhurst et al. 1995). Time spent preparing and anesthetizing animals, cleaning up, and disposing of cadavers are all eliminated, freeing time for more productive learning. Overall, existing studies demonstrate that humane alternatives generally provide time and cost advantages (Annandale et al. 2020; Oviedo-Peñata et al. 2020). After being developed for several decades, many thousands of alternatives now exist and are widely available, with details and suppliers available in alternatives databases such as those at www.humanelearning.info and www.interniche.org.

## Legislative Requirements

The interests of both animals and students who do not wish to harm them are protected by animal welfare and human rights legislation in various countries.

### Protection of Animals

The use of animals for educational purposes frequently falls under the purview of animal welfare legislation or codes of practice covering scientific animal use. Within the United States, the main federal law intended to protect animals is the Animal Welfare Act (AWA) (Animal Welfare Act 1985), which is administered by the US Department of Agriculture (USDA). Its scope includes any living or dead dog or cat or warm-blooded animal (excluding birds, mice or rats bred for research, and animals used for the production of food or fiber) that is used for research, teaching, testing, or that is a "pet." The Act requires the principal investigator in an experiment or procedure to investigate the use of humane alternatives. This would include teachers in charge of educational activities involving animals. The Act requires such principal investigators or educators to submit protocols describing intended animal use to Institutional Animal Care and Use Committees (IACUCs), and to demonstrate that they have considered alternatives to procedures that may be potentially painful or distressing. This is commonly indicated by stating that a scientific literature search for alternatives has been conducted (Lairmore and Ilkiw 2015). State animal protection legislation may also be applicable. However, precollege use is not covered by the AWA.

Within Australia, the National Health and Medical Research Council (NHMRC) *Australian Code of Practice for the Care and Use of Animals for Scientific Purposes* (National Health and Medical Research Council 2013) governs all use of living nonhuman vertebrates in research and teaching. It similarly states:

> 1.5 Evidence to support a case to use animals must demonstrate that:
>
> (i) the project has scientific or educational merit ...
> (ii) the use of animals is essential to achieve the stated aims, and suitable alternatives to replace the use of animals to achieve the stated aims are not available

> 4.3 Institutions must ensure that animals are used for teaching only when their use is essential to achieve an educational outcome in science, as specified in the relevant curriculum or competency requirements, and suitable alternatives to replace the use of animals to achieve the educational outcome are not available (see Clause 1.5).

By 2001, the NHMRC Code was legally enforceable in almost all Australian states and territories.

Unfortunately, the widespread ongoing educational use of animals via harmful procedures, despite the existence of educationally effective and available alternatives, demonstrates that compliance with such requirements to search for, consider, and implement appropriate alternatives is often lacking. Indeed, within the United States, USDA inspectors have previously cited a large number of veterinary schools for noncompliance with provisions of the AWA requiring such consideration of alternatives (Willems 2007).

### Protection of Students

International human rights legislation, as well as the laws of several countries, e.g. Argentina, Italy, the Slovak Republic, and the United States, support the rights of students to decline to participate in educational activities that conflict with their conscientiously held beliefs (Knight 2014). Such provision for the exercise of conscientiously held beliefs is recognized as an essential pillar of democracies.

Another example is provided by the Western Australian Equal Opportunity Act (1984) (Commissioner for Equal Opportunity n.d.), which in some circumstances outlaws discrimination in education on the grounds of belief. This Act was used by one of us (AK) to uphold his rights not to harm animals as a veterinary student. Within the United States, several students have successfully used the First Amendment to the United States Constitution to sue colleges that initially penalized them for refusing to participate in harmful animal usage. By 2021, Student Choice laws protecting the rights of students up to Grade 12 not to dissect or, in some cases, engage in other harmful animal usage, had been passed in 22 states (American Antivivisection Society 2021).

## Veterinary Professional Positions

The positions of veterinary professional associations with respect to harmful educational animal use have evolved over the past 50 years, following changing societal views about the acceptability of such animal use.

In the 1990s, the American Veterinary Medical Association (AVMA) Council of Research created a panel to develop guidelines for performing animal surgery within teaching or research. These were refined by the American Society of Laboratory Animal Practitioners and duly published (Brown et al. 1993). In veterinary schools within the United States and elsewhere, students opposed to the reuse of animals in multiple, consecutive, survival surgical laboratories within their surgical courses, campaigned for terminal single surgical exercises. In some cases, student lawsuits resulted in schools being required to develop academically sound alternative surgical exercises (Greenfield et al. 1995b).

By 2000, the veterinary profession was questioning whether even terminal surgical laboratories would continue. The American College of Veterinary Surgeons called for animal use to be reserved for occasions when acceptable alternatives were lacking. However, the AVMA defended and promoted the use of animals in research, testing, and education, while calling for the exercise of "proper stewardship" (Kahler 2000). The AVMA's Council on Education (COE), which accredits veterinary schools, notes in its requirements that, "Normal and diseased animals of various domestic and exotic species must be available for instructional purposes, either as clinical patients or provided by the institution" (American Veterinary Medical Association 2020). There is no mention of nonanimal teaching methods.

At the time of writing, the AVMA (2021) continues to support "the judicious use of animals in meaningful research, testing, and education programs," while concurrently endorsing the Three Rs (Russell et al. 1959) citing the need for "replacement of animals with non-animal methods wherever feasible." As we have demonstrated previously, alternatives have been developed and are available for virtually every type of educational animal use, and well-designed alternatives normally produce learning outcomes equal or superior to those produced by harmful animal use, including within veterinary surgical training (Zemanova and Knight 2021). Accordingly, some veterinarians have called for an end to harmful educational animal use. As noted by Abood and Siegford (2012), the veterinarian's role is to uphold animal welfare, embodying the duty of care to relieve pain and suffering. The harmful use of animals is contrary to providing them with good welfare, and hence is fundamentally contrary to what should be the ethics of the veterinary profession.

## Recommendations for Students

Unfortunately, implementation of humane teaching methods within veterinary schools remains variable, with harmful animal use still required of students. Accordingly, students who do not wish to engage in harmful animal use should proceed with care. Advice for such students is available within Francione and Charlton (1992) and Knight (2004), and at www.humanelearning.info and www.interniche.org. Interested students should consider implementing the following steps:

1. *School selection.* Veterinary school admission is highly selective, and students might reasonably be worried that voicing concerns about curricular animal use in schools where harmful animal use continues could prejudice their entry chances. Hence, in such cases, prior inquiries about curricular animal use should possibly be made anonymously. If harmful animal use remains part of the required curriculum, and alternatives are not available, students can either seek alternative schools or seek admission with a view to aiming to change institutional policy and practice regarding animal use and alternatives.

2. *Start early.* Enrolled students are usually in a much stronger position to campaign for alternatives than people external to a veterinary school. However, it can take a lot of time to educate oneself about humane alternatives, to prepare a submission describing specific alternatives aimed at achieving comparable learning objectives, and to negotiate with one's university. Hence it is wise to start as early as possible. However, veterinary students are extremely busy, and such prior preparation is not always possible. Many students have commenced alternatives campaigns only after animal laboratories were underway and have still been successful.

3. *Gather information.* If not already known, students should determine what use of animals or animal tissues, living or dead, is required, what their sources are, and what noninvasive or nonanimal alternatives are available. Students wishing to

establish new alternatives will also need to determine the learning objectives of the practical sessions involving animal use.

4. *Determine one's position.* Students should carefully consider which kinds of animal use will be acceptable to them. Depending on the kinds of animal use within the curriculum, students may need to consider harmful or terminal procedures on not only vertebrates, but also invertebrates. Students may need to consider their position on minimally invasive or noninvasive procedures such as blood or urine sampling (which would, of course, be part of routine veterinary practice). Students may need to consider use of cadavers, body parts, or tissues sourced from animals killed primarily for teaching purposes, or for reasons that, although of questionable ethics, are unrelated to teaching. These may include animals used or surplus to needs within animal research, greyhounds killed due to poor racing performance or injury, dogs and cats killed due to pet overpopulation, and slaughterhouse "by-products."

Next, students should consider what sacrifices they are prepared to make to maintain that position. Previously, such students have been ostracized by and faced hostility from classmates and some faculty members. They have been academically penalized, and even failed. Some have pursued their cases legally, through mass media exposure of curricular animal killing, or other external forms of pressure. One of us (AK) has experienced all of these consequences while a veterinary student, and other students have as well. It is important to consider such matters, and to determine one's position, before very considerable pressure may be brought to bear by one's veterinary school. One should ensure one's position is well reasoned and evidence-based, and one should be able to communicate and defend it.

5. *Request alternatives.* If students do not provide their universities with sufficient time to organize and prepare alternatives not yet in use, universities might reasonably argue this is not possible, or alternatives provided might be suboptimal. Accordingly, students should formally request alternatives as early as possible – ideally, well prior to the start of the relevant semester. Students should also be clear about what kinds of alternatives or animal use they would be prepared to accept. Of course, if a university fails to publicize sufficient information to the student body about animal use far enough in advance, along with a request for students to notify them if they feel unable to participate, this can be used as a defense for failure to provide reasonable notice.

It can be wiser to submit a simple, written statement that one is unable to participate in the relevant activities due to conscientiously held beliefs, and request alternatives, rather than engaging in detailed discussions concerning reasons, unless the faculty is supportive. The experience of one of us (AK) and students with similar experiences internationally have shown that unsupportive faculty are unlikely to change their views, and, if they can find real or imagined flaws in one's reasoning, may use these as a reason to deny requests for alternatives. However, the jurisprudential foundations for legal protection of conscientiously held beliefs are very clear that their protection does not rely on the views of others about the rationality of the protected beliefs (Knight 2014). It is acceptable for faculty to ask questions to determine the genuineness of beliefs, but universities must not unduly cross-examine students, harass them, or seek to alter their conscientiously held beliefs.

Any alternatives provided should be of approximately equal difficulty, and in particular should *not* be punitively difficult. A reasonable level of compromise may be required, however.

6. *Be prepared to assist.* Students should be prepared to present ideas for alternatives, or even a detailed submission. The latter could describe existing laboratories, learning outcomes, alternative suggestions, any evidence of educational efficacy, and examples of courses elsewhere where these have been successfully implemented. Several examples are available at www.humanelearning.info. Examples of suitable alternatives may be compiled using the Internet alternatives databases such as those available via www.humanelearning.info and www.interniche.org. Besides presenting alternatives submission(s) to one's faculty, students may also wish to present these to IACUCs or animal ethics committees. These are required to oversee and approve all animal use.

7. *Exhaust internal avenues.* If initial requests are unsuccessful, students may need to go up the academic chain of command. Appeals could be considered to any applicable committees, department or school chairs/heads, deans, provosts, vice-chancellors, presidents, and, finally, the board of trustees. The support of student organizations may be sought. Every approach and response should be logged within a diary and details of communications filed in case these are needed to support further action.

8. *Create new avenues and apply pressure.* Pressure for change can be built through engaging the support of external organizations, and through actions such as letter writing appeals and petitions, lawsuits, and media coverage. Some students including one of us (AK) have successfully utilized such strategies, when prior steps were not successful.

Students may also create new avenues to support the case for change. Along with media exposure, a 1999 survey was highly successful in facilitating the rapid termination of all invasive animal physiology laboratories at the University of Illinois College of Veterinary Medicine in 2000, saving well over 100 animals annually. Another survey conducted in 2001 was similarly successful in ending invasive animal physiology laboratories in which 68 sheep were killed annually at the Massey University Institute of Veterinary and Biomedical Sciences in New Zealand. These surveys explored the extent to which veterinary students felt these laboratories were beneficial for their learning and were worth the animal and other resources consumed. The results clearly indicated that these laboratories should cease. These surveys were student-led. One of them is available as an example at www.humanelearning.info. Numerous inspirational narratives describing successful student alternatives campaigns are available at www.interniche.org. Some provide additional ideas for helping introduce humane teaching methods and aiding such campaigns.

## Recommendations for Veterinary Schools and Universities

Well-designed humane teaching methods generally achieve learning outcomes as good as or better than methods reliant on harmful animal use, increase compliance with applicable legislation and codes of practice covering educational animal use, and may also bring time and cost savings. Accordingly, ongoing harmful animal use should be replaced with humane alternatives.

To date, many universities have adopted an ad hoc approach to handling student claims of conscientious objection, where harmful animal use remains. As we described elsewhere (Knight 2014), this brings a range of potential problems. Lack of early information provision to students frequently results in student requests for humane alternatives being made at late notice. This increases the risk such requests cannot be accommodated, and the chances of subsequent conflict. Consequently, alternatives provided may be suboptimal. To minimize risks of such outcomes, a formal conscientious objection policy and process is recommended.

Some veterinary schools and universities have now implemented policies allowing and formalizing the process of student conscientious objection to animal use considered harmful or objectionable. These have been termed "conscientious objection" or "student choice" policies, with the latter being more common in North America. The first formal, written policy adopted in an Australian veterinary school appears to have been that adopted by Australia's Murdoch University in 1998 (which has since been progressively updated; Knight 2014), following a student campaign by one of us (AK) for humane teaching methods. Consistent with the university's policies respecting student diversity, the scope of this policy was not restricted to animal use but covered any teaching or assessment activities to which students might conscientiously object. It is applicable to the university at large. Similar policies have since been adopted at other veterinary schools within Australia and abroad, such as those at the Universities of Sydney (McGreevy et al. 2005), Illinois at Urbana-Champaign (Knight 2007b), Queensland (University of Queensland School of Veterinary Science 2008), and Adelaide (Whittaker and Anderson 2013) as well as by several other universities lacking veterinary faculties. Examples of several such policies are available at www.humanelearning.info.

Such policies allow students to lodge formal requests for alternative learning and assessment activities when faced with educational activities that violate conscientiously held beliefs. Alternative educational experiences and assessments should aim to provide equivalent outcomes in terms of knowledge and/or ability. These should require approximately equal commitments of time and effort, and in particular, should not be punitively burdensome.

Details of such policies, and of the procedure for submitting and assessing claims, along with information about animal use and available alternatives, should be published within student handbooks, curricular and course guides, etc. well prior to the commencement of any course in which animals are used. Students should be advised to seek information as early as possible about educational activities to which they might conscientiously object, and to submit claims sufficiently early for these to be assessed, and for alternatives to be sourced and prepared if necessary.

To facilitate this process, course and curricular materials should summarize information on potentially objectionable animal use. This information is provided in Table 18.2.

There are reasonable and legal constraints on conscientious objection. Not all requests should be accommodated, e.g. demands for racial segregation due to beliefs based on racism.

Finally, an appeals process should be available in the event that a student's request is denied, or the student is unsatisfied with the alternatives offered. We have provided detailed advice elsewhere (Knight 2014) for the optimal establishment of conscientious objection policies and procedures.

**Table 18.2** Minimum information about curricular animal use universities should disclose to students.

- Which courses animals are used in
- Species and numbers of animals used
- How the animals are sourced
- Summary of the procedures to be carried out (e.g. dissection, experimentation on living animals, terminal surgery)
- Why the animals are considered necessary
- Refinement methods used (to decrease suffering, and maximize well-being, such as analgesics or environmental enrichment)
- Details of other welfare determinants, including of their transportation and confinement
- Whether and how the animals are to be killed and disposed of
- Details of any university conscientious objection policy, including processing for submitting claims and appealing against decisions
- Contact points for further questions and support

## Recommendations for Veterinary Professional Associations

As long as veterinary schools produce graduates demonstrably competent in specified skills ("Day one competencies"), institutions often have considerable freedom about how to teach them. The Australasian Veterinary Boards Council, for example, which accredits Australian and New Zealand veterinary schools, provides generic guidelines, such as: "Institutions need to demonstrate that students have supervised, intramural exposure to the major production and companion animal species relevant to veterinary professional activities in Australasia" (Australasian Veterinary Boards Council 2010). The equivalent US organizations – the Association of American Veterinary Medical Colleges and the AVMA COE – should support and promote best practices in the humane care and appropriate use of animals in education, as it looks to the future (Lairmore and Ilkiw 2015).

We noted previously that the AVMA (2021) continues to support the use of animals in teaching, while concurrently endorsing the Three Rs and, in particular, replacement with alternatives wherever possible. Such replacement is now possible for virtually all harmful educational animal use. To date, veterinary professional associations have not prominently called for the ending of harmful animal use within veterinary curricula. It is now time that they did so.

## Conclusions

Mullan and Main (2001) describe key steps within ethical decision-making as "identification of possible courses of action, consideration of all interested parties (including any related legal or professional guidance), formulating a decision and minimizing any negative consequences of the decision." With respect to the harmful use of animals within veterinary education, the main choices are whether to continue with the status quo, or to implement alternatives. The main interested parties are the animals themselves, the students, their educators, and universities concerned about their reputations, resources, and educational outcomes. Animals are clearly harmed by present educational uses and, as we've shown, in large numbers. The rationale for using animals is to provide students with vital education in clinical and surgical skills, along with animal handling, and demonstration of scientific knowledge in preclinical subjects such as anatomy, physiology, and biochemistry. However, humane alternatives generally appear at least as effective. There are now at least 50 studies assessing the educational efficacy of humane alternatives in comparison with harmful animal use, covering virtually all educational subjects and levels at which animals are used, and especially veterinary surgical training. Among the 50 studies located in our systematic review (Zemanova and Knight 2021), humane alternatives provided outcomes that were superior (30%), equivalent (60%), and inferior (10%) to those provided by harmful animal use.

It is clear that well-designed alternatives generally perform at least as well, and often better, as educational tools. These are readily available and often confer educational, time, and cost benefits, as well as directly preventing animal stress, pain, and unjustified death, mitigating student moral stress, and increasing compliance with animal welfare legislation and codes of practice. These are also often required by the policies of veterinary professional associations. International and in some cases national and state human rights legislation upholds the rights of students to receive an education that does not require them to violate conscientiously held beliefs – in this case, beliefs against harming animals without overwhelming necessity. In short, when considering the key steps within ethical decision-making as described by Mullan and Main (2001), the correct choice on this issue is clear: harmful animal use should be replaced by humane alternatives within veterinary education. This is also true within other educational disciplines, to which most of the above reasoning also applies.

## Acknowledgment

Figures 18.1–18.21 were originally published in Knight (2012), which was published under a Creative Commons CC-BY license.

## References

Abood, S.K. and Siegford, J.M. (2012). Student perceptions of an animal-welfare and ethics course taught early in the veterinary curriculum. *Journal of Veterinary Medical Education* 39: 136–141.

Abutarbush, S.M., Naylor, J.M., Parchoma, G. et al. (2006). Evaluation of traditional instruction versus a self-learning computer module in teaching veterinary students how to pass a nasogastric tube in the horse. *Journal of Veterinary Medical Education* 33: 447–454.

Akbarsha, M.A., Zeeshan, M., and Meenakumari, K.J. (2013). Alternatives to animals in education, research, and risk assessment: An overview with special reference to Indian context. *ALTEX Proceedings* 2: 5–19.

American Antivivisection Society (2021). Student choice laws. https://aavs.org/animals-science/laws/student-choice-laws (accessed 26 March 2021).

American Veterinary Medical Association (AVMA) (2020). COE accreditation policies and procedures: Requirements. https://www.avma.org/education/accreditation/colleges/coe-accreditation-policies-and-procedures-requirements (accessed 3 April 2021).

American Veterinary Medical Association (AVMA) (2021). Use of animals in research, testing, and education. https://www.avma.org/resources-tools/avma-policies/use-animals-research-testing-and-education (accessed 26 March 2021).

Andrade, E.F., Zaine Teixeira Debortoli, G., Gomes Batista, V.L. et al. (2020). Learning perception of veterinary students about cardiovascular physiology using a functional model. *Journal of Biological Education* 1–9. https://doi.org/10.1080/00219266.2020.1769705

Annandale, A., Scheepers, E., and Fosgate, G.T. (2020). The effect of an ovariohysterectomy model practice on surgical times for final-year veterinary students' first live-animal ovariohysterectomies. *Journal of Veterinary Medical Education* 47: 44–55.

Anon. (2004). Comparison of alternatives offered by veterinary schools. https://www.hsvma.org/assets/pdfs/alternativeschart_final_3.pdf (accessed 21 April 2021).

Arluke, A. and Hafferty, F. (1996). From apprehension to fascination with "dog lab": The use of absolutions by medical students. *Journal of Contemporary Ethnography* 25: 201–225.

Atkins, C.E. and Ames, M.K. (2018). Digitalis, positive inotropes and vasodilators. In: *Veterinary Pharmacology and Therapeutics*, 10e. (eds. J.E. Riviere and M.G. Papich). Hoboken, NJ: Wiley-Blackwell.

Australasian Veterinary Boards Council (2010). *AVBC – Policies, Procedures and Standards*. Melbourne, Australia: AVBC.

Bauer, M.S. (1993). A survey of the use of live animals, cadavers, inanimate models, and computers in teaching veterinary surgery. *Journal of the American Veterinary Medical Association* 203: 1047–1051.

Bhat, D., Chittoor, H., Murugesh, P. et al. (2019). Estimation of occupational formaldehyde exposure in cadaver dissection laboratory and its implications. *Anatomy & Cell Biology* 52: 419–425.

Brown, A.J., Phillip, T., Pearson, D. et al. (1993). Guidelines for animal surgery in research. *American Journal of Veterinary Research* 54: 1544–1559.

Capaldo, T. (2004). The psychological effects on students of using animals in ways that they see as ethically, morally or religiously wrong. *Alternatives to Laboratory Animals* 32: 525–531.

Carpenter, L.G., Piermattei, D.L., Salman, M.D. et al. (1991). A comparison of surgical training with live anesthetized dogs and cadavers. *Veterinary Surgery* 20: 373–378.

Clarke, K. (1987). The use of microcomputer simulations in undergraduate neurophysiology experiments. *Alternatives to Laboratory Animals* 14: 134–140.

Colombo, E.S., Pelosi, A., and Prato-Previde, E. (2016). Empathy towards animals and belief in animal-human-continuity in Italian veterinary students. *Animal Welfare* 25: 275–286.

Commissioner for Equal Opportunity (n.d.). *Equal Opportunity Act 1984 Reference Guide*. Perth, Australia: Equal Opportunity Commission.

Craven, S. and Goh, A.C. (2018). Animal laboratory training: Current status and how essential is it? In: *Robotics in Genitourinary Surgery* (eds. A.K. Hemal and M. Menon), 175–182. London: Springer International Publishing.

Davy, R.B., Hamel, P.E., Su, Y. et al. (2019). Evaluation of two training methods for teaching the abdominal focused assessment with sonography for trauma technique (A-FAST) to first- and second-year veterinary students. *Journal of Veterinary Medical Education* 46: 258–263.

Dewhurst, D.G., Hardcastle, J., Hardcastle, P.T. et al. (1994). Comparison of a computer simulation program and a traditional laboratory practical class for teaching the principles of intestinal absorption. *Advances in Physiology Education* 267: S95.

Dewhurst, D.G. and Jenkinson, L. (1995). The impact of computer-based alternatives on the use of animals in undergraduate teaching. *Alternatives to Laboratory Animals* 23: 521–530.

Dilly, M., Read, E.K., and Baillie, S. (2017). A survey of established veterinary clinical skills laboratories from Europe and North America: Present practices and recent developments. *Journal of Veterinary Medical Education* 44: 580–589.

Eichel, J.E., Korb, W., Schlenker, A. et al. (2013). Evaluation of a training model to teach veterinary students a technique for injecting the jugular vein in horses. *Journal of Veterinary Medical Education* 40: 288–295.

Engel, R.M., Silver, C.C., Veeder, C.L. et al. (2020). Cognitive dissonance in laboratory animal medicine and implications for animal welfare. *The Journal of the American Association for Laboratory Animal Science* 59: 132–138.

European Commission (2020). 2019 report on the statistics on the use of animals for scientific purposes in the Member States of the European Union in 2015–2017. https://eur-lex.europa.eu/legal-content/EN/TXT/?qid=1581689520921&uri=CELEX:52020DC0016 (accessed 18 April 2021).

Francione, G.L. and Charlton, A.E. (1992). *Vivisection and Dissection in the Classroom: A Guide to Conscientious Objection*. Philadelphia, PA: American Anti-Vivisection Society.

French, E.D., Griffon, D.J., Kass, P.H. et al. (2021). Evaluation of a laparoscopic abdominal simulator assessment to test readiness for laparoscopic ovariectomy in live dogs. *Veterinary Surgery* 50: 49–66.

Giese, H., Dilly, M., Gundelach, Y. et al. (2018). Influence of transrectal palpation training on cortisol levels and heart rate variability in cows. *Theriogenology* 119: 238–244.

Greenfield, C.L., Johnson, A.L., Smith, C.W. et al. (1994). Integrating alternative models into the existing surgical curriculum. *Journal of Veterinary Medical Education* 21: 23–24.

Greenfield, C.L., Johnson, A.L., Schaeffer, D.J. et al. (1995a). Comparison of surgical skills of veterinary students trained using models or live animals. *Journal of the American Veterinary Medical Association* 206: 1840–1845.

Greenfield, C.L., Johnson, A.L., Klippert, L. et al. (1995b). Veterinary student expectations and outcomes assessment of a small animal surgical curriculum. *Journal of the American Veterinary Medical Association* 206: 778–782.

Griffon, D.J., Cronin, P., Kirby, B. et al. (2000). Evaluation of a hemostasis model for teaching ovariohysterectomy in veterinary surgery. *Veterinary Surgery* 29: 309–316.

Hage, M.C., Massaferro, A.B., Lopes, É.R. et al. (2016). Value of artisanal simulators to train veterinary students in performing invasive ultrasound-guided procedures. *Advances in Physiology Education* 40: 98–103.

Hellyer, P., Frederick, C., Lacy, M. et al. (1999). Attitudes of veterinary medical students, house officers, clinical faculty, and staff toward pain management in animals. *Journal of the American Veterinary Medical Association* 214: 238–244.

Howe, L.M. and Slater, M.R. (1997). Student assessment of the educational benefits of a prepubertal gonadectomy program (preliminary findings). *Journal of Veterinary Medical Education* 24: 12–17.

Jensen, K.K. (2017). How should death be taken into account in welfare assessments? *Journal of Agricultural & Environmental Ethics* 30: 615–623.

Jones, J.L., Rinehart, J., and Englar, R.E. (2019). The effect of simulation training in anesthesia on student operational performance and patient safety. *Journal of Veterinary Medical Education* 46: 205–213.

Kahler, S.C. (2000). Will nonrecovery surgery courses survive? *Journal of the American Veterinary Medical Association* 216: 1201–1204.

Kipperman, B., Morris, P., and Rollin, B. (2018). Ethical dilemmas encountered by small animal veterinarians: Characterisation, responses, consequences and beliefs regarding euthanasia. *Veterinary Record* 182 (19): 548.

Kipperman, B., Rollin, B., and Martin, J. (2020). Veterinary student opinions regarding ethical dilemmas encountered by veterinarians and the benefits of ethics instruction. *Journal of Veterinary Medical Education* 48: 330–342.

Knight, A. (2004). Learning without killing: A guide to conscientious objection. www.humanelearning.info (accessed 9 March 2021).

Knight, A. (2007a). The effectiveness of humane teaching methods in veterinary education. *ALTEX* 24: 91–109.

Knight, A. (2007b). Humane teaching methods in veterinary education. *Australian Veterinary Journal* 85: N28–N29.

Knight, A. (2008). Advancing animal welfare standards within the veterinary profession. *Revista Electrónica de Veterinaria* 9: 1–17.

Knight, A. (2011). *The Costs and Benefits of Animal Experiments*. London: Palgrave Macmillan.

Knight, A. (2012). The potential of humane teaching methods within veterinary and other biomedical education. *ALTEX Proceedings* 1: 365–375.

Knight, A. (2014). Conscientious objection to harmful animal use within veterinary and other biomedical education. *Animals* 4: 16–34.

Kumar, A.M., Murtaugh, R., Brown, D. et al. (2001). Client donation program for acquiring dogs and cats to teach veterinary gross anatomy. *Journal of Veterinary Medical Education* 28: 73–77.

Lairmore, M.D. and Ilkiw, J. (2015). Animals used in research and education, 1966–2016: Evolving attitudes, policies, and relationships. *Journal of Veterinary Medical Education* 42: 425–440.

Langebæk, R., Toft, N., and Eriksen, T. (2015). The SimSpay – Student perceptions of a low-cost build-it-yourself model for novice training of surgical skills in canine ovariohysterectomy. *Journal of Veterinary Medical Education* 42: 166–171.

Levi, O., Shettko, D.L., Battles, M. et al. (2019). Effect of short-versus long-term video game playing on basic laparoscopic skills acquisition of veterinary medicine students. *Journal of Veterinary Medical Education* 46: 184–194.

Lutterschmidt, W. and Lutterschmidt, D. (2008). *Laboratory Exercises in Human Physiology: A Clinical and Experimental Approach with Ph.I.L.S. 3.0 CD*. New York: McGraw-Hill Education.

McCool, K.E., Bissett, S.A., Hill, T.L. et al. (2020). Evaluation of a human virtual-reality endoscopy trainer for teaching early endoscopy skills to veterinarians. *Journal of Veterinary Medical Education* 47: 106–116.

McGreevy, P.D. and Dixon, R.J. (2005). Teaching animal welfare at the University of Sydney's Faculty of Veterinary Science. *Journal of Veterinary Medical Education* 32: 442–446.

McReynolds, T. (2021). CSU moving to eliminate terminal surgeries from DVM program. https://www.aaha.org/publications/newstat/articles/2021-03/csu-moving-to-eliminate-terminal-surgeries-from-dvm-program (accessed 27 April 2021).

Mullan, S. and Main, D. (2001). Principles of ethical decision-making in veterinary practice. *In Practice* 23: 394–401.

Nagel, C., Ille, N., Aurich, J. et al. (2015). Teaching of diagnostic skills in equine gynecology: Simulator-based training versus schooling on live horses. *Theriogenology* 84: 1088–1095.

National Health and Medical Research Council (2013). *Australian Code of Practice for the Care and Use of Animals for Scientific Purposes, 8th Edition*. Canberra: NHMRC.

Olsen, D., Bauer, M.S., Seim, H.B. et al. (1996). Evaluation of a hemostasis model for teaching basic surgical skills. *Veterinary Surgery* 25: 49–58.

Oviedo-Peñata, C.A., Tapia-Araya, A.E., Lemos, J.D. et al. (2020). Validation of training and acquisition of surgical skills in veterinary laparoscopic surgery: A review. *Frontiers in Veterinary Science* 7: 306.

Paul, E.S. and Podberscek, A.L. (2000). Veterinary education and students' attitudes towards animal welfare. *Veterinary Record* 146: 269–272.

Pavletic, M.M., Schwartz, A., Berg, J. et al. (1994). An assessment of the outcome of the alternative medical and surgical laboratory program at Tufts University. *Journal of the American Veterinary Medical Association* 205: 97–100.

Pereira, G.D., Dieguez, J., Demirbas, Y.S. et al. (2017). Alternatives to animal use in veterinary education: A growing debate. *Ankara University Faculty of Veterinary Medicine* 64: 235–239.

Russell, W.M.S. and Burch, R.L. (1959). *The Principles of Humane Experimental Technique*. London: Methuen.

Self, D.J., Schrader, D.E., Baldwin, J.D.C. et al. (1991). Study of the influence of veterinary medical education on the moral development of veterinary students. *Journal of the American Veterinary Medical Association* 198: 782–787.

Silva, L.J., Cordeiro, C.T., Cruz, M.B. et al. (2021). Design and validation of a simulator for feline cephalic vein cannulation – A pilot study. *Journal of Veterinary Medical Education* 48: 276–280.

Smeak, D.D., Hill, L.N., Beck, M.L. et al. (1994). Evaluation of an autotutorial-simulator program for instruction of hollow organ closure. *Veterinary Surgery* 23: 519–528.

Taylor, K. and Alvarez, L.R. (2019). An estimate of the number of animals used for scientific purposes worldwide in 2015. *Alternatives to Laboratory Animals* 47: 196–213.

University of Queensland School of Veterinary Science (2008). *University of Queensland School of Veterinary Science Guidelines on Ethical Concerns on Use of Animals in Teaching*. Gatton, Australia: University of Queensland School of Veterinary Science. http://www.humanelearning.info/resources/conscientious_objection.htm (accessed 3 November 2013).

van Vollenhoven, E., Fletcher, L., Page, P.C. et al. (2017). Heart rate variability in healthy, adult pony mares during transrectal palpation of the reproductive tract by veterinary students. *Journal of Equine Veterinary Science* 58: 68–77.

Webster, J. (1994). *Animal Welfare: A Cool Eye Towards Eden*. Oxford, UK: Blackwell Publishing.

Western University of Health Sciences (2020). Doctor of Veterinary Medicine (DVM). https://prospective.westernu.edu/veterinary/dvm (accessed 27 April 2021).

Whittaker, A.L. and Anderson, G.I. (2013). A policy at the University of Adelaide for student objections to the use of animals in teaching. *Journal of Veterinary Medical Education* 40: 52–57.

Willems, R.A. (2007). Animals in veterinary medical teaching: Compliance and regulatory issues, the US perspective. *Journal of Veterinary Medical Education* 34: 615–619.

Williamson, J.A., Brisson, B.A., Anderson, S.L. et al. (2019). Comparison of 2 canine celiotomy closure models for training novice veterinary students. *Veterinary Surgery* 48: 966–974.

Winder, C.B., LeBlanc, S.J., Haley, D.B. et al. (2018). Comparison of online, hands-on, and a combined approach for teaching cautery disbudding technique to dairy producers. *Journal of Dairy Science* 101: 840–849.

Yeates, J.W. (2010). Death is a welfare issue. *Journal of Agricultural & Environmental Ethics* 23: 229–241.

Zemanova, M.A. and Knight, A. (2021). The educational efficacy of humane teaching methods: A systematic review of the evidence. *Animals* 11: 114.

Zemanova, M.A., Knight, A., and Lybæk, S. (2021). Educational use of animals in Europe indicates a reluctance to implement alternatives. *ALTEX* 38(3): 490–506.

## Legislation

Animal Welfare Act (1985). Amendment of title XVII, subtitle F, ss 1751–1759, US Statutes at Large 99:50

# 19

# Animal Pain

*Bea Monteiro and Sheilah Robertson*

## Introduction

Pain is a personal, complex experience influenced by biological, psychological, and social factors. The International Association for the Study of Pain (IASP) defines pain as "an unpleasant sensory and emotional experience associated with ... actual or potential tissue damage" acknowledging that animals learn concepts, including that of pain, and the inability to communicate through language does not negate the possibility that an animal is experiencing pain (Raja et al. 2020).

The sensory component of pain, resulting from activity in specialized neurons, refers to "what it feels like" (i.e. perceptual qualities such as mild, severe, burning, tingling, etc.). The emotional component of pain refers to "how it makes one feel" (i.e. fearful, frustrated, anxious). Pain burden refers to the negative effects of pain for the animal and the owner/caregiver. For the animal, pain has a negative impact on physical health and function, nutrition, behavior, socialization, and mental state (Steagall et al. 2021). Pain has negative effects on production (i.e. animals raised for human consumption may have decreased food intake, impaired growth, and reproduction) and quality of research studies (i.e. pain in laboratory animals may produce erroneous results). The pet–owner relationship may be taxed or broken (i.e. pets with chronic pain require significant financial, time, and physical commitments from owners, and caring for them can be emotionally demanding; Spitznagel et al. 2018). An overlooked issue is the impact that painful animals can have on veterinary team members, including emotional distress and compassion fatigue.

## Understanding the Difference Between Nociception and Pain

Pain and nociception are different. Nociception refers to the neural processing of noxious stimuli that could or does cause tissue damage (Sneddon 2018). It occurs without conscious perception and can result in reflex withdrawal. The "pain pathway" comprises four main steps. The first step is *transduction* – activation of peripheral nociceptors located in the skin, muscles, joints, and viscera, by noxious or potentially damaging stimuli. Such stimuli cause depolarization of nerve cell membranes with generation of an action potential. Step 2 is *transmission* from the periphery to the dorsal horn of the spinal cord in the central nervous system. The third step is *modulation* – the nociceptive

*Ethics in Veterinary Practice: Balancing Conflicting Interests*, First Edition. Edited by Barry Kipperman and Bernard E. Rollin.

signal can be amplified (pain facilitation) or decreased (pain inhibition) by various mechanisms. Thus, nociception comprises steps 1 to 3. The fourth step is *perception* – the nociceptive signal is integrated in the cerebral cortex and emotional attributes are incorporated with sensory signals (i.e. pain is consciously perceived) (Klinck and Troncy 2016). It is only when the nociceptive signals reach the conscious brain that it can be called "pain." For example, in an anesthetized patient, nociception is occurring, but there is no conscious experience of pain. Once the patient recovers from anesthesia and regains consciousness, the nociceptive stimuli (e.g. peripheral and/or central sensitization) will be perceived. That is why pain must be prevented and treated when patients are under general anesthesia and painful procedures are being performed.

## Types of Pain

Adaptive or acute pain refers to pain that is protective, either to protect a healthy area from injury or a damaged area from further injury. The severity of adaptive pain correlates with the degree of injury (e.g. minor or major surgery, trauma, wounds, burns, intestinal obstruction, and pancreatitis). Although usually self-limiting, adaptive pain should be treated. Maladaptive or chronic pain refers to pathological pain that serves no biological function. Maladaptive pain does not always correlate with the inciting lesion or disease severity (e.g. osteoarthritis, invasive tumors, periodontal disease). Maladaptive pain can develop from adaptive pain (e.g. due to inadequate perioperative pain management or in conditions with extensive damage to soft tissues, bone, and neural tissues) resulting in persistent postsurgical pain (e.g. following amputations including tail docking and onychectomy). Finally, maladaptive pain can occur without any identifiable primary cause (i.e. maladaptive pain is a disease in its own right).

Pain can be categorized in different ways including:

- Nociceptive pain: protects from self-harm. Examples: contact with a hot object (thermal nociception), pressure against a sharp surface (mechanical nociception).
- Inflammatory pain: occurs in adaptive or maladaptive pain when there is a tissue lesion, release of inflammatory cytokines, and sensitization of sensory nerves. Examples: postoperative pain, trauma, osteoarthritis, chronic periodontal disease, wounds, and otitis.
- Neuropathic pain occurs when there is a lesion or disease of the somatosensory system: it may be peripheral and/or central. Examples: intervertebral disc disease, nerve sheath tumors.
- Cancer pain: arises from cancers resulting in the release of chemicals that contribute to cancer growth and the generation and maintenance of pain. Additional pain may be induced by treatments, e.g. radiation therapy or surgery.
- (Dys)functional pain: disorders for which no organic disease can be identified despite comprehensive investigation, i.e. feline idiopathic cystitis.

Pain can be spontaneous due to natural disease or induced by humans caring for animals or by veterinary health professionals during medical interventions. Examples of spontaneous pain include acute pancreatitis, degenerative diseases (e.g. osteoarthritis), stomatitis, and wounds. Examples of induced pain include pain due to inappropriate handling or equipment (e.g. a harness that causes chronic wounds), inadequate housing conditions (e.g. restricted movement causes musculoskeletal pain; inappropriate flooring contributes to lameness), and genetic selection (e.g. broiler chickens selected for fast growth suffer from lameness, mobility impairment, and even fractures because their skeletal growth does not keep pace with their muscle growth) (Nalon and Stevenson 2019). Examples of induced pain caused by medical interventions include procedures performed in laboratory animals for the study of pain (e.g. nerve constriction for induction of neuropathic pain, transection of the cranial cruciate ligament for induction of osteoarthritis), and common veterinary procedures such as neutering surgeries, wound management, and diagnostic procedures.

## Pain and Emotions

Pain may have far-reaching and long-term consequences. The pain experience is modulated by the neurobiology of the individual, past experiences, environmental and social factors, and emotions. There is a complex bidirectional interrelationship between pain and emotions.

Long-term pain negatively impacts cognitive functioning and produces anxiety-like behaviors weeks to months after initial injury (Bushnell et al. 2015). Pain causes negative emotions, whereas emotions modulate the pain experience. Emotions from higher brain centers modulate nociceptive signals in the spinal cord and can decrease or increase this signal before it reaches the brain where it is perceived. Overall, *positive emotions decrease pain perception and negative emotions increase pain perception* (Finan and Garland 2015; Hanssen et al. 2017). Therefore, if we promote positive experiences, we can refocus the patient's attention to pleasurable and rewarding experiences helping them build emotional resilience and coping abilities (Finan and Garland 2015; Mills et al. 2020). Optimizing the animal's environment to provide opportunities for performance of species-specific motivated behaviors (e.g. rewarding experiences such as play, appropriate socialization, and exploratory or predatory behaviors) can decrease the pain experience (Bushnell et al. 2015).

Not only is pain unpleasant to the individual experiencing it, pain in conspecifics is also unpleasant and laboratory studies show emotional contagion and social modulation of pain. For example, pain behaviors increase when cage mate mice are exposed to a painful stimulus together, and pain behaviors decrease when nonpainful mice spend more time near a painful cage mate (Langford et al. 2006, 2010; Mogil 2019).

Another interesting relationship between pain and emotions is that fear and stress can cause painful conditions. A classic example is idiopathic cystitis in domestic cats, which is associated with poor emotional health due to potential threats to their perception of control (Buffington and Bain 2020).

## The Debate of the Pain Experience in Animals

The neurobiology of pain is similar among mammalian species. Some of these similarities include anatomy, peripheral nociceptors and their electrophysiological properties, mechanisms of pain modulation, and peripheral and central sensitization

(Sneddon 2018). The clinical symptomatology and response to therapy of conditions affecting humans and other mammals are also similar. Indeed, animals have been crucial for our understanding of pain as attested by their widespread use in translational pain research (Mogil 2019). For example, osteoarthritis is biomechanically, histologically, and molecularly similar between dogs and people (McCoy 2015). Dogs and cats with spontaneous osteoarthritis develop peripheral and central sensitization in addition to negative effects on their quality of life including decreased physical activity and sleep disturbances, which are also reported in humans with osteoarthritis (Knazovicky et al. 2016; Monteiro et al. 2020). Osteosarcoma, a very painful bone cancer, is biologically similar in children and dogs (Simpson et al. 2017).

The debate as to whether invertebrates and nonmammalian vertebrates experience pain (and not only nociception) is ongoing: yet scientific evidence from physiological (Sneddon 2018) and behavioral observations strongly suggest an affective pain experience (Baker et al. 2019; Crook 2021). For example, animals display species-specific changes in behavior related to pain (e.g. grooming in octopuses, tail beating in zebrafish) and are motivated to avoid locations previously associated with pain, which indicates they learn from a painful experience, one of the key points in the IASP's definition of pain (Raja et al. 2020). Pain-related behaviors are not seen in the absence of painful stimuli and resolve when analgesics are given. Together, these observations indicate that these animals experience negative emotions associated with pain (i.e. the experience is not only sensorial: a negative emotion is attached to it that affects their present and future behaviors to avoid the experience).

From an evolutionary perspective, pain most likely did not appear de novo in humans: the functions and mechanisms of pain are products of prior evolution (Walters and Williams 2019). However, the clinically oriented definition of pain in humans has profound legal and ethical implications in protecting animals because producing compelling evidence of conscious pain perception in nonhuman animals is a complicated task (Walters and Williams 2019). This is a topic of debate among scientists studying animal behavior while aiming to avoid anthropomorphism and skeptics insisting on anthropodenial. Differences in neurobiology among species such as humans and rodents are of quantity and not quality (Mogil 2019) and complex social/cognitive phenomena occur similarly between such species.

If we describe sentience as "feelings that matter" (positive and negative) and state that the prerequisites for suffering are sentience and consciousness, our task is to define how sentience is experienced in animals of different taxa and under different circumstances. Indeed, animal sentience and capacity to suffer are the basis of animal welfare science and available frameworks for welfare assessment (UK Farm Animal Welfare Council 1979; Mellor et al. 2020). Comparative and translational pain research is focused on similarities among different species, particularly with regard to the affective component of pain, and is likely to contribute substantially to ethical discussions related to pain in animals and their consequent legal protection. When we look at the many shortcomings of current animal welfare legislation it is sobering to reflect that it was in 1789 that the British philosopher Jeremy Bentham stated (referring to animals) "The question is not can they reason? Nor can they talk? But can they suffer?" (Bentham 2000). Based on such an expansive body of evidence, it is reasonable to assume that what is painful for humans is painful for animals.

## Laws, Regulations, Policies, and Guidelines Pertaining to Pain Management in Domestic Animals

### Relationship Between Animal Welfare Science, Ethics, and Law

There is a clear link between animal welfare science, ethics, and law. Scientific research provides understanding about important issues such as pain management, which influences ethical debate and public opinion. The latter influences public policy to be converted into law by legislative processes. Laws and regulations usually represent minimum standards and often fall short of societal expectations. Many guidelines exist to aid veterinarians in the prevention and alleviation of pain, but these are not legally enforceable (e.g. Pain Management Guidelines for Dogs and Cats; Epstein et al. 2015).

The science–policy gap (i.e. the inconsistency of translating science into policy) is a well-recognized problem with numerous challenges (Bradshaw and Borchers 2000). We must accept there is scientific uncertainty; for example, if we look at the issue of elective amputations such as tail docking in dogs (for cosmetic reasons) and pigs (to prevent tail biting in confined housing), or onychectomy in cats (to avoid scratching of household items), several scientific questions remain, including the prevalence and severity of persistent postoperative pain, the animal production benefits, the influence on relinquishment of cats, etc. Scientific uncertainty muddies the waters when attempting to educate both the public and those involved in animal care to form ethical opinions about issues.

The public is largely unaware about painful procedures in animals. For example, approximately 40% of people viewing pictures of dogs with docked tails believed this was a result of genetics and the breed's natural characteristics and did not know that docked tails are the result of humans surgically removing them from puppies (Mills et al. 2016). Similarly, it is not known how much the public, even cat owners, understand about what is involved in onychectomy. The use of the lay term "declawing" is misleading – it suggests that only the claws are removed rather than the bony digits. Despite being illegal in most countries, onychectomy is socially accepted and widely performed across the United States and Canada where it remains legal in most jurisdictions (AVMA n.d.a; CVMA 2017). It is only through science and knowledge that people can form sound ethical views about a subject and use this to advocate for legislative reforms to protect animals.

### Laws Protecting Animals

The importance of protecting animals has been the subject of official government documents for nearly two centuries since the Martin's Act of 1822 in the UK, which led to the first legislation to protect animals from cruelty (UK Parliament 1822). However, it was only in 2007 that animal sentience was recognized officially in the European Union (EU) Treaty of Lisbon (EUR-Lex 2007). In the United States, the Animal Welfare Act (AWA) is a federal law that sets minimum acceptable standards and regulates the care of animals in research, exhibition, transport, and by dealers (USDA n.d). It has been expanded and amended since its creation in 1966 with the last edition in 2013. The AWA is administered and enforced by the Animal and Plant Health Inspection Service

(APHIS) agency of the US Department of Agriculture (USDA). A common criticism of the AWA relates to which species are protected. It defines "animals" as "any live or dead dog, cat, nonhuman primate, guinea pig, hamster, rabbit, or any other warm-blooded animal used for research, teaching, testing, experimentation or exhibition purposes, or as a pet." It excludes rats, mice, and birds used for research, horses not used for research purposes, and other farm animals such as livestock or poultry used in agriculture. This means that most animals used in research (rats and mice) and all animals raised for food and fiber are not protected under this federal law (USDA 2009).

Laws that impact the protection of animals exist in all 50 states, but with large discrepancies between them (Animal Law Research Center 2021). It should be noted that there is a clear distinction between animal welfare legislation, which protects animals from suffering and seeks to promote a good quality of life (i.e., imposes positive duties and obligations on those responsible for animals), and animal cruelty legislation, which empowers enforcement agencies to punish perpetrators only when animal suffering can be demonstrated beyond any reasonable doubt (i.e., does not protect animals from suffering). Despite being frequently available for common domestic species used in animal production, welfare codes of practice are not legally binding; if one fails to comply with a welfare code that does not constitute an offense.

## Animals Used for Research

It is estimated that in 2015 approximately 79.9 million animals including mammals, birds, reptiles, amphibians, fish, and cephalopods were used for research in the United States that involved procedures which likely caused pain, suffering, distress, or lasting harm (Taylor and Alvarez 2019). In the United States, laboratory animals are protected by two overlapping regulations. The AWA regulates the use of covered animal species in any research, whereas research involving public funds by the National Institutes of Health requires adherence to the Public Health Service Policy as stipulated by the Health Research Extension Act (HREA). The AWA outlines the role of Institutional Animal Care and Use Committees, defines requirements for veterinarians, provides standards for care, housing, and transportation, and defines reporting requirements to the APHIS. The HREA mandates that research institutions use the *Guide for the Care and Use of Laboratory Animals*, also known as the "Guide" (National Research Council 2011). The Guide has different scope and recommendations from the AWA. It covers all vertebrate animals, requires that a cost–benefit analysis be done for study protocols, and stipulates that euthanasia be conducted in accordance with the American Veterinary Medical Association (AVMA) Guidelines for the Euthanasia of Animals (Leary et al. 2020).

In the EU, Directive 2010/63/EU regulates the use of laboratory animals, which covers live nonhuman vertebrates, independently feeding larval forms, fetal forms of mammals (last third of development), and live cephalopods (European Parliament and the Council 2010). The EU directive relies heavily on the principles of the Three Rs (Replacement, Reduction, and Refinement) and allows the legislation to be updated frequently according to progress in animal welfare or laboratory animal science. Since leaving the EU, the UK follows similar directives. China, Japan, and the United States are by far the three main countries using animals in research and, unfortunately, they do not have such comprehensive legislation as the EU (Taylor and Alvarez 2019).

Regardless of the country, animal research is reviewed and approved in some form by Ethics Committees or Institutional Animal Care and Use Committees (IACUCs). The roles of IACUCs are to review and approve all animal activities (i.e. study protocol), inspect facilities, and investigate animal welfare concerns. They also determine that the proposed activities in the study protocol meet requirements for the avoidance or minimization of discomfort, distress, and pain to the animals, and if animals experience severe or chronic pain that cannot be relieved, they are euthanized during or at the end of the procedure. Particularly, they are expected to perform harm–benefit analysis for which a joint effort from the American Association for Laboratory Animal Science and the Federation of European Laboratory Animal Science Associations produced extensive guidelines (Bronstad et al. 2016; Laber et al. 2016). Pain and distress are the most relevant potential harms for laboratory animals, and these are weighed against the potential benefits of the research. In the harm–benefit analysis, the level of harm is discriminated according to severity classification that considers the level and duration of pain ("quantity of pain") as well as the provision of analgesia and/or anesthesia. It is the duty of the investigators and IACUC committees to determine "humane endpoints": however, there is a great need to determine specific and objective measures of suffering. In addition, even though pain can compromise research findings, pain management may still be withheld if it is deemed to interfere with experimental results (Larry 2019). Painful procedures in animals have been a major concern in the public forum (Lund et al. 2014).

### Farmed Animals and Pain Management

While the numbers of animals used in research are staggering, these are nowhere near the estimated number of animals produced globally for human consumption, which is well over 50 billion per year, including poultry, pigs, ruminants, fish, etc. (FAOSTAT 2021). In the United States, farmed animals are not protected under federal laws despite routinely being subjected to painful procedures without the provision of anesthesia and/or analgesia (Steagall et al. 2021).

### Companion Animals

There is minimal oversight of pain management in clinical practice, therefore veterinarians decide what is appropriate for their patients. There is no doubt that many patients receive inadequate pain relief because of gaps in education and training on state-of-the-art pain management, lack of standardized objective pain assessment tools, and lack of accountability for the undertreatment of pain (Carvalho et al. 2018). For example, clients might be given the option to choose or decline analgesics for painful conditions or procedures in their pets to save money. This is highly inappropriate, and this choice should not be offered by veterinarians as clients are not educated to make such decisions and do not understand the negative consequences of inadequate pain management (Simon et al. 2017).

## Ethical Duty of Veterinary Professionals to Manage Pain

Veterinarians have an ethical and medical duty to prevent, diagnose, and treat pain. The ethical responsibilities are stated in the AVMA Veterinarian's Oath. Although the word "pain" does not specifically appear, it is implied within the concept of "suffering": "prevention and relief of animal suffering" (AVMA n.d.c). Furthermore, the AVMA Principles of Veterinary Medical Ethics state that the practice of veterinary medicine requires one to "diagnose, prognose, treat, correct, change, alleviate, or prevent ... pain" (AVMA n.d.d). Similarly, the Veterinary Technician Code of Ethics states that professionals "shall prevent and relieve the suffering of animals with competence and compassion" (NAVTA 2007). Violation of the AVMA Principles of Veterinary Medical Ethics might result in disciplinary action or legal prosecutions: however, this rarely happens when substandard pain management is identified since punishment requires substantial proof of misconduct, animal cruelty, or neglect. The AVMA has numerous policies related to pain management in several species. Voluntary adherence to such policies is encouraged but does not supersede laws or regulations.

The medical obligations refer to the fact that pain has negative consequences including activation of the sympathetic nervous system, increased secretion of stress hormones, immunosuppression, decreased food intake, altered function (e.g. lameness), impaired healing, increased morbidity, etc. (Steagall and Monteiro 2019; Steagall et al. 2021).

It is curious that despite these ethical and medical duties of veterinarians, there is a general acceptance of painful procedures in farm animals without mitigation of pain (i.e. speciesism). A classic example is the castration of piglets without anesthesia/analgesia (Yun et al. 2019). One could argue that in such circumstances, a veterinarian is disrespecting the oath and their medical responsibilities (i.e. pain is not being prevented or treated). Nevertheless, the issue is not that simple: it is one of cultural and societal norms, and the triad relationships between the animal, veterinarian, and client. A veterinarian may well face an ethical dilemma if the farmer refuses to pay for effective anesthetics/analgesics for piglet castration (Scollo et al. 2021) (i.e. protecting the animal versus complying with the client's request). This can be approached from a principlist theory based on respect for autonomy, nonmaleficence, beneficence, and justice (Beauchamp 2016). In this example, the veterinarian must: respect a client's autonomy; abstain from causing harm; act for another's benefit (to prevent harm and heal when harm has occurred); and consider the moral rules of justice according to what is fair, due, or owed. Based on the principlist theory, the Veterinarian's Oath, and the Principles of Veterinary Medical Ethics, prevention of animal suffering should, in this example, prevail over the client's wishes, but often does not.

Ethical conflicts are part of everyday veterinary practice and different stakeholders must be considered including but not limited to the animal, owner/caretaker, attending veterinarian, policy makers, and the public. Using the same example of castration in piglets, we might analyze the situation using different ethical theories (see Chapter 4). From a contractarian view, a person's own interest is what matters most. For a contractarian, piglets are not moral subjects and are not worthy of moral concern including treatment of pain (Gjerris et al. 2013). From an animal rights view, there are things that you simply cannot do to animals. Animals, like people, have rights. Rights are moral constraints ("subject-of-a-life"), and it is simply wrong to violate one's rights, which includes castration. A utilitarian view is based on maximizing welfare for the largest number of individuals, even if it means that some will suffer to benefit the most. This approach is often referred to as "the end justifies the means." The impact of choices on the welfare of all concerned parties is taken into consideration. While the goal is to choose the course of action that will result in the largest total sum of welfare, in most cases, the interests of humans supersede those of animals (Gjerris et al. 2013). Despite different ethical views, the Veterinarian's Oath should prevail and guide decision making with a focus on preventing animal suffering and protecting animal welfare above all else.

Other examples of common ethical issues in veterinary pain medicine include: onychectomy in cats (amputation of the last digits of the front and/or hind limbs); "cosmetic" or "convenience" surgeries in dogs (ear cropping and caudectomy); devocalization in dogs; debeaking in chickens; and castration, tail docking, dehorning/disbudding, branding, ear notching/tagging, and nose ringing in pigs, cattle, and/or sheep. In farm animals, painful procedures are generally performed for human safety (e.g. dehorning), identification (e.g. branding, tagging), or preventing problems usually caused by inadequate housing and/or environmental conditions (e.g. tail biting, feather pecking). The ethical issues in these examples are twofold: one because these procedures are not usually medically justified; and two because frequently pain management is either omitted or inadequate. Extensive literature demonstrates that these animals display pain behaviors during and after these procedures and that such behaviors subside with multimodal pain management (Steagall et al. 2021).

Measures to avoid painful procedures in farm animals already exist or are being studied and include but are not limited to: genetic selection of cattle without horns; production of pigs without castration (slaughter at a younger age before boar taint occurs); improving housing, handling, and environmental enrichment of animals to improve welfare and remove the need for tail docking or debeaking; and attaching sensors or collars for animal identification to avoid branding or tagging. In companion animals, there is a need to change breed standards to avoid ear cropping and tail docking in dogs and to promote owner education regarding feline behavior to avoid onychectomy.

## Provision of Futile Care in Companion Animal Practice

Small animal veterinarians are for the most part free to perform procedures on animals with minimal oversight or risk of whistleblowing. Although specialized training and certification is available (e.g. surgery), it is not mandatory, resulting in some practitioners performing procedures beyond their technical expertise. There is no governing body in veterinary medicine that mandates benchmarking (i.e. what outcomes should look like) or performs clinical audits; there are no clinical registers for specific procedures, and perioperative morbidity and mortality reporting is not mandated.

An emerging and growing cause of ethical conflict in companion animal practice relates to overtreatment. This revolves around the statement "just because we can, should we?". Discussions on "drawing the line in clinical treatment" (Grimm et al. 2018) and recognizing the boundary between heroism and futility (Clutton 2017) are increasing in the veterinary community. Animals are considered property in legal terms, so despite a veterinarian's wish to end suffering or not to perform a procedure they think will compound suffering, this may conflict with the owner's rights. There are also veterinarians who will proceed with novel or radical procedures and invasive testing because of ego ("I can"), fear of failure ("there must be more I can do"), or because it may be self-fulfilling to do so (i.e. "the cool factor") (Yeates 2016). In addition, a clinician's motivation for performing a procedure may be linked to financial gain or reputation (Grimm et al. 2018). The reason for performing a procedure requires self-reflection. Defensive medicine (the practice of ordering tests, procedures, and other medical care that may not benefit the patient, solely to reduce the threat of litigation) is no longer restricted to human medicine.

With advances in available treatment options, pets being considered family members or child substitutes, the client's willingness to pay for veterinary care, and an increase in the number of owners who purchase pet insurance, it is likely that animals might undergo invasive and painful procedures despite a poor prognosis and/or short life expectancy. Surgical oncology is one area where overtreatment may occur. For example, is it ethical to perform an invasive oncologic surgery in a dog when it is not likely that survival time will be prolonged, quality of life will be improved, and complications will not arise? Examples such as this demand a reflection on which treatments are morally justified. Once again, the subjective nature of assessing an animal's current and projected well-being is a barrier to decision making. Primary clinicians, support clinicians (e.g. anesthesiologists), staff (e.g. nurses and technicians), and owners may not agree with each other regarding treatment of a patient (Lehnus et al. 2019). In human medicine, third-party clinical ethics review committees can be called upon to review individual cases: in veterinary clinical medicine such committees are rare (Rosoff et al. 2018).

### Framing

How information is presented to clients is important and it can be difficult to avoid unconscious bias that influences clients' decisions (Yeates and Main 2010). Framing is defined as "the presentation of two equivalent situations, where one is presented in positive or gain terms and the other in negative or loss terms" (Garcia-Retamero and Galesic 2010). How we frame our conversation can alter the choice an owner makes; for example, when discussing a procedure for which there is a large body of information on its success and failure rate, there are two options. Option 1 is to say, "There is a 70% success rate," but option 2 is to state that "There is a 30% mortality or failure rate." Both statements are true but framing the outcome in a positive way is more likely to get owners to agree to treatment (Garcia-Retamero and Galesic 2010). It has been our experience that practitioners tend to diminish the degree of expected or experienced pain in patients when communicating with clients. This results in owners not requesting analgesia and not knowing what to expect or how to monitor their animals for the presence of pain-related behaviors, and, consequently, animals can suffer from untreated pain.

## Assessing and Treating Pain in Animals

The first steps in treating pain are to anticipate it, look for it, recognize it, and in some way quantify it. Methods of pain assessment range from the highly subjective (i.e. opinion) to sophisticated and objective analysis of activity, body posture, and facial expressions. Pain assessment in animals can be performed using different methods such as observing behavior, quantitative sensory testing, biomarkers, etc. Although physiological parameters such as heart and respiratory rates or levels of cortisol have been used to assess pain, these are nonspecific, are influenced by fear and anxiety, and should not be relied upon for the evaluation of pain (Quimby et al. 2017). In practice, assessment usually relies on the observation of pain-related behaviors.

An important aspect of pain assessment is to evaluate the behaviors of animals *before* a painful insult such as surgery. Pain assessment can be particularly challenging in animals with shy or fearful temperaments: therefore, knowing the normal behavior of an animal before surgery can help with interpretation of pain-related behaviors following surgery (Steagall and Monteiro 2019). The most common abnormal behaviors observed in animals with acute pain are noted in Table 19.1. Chronic pain has been less

# The Past and Future of Veterinary Pain Management

## The Past

Old myths such as "animals do not feel pain" have been dispelled by comparative anatomy and neurophysiologic studies. In addition, there are pain-specific behaviors that are measurable. The outdated notion that "pain is desirable after surgery because it restricts the patient's activity and prevents further damage" has been disproved by studies showing pain delays healing and return of function and causes negative emotions. Restricted exercise is often prudent after some procedures but can be achieved with stall or cage rest and supervised activity: in some cases, this is facilitated when sedatives are prescribed (Gruen et al. 2014). Misconceptions about the use of opioids in cats can be traced back to reports of undesirable "manic" behaviors that were caused by doses 10 to 20 times greater than today's recommended analgesic doses.

## The Future of Pain Management

A sound knowledge of pain management must be a day-one competency for veterinarians. Although there are veterinary specialists in this field, every clinician sees painful patients on a regular basis. To assist practitioners in keeping abreast of new information, organizations such as the World Small Animal Veterinary Association created a Global Pain Council to improve the treatment of acute and chronic pain globally. The International Veterinary Academy of Pain Management (ivapm.org) is a forum and educational resource for veterinary professionals and pet owners interested in animal pain, prevention, and treatment.

Education on pain management has improved within the veterinary curriculum (AVMA n.d.b), as societal concerns related to pain and the promotion of animal welfare have increased (Steagall et al. 2017; Simon et al. 2018). As animals live longer due to preventive care and new therapies, we need to learn more about pain management in older populations where comorbidities exist with pain. The future of pain management for animals is cautiously optimistic but requires a concerted effort by motivated researchers and clinicians; areas for focus include improvement of species-specific pain and quality of life assessment tools with clinical utility, assessment of new targeted drug and biological therapies, global education, and ethical decision making in all pain management curricula.

# References

American Veterinary Medical Association (AVMA) (n.d.a). Declawing of domestic cats. https://www.avma.org/resources-tools/avma-policies/declawing-domestic-cats (accessed 23 April 2021).

American Veterinary Medical Association (AVMA) (n.d.b). Joint AVMA-FVE-CVMA statement on veterinary education. https://www.avma.org/resources-tools/avma-policies/joint-avma-fve-cvma-statement-veterinary-education (accessed 23 April 2021).

American Veterinary Medical Association (AVMA) (n.d.c). Veterinarian's Oath. https://www.avma.org/resources-tools/avma-policies/veterinarians-oath (accessed 23 April 2021).

American Veterinary Medical Association (AVMA) (n.d.d). Principles of Veterinary Medical Ethics of the AVMA. https://www.avma.org/resources-tools/avma-policies/principles-veterinary-medical-ethics-avma (accessed 9 April 2021).

Animal Law Research Center (2021). Search laws. http://animallaw.com/Laws.cfm (accessed 9 April 2021).

Baker, B.I., Machin, K.L., and Schwean-Lardner, K. (2019). When pain and stress interact: Looking at stress-induced analgesia and hyperalgesia in birds. *World's Poultry Science Journal* 75 (3): 457–468.

Beauchamp, T.L. (2016). Principlism in bioethics. In: *Bioethical Decision Making and Argumentation* (eds. P. Serna and J.A. Seoane), 1–16. International Library of Ethics, Law, and the New Medicine, Vol. 70. Cham, Switzerland: Springer.

Belshaw, Z. and Yeates, J. (2018). Assessment of quality of life and chronic pain in dogs. *Veterinary Journal* 239: 59–64.

Bentham, J. (2000). Of the limits of the penal branch of jurisprudence. In: *An Introduction to the Principles of Morals and Legislation* (ed. J. Bentham), 224–238. Kitchener, Ontario: Batoche Books.

Bradshaw, G.A. and Borchers, J.G. (2000). Uncertainty as information: Narrowing the science-policy gap. *Conservation Ecology* 4 (1): 7.

Bronstad, A., Newcomer, C.E., Decelle, T. et al. (2016). Current concepts of harm-benefit analysis of animal experiments – Report from the AALAS-FELASA Working Group on Harm-Benefit Analysis – Part 1. *Laboratory Animals* 50 (1): 1–20.

Brown, D.C., Boston, R., Coyne, J.C. et al. (2009). A novel approach to the use of animals in studies of pain: Validation of the Canine Brief Pain Inventory in canine bone cancer. *Pain Medicine* 10 (1): 133–142.

Buffington, C.A.T. and Bain, M. (2020). Stress and feline health. *Veterinary Clinics of North America – Small Animal* 50: 653–662.

Bushnell, M.C., Case, L.K., Ceko, M. et al. (2015). Effect of environment on the long-term consequences of chronic pain. *Pain* 156: S42–S49.

Canadian Veterinary Medical Association (CVMA). (2017). Partial digital amputation (onychectomy or declawing) of the domestic felid – Position statement. https://www.canadianveterinarians.net/documents/partial-digital-amputation-onychectomy-or-declawing-of-the-domestic-felid-position-statement (accessed 23 April 2021).

Carvalho, A.S., Martins Pereira, S., Jácomo, A. et al. (2018). Ethical decision making in pain management: A conceptual framework. *Journal of Pain Research* 11: 967–976.

Clutton, R.E. (2017). Recognising the boundary between heroism and futility in veterinary intensive care. *Veterinary Anaesthesia and Analgesia* 44 (2): 199–202.

Crook, R.J. (2021). Behavioral and neurophysiological evidence suggests affective pain experience in octopus. *iScience* 24 (3): 102229.

Davies, V., Reid, J., Wiseman-Orr, M.L. et al. (2019). Optimising outputs from a validated online instrument to measure health-related quality of life (HRQL) in dogs. *PLoS ONE* 14 (9): e0221869.

Epstein, M., Rodan, I., Griffenhagen, G. et al. (2015). 2015 AAHA/AAFP Pain Management Guidelines for Dogs and Cats. *Journal of the American Animal Hospital Association* 51 (2): 67–84.

EUR-Lex (2007). Treaty of Lisbon amending the Treaty on European Union and the Treaty establishing the European Community. https://eur-lex.europa.eu/legal-content/EN/TXT/?uri=CELEX%3A12007L%2FTXT (accessed 6 April 2021).

European Parliament and the Council (2010). DIRECTIVE 2010/63/EU. https://www.
legislation.gov.uk/eudr/2010/63 (accessed 23 April 2021).

Evangelista, M.C., Monteiro, B.P., and Steagall, P.V. (2021). Measurement properties of
grimace scales for pain assessment in non-human mammals: A systematic review. *Pain*
online early. doi:10.1097/j.pain.0000000000002474.

Finan, P.H. and Garland, E.L. (2015). The role of positive affect in pain and its treatment.
*The Clinical Journal of Pain* 31 (2): 177–196.

Food and Agriculture Organization of the United Nations (FAOSTAT) (2021). FAOSTAT.
http://www.fao.org/faostat/en/#data/QL (accessed 9 April 2021).

Garcia-Retamero, R. and Galesic, M. (2010). How to reduce the effect of framing on
messages about health. *Journal of General Internal Medicine* 25 (12): 1323–1329.

Gjerris, M., Nielsen, M., and Sandøe, P. (2013). Part II: The Right. In: *The Good, the Right
and the Fair. An Introduction to Ethics*, 1e (eds. M. Gjerris, M. Nielsen, and P. Sandøe),
67–133. Milton Keynes, UK: Lightning Source.

Grimm, H., Bergadano, A., Musk, G.C. et al. (2018). Drawing the line in clinical treatment
of companion animals: Recommendations from an ethics working party. *Veterinary
Record* 182 (23): 664.

Gruen, M.E., Roe, S.C., Griffith, E. et al. (2014). Use of trazodone to facilitate postsurgical
confinement in dogs. *Journal of the American Veterinary Medical Association* 245 (3):
296–301.

Hanssen, M.M., Petters, M.L., Boselie, J.J. et al. (2017). Can positive affect attenuate
(persistent) pain? State of the art and clinical implications. *Current Rheumatology
Reports* 19: 80.

Klinck, M.P. and Troncy, E. (2016). The physiology and pathophysiology of pain. In:
*BSAVA Manual of Canine and Feline Anaesthesia and Analgesia*, (eds. T. Duke-
Novakovski, M. de Vries and C. Seymour), 3e, 97–112. Gloucester, UK: BSAVA.

Knazovicky, D., Helgeson, E.S., Case, B. et al. (2016). Widespread somatosensory
sensitivity in naturally occurring canine model of osteoarthritis. *Pain* 157 (6): 1325–
1332. https://doi.org/10.1097/j.pain.0000000000000521.

Laber, K., Newcomer, C.E., Decelle, T. et al. (2016). Recommendations for addressing
harm-benefit analysis and implementation in ethical evaluation – Report from the
AALAS-FELASA working group on harm-benefit analysis – Part 2. *Laboratory Animals*
50 (1): 21–42.

Langford, D.L., Crager, S.E., Shehzad, Z. et al. (2006). Social modulation of pain as
evidence for empathy in mice. *Science* 312: 1967–1970.

Langford, D.J., Tuttle, A.H., Brown, K. et al. (2010). Social approach to pain in laboratory
mice. *Social Neuroscience* 5 (2): 163–170.

Larry, C. (2019). Ethical and IACUC considerations regarding analgesia and pain
management in laboratory rodents. *Comparative Medicine* 69 (6): 443–450.

Leary, S., Underwood, W., Anthony, R. et al. (2020). AVMA guidelines for the euthanasia
of animals: 2020 edition. https://www.avma.org/sites/default/files/2020-02/Guidelines-
on-Euthanasia-2020.pdf (accessed 9 April 2021).

Lehnus, K.S., Fordyce, P.S., and McMillan, M.W. (2019). Ethical dilemmas in clinical
practice: A perspective on the results of an electronic survey of veterinary anaesthetists.
*Veterinary Anaesthesia and Analgesia* 46 (3): 260–275.

Luna, S.P.L., de Araújo, A.L., da Nóbrega Neto, P.I. et al. (2020). Validation of the UNESP-
Botucatu pig composite acute pain scale (UPAPS). *PLoS ONE* 15: e0233552.

Lund, T.B., Morkbak, M.R., Lassen, J. et al. (2014). Painful dilemmas: A study of the way the public's assessment of animal research balances costs to animals against human benefits. *Public Understanding of Science* 23: 428–444.

Mathews, K., Kronen, P.W., Lascelles, D. et al. (2014). Guidelines for recognition, assessment and treatment of pain. *Journal of Small Animal Practice* 55 (6): E10–E68.

McCoy, A.M. (2015). Animal models of osteoarthritis: Comparisons and key considerations. *Veterinary Pathology* 52 (5): 803–818.

Mellor, D.J., Beausoleil, N.J., Littlewood, K.E. et al. (2020). The 2020 Five Domains Model: Including human–animal interactions in assessments of animal welfare. *Animals* 10 (10): 1870.

Mills, D.S., Demontigny-Bédard, I., Gruen, M. et al. (2020). Pain and problem behavior in cats and dogs. *Animals* 10 (2): 318.

Mills, K.E., Robbins, J., and von Keyserlingk, M.A.G. (2016). Tail docking and ear cropping dogs: Public awareness and perceptions. *PLoS ONE* 11 (6): e0158131.

Mogil, J.S. (2019). The translatability of pain across species. *Philosophical Transactions of the Royal Society B* 374: 20190286.

Monteiro, B.P., Lorimier, L.P., Moreau, M. et al. (2018). Pain characterization and response to palliative care in dogs with naturally-occurring appendicular osteosarcoma: An open label clinical trial. *PLoS ONE* 13 (12): e0207200.

Monteiro, B.P., Otis, C., del Castillo, J.R.E. et al. (2020). Quantitative sensory testing in feline osteoarthritic pain – A systematic review and meta-analysis. *Osteoarthritis Cartilage* 28 (7): 885–896.

Monteiro, B.P. and Steagall, P.V. (2019). Chronic pain in cats: Recent advances in clinical assessment. *Journal of Feline Medicine and Surgery* 21 (7): 601–614.

Nalon, E. and Stevenson, P. (2019). Addressing lameness in farmed animals: An urgent need to achieve compliance with EU Animal Welfare Law. *Animals* 9 (8): 576.

National Research Council (US) Committee for the Update of the Guide for the Care and Use of Laboratory Animals. (2011). *Guide for the Care and Use of Laboratory Animals*, 8e. Washington, DC: National Academies Press.

North American Veterinary Technician Association (NAVTA) (2007). Veterinary Technician Code of Ethics. https://cdn.ymaws.com/www.navta.net/resource/collection/946E408F-F98E-4890-9894-D68ABF7FAAD6/navta_vt_code_of_ethics_07.pdf (accessed 23 April 2021).

PennVet (n.d.). Canine Brief Pain Inventory. https://www.vet.upenn.edu/research/clinical-trials-vcic/our-services/pennchart/cbpi-tool. (accessed 25 October 2021).

Quimby, J.M., Smith, M.L., and Lunn, K.F. (2017). Evaluation of the effects of hospital visit stress on physiologic parameters in the cat. *Journal of Feline Medicine and Surgery* 13: 733–737.

Raja, S.N., Carr, D.B., Cohen, M. et al. (2020). The revised International Association for the Study of Pain definition of pain: Concepts, challenges, and compromises. *Pain* 161: 1976–1982.

Rosoff, P.M., Moga, J., Keene, B. et al. (2018). Resolving ethical dilemmas in a tertiary care veterinary specialty hospital: Adaptation of the Human Clinical Consultation Committee Model. *American Journal of Bioethics* 18 (2): 41–53.

Scollo, A., Contiero, B., De Benedictis, G.M. et al. (2021). Analgesia and/or anaesthesia during piglet castration – Part I: Efficacy of farm protocols in pain management. *Italian Journal of Animal Science* 20 (1): 143–152.

Simon, B.T., Scallan, E.M., Carroll, G. et al. (2017). The lack of analgesic use (oligoanalgesia) in small animal practice. *Journal of Small Animal Practice* 58 (10): 543–554.

Simon, B.T., Scallan, E.M., Von Pfeil, D.J.F. et al. (2018). Perceptions and opinions of pet owners in the United States about surgery, pain management, and anesthesia in dogs and cats. *Veterinary Surgery* 47 (2): 277–284.

Simpson, S., Dunning, M.D., de Brot, S. et al. (2017). Comparative review of human and canine osteosarcoma: Morphology, epidemiology, prognosis, treatment and genetics. *Acta Veterinaria Scandinavica* 59 (1): 71.

Sneddon, L.U. (2018). Comparative physiology of nociception and pain. *Physiology* 33 (1): 63–73.

Spitznagel, M.B., Jacobson, D.M., Cox, M.D. et al. (2018). Predicting caregiver burden in general veterinary clients: Contribution of companion animal clinical signs and problem behaviors. *The Veterinary Journal* 236: 23–30.

Steagall, P.V., Bustamante, H., Johnson, C.B. et al. (2021). Pain management in farm animals: Focus on cattle, sheep and pigs. *Animals* 11: 1483.

Steagall, P.V., Monteiro, B.P., Ruel, H.L.M. et al. (2017). Perceptions and opinions of Canadian pet owners about anaesthesia, pain and surgery in small animals. *Journal of Small Animal Practice* 58 (7): 380–388.

Steagall, P.V. and Monteiro, B.P. (2019). Acute pain in cats: Recent advances in clinical assessment. *Journal of Feline Medicine and Surgery* 21 (1): 25–34.

Taylor, K. and Alvarez, L.R. (2019). An estimate of the number of animals used for scientific purposes worldwide in 2015. *Alternatives to Laboratory Animals* 47 (5–6): 196–213.

Tomacheuski, R., Monteiro, B., Evangelista, M. et al. (2021). Measurement properties of pain scoring instruments in farm animals: A systematic review protocol using the COSMIN checklist. *PLoS ONE* 16 (5): e0251435.

UK Farm Animal Welfare Council (1979). Five Freedoms. https://webarchive. nationalarchives.gov.uk/20121010012427/http://www.fawc.org.uk/freedoms.htm (accessed 20 April 2021).

UK Parliament (1822). Martin's Act 1822: Act to Prevent the Cruel and Improper Treatment of Cattle. https://en.wikisource.org/wiki/Martin%27s_Act_1822 (accessed 22 September 2021).

United States Department of Agriculture (2009). Code of Federal Regulations. Title 9: Animals and Animal Products, subchapter A – Animal Welfare. https://www.govinfo. gov/content/pkg/CFR-2009-title9-vol1/xml/CFR-2009-title9-vol1-chapI-subchapA.xml (accessed 12 April 2021).

United States Department of Agriculture (USDA) (n.d). Animal Welfare Act. https:// www.nal.usda.gov/animal-health-and-welfare/animal-welfare-act (accessed 6 April 2021).

Walters, E.T. and Williams, A.C.C. (2019). Evolution of mechanisms and behaviour important for pain. *Philosophical Transactions of the Royal Society B* 374: 20190275.

Yeates, J.W. (2016). Ethical principles for novel therapies in veterinary practice. *Journal of Small Animal Practice* 57 (2): 67–73.

Yeates, J.W. and Main, D.C. (2010). The ethics of influencing clients. *Journal of the American Veterinary Medical Association* 237 (3): 263–267.

Yun, J., Ollila, A., Valros, A. et al. (2019). Behavioural alterations in piglets after surgical castration: Effects of analgesia and anaesthesia. *Research in Veterinary Science* 125: 36–42.

## 20

# Animal Maltreatment

*Martha Smith-Blackmore*

## Introduction

Approximately 85% of veterinarians have seen cases of suspected or confirmed animal abuse (Kogan et al. 2017; Joo et al. 2020). A retrospective study of over 13,000 necropsies of dogs and cats concluded that 1% had signs suggestive of abuse (Almeida et al. 2018). Veterinarians are likely to find themselves at a perceived crossroads of duty when a case of suspected animal abuse arrives at their practice. Questions may come to mind that don't have obvious answers. What regard do I owe my client? What protections do I owe my patient? When is a situation amenable to treatment and counseling? Am I required to make a report? When does the lack of care or question of what really happened rise to the level that a report must be made? What about the client–veterinarian relationship and confidentiality? When is an animal's poor condition a crime? Who makes that determination? What is the veterinarian's responsibility to family health and safety as "the other family doctor"? Further, what is the veterinarian's obligation when accepting a role as an expert for either the defense or prosecution in a legal matter involving an animal?

### Terminology

The terms animal cruelty, abuse, and neglect are often used interchangeably but, depending on context, they may have specific meanings and weight, particularly in a court of law, and legal definitions vary by jurisdiction. Rowan (1999) distinguishes "cruelty," "abuse," and "neglect," where cruelty is the intention to derive pleasure from inflicting harm to another, abuse is leveraging physical power and inappropriate force on an animal, and neglect is a failure to provide an animal with care to an extent that it harms an animal whether intentional or not.

It may be helpful to think of cruelty as deliberate harm, abuse as a deliberate act (where the action that ultimately harms the animal is intended but the resulting injuries were not necessarily part of the plan), and neglect as a passive failure (and the injuries caused by failure to act may or may not be deliberate). However, it must be acknowledged that animals who have been neglected often live tortured existences, and not all forms of cruelty and abuse share the same level of harms. Injuries resulting from a failure to act are also considered nonaccidental injuries.

Because laws vary, the United States Department of Justice uses the following definition of animal cruelty for the purposes of data collection:

*Ethics in Veterinary Practice: Balancing Conflicting Interests*, First Edition. Edited by Barry Kipperman and Bernard E. Rollin.

Intentionally, knowingly, or recklessly taking an action that mistreats or kills any animal without just cause, such as torturing, tormenting, mutilation, maiming, poisoning, or abandonment. Included are instances of duty to provide care, e.g., shelter, food, water, care if sick or injured; transporting or confining an animal in a manner likely to cause injury or death; causing an animal to fight with another; inflicting excessive or repeated unnecessary pain or suffering, e.g., uses objects to beat or torture an animal. This definition does not include proper maintenance of animals for show or sport; use of animals for food, lawful hunting, fishing, or trapping.

*(FBI n.d.)*

A felony law for animal maltreatment exists in all 50 states (Randour 2004). In some states, cruelty is a felony crime, and neglect may only be prosecuted as a misdemeanor. In some places, the *mens rea*, or "state of mind" of the offender must be proven – that the harm to the animal was intended. In other states, only the intent to commit the act that harms the animal must be proven, which is one step away from intending to hurt the animal. Whether the animal survived the abuse may determine decisions on how to charge a crime. Restraining an animal by a leash while kicking them is an indication of *mens rea* – by restricting the animal's movement and preventing escape, the abuser ensures the blows will land.

The animal hoarder who keeps animals in cages long term intends to keep the cage doors shut and intends to restrict the animals to their limited and often filthy space, but they may not intend the specific harms of nutritional deprivation, dehydration, dermatitis, or psychological distress. Another abuser might lock an animal away in retaliation for perceived bad behavior or out of revenge toward another person who cares about the animal, deliberately denying access to food and water until they starve or dehydrate to death. The difference between the two is known as "general intent" versus "specific intent." The hoarder intended to lock the animals up and the vengeful person had specific intent to cause suffering through starvation abuse.

Because abuse, cruelty, and neglect can have either specific or ambiguous interpretations in the law depending on the context and the perception of those terms by different individuals, some prefer to use the umbrella term "animal maltreatment" when referring to all nonaccidental harms to animals. This parallels the widely used term "child maltreatment."

## Animal Hoarding

Animal hoarding is a specific type of animal maltreatment that straddles the definitions of abuse and neglect. Animal hoarding may be passive accrual of animals due to unintended accumulation or breeding, or active accrual secondary to "rescue" efforts, or intentional, intensive but poorly managed breeding for profit.

Animal hoarding is defined by Patronek (1999) as having more than the typical number of companion animals; failing to provide even minimal standards of care, with this neglect often resulting in illness, suffering, and death. Additionally, hoarders often deny their inability to provide this minimum care and the impact of that failure on the animals and human occupants of the dwelling. There may be persistence, despite this failure, in accumulating and controlling animals. The accumulation and even caging of animals may be deliberate, but the failure to provide the population of animals with adequate care is generally an unintended sequela. The person with animal hoarding disorder either does not recognize the poor conditions, or they may simply not care (Ferreira et al. 2017). Hoarders are now believed to possibly suffer from a number of psychiatric disorders (Ferreira et al. 2017).

The suffering in animal hoarding far exceeds the benign picture of the "crazy cat lady." Stressed, crowded animals living in filth have reduced immunity and may incubate more intense forms of infectious disease. Inadequate grooming may lead to painful matting that strangulates limbs, forms fecal dams, or even leads to ocular rupture. Ammonia and toxic bioaerosols render the air unbreathable. There is intense mental anguish caused by overly dense or restrictive housing, competition for resources, an inability to escape filth or find a comfortable position, and other stressors.

## Animal Maltreatment Is Underrecognized

Official reports of animal maltreatment far undercount the number of cases that occur each year. Every locality has animals exempt from cruelty laws, whether it is animals used in agriculture, wildlife, research, or animals of certain species. It must be acknowledged that egregious animal maltreatment does occur within these "extra-label" settings, but they are currently beyond the reach of the criminal justice system.

Beyond the exemptions for enforcement, potentially prosecutable cases of animal cruelty go unrecognized, and therefore unreported. Deceased animals found on public streets, lands, or in bodies of water, are often picked up and disposed of without examination. In other communities, dogs and cats found dead may be photographed for potential future owner identification but the animals are not examined for evidence of nonaccidental injury. While it is often assumed the deceased animals are victims from hit by car, a certain percentage died for other reasons.

The Department of Justice maintains a National Incident Based Reporting System (NIBRS) and counts animal maltreatment in the four categories of intentional abuse, neglect, animal sexual abuse, and organized abuse (animal fighting). These incidents are recorded if the report of suspected animal maltreatment is made to an investigating agency with an Originating Agency Identification (ORI) number. It is estimated that approximately 55% of animal control officers are employed by agencies without an ORI number (e.g. Department of Agriculture, Department of Public Health, or a private humane agency) (M.L. Randour and L.A. Addington, Summary of Survey to Animal Control Agencies on Animal Cruelty Crime Statistics, 2011, unpublished). Only law enforcement agencies can report data to the NIBRS. If data are collected by an animal control agency, humane society, or other municipal or government office that is not in some way associated with law enforcement, the data may not end up in the NIBRS data submission to the Federal Bureau of Investigation (Palais 2021).

## Crimes of Commission Versus Crimes of Omission

The distinction of abuse as a crime of commission and neglect as a crime of omission is a helpful one. These are sometimes also referred to as active and passive abuse. There may be distinctions that are of value from a sociological, psychological, or criminological perspective. However, whether the abuser intended the harm or not, and whether they performed an act that harmed an animal or failed to intervene in a situation that would have prevented suffering does not matter to the veterinarian. The veterinarian's job is to effectively document and capture the animal's physical condition and any statements made related to the animal's condition. Understanding common motives underlying animal cruelty can aid the veterinarian in asking appropriate questions when gathering a history (Lockwood and Arkow 2016).

## Who Maltreats Animals, and Why?

Any profile of person may maltreat an animal or animals: however, there are certain trends. Animal hoarders are more likely to be single, older, socioeconomically disadvantaged women who live alone (Patronek 1999; Ferreira et al. 2017; Elliott et al. 2019). Poisoners are more likely to be neighbors and usually target a single animal one time rather than continuing a pattern of poisoning, but they can be strangers who are indiscriminate poisoners (Gwaltney-Brant 2007). Perpetrators who are intimate partners or family members of the owner of the animal are more likely to demonstrate active cruelty such as kicking or blunt-force injuries, while owners themselves are more likely to evidence forms of neglect. Interpersonal relationships and the types of animal maltreatment perpetrated are more complex than previously understood, as are the motivations to maltreat animals. Actions taken to reduce harms to animals must be multipronged and consider these variations (Richard and Reese 2019).

While the reasons for any criminal conduct can be complex and multifactorial, it is helpful to understand generalities of criminal motivations. Reasons for harming animals include: a need or desire to control or punish human partners; frustration over a pet's actions; retaliation against a particular animal; retaliation against a person; satisfying a prejudice against a certain species or breed of animal; enhancing one's personal aggressive persona; entertainment; and sadism (Kellert and Felthous 1985). Animal abusers are bullies who seek to harm and intimidate vulnerable animals and the people who care about them.

"The Link" refers to the strong association between animal maltreatment and human violence, especially toward women and children (Newberry 2017). This knowledge has been the driving force behind legislation to include animals in protective orders and mandatory cross-reporting of animal and child abuse (Gentry 2001; Flynn-Poppey et al. 2016). Animal maltreatment may occur in the context of human maltreatment within an interpersonal relationship or household. Interestingly, perpetrators of intimate partner violence who also abuse animals have a likelihood of more intense forms of domestic violence (DV). In a survey of violent acts perpetrated in a home setting, 8% of DV abusers committed acts of forced sex, but 26% of those who had also abused pets forced sex on their human partners (Campbell et al. 2021). Forty-seven percent of DV abusers had attempted strangulation of their victim, but 76% of the DV/animal abusers had done so. Thirty-five percent of DV victims reported they feared their abuser would kill them, but 78% of those abused by a person with animal abuse history thought their life was at risk. This study suggests that DV perpetrators with a history of animal abuse are significantly more dangerous than DV perpetrators who have not abused animals.

A person may redirect misplaced aggression on an animal out of frustration at not being able to act against their actual target (Kellert and Felthous 1985). They may be thrill-seeking, alleviating boredom, or harming animals for shock value (Hensley et al. 2011). Children may commit animal abuse as a response to violence within the home

(Ascione 2001) or they may use animal cruelty as a form of "dirty play" that allows them to explore aspects of adult life by acting independently of adult monitoring, or to exert control and dominance over their environment (Arluke 2002).

Animal neglect may occur because an individual overestimates an animal's ability to care for itself. A person who self-neglects will likely fail to provide adequate care to animals in their control as well, usually secondary to cognitive decline or distortion from mental illness (Nathanson 2009).

Animals may be sexually abused for reasons of perversion (Beirne 1997). Animals may be criminally abused for financial gain, through intensive breeding operations without regard for the experience of the animal that fail to provide a life worth living for the breeding animals. The environment and animals both suffer when animals are poached for the dollar value of their meat, fur, hides, or other body parts.

Dogfighters may have financial and other motivations including membership in a group bonded by shared clandestine activity, or the machismo bragging rights of owning a vicious and dangerous winner. Likewise, should the dog shame the dogfighter by losing, the dogfighter may dispatch the animal in a cruel manner to save face (Ortiz 2010).

### Mental Capacity and Burden of Proof

Law enforcement investigates crimes regardless of questions about the accused person's mental capacities. In a prosecution, it is up to the defense to argue that the accused lacks mental competence and cannot bear criminal responsibility. For similar reasons, veterinarians should not avoid reporting suspicions of animal maltreatment out of feelings of sympathy for an animal abuser. A veterinarian's report simply ensures that the legal system is allowed to perform investigations and decide about appropriate next steps.

The criminal justice system has increasing levels of certainty needed at various steps. For instance, a police officer may detain someone briefly for questioning based on "reasonable suspicion." They only need to have "probable cause" that a suspect committed a crime to arrest a person: probable cause is present when an officer has 51% or higher certainty. For this reason, probable cause can exist even where there is some doubt. Conversely, the burden of proof for a judge or jury is that they must have "certainty beyond a reasonable doubt" to affirm a criminal conviction of a defendant. A veterinarian's report of suspected animal cruelty is at the lowest level of the burden of proof pyramid (Figure 20.1).

In cases of borderline care verging on neglect, it is appropriate for a veterinarian to counsel their client before reporting suspicions of maltreatment. Advice given for improving care should be noted in the animal's record and a recheck appointment scheduled. It may be appropriate to advise the client that if they do not follow up or if the animal is not improved at recheck, the veterinarian will have an obligation to make a report of suspected animal neglect.

## Veterinarians Are Obligated to Recognize and Report Suspected Animal Maltreatment

Currently, about 20 states require veterinarians to report suspicions of animal abuse or neglect, and nine states include mandates for veterinary technicians, assistants, or

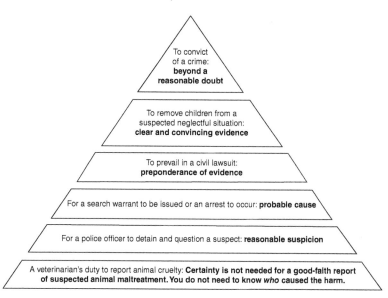

**Figure 20.1** Pyramid of the burden of proof in the criminal justice system, from lowest to highest.

other employees working for veterinarians to do so (Wisch 2020). Twenty-nine states provide for civil immunity from lawsuits for reports of suspected animal cruelty that are made in good faith, meaning an individual cannot sue a veterinarian for reporting their concerns, regardless of whether a criminal process ensues. Nine states mandate reporting of suspicions of animal cruelty but do not specifically provide civil immunity (ALDF 2020; Wisch 2020; American Veterinary Medical Association [AVMA] 2021). It is not clear whether veterinary malpractice insurance will cover a veterinarian if sued for making a good-faith report in a state where civil immunity is not articulated by law. For that reason, veterinarians are encouraged to discuss this situation with an insurance agent and may want to obtain umbrella coverage.

The veterinarian should have a general awareness of the animal maltreatment laws (often referred to as "cruelty laws") in the jurisdictions where they practice, and if the practice sees patients from adjoining states, they should be familiar with the applicable laws there as well. A general awareness means knowing how that state defines "animal" for the purposes of the applicable law (i.e. what species are covered), and the general language, and what agency receives reports of suspected animal cruelty.

It is important to know that although a statutory law (the written law in the books) may be constructed from what seems like ancient language, the interpretation of statutory law is modified by subsequent appeals decisions. This is known as "common law," which is the reliance on successive court rulings for the interpretation and application of the statutory law. Decisions about current cases therefore reflect historical judicial rulings. This means the law may be interpreted by the courts in a manner that is different than is understood when the statute is read by the lay person. Most state bar associations have an animal law section, which can be a resource for learning how the animal maltreatment laws work and how they are applied in a particular state. Reports of suspected animal maltreatment should be made in the state and jurisdiction where patients are thought to have been harmed.

Regardless of local law, veterinarians have an ethical responsibility to report suspicions of animal maltreatment. The AVMA (n.d.a) holds that "prompt disclosure of abuse is necessary to protect the health and welfare of animals and people." The veterinarian is seen by the public as "the other family doctor" (Gooding 2008). By reporting suspected animal cruelty, veterinarians fulfill a public health and safety role, and societal expectations for our profession.

Certainly, veterinarians cannot report animal abuse if they do not recognize it. It is incumbent upon the veterinarian to seek training in recognizing signs of nonaccidental injury and to maintain nonaccidental injury and failure to provide adequate care on their list of differential diagnoses. It can be difficult to fathom how a person could be so callous as to hurt their own animal and yet also care enough to bring them in for veterinary care. Pediatricians used to hold the same expectations that parents would not harm their own children and still bring them in for medical evaluation. This type of thinking has since been debunked (Munro 1996).

As one of the few persons likely to interact with an abused animal, the veterinarian is in a unique position to recognize and identify animal abuse (Benetato et al. 2011). A veterinarian suspecting animal maltreatment, and struggling with a decision to report should ask themselves, "If not me, then who will speak up for this animal?"

Having an awareness of animal abuse or suspected animal maltreatment is a type of psychological trauma (Randour et al. 2021). Reporting suspicions can mitigate moral distress (see Chapter 22) for the veterinarian. Not reporting suspicions of animal maltreatment allows for ongoing feelings of misgiving and concern. Making the report terminates the internal struggle of "To report or not report?" and can help protect the veterinarian's mental health.

It is not incumbent upon the veterinarian to determine *mens rea* or motivations – leave that to the investigator. It is not the veterinarian's responsibility to determine whether all necessary elements of a crime are present – leave that to the prosecutor. However, the veterinarian may have insight that helps to underscore the intentionality or nonaccidental characteristics of an animal's injuries.

What is most imperative when nonaccidental injury is suspected is that a report is made so an investigation can ensue. Proper, detailed medical records must be maintained to appropriately memorialize any statements made, the animal's presenting condition, and response to treatment. The veterinarian is also responsible for understanding how to differentiate accidental and nonaccidental injury, whether resulting from an act (commission) or a failure to act (omission). Importantly, the veterinarian need not be certain an injury or condition is nonaccidental to be sufficiently suspicious to make a report of their concerns. Nonaccidental injury does not have to be a definitive diagnosis to make a report of suspected animal maltreatment. When a veterinarian chooses not to make a report, they are an effective gatekeeper, preventing investigation. When a veterinarian prevents an investigation into suspected animal cruelty, they are potentially preventing the relief of animal suffering and perhaps allowing unmitigated co-occurring human suffering as well (Case Study 20.1).

---

**Case Study 20.1 A reporting quandary: Cats and your client in poor condition**

Dr. S has been treating three cats belonging to an elderly owner, Mrs. J. Over the years, Mrs. J has brought all her cats to Dr. S's veterinary practice, and Mrs. J always follows the recommendations for treatment of various conditions, and dutifully presents the cats for annual examinations. Each cat is brought in individually as Mrs. J uses public transportation. Medical records document steadily increasing weights of all cats for the past few years. At the most recent annual visits, the cats are all noted to be obese, with body condition scores (BCS) of 8 or 9 out of 9 on the Purina BCS scoring system. All the cats have heavy amounts of dandruff and greasy hair coats.

The heaviest cat, Fiona, a 13-year-old spayed female domestic long-haired cat, has a fetid, urine-soaked hair mat adhered to her hind end that obscures her anus. The other two cats also had a distinct odor, with yellow-brown staining of white fur on their feet. The other two cats are shorthaired but had large mats of fur on their backs. Mrs. J was unaware of the mats until they were pointed out to her.

Dr. S notices that, while Mrs. J is wearing a matching dress and jacket, the hems are frayed and Mrs. J also emits a foul odor of filth. Mrs. J agrees to hospitalization of Fiona so that she can be sedated, shaved, and bathed, and she agrees to send her adult son Bill (who lives in the house) in the following day to pick Fiona up. The receptionist reports that Mrs. J rummaged through wrinkled and dirty papers in her purse while looking for her wallet. After sedating Fiona and shaving the mat it is apparent that she has a severe perineal dermatitis and obstipation, which were treated.

Dr. S's practice is in a state with a law mandating veterinarians to report suspicions of animal cruelty. Dr. S's lead veterinary technician, Amanda, who was working on Fiona, requests that Dr. S initiate a report. Dr. S replies she isn't sure that the situation rises to the level of animal cruelty.

**What should Dr. S do?**
Interests include:

1) Fiona and the other two cats:
   - To avoid suffering.
   - To have the opportunity to live a good quality of life in a sanitary environment.
   - To minimize fear and distress including major disruptions to their environment.
2) Mrs. J:
   - To continue living her life with her three cats.
   - To feel she is providing her cats with excellent care.
   - To avoid being embarrassed.
   - To avoid being reported to authorities.
3) Bill and the neighbors:
   - To live in a safe and healthy environment.
4) Dr. S:
   - To avoid interpersonal conflicts regarding how to address patient welfare concerns.
   - To avoid the distress of legal cases.
   - To preserve practice income and reputation.

- To adhere to local laws.
- To promote public health.
- To avoid contributing to unnecessary suffering.
- To continue a positive long-term relationship with a client and her pets.

5) The rest of the veterinary team:
- To feel they have advocated for the welfare of their patients.
- To mitigate moral stress (see Chapter 22).

Options:

Dr. S has various options:

1) Ignore the welfare concerns.
2) Provide the client with weight management nutrition and counseling for the cats, with frequent scheduled rechecks and provide Mrs. J with a referral to a local cat groomer.
3) Discuss the concerns with Bill.
4) Report the owner to the authorities.

Ethical analysis:

Choosing not to address this situation avoids disruptions to Mrs. J's, Bill's, and the cats' lives, but may allow continued deteriorating living conditions for them. Abutting neighbors may have concerns about odors or even risks of fire, which is a common hazard in object hoarding homes. This decision may incur moral stress for Dr. S or her team and may create the perception among Dr. S's team of Dr. S not being an animal welfare advocate, leader, or role model.

Simply advising that the cats lose weight and be groomed regularly may improve their condition and quality of life. This is an appealing solution because Mrs. J is a compliant client and will likely follow through. However, this limited solution is problematic because it does not address the other problems, such as an unhealthy or unsafe living situation for the cats, Mrs. J, and Bill. Ideally, intervention for weight control should have been implemented sooner before the cats were obese.

Choosing to have a conversation with Bill about the various concerns and bypassing directly discussing the situation with Mrs. J could cause her to feel upset or excluded. Also, Mrs. J. is Dr. S's client, not Bill. Talking with Bill may violate client confidentiality. In this case, Bill has been living with the cats as well, and he apparently did not have concerns, at least not enough to point them out to his mother. Or perhaps he did point them out, but she either feigned ignorance or lacks the mental capacity to recognize her cats' increasingly poor conditions. Living in filthy conditions may be the result of self-neglect secondary to cognitive disorders. Hoarding disorder appears to have a heritable cause, so Mrs. J. and Bill may share similar cognitive processing challenges.

In some cases, it can be appropriate to first counsel a client to correct a neglectful situation, but in this case, the neglect goes beyond involving only the cats. Veterinary professionals must consider their duties to both public health and patient welfare. If a report of concerns about the cats' living conditions is made to the proper authorities, whether that is the police, an animal control officer or some other agency, an investigation can ensue to determine whether the living conditions are safe for Mrs. J., Bill, and the cats. In this case, the report should be made.

> This report will not necessarily result in criminal prosecution, or even removal of Mrs. J., Bill, or the cats from the environment, but it will ensure that the veterinary practice is not turning its back on a potentially dangerous situation resulting in poor welfare. Although anyone can file a report, veterinarians are more likely to be protected from legal liability than paraprofessionals, so they are better suited to initiate concerns of animal maltreatment. Dr. S. should not be a gatekeeper who prevents social services from assisting the family or their neighbors.

### Barriers to Veterinarians Recognizing and Reporting Maltreatment

Concerns veterinarians may have about reporting animal maltreatment include possible reprisal or lost income from a reported client, loss of business and income from other clients if accusations are made on social media, criminal or civil liability if a good-faith report proves to be unfounded, the belief that paying clients would not abuse their animals, and breach of client confidentiality. Reasons cited by veterinarians for reluctance to report included lack of training in recognizing and reporting abuse, uncertainty regarding whether abuse occurred, a desire to educate clients rather than report them, and feeling discouraged to make a report by their superior (Kogan et al. 2017). Perhaps because of these concerns, 44% of US veterinarians indicated not reporting an encountered case of animal abuse (Kogan et al. 2017) and 50% of practitioners in South Korea noted that they were reluctant to report (Joo et al. 2020).

### The Importance of Courage

There may be trepidation or fear associated with reporting potential animal abuse, either relative to the process that will follow, fallout from making the report, or out of fear of how the potential abuser may react or for other reasons. A veterinarian must exercise courage in the face of this discomfort. Fear that is predicated on real or imagined potential negative outcomes likely puts the veterinarian's interests before those of the animal and society. Ethical behavior often requires action even if it is not necessarily in one's immediate best interest to do so. As noted by Hernandez et al. (2018), "Advocating for animal welfare may not be comfortable and may, at times, require courage."

Courts generally accept veterinarians as experts on animal health and welfare. Unlike other witnesses in a trial, an expert witness has the freedom to express opinions when testifying. Veterinarians can formulate plausible theories of harm and interpret the animal's experience for the court. This is a privilege that must be exercised – if veterinarians do not embrace this role, no one else will and no one else can with that specific skillset. Equally important, veterinarians may have insight that can exonerate an individual accused of animal maltreatment.

Understanding how other professionals make mandated reports of suspected crimes, such as child maltreatment, can help veterinarians develop the courage to make reports of suspected animal maltreatment. Some social workers will make a call to report families where child maltreatment is suspected, with the family in the room, and after discussing the reasons why a report is being made.

## Recognizing Abused Animals and Documentation

Like child abuse, indicators of animal abuse include an animal presented with a history that is inconsistent with the extent or severity of the injuries (Woolf 2020). Alternatively, discrepant histories may be provided, with different stories told to various staff members or versions that do not match what other household members have reported. Factors that should raise suspicion include changes in an animal's behavior such as new aggression or submissive behavior, especially in the presence of a particular household member, or visible relief when separated from a suspected abuser. A history of unexplained injuries or deaths of other animals in the household is also a warning sign (Munro and Thrusfield 2001).

Other signs include the type of injury an animal has sustained, particularly a history of repetitive injuries, and old unrelated injuries (Table 20.1). In a blind retrospective study of radiological findings of accidental versus nonaccidental orthopedic injuries in dogs, the following distinctions in fracture characteristics were noted: abused dogs often had multiple fractures; abused dogs were more likely to have fractures in multiple regions (forelimbs, hindlimbs, or axial); cases presented in a later stage of healing; and the presence of fractures in two or more distinct stages of healing (Tong 2014). In a similar study examining medical records of dogs and cats treated for either motor vehicle accidents or nonaccidental injury, the skeletal injuries associated with nonaccidental cases were skull fractures, teeth fractures, rib fractures, and vertebral fractures (Intarapanich et al. 2016). Cats, younger, and smaller animals were also more likely to experience nonaccidental injuries (Intarapanich et al. 2016).

The clinical or postmortem exam of a suspected abused animal requires attention to detail and detailed record keeping. Any case may eventually end up in court if there is a civil charge of malpractice against a veterinarian, so every medical record should be

**Table 20.1** Signs suggestive of nonaccidental injury (Munro et al. 2001; Tong 2014; Intarapanich et al. 2016).

| |
|---|
| Animal presented with history inconsistent with injuries |
| Different histories relayed by different members of the household |
| Skull or teeth fractures or scleral hemorrhage |
| Mid-rib fractures or bilateral rib fractures |
| Injuries on multiple areas of the body |
| Fractures in various states of healing |
| Repetitive injuries (the same injury occurring over and over again) |
| Multiple types of injuries (e.g. burns, blunt and sharp trauma) in one pet |
| Delayed presentation for care (longstanding injuries) |
| History of multiple unexplained injuries of different types |
| Frequent presentation of new juvenile pets, prior pets disappear |
| New aggression or submissive behavior in the presence of one person |
| Presentations of numerous pets, each only seen one time |
| Presenting pets in poor nutritional or grooming condition |
| Presenting multiple pets with various infectious or parasitic conditions |

carefully reviewed. However, in cases involving questionable circumstances, the stakes are even higher, calling for more documentation via notes, sketches, and photography. Photos are essential and provide a body of information that helps other experts and investigators see what you saw. Performing photography in all cases helps to make it a part of all standard examinations: however, a veterinarian can articulate in court that they took photographs because they had an index of suspicion of nonaccidental injury. The client does not have to be informed that photography is taking place.

In some cases, additional diagnostic procedures or tests will help a veterinarian determine nonaccidental harm. If a client declines tests such as laboratory work or imaging and the veterinarian suspects animal maltreatment, now is the time to make a report. The investigating agency may take responsibility for the case at that point and authorize and pay for such tests. A veterinarian may offer to take radiographs or do testing "on the house" but should not do so if the client continues to decline. At that point, a legal entity may need to be consulted so they can impound the animal and pursue testing. Another tactic is the "don't ask" policy. If the animal is taken from the client for urgent examination and stabilization, and nonaccidental injury is suspected, radiographs or lab work may be performed as part of the stabilization. This runs the risk that the client will balk at the cost of tests performed without first consenting to them. Restitution for the testing may be ordered at the end of a legal process. Alternatively, the veterinarian could perform radiographs of the whole body on a small patient to expand the evaluation when a regional radiograph had been approved.

## Reporting

One of the most important steps a veterinarian can take to help ensure a positive outcome in abuse cases is to prepare for this possibility in advance by having a clinic policy. The policy should address factors such as determining whether reporting is mandated or protected in that state and knowing the correct agency to which abuse should be reported. When unsure about an abuse case, physicians have been advised to consult with others so that any decision to report originated from a group rather than an individual, thereby avoiding any possible negative reprisals against a particular physician (Kogan et al. 2017).

The state veterinary medical association may be able to advise on the appropriate agency for reporting suspicions of animal maltreatment. The National Link Coalition maintains a national directory listing where a report should be made, along with contact information (National Link Coalition n.d.). The reporting veterinarian does not need to gain permission from the practice owner or manager to make the report, but they should consider informing them so that subsequent inquiries and subpoenas from law enforcement do not arrive as a surprise. A veterinarian does not have to inform a client they are going to call authorities but doing so is recommended because it is honest and may solicit information that may be helpful in learning the truth about the incident.

A veterinarian suspecting animal maltreatment should summarize the salient findings in a written report. This report should be written in clearly understood lay terms detailing the reasons the veterinarian believes the injuries are nonaccidental and outlining the degree and duration of suffering of the animal. This report will assist the agency receiving the report of suspected animal maltreatment in understanding what the animal endured and why there may be substantial and potentially criminal concerns related to the animal's condition.

When reporting suspected nonaccidental injury to an animal the veterinarian should focus on the injury and why it is inconsistent with an accidental injury. Who caused the injury is less important or may even be irrelevant. Verbally articulating that an injury of such characteristics appears nonaccidental or is inconsistent with the provided history may elicit further (and sometimes varying) explanations of circumstances related to how the animal was harmed from the presenting party.

In some circumstances it may be appropriate to make a verbal report with the client present. One technique borrowed from human social work is to describe a strength in the family, report the failure of adequate care, followed by another strength. A statement a veterinarian might make could be something like "Oreo's owner clearly loves Oreo as exhibited by them bringing Oreo in for care. Since counseling them on specific care needs for Oreo, I am concerned about their ability to provide adequate care as they have not improved Oreo's grooming or skin condition and Oreo is suffering. Oreo's owner has made strides with regards to providing better nutrition." This reporting technique exhibits the veterinarian's concern for the animal while recognizing positive attributes of the owner and makes the report a collaboration. A report such as this may get animal control officers involved in a monitoring role and shifts the responsibility for ongoing investigation and monitoring to the animal control agency without necessarily triggering criminal charges.

It is possible a client will bring a nonaccidentally injured animal to a veterinarian with the hopes the veterinarian will make the report of maltreatment that the client is afraid to make themselves. This can happen in cases of DV, and the client may express relief that a report is going to be made. In other cases, the client may implore the veterinarian to not make the report out of fear for their own safety. In such cases it may be helpful to encourage the client to seek services from a DV helpline, or even the police at that time, even before leaving the veterinary practice.

Once a veterinarian has decided to make a report of their suspicion of animal maltreatment, they should identify the appropriate authority to receive the report. Reporting suspected animal maltreatment may or may not be as straightforward as calling your local police department. Reports should be made to the appropriate investigating agency in the jurisdiction where the harm is thought to have occurred. In various communities this may be animal control services, the police, the sheriff's office, the department of agriculture, code enforcement, environmental services, community dispatch, or others.

It is reasonable for a veterinarian to include the animal's veterinary records when making a mandated report of suspected animal maltreatment as the record is supporting documentation for the suspicion. When law enforcement requests veterinary records during an animal maltreatment investigation that the veterinarian did not initiate, veterinarians should request a subpoena before releasing the records. Even in states without veterinary-client confidentiality laws, requesting a subpoena ensures the veterinarian protects the client's confidentiality expected in a state's practice act to the best of their ability. Requesting a subpoena also protects the veterinarian against client reprisal and potential liability.

Veterinarians can become more confident about reporting suspicions of animal cruelty by seeking further education. Such subject matter is regularly covered at veterinary conferences, in veterinary journals, and in online continuing education courses. Practices should include nonaccidental injury as a differential in rounds in cases of trauma or animals in poor condition. Educators should include identifying nonaccidental injury in veterinary school curricula. State veterinary medical associations can include case reports of successfully reported suspected animal cruelty cases in newsletters.

## Ethical Guidance for the Forensic Veterinarian

There are an increasing number of veterinarians applying their medical expertise to gather and interpret evidence in civil and criminal court cases that involve animals. Some end up in the field as part of their duties at an animal shelter or as a veterinary pathologist. Others may be private practitioners with an interest in supporting local investigations of animal cruelty.

There is currently no AVMA-credentialed or accepted training path for a veterinarian to be considered an expert in forensics. If a veterinarian is going to represent themselves as an expert in veterinary forensics, they must seek further education and adhere to informed and ethical conduct in that role. Veterinarians may engage in an online certificate training or undertake a Master's degree in veterinary forensics. There are multiple textbooks on veterinary forensics (Merck 2013; Bailey 2016; Brooks 2018; Rogers and Stern 2018). A small number of veterinarians have "hung a shingle" by seeking further education and establishing a private consulting business, and more and more are doing so (Parry and Stoll 2020). Guidance for the appropriate conduct of a clinical (Touroo et al. 2020) and postmortem forensic examination (McEwen et al. 2019) has been published and should be consulted.

### Responsibilities of an Expert Witness

Veterinary forensics, being a relatively nascent field, is in a developmental phase in the realm of ethics and accepted conduct for expert witnesses at trial. Any veterinarian can serve as an expert witness. Veterinarians have been accepted as experts at trials involving matters related to animals for a long time, but the field does not have explicit ethical direction for trial testimony. The primary purpose of a trial is to ascertain the truth, and the central obligation of expert witnesses providing opinion at trial is to provide adequate, unbiased justification for their position.

An expert witness veterinarian must formulate opinions and testify truthfully at trial, regardless of whether testifying on behalf of the prosecution or defense. The AVMA Veterinarian's Oath (AVMA n.d.b) references Principles of Veterinary Medical Ethics, which provide general guidance to the veterinarian on professional conduct but do not address conduct as an expert witness. Given the lack of specific professional conduct guidance for expert testimony in veterinary forensic medicine, we can benefit from looking to other fields for direction.

For example, the American Academy of Psychiatry and the Law (AAPL) in its ethics guidelines calls upon witnesses to "consider all relevant data ... and analyze it objectively in formulating conclusions" and to perform only as they "would routinely perform in the course of normal professional duties" (AAPL n.d). In other words, the expert must employ the "same intellectual rigor" with respect to their courtroom testimony that they would with respect to their everyday work (Kumho Tire Co. vs. Carmichael).

The expert witness is not simply representing themselves, but the knowledge their field has about some topic. Their role is to provide specialized knowledge that "will assist the trier of fact to understand the evidence" (US Government Publishing Office 2010). To preserve justice in our criminal justice system, the single most important obligation of an expert witness is to approach every question with independence and objectivity.

The forensic veterinarian has an obligation to develop familiarity with the criminal justice system and process in their area. They should produce written opinion reports in clear, fact-based lay language. It is essential that veterinarians do not overstate expertise or overreach in their work. If a forensic veterinarian is not accustomed to working on a particular species, they are advised to partner with a species expert or fully refer the case to a more appropriate expert. Veterinarians must limit their opinions to veterinary practice, and not opine on matters that are the domain of other forensic specialists or scientists (e.g. blood spatter evidence, fingerprint evidence).

While collegiality is important, forensic veterinarians should not be reluctant to participate in veterinary malpractice cases. Part of our responsibility to society includes protecting clients and animals from poor veterinary practice. Providing testimony in such civil matters is not a violation of collegiality, but rather another way of advocating for justice and endorsing the trustworthiness of veterinary medicine as a profession.

### Avoiding Biases

We all hold biases, both explicit and implicit. It is imperative that the forensic veterinarian be aware of biases and assiduously avoid confirmation bias. Confirmation bias is a pervasive psychological phenomenon: it is the tendency of people to seek, perceive, interpret, and create new evidence in ways that verify their pre-existing beliefs (Kassin et al. 2013). As such, confirmation bias can be seen as a type of prejudice in gathering and analyzing evidence and drawing certain conclusions.

Veterinarians conducting clinical and postmortem examinations must seek the truth and avoid an a priori "think dirty" stance (McDonough and McEwen 2016). In the past, forensic pathologists and other death investigators often assumed that a death was unnatural until proven otherwise, particularly in specific scenarios, such as the deaths of infants and children. This "thinking dirty" led to wrongful convictions and undermined the professional reliability of forensic pathology (Pollanen 2016). It is vital that veterinarians working in forensics avoid similar mistakes.

For a greedy and/or ethically unprincipled expert witness veterinarian, testimony may be shaped to match the desires of those who are paying them to testify. This may mean incremental statements are made, each one on its face the truth, but when considered altogether sum to a totality that is far from the truth: "The worst that can be said about an expert opinion is not that it is a lie – that criticism is often beside the point – but that it is unreasonable, that no competent expert in the field would hold it" (Gross 1991).

A deliberate misapplication of multiple facts out of context to the case is worse than a lie because it is an expert clouding fact finders' ability to discern the whole truth. When testifying in court, the expert witness veterinarian's duty is to bring clarity to the process, not obfuscation. Veterinary medicine would benefit from developing ethical training and guidance for expert witness veterinarians. This would help ensure our scientific knowledge and skills are used for the benefit of society, and the health and welfare of animals, in accordance with our professional oath. The forensic veterinarian is a truth seeker and advocate for justice, not an advocate for a particular animal, defendant, or outcome.

## Possible Outcomes of the Criminal Justice Process

Once a veterinarian has documented a case of suspected animal maltreatment, delivered evidence to the investigating agency, and perhaps testified at trial, the decision is in the hands of the legal system. Potential outcomes may include pretrial resolutions such as a guilty plea to the original charge, or to a lesser charge. Or the defendant may receive a "continued without a finding" decision. They may "admit to sufficient facts" that if a trial were to be held, they would likely be found guilty, while still maintaining their innocence – this is known as an "Alford plea," a plea of guilty containing a protestation of innocence. If the burden of proof (beyond a reasonable doubt) is not met, the defendant will be found not guilty. If the defendant is found guilty through either a pretrial or trial process, a sentence will be issued.

Veterinarians should understand that sentences are delivered in context of the offender's prior acts, within sentencing guidelines, and in context of sentences for similar crimes committed on human victims. Sentencing may include imprisonment in a state prison or house of corrections, fines, ownership bans, counseling, community service and supervision (probation), or other diversionary programs. A split sentence means some time to serve, and the balance is time on probation. When on probation, if a convict reoffends, they may be required to serve the remainder of the sentence in jail. With a suspended sentence, the convict is not required to go to jail but, similarly, violations of probation may result in jail time.

In most states, a person whose animal has been killed or injured may have an opportunity to make a victim impact statement after the defendant is convicted but before they are sentenced. In cases where there is no owner, a veterinarian can prepare a victim impact statement that details the suffering of an animal. The statement should be concise but realistic. If the animal struggled to breathe, or if there was marked blood loss, or if the duration of suffering was prolonged, or the pain was likely to have been intense, now is the time to state that. The victim impact statement should not repeat the facts already presented in court, and veterinarians must assiduously avoid taking a posture of vigilantism. It is important that the focus of the statement be factual and not vengeance seeking. It is simply time to ensure the judge understands what the animal endured. A victim impact statement provided by a veterinarian may not be admitted into the record, but it still helps to inform the court.

Restorative justice is an alternative to a carceral or punitive response. The aim is to have the offender acknowledge the harm they have caused and try to address the harm caused to victims and their communities through rehabilitation, reconciliation, and restoration. One program that has been used is the Benchmark Animal Rehabilitative Curriculum program (BARC n.d.). The court-ordered curriculum is intended to create a positive change in behavior by increasing awareness of the value and needs of all sentient beings, and an understanding of the potential consequences of failing to meet those needs. Veterinarians should understand that sentences are decided by judges with perspective on all manner of crime and justice. It is not appropriate for a veterinarian who has worked as an expert in a case to publicly denigrate the judge or outcome of the process.

## All Veterinarians Must Be Prepared to Document Cases and Make Reports

The availability of forensic veterinarians does not minimize the ongoing role of the private practitioner, veterinary pathologist, or shelter veterinarian to recognize, document, and report suspected animal cruelty. The services of the forensic veterinarian can complement but not replace the work of other veterinarians.

When there are challenging cases with critical diagnoses, complex scenes, and related court appearances, the availability of a forensic veterinarian for consultation or case referral may be an option. The forensic veterinarian can serve other veterinarians in such roles similarly to subspecialists in internal medicine, neurology, or dermatology. A forensic expert may review records kept by another veterinarian and provide a summary report of their opinion. In such cases, the prosecution and defense may stipulate the content of the record, and the forensic veterinarian may provide expert opinion, sparing the examining veterinarian much of the court responsibility.

In some areas of the United States, responsibility for frontline enforcement of animal cruelty laws has predominantly fallen to private police forces at organizations such as Societies for the Prevention of Cruelty to Animals (SPCAs) and humane societies, and nonprofits, which depend on donations and fundraising. There are compelling ethical, human safety, health, feminist, and workers' rights reasons for governments to be investing in animal cruelty investigations (Coulter and Campbell 2020). The enforcement of laws should not be delegated to special interest groups. Veterinarians are encouraged to engage within their communities to increase the provision of veterinary expertise in criminal justice matters involving animal maltreatment investigated by local law enforcement. This allows the data to be recorded by the Department of Justice and helps to ensure that other co-occurring crimes will be identified.

## References

Almeida, D.C., Torres, S.M., and Wuenschmann, A. (2018). Retrospective analysis of necropsy reports suggestive of abuse in dogs and cats. *Journal of the American Veterinary Medical Association* 252 (4): 433–439.

American Academy of Psychiatry and the Law (AAPL) (n.d.). Ethics guidelines for the practice of forensic psychiatry. https://www.aapl.org/ethics.htm (accessed 3 November 2021).

American Veterinary Medical Association (AVMA) (n.d.a). Animal abuse and animal neglect. https://www.avma.org/resources-tools/avma-policies/animal-abuse-and-animal-neglect (accessed 30 October 2021).

American Veterinary Medical Association (AVMA) (n.d.b). Veterinarian's Oath. https://www.avma.org/KB/Policies/Pages/veterinarians-oath.aspx (accessed 10 October 2021).

American Veterinary Medical Association (AVMA) (2021). Reporting requirements for animal abuse summary report. https://www.avma.org/resources/animal-health-welfare/abuse-reporting-requirements-state (accessed 25 October 2021).

Animal Legal Defense Fund (ALDF) (2020). Laws in favor of veterinary reporting of animal cruelty. U.S. animal protection laws state rankings. https://aldf.org/project/veterinary-reporting (accessed 30 October 2021).

Arluke, A. (2002). Animal abuse as dirty play. *Symbolic Interaction* 25: 405–430.

Ascione, F.R. (2001). Animal abuse and youth violence. *Juvenile Justice Bulletin* September: 1–15.

Bailey, D. (2016). *Practical Veterinary Forensics*. Wallingford, UK: CAB International.

Beirne, P. (1997). Rethinking bestiality: Towards a concept of interspecies sexual assault. *Theoretical Criminology* 1 (3): 317–340.

Benchmark Animal Rehabilitative Curriculum (BARC) (n.d.). Online Animal Cruelty Prevention and Education Course. http://barceducation.org (accessed 29 October 2021).

Benetato, M.A., Reisman, R., and McCobb, E. (2011). The veterinarian's role in animal cruelty cases. *Journal of the American Veterinary Medical Association* 238: 31–34.

Brooks, J.W. (ed.) (2018). *Veterinary Forensic Pathology*, Vols. 1 and 2. Cham, Switzerland: Springer.

Campbell, A.M., Thompson, S.L., Harris, T.L. et al. (2021). Intimate partner violence and pet abuse: Responding law enforcement officers' observations and victim reports from the scene. *Journal of Interpersonal Violence* 36 (5–6): 2353–2372.

Coulter, K. and Campbell, B. (2020). Public investment in animal protection work: Data from Manitoba, Canada. *Animals* 10 (3): 516.

Elliott, R., Snowdon, J., Halliday, G. et al. (2019). Characteristics of animal hoarding cases referred to the RSPCA in New South Wales, Australia. *Australian Veterinary Journal* 97 (5): 149–156.

Federal Bureau of Investigation (FBI) (n.d.). UCR Program: Criminal Information Service Division. https://ucr.fbi.gov/ucr-program-quarterly/ucr-quarterly-january-2015 (accessed 21 October 2021).

Ferreira, E.A., Paloski, L.H., Costa, D.B. et al. (2017). Animal hoarding disorder: A new psychopathology? *Psychiatry Research* 258: 221–225.

Flynn-Poppey, E., Atkins, E., Smith-Blackmore, M. et al. (2016). Massachusetts Animal Cruelty and Protection Task Force: Findings and recommendations. https://malegislature.gov/Bills/189/SD2649.pdf (accessed 3 November 2021).

Gentry, D.J. (2001). Including companion animals in protective orders: Curtailing the reach of domestic violence. *Yale JL & Feminism* 13: 97.

Gooding, B.C. (2008). Veterinary public health collaborations: An essential component of future public health preparedness. Master's thesis. University of North Carolina. https://doi.org/10.17615/b1z7-j995.

Gross, S.R. (1991). Expert evidence. *Wisconsin Law Review* 6: 1113–1232.

Gwaltney-Brant, S.M. (2007). Patterns of non-accidental injury: Poisoning in veterinary forensics. In: *Veterinary Forensics: Animal Cruelty Investigations* (ed. M.D. Merck), 185–205. Oxford, UK: Blackwell Publishing.

Hensley, C., Tallichet, S.E., and Dutkiewicz, E.L. (2011). Examining demographic and situational factors on animal cruelty motivations. *International Journal of Offender Therapy and Comparative Criminology* 55 (3): 492–502.

Hernandez, E., Fawcett, A., Brouwer, E. et al. (2018). Speaking up: Veterinary ethical responsibilities and animal welfare issues in everyday practice. *Animals* 8 (1): 15.

Intarapanich, N.P., McCobb, E.C., Reisman, R.W. et al. (2016). Characterization and comparison of injuries caused by accidental and non-accidental blunt force trauma in dogs and cats. *Journal of Forensic Sciences* 61 (4): 993–999.

Joo, S., Jung, Y., and Chun, M.S. (2020). An analysis of veterinary practitioners' intention to intervene in animal abuse cases in South Korea. *Animals* 10 (5): 802.

Kassin, S.M., Dror, I.E., and Kukucka, J. (2013). The forensic confirmation bias: Problems, perspectives, and proposed solutions. *Journal of Applied Research in Memory and Cognition* 2 (1): 42–52.

Kellert, S. and Felthous, A. (1985). Childhood cruelty toward animals among criminals and noncriminals. *Human Relations* 38: 1113–1129.

Kogan, L.R., Schoenfeld-Tacher, R.M., Hellyer, P.W. et al. (2017). Survey of attitudes toward and experiences with animal abuse encounters in a convenience sample of US veterinarians. *Journal of the American Veterinary Medical Association* 250 (6): 688–696.

*Kumho Tire Co. vs. Carmichael*, 526 US 137, (1999).

Lockwood, R. and Arkow, P. (2016). Animal abuse and interpersonal violence: The cruelty connection and its implications for veterinary pathology. *Veterinary Pathology* 53 (5): 910–918.

McDonough, S.P. and McEwen, B.J. (2016). Veterinary forensic pathology: The search for truth. *Veterinary Pathology* 53 (5): 875–877.

McEwen, B.J., Stern, A.W., Viner, T. et al. (2019). Veterinary Forensic Postmortem Examination Standards. https://www.ivfsa.org/wp-content/uploads/2020/12/IVFSA-Veterinary-Forensic-Postmortem-Exam-Standards_Approved-2020_with-authors.pdf (accessed 3 November 2021).

Merck, M. (2013). *Veterinary Forensics: Animal Cruelty Investigations*. Ames, IA: John Wiley & Sons.

Munro, H.M. (1996). Battered pets. *Veterinary Record* 138 (23): 576.

Munro, H.M.C. and Thrusfield, M.V. (2001). "Battered pets": Non-accidental physical injuries found in dogs and cats. *Journal of Small Animal Practice* 42: 279–290.

Nathanson, J.N. (2009). Animal hoarding: Slipping into the darkness of comorbid animal and self-neglect. *Journal of Elder Abuse & Neglect* 21 (4): 307–324. doi:10.1080/08946560903004839.

National Link Coalition (n.d.). The National Directory of Abuse Investigation Agencies. https://nationallinkcoalition.org/how-do-i-report-suspected-abuse (accessed 25 October 2021).

Newberry, M. (2017). Pets in danger: Exploring the link between domestic violence and animal abuse. *Aggression and Violent Behavior* 34: 273–281.

Ortiz, F. (2010). Making the dogman heel: Recommendations for improving the effectiveness of dogfighting laws. *Stanford Journal of Animal Law and Policy* 3: 1–75.

Palais, J.M. (2021). Using the national incident-based reporting system (NIBRS) to study animal cruelty: Preliminary results (2016–2019). *Social Sciences* 10 (10): 378.

Parry, N.M. and Stoll, A. (2020). The rise of veterinary forensics. *Forensic Science International* 306: 110069–110069.

Patronek, G.J. (1999). Hoarding of animals: An under-recognized public health problem in a difficult-to-study population. *Public Health Reports* 114 (1): 81.

Pollanen, M.S. (2016). The rise of forensic pathology in human medicine: Lessons for veterinary forensic pathology. *Veterinary Pathology* 53 (5): 878–879.

Randour, M.L. (2004). Including animal cruelty as a factor in assessing risk and designing interventions. Proceedings of Persistently Safe Schools, Washington, DC.

Randour, M.L., Smith-Blackmore, M., Blaney, N. et al. (2021). Animal abuse as a type of trauma: Lessons for human and animal service professionals. *Trauma, Violence, & Abuse* 22 (2): 277–288.

Richard, C. and Reese, L.A. (2019). The interpersonal context of human/nonhuman animal violence. *Anthrozoös* 32 (1): 65–87.

Rogers, E. and Stern, A.W. (eds.) (2018). *Veterinary Forensics: Investigation, Evidence Collection, and Expert Testimony*. Boca Raton, FL: CRC Press.

Rowan, A.N. (1999). Cruelty and abuse to animals: A typology. In: *Child Abuse, Domestic Violence, and Animal Abuse: Linking the Circles of Compassion for Prevention and Intervention* (eds. F.R. Ascione and P. Arkow), 328–334. West Lafayette, IN: Perdue University Press.

Tong, L. (2014). Fracture characteristics to distinguish between accidental injury and non-accidental injury in dogs. *The Veterinary Journal* 199 (3): 392–398.

Touroo, R., Baucom, K., Kessler, M. et al. (2020). Minimum standards and best practices for the clinical veterinary forensic examination of the suspected abused animal. *Forensic Science International: Reports* 2: 100150.

US Government Publishing Office (2010). Federal Rules of Evidence. Rule 702. https://www.govinfo.gov/app/details/USCODE-2010-title28/USCODE-2010-title28-app-federalru-dup2-rule702 (accessed 3 November 2021).

Wisch, R.F. (2020). Table of veterinary reporting requirement and immunity laws. https://www.animallaw.info/topic/table-veterinary-reporting-requirement-and-immunity-laws (accessed 25 October 2021).

Woolf, J. (2020). Identifying signs of animal abuse. *Today's Veterinary Practice* July.

## 21

## Death

*James W. Yeates*

### Introduction

All veterinary patients die. Veterinarians may save lives, deliberately or unintentionally end them, or support practices that involve an animal's premature death. Legally and culturally, the veterinary profession is the only one authorized to or that regularly kills its patients. This might be seen as contrary to, or as part of the veterinary professional's role as a helper or healer. This chapter considers death in the context of veterinary ethics. It describes differing types of death and considers a range of ways in which death might be ethically significant for veterinarians or clients. The first sections are quite philosophical (more practically minded readers might choose to start later on and come back to them). Later sections consider the general types of ethical dilemmas veterinarians face in relation to death. Finally, some approaches to ethical decision-making are described and then applied to a specific example.

### Types of Death

We might differentiate death according to its method, context, and aim or purpose. For example, "humane slaughter" relates to (i) painless active killing of (ii) farmed animals for (iii) consumption.

Similarly, veterinary professionals might define euthanasia as death that (i) minimizes suffering, (ii) is in the animal's interests, and/or (iii) is caused intentionally for the animal's benefit. The American Veterinary Medical Association (AVMA) defines euthanasia as "the humane termination of an animal's life" and more precisely as "A method of killing that minimizes pain, distress, and anxiety experienced by the animal prior to loss of consciousness" (AVMA 2020). The second criterion (ii) is often considered in terms of avoiding later illness. For example, the Royal College of Veterinary Surgeons (RCVS) defines euthanasia as "painless killing to relieve suffering" (RCVS 2021). More widely, veterinary professionals might say euthanasia avoids life that would have overall negative value. The third criterion (iii) would mean that, for example, "humane slaughter" would not count as euthanasia even when it is humane and prevents an animal from continuing a miserable existence on a farm because the aim is not for the animal's benefit.

The term euthanasia is used in a wider range of cases than the above. It is applied to the killing of laboratory animals who are "surplus" or after use (which may be done

*Ethics in Veterinary Practice: Balancing Conflicting Interests*, First Edition. Edited by Barry Kipperman and Bernard E. Rollin.
© 2022 John Wiley & Sons, Inc. Published 2022 by John Wiley & Sons, Inc.

humanely, but often is arguably not; Ambrose et al. 2000), of healthy animals per owner requests, and killing animals in shelters where intake exceeds expected rehoming opportunities. Whether these constitute euthanasia obviously depends on the criteria used and the case. The use of the term creates risks of misunderstanding and of killing being justified as euthanasia when it fulfills only one of the above criteria, such as use of humane methods.

These etymological complexities have real-life implications. Using the term euthanasia might make us feel better about doing it, reducing moral stress. But it might also hide some moral concerns, insofar as "euthanasia" is a label that implies morally acceptable (or even laudable) killing. In cases that stretch or miss that definition, this might mislead people, and diminish the inclination to consider the moral aspects of the decision, making the thus-labeled killing more prevalent.

We might also differentiate whether the method of killing is *active* killing/euthanasia (e.g. a percussive blow or barbiturate overdose) or *passive* (e.g. withholding treatment). Sometimes owners also make the distinction between killing as an intervention and "natural" death due to biological processes. In many cases, a passive, natural death may be expected to involve greater suffering than an active intervention.

We might further categorize different active methods of killing (percussion, anoxia, toxic, chemical, etc.), which can have different welfare effects. Some common methods cause significant suffering (e.g. $CO_2$ insufflation) but may be more convenient or less unpleasant for humans (AVMA 2020).

We might also classify death in terms of the authority for the killing. While this authority might be based on the animal's expected quality of life (e.g. veterinarians may be able to morally legitimize killing any animal to avoid severe suffering), the legal situation may differentiate killing based on whether it has the owner's permission.

## Ethical Significance of Death

We might think of death as ethically important in different ways and for different individuals. While veterinary professionals might believe that only their view is morally relevant, it is important to consider and understand other stakeholders' views and to identify potential biases in our decision-making.

### Death as a Welfare Concern for the Patient

#### As Indicator of Prior Suffering

The process or cause of dying may be associated with unpleasant experiences or be caused by long-term conditions that involve suffering. Veterinary professionals might therefore see death as an indicator or symptom of (previous) welfare problems, and so avoid or reduce death in association with preventing its causes (e.g. reducing mortality rates by tackling flock diseases).

#### As the Avoidance of Continued Life

Another approach is to consider death in terms of what life it excludes (Yeates 2010a). Where it prevents suffering, it can be considered to be beneficial. Where death prevents enjoyable life, it represents an opportunity cost or deprivation. This approach may be linked to a common intuition that killing a "healthy" animal seems worse than killing an "unhealthy" one (although the term "healthy" can be ambiguous, especially with regard to mental health). These ideas are often considered in terms of whether an animal's life is (or was or is going to be) "worth living" or "worth avoiding" for the animal (Yeates 2011; Mellor 2016).

Defining when an animal's life is worth living or worth avoiding is difficult, involving complex predictions and subjective judgments. In practice, there may be some considerable gray zone between lives veterinary professionals can confidently say are worth living or avoiding for the animal. Nevertheless, many of us feel those judgments can be made at least in some cases.

We might also differentiate cases where the animal *cannot* conceivably have a good future quality of life (e.g. some incurable, painful condition) versus those in which the patient *could have* had a good quality of life, but the circumstances mean this is effectively not an available option for the veterinarian (not without undue sacrifices by the vet, for example by providing extensive free treatment).

### As Frustration of Preferences for Life

Another way in which veterinary professionals might consider death is in terms of whether it fulfills or prevents the satisfaction of the animal's preference. There is limited evidence that veterinary patients have life/death preferences or the cognitive abilities needed for a life/death preference such as a concept of one's self, but veterinary professionals might consider animals as having preferences for which life is necessary (Simmons 2009), and death prevents the fulfillment of those desires.

## Death as a Nonwelfare, Animal-Based Ethical Concern

### Value of Life

Another paradigm is to consider that life has intrinsic value, and its shortening therefore destroys that value (Taylor 1983; Butterworth and Yeates 2018). It is hard to say here for *whom* the life has value. If it is for the animal, then the deprivation-based approach noted above seems more germane. If not for the animals, then this approach might conflict with concerns for the animal (e.g. that veterinary professionals should keep animals alive even when they would be "better off dead"). Veterinarians tend not to talk about an inherent value of life for animals (Rathwell-Deault et al. 2017a, 2017b).

### Right to Life

A related model is to consider that animals have a right to life, either a positive right to be kept alive or a negative right not to be killed. This right might be limited to those animals who can conceivably *claim* this right, which would exclude veterinary patients (and, arguably, neonatal humans). Alternatively, this right might be afforded only to animals who are the "subject-of-a-life" (Regan 2017 [1983], 1997). Another paradigm is to generalize from concepts applied to humans based on animals' reasoning (Pluhar 1995).

## Ethical Concerns in Relation to Other Stakeholders

While death relates primarily to the animals who die, it also affects other stakeholders.

### Owner and Client Preferences

Owners might have a preference as to whether their animal lives or dies. Veterinary professionals might think owners have a moral right to decide, since the animal is their property, because they are best placed to make decisions in their animal's best interests, or because veterinary professionals have a contractual relationship with them. Often these factors get combined or conflated, but differentiating them may help us make decisions in difficult cases such as when owners are absent or seem irresponsible.

### Impacts on Owners and Others Who Work with Animals

Death might cause human caregivers grief and loss of companionship. Ongoing life might necessitate their expenditure of money or time, affecting their own quality of life (Christiansen et al. 2013), or give them enjoyment or profit. Veterinary professionals might think such concerns should factor into their decisions alongside the animal's interests, or that veterinary professionals should prioritize the patient's interests (e.g. not keep a suffering animal alive for the owner's profit). Studies have documented a high prevalence of occupational stress and euthanasia-related strain among people working in animal shelters, veterinary clinics, and biomedical research facilities (Scotney et al. 2015; LaFollette et al. 2020).

### Impacts on Veterinarians' Interests

We might similarly be concerned with the impact of euthanasia on veterinary professionals (Rathwell-Deault et al. 2017a, 2017b). Veterinary professionals might find saving animals to be rewarding or beneficial to their self-image, morale, reputation, research, or career, although it can be argued that veterinary professionals should morally not take such factors into account in most cases (e.g. not keep animals alive to boost practice profit). Veterinary professionals may experience negative emotional effects related to various aspects of death due to:

- Their frequent exposure to death (Hart et al. 1987; Fogle and Abrahamson 1990; Nett et al. 2015).
- Avoidable suffering can be stressful to observe and can relate to feelings of powerlessness or compassion fatigue.
- Making decisions about euthanasia can cause moral stress (Bartram and Baldwin 2010; Morris 2012a; Kipperman et al. 2018).
- The act of killing animals can involve anxiety or lead to guilt (Herzog et al. 1989; Cholbi 2017).
- The emotional energy expended in counseling and navigating owner decision-making (Morris 2012b).
- Whether or not to report owners when they will not allow suffering animals to be euthanized.
- Killing animals might also be linked to attitudes to suicide, although this may be less due to the act than the stressful dilemmas (Bartram and Baldwin 2010; Platt et al. 2012).

Even if veterinary professionals do not factor these into patient decisions, the profession should aim to minimize their negative effects.

### Death as Indicator of Owner/Vet Attitudes

We might also see death as an indicator of the veterinarian's, or owner's, values. Some owners seem to think that providing more treatment or declining euthanasia somehow shows they love their animal more. Vets might view euthanasia as evidence of failure and treatment as more heroic. Some owners seem reluctant to euthanize their animal for problems that they have caused or failed to prevent, as if that would mean their failure is less severe (or at least recognize it as such). One might also see euthanasia as taking responsibility (rather than ducking it).

### Death as a Cause of Owner/Veterinarian Attitudes

Another idea is that killing animals somehow desensitizes the killer to killing. This might be linked to explicit acceptance or rationalization of killing in general and/or to cognitive biases that defend previous acts of killing to avoid cognitive dissonance. There are some data suggesting that vets become more at ease with killing animals with time (Ogden et al. 2012). This may provide a useful coping mechanism for the stresses of practice that helps veterinary professionals' mental health and resilience. Conversely, it may make us less likely to reconsider our ethics and perhaps more likely to engage in killing that we believe is morally wrong.

### Societal Impacts

We might also worry that killing animals might promote or reinforce societal attitudes that animals are unimportant or disposable. Veterinary professionals might also worry that a lack of regard for animal life could also encourage a lack of concern for, say, animal suffering or responsible ownership. Conversely, refusing to kill an animal might make a difference in terms of how owners see animals, e.g. in promoting responsibility.

### Reputation of the Veterinary Profession

Killing animals may detract from veterinary professionals' image as healers or make us seem uncaring. Conversely, attempting to save animals through expensive treatment may be perceived as profiteering and clients may see vets as incompetent or exploitative if the animal still dies. Vets might also be criticized for seeming to "coerce" owners into or against euthanasia unduly. Ignoring clients' wishes might conceivably make owners less willing to present animals for treatment. Veterinary professionals might think that the best reputation for the profession is to be known to always do what is right, regardless of the reputational element – but veterinary professionals know what is right is not always perceived as such by others.

## Veterinary Roles and Dilemmas

Veterinarians in practice have a variety of roles and face various ethical dilemmas related to end-of-life decisions. These can often involve (combinations of) the following:

### Shortening Animals' Lives

Veterinarians often face dilemmas regarding whether to kill an animal actively. In other cases, vets have to make the difficult decision on whether to provide a treatment that may reduce an animal's longevity (e.g. providing analgesics that may quicken renal deterioration or surgery that has a risk of perioperative death). Some cases may seem easy (e.g. euthanasia with owner permission to avoid extreme suffering in a terminal case): others may involve more complicated trade-offs (e.g. the choice is between a short, happier life and a longer, less happy one), prompting the question of whether the "total happiness" is better overall.

A secondary dilemma may relate to the method of death. It can be hard to evaluate what method is always best, although some clearly cause considerable pain or suffering (e.g. hypercapnia and asphyxiation). In practice, this dilemma may simply be a predictive factual question of which method would cause the least suffering. Veterinary professionals might also reframe some dilemmas about whether to kill or allow an animal to die "naturally" in terms of the method and the suffering involved. A "natural" death may involve considerably more suffering, so a dilemma over whether to kill might reflect, on one side, a motivation not to actively kill an animal and, on the other, a desire to prevent a longer dying process involving considerably more suffering.

## Saving Lives

Other dilemmas concern whether to save an animal from dying. Considering the animal, the outcome of death is the same. However, veterinarians might feel that there is a difference insofar as killing involves a deliberate act, whereas failing to save is an omission. Vets might intuitively feel they have less responsibility to extend lives than to avoid shortening them (and so veterinary professionals feel less guilty when patients die than if they killed them), especially knowing it is impossible for us to save every patient, whereas it is possible to kill none of them.

## Interacting with Owners

Human medicine differentiates euthanasia based on whether it is voluntary (patient consent), involuntary (contrary to the patient's wishes), or nonvoluntary (patient has no expressed wishes). The questions around animals' concepts of death mean these definitions are unhelpful when applied to the patient (Persson et al. 2020), but veterinary professionals might apply them to the owner: for example, if veterinary professionals think owners should be able to insist on and/or refuse euthanasia (but not necessarily both), or to consider cases where an owner is not available and in which it might seem illogical not to euthanize a suffering animal in the absence of consent.

Veterinarians have a duty to guide pet owners facing the loss of their animal (Fernandez-Mehler et al. 2013). While this chapter is not about owners' decisions per se, it is worth noting that veterinarians may have very different views from other people (Duerr et al. 2011); owners may choose euthanasia because they feel morally "overwhelmed" (Rohrer Bley 2018), or because death is irreversible and therefore "final," and veterinary professionals can help owners to avoid biases such as that euthanasia indicates less love than life-saving treatment (Yeates 2013).

At the same time, owners can apply considerable moral pressure on veterinarians. They may request euthanasia for an animal that the veterinary professional considers could have a life worth living. They may try to make us feel guilty for not offering free or subsidized treatment. They may threaten public criticism, litigation, or official complaints. They may simply make discussions unnecessarily challenging or unpleasant. In all cases, veterinary professionals might feel they should simply do what is right. Sometimes, veterinary professionals might legitimately take such risks into account (although doing so can seem unfair insofar as such clients then benefit from such behavior whereas "nicer" clients do not). Other times, veterinary professionals should stand steadfast with integrity.

Another veterinary role is to moderate the emotional impacts of death on owners, particularly in their feelings of loss and bereavement. Veterinary professionals might also consider factors such as owners having "a chance to say goodbye" and practical considerations (e.g. before a weekend). Most owners now stay with their pet during euthanasia (Dickinson et al. 2014), so veterinary professionals can reduce owners' distress by performing euthanasia well (Brackenridge and Shoemaker 1996; Endenburg et al. 1999). Owners value support from veterinarians after their animal's death (Adams et al. 2000). Practices may also direct clients to grief support services (Dickinson et al. 2014). Veterinarians and veterinary nurses can play particularly important roles in supporting owners to feel that their decision was the correct one, and validating their feelings of loss.

## Managing Our Emotions

It is quite logical to presume that frequent exposure to death and end-of-life decisions would cause anxiety and moral stress for veterinary professionals (Rollin 2011; Morris 2012a), and many veterinarians have some discomfort with killing in some scenarios (Hartnack et al. 2016; Persson et al. 2020). Some veterinarians report feeling coerced by their employer or practice manager to proceed with euthanasia decisions they do not feel serve the patient's best interest (Kipperman 2017). The veterinary or shelter team can be an important source of mutual support (Anderson et al. 2013; Hartnack et al. 2016) (see Chapter 22 for a discussion of emotional self-care).

## Handling of Cadavers

Many societies ascribe value to how cadavers are treated. Owners may wish to have bodies or ashes back or be opposed to postmortems or educational uses for spiritual or psychological reasons. More broadly, veterinary professionals might feel there is something wrong with "disrespectful" handling of cadavers, not in terms of its impact on the animal (who cannot experience such handling and probably had no predeath preferences on their postmortem disposal), but in terms of indirectly indicating or encouraging negative attitudes or lack of respect for owner wishes.

## Euthanasia Fees

While euthanasia may allow a fee, veterinarians arguably often undercharge for euthanasia services, given the time veterinary professionals can spend on doing it well and sympathetically. However, charging for euthanasia may discourage presentation (e.g. by members of the public finding casualty wildlife) or lead owners to choose less humane options.

## Improving Decision-making

Available quality-of-life assessment tools include scoring systems (Morton 2007), checklists (Yeates 2013), and frameworks (Morgan 2005; van Herten 2015). Information on communication skills related to end-of-life decisions can be found in Shaw et al. (2007) and Nogueira Borden et al. (2010). Perhaps the most valuable method is discussion with other colleagues. Historically, euthanasia ethics was insufficiently discussed (Fogle and Abrahamson 1990) but now that its importance is recognized, peer discussions are more obviously legitimate and beneficial.

End-of-life decisions for veterinarians may be helped by training in ethical thinking and communication, end-of-life protocols, consent form templates and resources for pet owners, psychological support of veterinarians, quality-of-life assessment and decision-making guides and tools, and updates in relevant legislation (Yeates 2010b; Rollin 2011; Knesl et al. 2018; Persson et al. 2020). Figure 21.1 is an algorithm to provide guidance regarding euthanasia decisions.

## Specific Scenarios

With this philosophical analysis to draw upon, we can consider some specific scenarios to imagine how veterinary professionals would personally address such cases.

### Ill Animals

In many cases, veterinarians face decisions about killing animals who have conditions that are expected to involve ongoing or future suffering, which can therefore be described as (genuine) euthanasia cases. Veterinarians may find some of these decisions morally relatively simple in terms of *whether* to euthanize an animal, even if it can be hard to know exactly *when* to euthanize an animal. These decisions may depend primarily on patient condition and prognostic factors (Mallery 1999), or on owner preferences.

### Lack of Consent for Euthanasia

We might feel that euthanasia would be best for a patient, but the owner might prefer continued life (Case Study 21.1). Sometimes this preference might be based on misunderstanding or the false hope that the veterinarian can "correct" the problem. Sometimes it may be that this disagreement is a "cover" from another concern (e.g. if the owner feels guilty for not having prevented the cause of the suffering that indicates euthanasia, then they may be disinclined toward euthanasia as it subconsciously confirms their self-perceived failure). Other times it may be a simple ethical disagreement about what is valuable (e.g. if they think life is sacred).

In such cases, euthanizing may be better for the animal but risks harm to the owner, and perhaps damage to the reputation of the profession. So, what veterinary professionals do may depend on their ethical views – whether and when duties to patients should outweigh the constraints of the doctrine of consent, within the relevant contemporaneous legal and regulatory context.

## Decision Tree

**This Decision Tree has been devised in order to give guidance to vets when faced with euthanasia as a management option for an animal under their care.**

It may be useful to consider the following scenarios when using the Decision Tree:

- Owned but unwanted healthy animal.
- Owned terminally ill, suffering animal; owner wants euthanasia.
- Owned terminally ill, suffering animal; owner refuses euthanasia.
- Owned terminally ill, mildly suffering animal; owner refuses euthanasia; owner very attached.
- Owned terminally ill, suffering animal; owner not available.
- Owned animal with illness with minor effect on quality of life — for example, mild heart failure; owner wants euthanasia.
- Owned healthy animal with incontinence/minor behavioural problem — owner requests euthanasia.
- Unowned wild animal with major injuries.
- Unowned wild non-indigenous species (for example, grey squirrel).
- Injured wild non-indigenous/pest species.

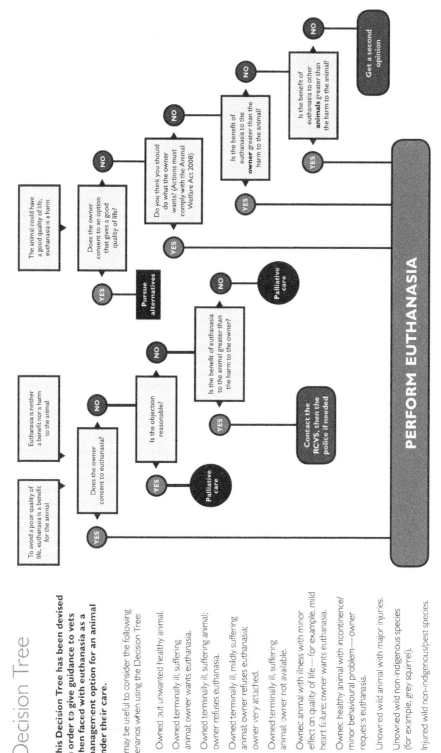

**Figure 21.1** Decision tree to provide guidance to veterinarians faced with euthanasia decisions (*Source:* British Veterinary Association [BVA] 2016).

We might also differentiate when an owner has not given consent (e.g. a stray's owner cannot be located) from when they have explicitly refused. Veterinary professionals might think euthanasia legitimate in the former setting but not the latter. A secondary related question is what effort and delay veterinary professionals should allow in trying to ascertain their preference or gain their permission.

Sometimes an owner might refuse euthanasia because they want an alternative option that the veterinarian believes is ethically wrong. For example, they might want more "invasive" or "intensive" treatment that veterinary professionals feel would cause unjustified suffering. Veterinary professionals should avoid being pressured into providing such "overtreatment" because clients will not allow euthanasia. Sometimes it may be better to be clear that such treatments are wrong, and this may help owners to realize that euthanasia is the best option.

### Convenience Requests and Owners Unwilling to Pay for Treatment

Owners may request that veterinarians kill animals for their own benefit or convenience. Usually in veterinary practice this is to avoid the cost or time of continued care. In some cases, veterinary professionals might worry that the animal will be otherwise killed in a way that causes greater suffering (Kipperman et al. 2018) and owners may sometimes explicitly threaten this. Veterinary professionals might think that the owner's motivation is ethically questionable or wrong, particularly when the owner could otherwise allow or help the animal to have an enjoyable life worth living. In some cases, veterinary professionals might be able to change the owner's preference, for example by providing information, offering free treatment, or "influencing" their decision-making. However, veterinary professionals would be naive or immodest to think they can achieve this in all cases (without threatening the financial sustainability of the practice). Veterinary professionals might feel they should not accede to such requests, because they are not worthy of our respect and/or we do not want to encourage such behaviors. While 80% of small animal veterinarians in a recent study indicated having declined a euthanasia request, these decisions were uncommon, with a median frequency of every few years (Kipperman et al. 2018).

Alternatively, veterinary professionals might separate their judgment about the owner from their decision about what to do: for example, veterinary professionals might recognize that an owner could do better but still feel that – if they cannot change the owner's decision – euthanasia is still the best option. For example, veterinary professionals might feel that an owner should fund veterinary treatment but if they will not (and veterinary professionals do not feel they should provide it for free), then euthanasia may be better than ongoing suffering. In such cases, a euthanasia decision might be contextually right even if veterinary professionals feel the owner's decision is not. Recognizing this may help us avoid inappropriate guilt, although providing euthanasia in such cases can still be stressful (Batchelor and McKeegan 2012; Tran et al. 2014).

### Destruction of Healthy Animals/Depopulation/Culling

Another scenario includes killing healthy animals for whom death is not indicated via euthanasia but where their death helps prevent risks to humans or other animals. These might include aggressive animals, situations of overpopulation, or to contain the spread of transmissible or zoonotic diseases. Veterinary professionals might think they should only kill an animal when in its best interests, which would preclude such culling. Alternatively, veterinary professionals might think that they should factor in the harms to the animals killed as part of an overall objective, which might be a utilitarian calculus or an anthropocentric prioritization of human interests.

## Slaughter

Slaughter is obviously the ending of animals' lives. Vets may only rarely be involved in routine slaughter but support industries that perform it. Vegans may object to this as unnecessary death (as might vegetarians, disregarding the slaughter of animals used in milk and egg production). Alternatively, veterinary professionals might feel that farming at least means the animals have some life – although this argument only works if the life is worth living, i.e. farming conditions provide overall enjoyable lives. Oddly, when farming conditions are worse, veterinary professionals can see slaughter as in the animal's interest as it avoids a longer life of suffering, although this should be more a motivation to improve conditions rather than a justification for the killing as a good. As another alternative, veterinary professionals might think that each batch of animal's deaths is necessary in practice for more animals to come into existence (otherwise farms would be unsustainable and overpopulated) and so they legitimize each animal's death as part of an overall system that gives animals good lives. Again, this argument only works if those lives are, in fact, enjoyable.

---

**Case Study 21.1   Unauthorized euthanasia of a dog in congestive heart failure**

Dr. G is treating Paco, a 12-year-old male Chihuahua hospitalized for congestive heart failure. His condition is critical due to labored breathing from fluid in his lungs, and Dr. G believes that euthanasia is in Paco's best interest. Dr. G informs the owner of Paco's diagnosis and prognosis, and the owner approves overnight care and oxygen support but refuses to consent to euthanasia and states that they never will. Dr. G considers reporting the owner to authorities but decides to wait and see how Paco fares overnight.

At 2 a.m., the on-site technician calls Dr. G at home to let her know that Paco's condition has declined despite therapy. The technician expresses that Paco is suffering from air hunger/dyspnea, is coughing up pink fluid, and appears to be suffering and in terminal extremis. Dr. G orders that the technician perform humane euthanasia, and tells the owner in the morning that Paco died of congestive heart failure.

Interests:

Paco:

- To avoid suffering.
- To have the chance for continued life (but this is considered very remote).

Owner:

- To keep their beloved pet slightly longer.
- To feel they have "done everything they can."

- To avoid making a difficult decision.
- To avoid being reported to authorities.

Vet team:

- To feel they have done the best for their patient.
- To avoid seeing or allowing unnecessary suffering.
- To avoid the distress of legal cases.
- To avoid losing their license for dishonesty.
- To mitigate moral stress (see Chapter 22).

Options:

Dr. G had various options:

Earlier:

1. Provide euthanasia there and then without permission and with the owner's knowledge.
2. Provide nonlethal treatment (in this case hospitalization).
3. Report the owner.
4. Refuse to be part of allowing suffering and refer Paco to another colleague or send Paco home.

That night:

a. Let Paco die.
b. Phone the owner to try (but probably fail) to obtain consent for euthanasia.
c. Euthanize Paco.
d. Give Paco a very high dose of analgesic and/or anxiolytic that was expected to be a lethal dose.

Ethical Analysis:

While this chapter is about death rather than communication, rarely (if ever) are death-related cases free from other moral concerns. In this case, the patient outcome aligned with Paco's best interest (as perceived by Dr. G) to avoid suffering and was equivalent to a passively allowed ("natural") death from the owner's perspective. Indeed, one could argue that Dr. G has taken on full responsibility for decision-making in the interests of her patient and achieved that end while also avoiding the owner having to suffer the distress of making a difficult decision or of being reported. The outcome was best for everyone (depending on definition of "best") – some might even call it a "win–win" – and Dr. G arguably was benevolent to both patient and client.

Conversely, if one considers that decision-making should be led primarily by owner wishes (e.g. because they have absolute rights over their property), then Dr. G has contravened their autonomous decision and expressed preference. It is not so clear that veterinary professionals can say that they should define what is best for their patient. Veterinary professionals might also consider that the duty to the patient should override the duty to the client. Ideally, Dr. G should have anticipated a decline in Paco's condition and set out a mutually agreed upon plan of action should this occur.

There is also the additional argument that ignoring client wishes in this way creates personal risks for Dr. G if reported by the technician, in particular losing her license, and client dissatisfaction has consequences of potential employer displeasure jeopardizing Dr. G's job security. In other contexts, taking risks for oneself to benefit others is considered admirable or heroic. Nonetheless, in this case, that outcome would also mean Dr. G would be unable in the future to help other patients. The risk of reduced client trust might also lead to owners not presenting animals for treatment, but there is limited evidence that such events would reduce the likelihood of owners presenting animals. In any case, these risks only crystallize if Dr. G is actually found out. There is also a concern regarding whether this decision impacts the technician's perception of Dr. G and the veterinary profession as being honest and trustworthy or has caused her moral stress, though it can be argued that Dr. G's decision spared the technician from the emotional trauma of being powerless to end Paco's suffering.

Reporting the owner to local authorities may have eventually led to euthanasia after considerable delay or pressured the owner into a decision sooner. Refusing to be part of allowing suffering and referring Paco to another hospital might have made Dr. G avoid feelings of complicity in prolonging suffering. This decision could risk Paco expiring from heart failure (an unpleasant death) during transport, which could have liability consequences for Dr. G as well as causing emotional trauma for the owner, who may witness Paco's demise.

In this case, Dr. G knowingly and deliberately caused Paco's death. Option D might have felt more acceptable, insofar as it was technically not intended to cause death – the intent was to alleviate anxiety. The dose may well have caused death, but this was only expected and not, strictly speaking, intended. One might say the painkillers would have had two effects: (i) an intended effect of reducing anxiety; and (ii) an unintended but foreseen effect of causing death. As such it was not deliberate killing. However, veterinary professionals might question whether this would have been different insofar as Dr. G did (also) want to cause death – so this approach may feel like mere sophistry. One might also question whether this satisfies the veterinary professional's concerns for owner autonomy (e.g. the validity of consent for analgesia if that was provided without the information that the dose could likely be lethal).

In this case, there are two connected but arguably independent decisions: whether to euthanize Paco without consent and what to tell the owner. We might agree with Dr. G on either, neither, or both. For example, we might think it is right to proceed against the owner's wishes on the euthanasia but not to misinform them, i.e. if we think that patient welfare should "trump" owner wishes, but our own interests should not.

# References

Adams, C.L., Bonnett, B.N., and Meek, A.H. (2000). Predictors of owner response to companion animal death in 177 clients from 14 practices in Ontario. *Journal of the American Veterinary Medical Association* 217: 1303–1309. doi: 10.2460/javma.2000.217.1303

Ambrose, N., Wadham, J., and Morton, D. (2000). Refinement of euthanasia. In: *Progress in the Reduction, Refinement and Replacement of Animal Experimentation* (eds. M. Balls, A.M. van Zeller, and M.E. Halder), 1159–1170. Amsterdam: Elsevier.

Anderson, K.A., Brandt, J.C., Lord, L.K. et al. (2013). Euthanasia in animal shelters: Management's perspective on staff reactions and support programs. *Anthrozoös* 26: 569–578. doi: 10.2752/175303713X13795775536057

American Veterinary Medical Association (AVMA) (2020). AVMA guidelines for the euthanasia of animals. https://www.avma.org/sites/default/files/2020-01/2020-Euthanasia-Final-1-17-20.pdf (accessed 1 May 2021).

Bartram, D.J. and Baldwin, D.S. (2010). Veterinary surgeons and suicide: A structured review of possible influences on increased risk. *Veterinary Record* 166: 388–397.

Batchelor, C.E.M. and McKeegan, D.E.F. (2012). Survey of the frequency and perceived stressfulness of ethical dilemmas encountered in UK veterinary practice. *Veterinary Record* 170: 19–22.

Brackenridge, S.S. and Shoemaker, R.S. (1996). The human/horse bond and client bereavement in equine practice. Part I. *Equine Practice* 18: 19–22.

British Veterinary Association (BVA) (2016). Guide to euthanasia. https://www.bva.co.uk/media/2981/bva_guide_to_euthanasia_2016.pdf (accessed 21 July 2021).

Butterworth, A. and Yeates, J. (2018). Longevity and brevity – Is death a welfare issue? In: *Animal Welfare in a Changing World* (ed. A. Butterworth), 190. Wallingford, UK: CAB International.

Cholbi, M. (2017). The euthanasia of companion animals. In: *Pets and People: The Ethics of Our Relationships with Companion Animals* (ed. C. Overall), 265–278. New York: Oxford University Press.

Christiansen, S.B., Kristensen, A.T., Sandøe, P. et al. (2013). Looking after chronically ill dogs: Impacts on the caregiver's life. *Anthrozoös* 26: 519–533.

Dickinson, G.E., Roof, K.W., Roof, P.D. et al. (2014). UK veterinarians' experiences with euthanasia. *Veterinary Record* 175 (7): 174.

Duerr, S., Fahrion, A., Doherr, M.G. et al. (2011). Acceptance of killing of animals: Survey among veterinarians and other professions. *Schweizer Archiv für Tierheilkunde* 153: 215–222.

Endenburg, N., Kirpensetijn, J., and Sanders, N. (1999). Equine euthanasia: The veterinarian's role in providing owner support. *Anthrozoös* 12: 138–142.

Fernandez-Mehler, P., Gloor, P., Sager, E. et al. (2013). Veterinarians' role for pet owners facing pet loss. *Veterinary Record* 172: 555–561.

Fogle, B. and Abrahamson, D. (1990). Pet loss: A survey of the attitudes and feelings of practicing veterinarians. *Anthrozoös* 3: 143–150. doi: 10.2752/089279390787057568

Hart, L. and Hart, B. (1987). Grief and stress from so many animal deaths. *Companion Animal Practice* 1: 20–21.

Hartnack, S., Springer, S., Pittavino, M. et al. (2016). Attitudes of Austrian veterinarians towards euthanasia in small animal practice: Impacts of age and gender on views on euthanasia. *BMC Veterinary Research* 12 (1): 1–14.

Herzog, H.A., Jr, Vore, T.L., and New, J.C., Jr. (1989). Conversations with veterinary students: Attitudes, ethics, and animals. *Anthrozoös* 2: 181–188. doi: 10.2752/089279389787058019

Kipperman, B. (2017). Ethical dilemmas encountered by small animal veterinarians: Characterization, responses, consequences and beliefs regarding euthanasia. MSc thesis. University of Edinburgh.

Kipperman, B., Morris, P., and Rollin, B. (2018). Ethical dilemmas encountered by small animal veterinarians: Characterisation, responses, consequences and beliefs regarding euthanasia. *Veterinary Record* 182 (19): 548.

Knesl, O., Hart, B.L., Fine, A.H. et al. (2018). Veterinarians and humane endings: When is it the right time to euthanize a companion animal? *Frontiers in Veterinary Science* 4: 45.

LaFollette, M.R., Riley, M.C., Cloutier, S. et al. (2020). Laboratory animal welfare meets human welfare: A cross-sectional study of professional quality of life, including compassion fatigue in laboratory animal personnel. *Frontiers in Veterinary Science* 7: 114.

Mallery, K.F. (1999). Factors contributing to the decision for euthanasia of dogs with congestive heart failure. *Journal of the American Veterinary Medical Association* 214 (8): 1201–1204.

Mellor, D.J. (2016). Updating animal welfare thinking: Moving beyond the "Five Freedoms" towards "a Life Worth Living". *Animals* 6 (3): 21.

Morgan, C. (2005). A guide to moral decision making for veterinarians. *Society for Veterinary Medical Ethics Newsletter* 12 (1): 3–4.

Morris, P. (2012a). *Blue Juice: Euthanasia in Veterinary Medicine*. Philadelphia, PA: Temple University Press.

Morris, P. (2012b). Managing pet owners' guilt and grief in veterinary euthanasia encounters. *Journal of Contemporary Ethnography* 42: 337–365.

Morton, D.B. (2007). A hypothetical strategy for the objective evaluation of animal well-being and quality of life using a dog model. *Animal Welfare* 16 (Suppl. 1): 75–81.

Nett, R.J., Witte, T.K., Holzbauer, S.M. et al. (2015). Risk factors for suicide, attitudes toward mental illness, and practice-related stressors among US veterinarians. *Journal of the American Veterinary Medical Association* 247 (8): 945–955.

Nogueira Borden, L.J., Adams, C.L., Bonnet, B.N. et al. (2010). Use of the measure of patient-centered communication to analyze euthanasia discussions in companion animal practice. *Journal of the American Veterinary Medical Association* 237: 1275–1287.

Ogden, U., Kinnison, T., and May, S.A. (2012). Attitudes to animal euthanasia do not correlate with acceptance of human euthanasia or suicide. *Veterinary Record* 171 (7): 174.

Persson, K., Selter, F., Neitzke, G. et al. (2020). Philosophy of a "good death" in small animals and consequences for euthanasia in animal law and veterinary practice. *Animals* 10 (1): 124.

Platt, B., Hawton, K., Simkin, S. et al. (2012). Suicidal behaviour and psychosocial problems in veterinary surgeons: A systematic review. *Social Psychiatry and Psychiatric Epidemiology* 47: 223–240. doi: 10.1007/s00127-010-0328-6

Pluhar, E.B. (1995). *Beyond Prejudice: The Moral Significance of Human and Nonhuman Animals*. Durham, NC: Duke University Press.

Rathwell-Deault, D., Godard, B., Frank, D. et al. (2017a). Expected consequences of convenience euthanasia perceived by veterinarians in Quebec. *Canadian Veterinary Journal* 58 (7): 723.

Rathwell-Deault, D.G., Doizé, B., and Frank, D. (2017b). Conceptualization of convenience euthanasia as an ethical dilemma for Quebec veterinarians. *Canadian Veterinary Journal* 58: 255–260.

Regan, T. (1997). The rights of humans and other animals. *Ethics & Behavior* 7 (2): 103–111.

Regan, T. (2017 [1983]). *The Case for Animal Rights*. 17–30. Abingdon, UK: Routledge.

Rohrer Bley, C. (2018). Principles for ethical treatment decision-making in veterinary oncology. *Veterinary and Comparative Oncology* 16 (2): 171–177.

Rollin, B.E. (2011). Euthanasia, moral stress, and chronic illness in veterinary medicine. *Veterinary Clinics of North America: Small Animal Practice* 41: 651–658.

Royal College of Veterinary Surgeons (RCVS) (2021). Euthanasia of animals. 8. Euthanasia of animals – Professionals. https://www.rcvs.org.uk/setting-standards/ advice-and-guidance/code-of-professional-conduct-for-veterinary-surgeons/supporting-guidance/euthanasia-of-animals (accessed 1 May 2021).

Scotney, R.L., McLaughlin, D., and Keates, H.L. (2015). A systematic review of the effects of euthanasia and occupational stress in personnel working with animals in animal shelters, veterinary clinics, and biomedical research facilities. *Journal of the American Veterinary Medical Association* 247 (10): 1121–1130.

Shaw, J.R. and Lagoni, L. (2007). End-of-life communication in veterinary medicine: Delivering bad news and euthanasia decision making. *Veterinary Clinics of North America: Small Animal Practice* 37 (1): 95–108.

Simmons, A. (2009). Do animals have an interest in continued life? In defense of a desire-based approach. *Environmental Ethics* 31: 375–392.

Taylor, P.W. (1983). In defense of biocentrism. *Environmental Ethics* 5: 237–243.

Tran, L., Crane, M.F., and Phillips, J.K. (2014). The distinct role of performing euthanasia on depression and suicide in veterinarians. *Journal of Occupational Health Psychology* 19 (2): 123–132.

van Herten, J. (2015). Killing of companion animals: To be avoided at all costs? In: *The End of Animal Life: A Start for Ethical Debate – Ethical and Social Considerations on Killing Animals* (eds. F. Meijboom and E. Stassen), 203–223. Wageningen, the Netherlands: Wageningen Academic Publishers.

Yeates, J.W. (2010a). Death is a welfare issue. *Journal of Agricultural & Environmental Ethics* 23 (3): 229–241.

Yeates, J. (2010b). Ethical aspects of euthanasia of owned animals. *In Practice* 32: 70–73.

Yeates, J.W. (2011). Is a life worth living a concept worth having? *Animal Welfare* 20 (3): 397–406.

Yeates, J. (2013). *Animal Welfare in Veterinary Practice*. Chichester, UK: Wiley-Blackwell.

## 22

# Moral Stress

*Carrie Jurney and Barry Kipperman*

## What Is Moral Stress?

The term moral stress (also referred to as moral distress) was introduced in the human nursing profession to describe a circumstance "when one knows the right thing to do, but institutional constraints make it nearly impossible to pursue the right course of action" (Jameton 1984). Moral distress has been defined as "The experience of psychological distress that results from engaging in, or failing to prevent, decisions or behaviors that transgress, ...personally held moral or ethical beliefs" (Crane et al. 2013). Moral stress is therefore recognized as a consequence of experienced conflicts involving work-related obligations or expectations that do not coincide with one's values (Rollin 2006; Fawcett and Mullan 2018).

## Moral Stress in the Veterinary Profession

Rollin (1987) introduced the concept of moral stress among veterinary professionals associated with the killing of animals for reprehensible reasons:

> The stress ... of killing healthy animals (or being asked to kill them even if one refuses to do so) is, in my experience, the most demoralizing part of [veterinary] practice. In fact, this stress is so qualitatively different from what is normally called occupationally "stressful" ... that I have called it *moral stress*, because it arises out of a fundamental conflict between one's reasons for going into animal work and what one is in fact doing or being asked to do.
>
> *(2006)*

Contributing factors to moral stress related to the killing or euthanasia of animals who could retain a good quality of life include a reverence for animals by those within the veterinary profession, the recognition that the affected animals are not benefiting from their death, the perception that one must suppress their moral outrage at those responsible for creating the ethical conflict, and a disinclination to discuss the problem with friends or family (Rollin 2011). In a study of small animal veterinarians, Morris discovered that interns experienced stress when they believed a high estimate of fees caused the client to elect for euthanasia, and nearly every veterinarian reported experiencing stress associated with frequent euthanasia procedures (Morris 2012). In

*Ethics in Veterinary Practice: Balancing Conflicting Interests*, First Edition. Edited by Barry Kipperman and Bernard E. Rollin.

accord with Rollin's observations, Morris (2012) notes that: "Veterinary work often causes distress for practitioners because it requires people who care strongly for animals to kill them when they are not sick enough to easily justify their death."

## Prevalence of Stress

There has been an increasing research interest examining the occurrence of stress within the veterinary profession and among those who work with animals. A literature review discovered a high prevalence of occupational stress and euthanasia-related strain among people working in animal shelters, veterinary clinics, and biomedical research facilities (Scotney et al. 2015). Veterinary technicians have been found to be particularly susceptible to occupational stress and burnout (Kogan et al. 2020; Hayes et al. 2020). Numerous studies have also documented moral stress among veterinary students (Yang et al. 2019; Kipperman et al. 2020; Lokhee and Hogg 2021).

Several studies have evaluated the prevalence of occupational stress among veterinarians. A recent investigation noted that 50% of veterinarians had high burnout scores (Ouedraogo et al. 2021). A study of small animal veterinarians found that 49% reported a moderate to substantial level of burnout (Kipperman et al. 2017). Another report found that when North American veterinarians were asked "How often have you felt distressed or anxious about your work?", 52% responded "often" or "always" (Moses et al. 2018). Veterinarians in the UK provided a mean score of over 4/5 when asked if veterinary work is stressful, and stress was thought to be one of the biggest difficulties in the profession (Institute for Employment Studies [IES] Report 2019). It's apparent that work-related stress is a significant challenge for the veterinary profession.

## Ethical Dilemmas and Moral Stress

A number of studies have investigated the association between specific types of ethical dilemmas and moral stress among veterinarians and veterinary students.

In one investigation, 52% of US small animal veterinarians reported that ethical dilemmas were the leading cause or were one of many equal causes of work-related stress (Kipperman et al. 2018). Veterinary students in the United States (Kipperman et al. 2020) classified almost all presented scenarios of potential ethical dilemmas with higher stress ratings than reported by small animal veterinarians (Kipperman et al. 2018). Veterinary surgeons in the UK assessed three ethical scenarios as "highly stressful": convenience euthanasia of a healthy animal, a client demanding treatment despite poor patient welfare, and financial limitations of clients compromising treatment options (Batchelor and McKeegan 2012). Among small animal veterinarians, 61% reported moderate to very high stress when encountering economic limitations compromising patient care (Kipperman et al. 2018), and 77% of small animal veterinarians in another study reported that the economic limitations of clients (see Chapter 8 for a more detailed discussion) were either a moderate or primary contributor to their burnout (Kipperman et al. 2017).

may spare the dogs from suffering in the future. In particular, severe dental disease can be a source of pain and can lead to starvation, and resolving aggressive behavior can be difficult. Moreover, the potential for the suitable adoption of two older dogs (one that is aggressive) ideally into the same household may seem remote, could result in a prolonged length of stay in a shelter, or may place potential adopters in jeopardy of being bitten. Euthanasia may therefore be perceived as an acceptable alternative to resolving a bad situation and one may believe that the identical outcome would occur were these dogs to be taken to a shelter. The utilization of temporary foster care of dogs who are not likely to be adopted because of their age or health has been shown to have a marked effect on improving odds of live release from shelters (Patronek and Crowe 2018).

Two studies have confirmed fear that the client may seek other options which could worsen the animal's welfare as rationales for veterinarians to proceed with euthanasia (Yeates and Main 2011; Kipperman et al. 2018). Given Mr. D's fragile emotional state, it is conceivable that euthanasia may spare the dogs from a less humane ending. This reasoning has to be balanced by the knowledge that we are responsible for our own choices, not for the decisions and actions of others. You as the attending veterinarian have to live with the consequences of *your* actions.

Informing the client that you are not comfortable complying with this request based on your belief that the dogs' present quality of life is still good, may be perceived as confrontational and jeopardize your and the practice's relationship with the client, is difficult to accomplish, and may be considered to place your job and financial security at risk if your employer is displeased. Providing parameters for when euthanasia should be considered is a reasonable course of action that respects both Mr. D's feelings and the dogs' interest in enjoying the remainder of their lives. What if you provide discrete criteria regarding symptoms of illness that justify euthanasia in the future, but Mr. D. does not recognize or chooses not to act when such symptoms arise? Sometimes, well intended choices can have unintended consequences for animal welfare.

Proposing adoption by another party would sever the bond the dogs have with the owner, may be viewed as impugning Mr. D's capacity as a caretaker, and adapting to a new environment would likely be traumatic for the dogs. Is some life better than a certain death? Some owners mistakenly believe that their pets could never be happy with another owner. Most would agree that quality of life is more important for animals than quantity. Animals can be quite adaptable to living in varied settings, but a successful adoption is by no means assured if the dogs are taken to a shelter.

Advising that Mr. D see another veterinarian may convince him that a euthanasia decision is inappropriate, only provided that another colleague would not proceed with euthanasia. If your colleague were to consent to this request, Mr. D may feel resentment about your unwillingness to accommodate his request and perceive you were insensitive to his emotional state. Perhaps for this reason, I have experienced colleagues defending euthanasia decisions reasoning that "If I don't do it, someone else will." Offering resources for financial assistance may be useful but doesn't address the emotional problems that Mr. D is experiencing, which may impact the dogs' welfare.

There are no easy answers to this challenging ethical dilemma with high potential to elicit moral stress.

## Consequences of Moral Stress

Studies in veterinary medicine have suggested or documented that moral distress is inversely associated with well-being and correlates with career dissatisfaction and attrition (Morris 2012; Chun et al. 2019). Rollin refers to emotional distancing as an adaptive mechanism for veterinary professionals to cope with moral stress:

> It is not surprising that some people in these fields protect themselves ... by abandoning the moral concern that is the chief source of the moral conflict that generates their stress, by thinking of themselves only as "scientists" ..., by taking the view that animals don't suffer or that their suffering doesn't matter.

> *(2011)*

The effects of work-related stress on mental health are well documented and include emotional exhaustion, anxiety, and depression (Ganster and Rosen 2013; Oh and Gastman 2015). A study has identified a correlation between stress and depression among veterinary students (Killinger et al. 2017). Moral stress has been associated with mental health problems in veterinarians including burnout (Kipperman et al. 2017) and compassion fatigue (Moses et al. 2018).

Numerous studies have documented high rates of suicidal ideation and suicide in the veterinary profession compared with those in the general population and other healthcare professionals (Nett et al. 2015; Volk et al. 2018; Tomasi et al. 2019; Witte et al. 2019). Some studies contend or conclude that moral stress may be a contributing factor to the high prevalence of suicide in the veterinary profession (Bartram and Baldwin 2010; Fink-Miller and Nestler 2018).

Let's now consider factors that may enhance one's susceptibility to experiencing moral stress.

## Demographic Risk Factors for Moral Stress

Numerous studies have concluded that younger, less experienced veterinarians have a higher prevalence of serious psychological distress or find ethical dilemmas more stressful compared with veterinarians as a whole (Nett et al. 2015; Kipperman et al. 2018; Volk et al. 2018). One might presume that with experience a practitioner would develop improved moral reasoning skills, which could moderate distress. However, a study documented no improvement in moral reasoning of veterinarians with experience, which disputes this assumption (Batchelor et al. 2015). The changes seen across age groups may instead represent enhanced coping strategies, which is supported by evidence that mental health of the public improves with age (Thomas et al. 2016). Alternatively, experienced practitioners over time may become desensitized to circumstances that novice colleagues may find ethically problematic and a source of moral stress.

Studies of veterinarians (Nett et al. 2015; Kipperman et al. 2018) and veterinary students (Killinger et al. 2017; Yang et al. 2019; Kipperman et al. 2020) have concluded that females experienced substantially greater levels of psychological distress and moral stress compared with males. Reports have also documented that female students in animal science and veterinary programs have greater empathy for animals than males (Hazel et al. 2011; Calderón-Amor et al. 2017) and that female veterinary students show more concern for animal welfare than their male counterparts (Cornish et al. 2016; Mariti et al. 2018). It seems reasonable to suggest that these characteristics would predispose an individual to experience moral stress.

## Environmental Risk Factors for Moral Stress

Autonomy "refers to decision latitude or skill discretion that reflects control over one's own work" (Wallace 2017) and is generally accepted as being associated with well-being (Kogan et al. 2020). Female practitioners and nonveterinary employees describe less autonomy and are less likely to be in a position of authority compared with male veterinarians (Wallace and Buchanan 2019). Reports have documented that lack of autonomy is a risk factor for burnout in female animal health technologists (Wallace and Buchanan 2019), and veterinary technicians (Kogan et al. 2020; Liss et al. 2020).

Perceived support in one's workplace has been shown to be an important factor influencing moral distress (Rushton 2016; Carse and Rushton 2017). The ability to speak up without fear of negative consequences reduces risk of moral distress. Therefore, organizational structures that encourage discussion of ethical dilemmas can decrease moral distress in healthcare settings (Vaclavik et al. 2018; Krautscheid et al. 2020).

Ambiguity has been defined as "vagueness and uncertainty" (Hancock et al. 2015). An increased likelihood of stress and burnout has been identified in general practitioner physicians in training with low tolerance of ambiguity (Cooke et al. 2013).

## Personality Risk Factors for Moral Stress

Perfectionism is a personality attribute in which there is a propensity for very high expectations of oneself and/or others (Holden 2020). Perfectionism has been established as a common attribute among veterinary students (Holden 2020). The competitive nature of being accepted into veterinary school likely selects for perfectionism as a necessary trait for a prospective veterinarian to be successful. Studies of veterinarians have concluded that perfectionism increases susceptibility to moral stress and psychological distress (Crane et al. 2015; O'Connor 2019). Perfectionism is therefore a double-edged sword, improving one's capacity to become a veterinarian, but also increasing one's vulnerability to moral stress as a consequence of the "imperfections" inherent in veterinary practice.

This dichotomy of adaptive and maladaptive perfectionism was first described as "normal and neurotic perfectionism" (Hamachek 1978). Neuroticism is the personality trait that describes "individual differences in negative emotional response to threat, frustration or loss" (Lahey 2009). Individuals with high levels of neuroticism have a tendency toward maladaptive emotional responses to stressful situations (Smith et al. 2014). Numerous authors have noted the relationship between neuroticism and perfectionism (Smith et al. 2014; Holden 2020). In a study of veterinary students, perfectionism significantly correlated with neuroticism, and neuroticism was found to have a negative correlation with resilience (Holden 2020). While both traits likely impact the experience of stress, neuroticism may play the greater role. A study of medical students showed that perfectionism alone was not a reliable predictor of stress, and some forms of perfectionism enhanced resiliency, whereas neuroticism was a robust predictor of stress (Enns et al. 2005).

The interplay of these personality types is relevant to veterinary professionals, as veterinarians have been found to have an increased incidence of perfectionism and neuroticism (Zenner et al. 2005; Strand 2019). Furthermore, these traits correlate with higher levels of occupational stress, burnout, and negative well-being (Crane et al. 2015; O'Connor 2019). Dr. Elizabeth Strand, Director of Veterinary Social Work at the University of Tennessee, suggests there are strategies available to mitigate the negative aspects of some personality types (Fender 2019). Let us now examine what can be done to alleviate both the occurrence and the pernicious effects of moral stress.

## Mitigation of Moral Stress

### Moral Resilience

Given the frequency of ethical dilemmas and the prevalence of moral stress reported in veterinary professionals, it seems prudent to implement coping strategies to address these issues within the workplace and as individuals. One author suggests that we endeavor to achieve moral resilience, defined as "the diligent, resolute and thoughtful ongoing effort to live in alignment with one's own principles and value commitments" which allows for the "ability to restore or sustain integrity under morally challenging circumstances" (Carse and Rushton 2017).

Moral resilience begins with understanding our moral landscape, or our personal and professional identity. This concept encompasses our perception of who we are, and what we believe is important in life as the basis for our moral view of the world (Rushton 2016). Within this process, a framework can facilitate addressing complex ethical dilemmas (see Tables 7.3 and 23.2). Once that problem solving has occurred, objective analysis, planning, and action are necessary in the resolution of moral distress. Due to the negative emotional impacts of moral distress, emotional regulation strategies, defined as the "processes through which individuals modulate their emotions to appropriately respond to environmental demands," are necessary to best achieve moral resilience (Aldao et al. 2010). Finally, seeking a sense of greater meaning and purpose, especially when ethical dilemmas are not sufficiently resolved, is an important strategy in attaining moral resilience (Rushton 2016).

### Understanding Our Moral Landscape

A reasonable place to start our journey toward moral resilience is to investigate and reflect on common ethical dilemmas in veterinary medicine (Moses et al. 2018; Kipperman et al. 2018) (see Table 7.2) and to identify our values or moral identity. Consideration of these dilemmas provides the practitioner with an opportunity to ponder solutions in advance of a potentially distressing situation. To that end, education in veterinary ethics seems a reasonable starting point. Unfortunately, ethics instruction is not a consistent component of veterinary education.

Only 30% of American Veterinary Medical Association-accredited veterinary schools in the United States that responded to a survey offered a formal course in ethics (Shivley et al. 2016). Other studies found that 51% of US small animal practitioners reported having received ethics training in their curriculum (Kipperman et al. 2018) and 29% of North American veterinarians received instruction in resolving conflicts about what is best care for patients (Moses et al. 2018). Supporting the value of ethics instruction, 84% of small animal veterinarians agreed that training in ethical theories and tools for addressing dilemmas was an effective strategy in reducing moral stress (Kipperman et al. 2018).

There are a number of online assessment tools available to assess core values, which are underlying beliefs about what is important in life. One resource can be found here: https://groups.lifevaluesinventory.org. People vary regarding how they identify with individual values. For example, one person may hold personal responsibility in the highest regard, while another views fairness as an essential quality. Knowledge of our values help inform conversations about our moral identity and therefore the situations that might cause us moral distress. In the above example, one person may feel significantly more distress when they are required not to fulfill an obligation, while another may be more distressed by inequality of time and resources for their patients.

An assessment of our personality traits may also be useful in understanding our individual reactions to ethical dilemmas, especially regarding factors that might increase our risk of moral distress. There are a number of validated scales for self-assessment of personality traits like neuroticism and perfectionism. A self-assessment of the big five personality traits can be found here: https://www.ocf.berkeley.edu/~johnlab/bfi.htm. Similarly, a self-assessment tool for perfectionism can be found here: https://www.idrlabs.com/multidimensional-perfectionism/test.php.

As we learn about our personality, we can start to explore coping strategies to help us compensate for the traits that hinder our capacity to adapt. Several coping techniques can mitigate risk factors for moral distress. For example, self-compassion exercises can help to address maladaptive perfectionism and therefore may have utility in reducing a practitioner's risk of moral distress (Smith et al. 2014). Self-compassion has also been linked to resiliency in veterinary students (McArthur et al. 2017).

## Ethical Mindfulness as a Framework for Addressing Moral Distress

Carse and Rushton (2017) define mindfulness as "an awareness of the present moment that emerges by purposefully paying attention to and not judging ones unfolding experience." Mindfulness has been suggested as a foundational skill to achieve moral resilience (Rushton 2016; Carse and Rushton 2017). Mindfulness has been linked to resiliency in veterinary students (McArthur et al. 2017). Importantly, this skill is trainable. In one study of graduate students, two months of mindfulness meditation improved moral reasoning and decision-making (Shapiro et al. 2012). A mindfulness-based program reduced the prevalence of distress in oncology nurses after experiencing an ethical dilemma from 88% to 44% (Vaclavik et al. 2018).

Guillemin and Gillam (2015) propose that the practice of ethical mindfulness in clinicians has five key features: recognition, acknowledgment, articulation, reflection, and courage. The first step in addressing moral distress is accurate identification of a state of negative arousal and discerning the underlying cause. We must recognize when we are experiencing negative emotions and acknowledge their relationship to an ethical dilemma. The recognition that we are experiencing distress is the cornerstone upon which all other actions arise. Mindfulness practice also centers on acknowledgment of our emotions.

Once the ethical dilemma is identified, we need to be able to articulate our feelings. This requires an emotional intelligence skill set as well as the time and a safe place to have these conversations. In a study of mindfulness interventions for moral distress in oncology nurses, the most impactful technique was the implementation of "Critical Debriefs," in which the staff met to discuss their concerns around a major clinical event, such as a death (Vaclavik et al. 2018). In making these meetings standard procedure, an organizational framework was provided to allow for mindfulness. If these spaces are not provided in one's workplace, individuals can join discussion groups, such as the Not One More Vet online support groups (https://nomv.org), or the discussion listserv for the Society for Veterinary Medical Ethics (https://svme.org).

As we explore these emotions, it is important to reflect on those feelings within the context of the situation and our own moral landscape. Previous experiences, moral identity, and personality types all inform and shape our emotional responses to morally distressing situations (Crane et al. 2013; Weber and Gray 2017). Veterinary professionals may experience moral distress in the same situation, but for different reasons based on their core values. For example, two veterinarians, Dr. Smith and Dr. Jones, share a core value regarding the relief of suffering. Charity is another core value for Dr. Smith while Dr. Jones highly values personal responsibility. They are presented with a patient that is suffering and needs care, but care is declined due to owner finances. They both feel moral distress because of the inability to relieve this patient's suffering. However, Dr. Smith's distress is compounded by her inability to fund care, while Dr. Jones is frustrated by a perceived lack of responsibility of the pet owner. Solutions to moderate Dr. Smith's distress could include connecting the pet owner with a charitable fund that assists with the cost of care, while Dr. Jones could recommend personal financing options. Dr. Smith's solution might not feel satisfactory to Dr. Jones, and vice versa. Prior work in understanding our own values helps inform this process and can lead us to solutions that are appropriate for the situation and our sense of moral well-being.

Finally, we must have the courage to act. In this last step of ethical mindfulness, moral action often requires people to speak up or act in uncomfortable and challenging situations (Hernandez et al. 2018). By stating this as integral from the beginning, it encourages the practitioner to engage with the morally distressing situation, rather than avoid or ignore it. Practice leadership has a clear role here in making sure these courageous acts are encouraged, rather than discouraged.

## Planning for Moral Action

Resilience theory defines two models of coping: problem-based coping, defined as strategies aimed at reducing or removing the cause of distress and emotional-based coping, which focuses on regulating the emotional responses to a problem (Lazarus and Folkman 1984). As expected, problem-based methods that directly deal with the cause of the stress are consistently found to be more effective in mediating distress (Morris 2012; Howlett et al. 2015). Rollin asserts that the only way to relieve moral stress is by way of moral action aimed at eliminating the source of the stress (Rollin 2006). An example of a problem-based coping strategy includes creation of hospital policies regarding common ethical issues.

The first step in problem-based coping is objective analysis of the situation. Once the practitioner has identified a situation that has caused distress, consider the following five questions: who is involved, what is contributing to this ethical dilemma, why did the dilemma arise, where is there room for compromise, and how will we find a solution?

Often morally distressing situations involve another person (Case Study 22.2) – for instance, an interaction with a client or a co-worker. Our analysis of the situation therefore naturally begins with: who are the morally relevant stakeholders in this conflict? Once identified, we need to define their perceived interests and consider their perspective. Without careful questioning, our previous experiences may bias us toward assumptions that lead us to moral distress, when in fact our moral boundaries have not been crossed. It may be via these questions that we uncover further information that resolves our distress.

---

**Case Study 22.2   Euthanasia request in a cat with ringworm**

Dr. G has diagnosed a cat with relapsing ringworm infection. She recommends a long course of oral antifungal medication. The owner declines treatment and requests euthanasia. Dr. G has recently had several clients refuse treatment because their cats are difficult to medicate. These experiences have led her to assume that this euthanasia decision is due to the inconvenience of administering oral medication. This is not a morally acceptable reason for euthanasia for Dr. G, and she feels distressed by the request. Dr. G could refuse the euthanasia request. However, this leaves her with unresolved emotions about being unable to help this cat and concern that the owner will seek euthanasia elsewhere.

Dr. G further questions the client as to why euthanasia has been requested. The client reveals their spouse is immunocompromised and has a serious fungal infection. The spouse's physician specifically asked that the cat be tested for ringworm as a possible source of the infection, which prompted the first appointment. The client justifiably believes repeated exposure to their cat is contributing to this potentially life-threatening infection in their spouse. The client's perspective is that they gave the first round of treatment a try in order to save the animal, but now that the infection has returned, they have to prioritize their spouse.

Discovering that the decision is based on a genuine medical concern for their family member and not on convenience mitigates Dr. G's feelings of moral distress. In this example we can see that by fully exploring the perspective of the other party, we can discover information vital to problem solving, correct our assumptions, and potentially resolve our distress.

The next step in our analysis is to define exactly what the dilemma entails. Our work on personal values is critical to this process as we need to identify which of our personal values are at stake. In the above example, Dr. G initially thought her value of selflessness was being violated. Pilling a cat is difficult but she would go to any inconvenience or effort to help a loved one. Her initial perception that her client wouldn't do the same caused distress. That same value helps her find resolution when Dr. G discovers that the owner is making a difficult decision to let go of a beloved pet for the health of their spouse.

Next, we consider why this dilemma has occurred. In the scenario in Case Study 22.2, this distressing situation has arisen because one of the clients has a serious illness, and the cat is likely the source. Emotions and conjecture are not helpful in this step. Sticking to the facts allows us to be more objective and helps in the next step, which is implementing a plan.

We need to think about how we might solve this problem. Not all problems can be resolved, so we may need to look for a utilitarian or "best outcome" solution or where there is room for compromise or alternative solutions. In Case Study 22.2, perhaps Dr. G is still not comfortable euthanizing the cat. However, our analysis has shown it's not realistic for this cat to stay in this household, which leads us to consider alternatives, such as rehoming the cat.

It's important to note that often in a clinical setting, the current dilemma needs to be addressed in a relatively short timeframe, for instance during an appointment. The solution in the moment may be unsatisfying, which makes following up with a long-term solution important. Perhaps in the weeks following the above scenario, Dr. G finds local rescue groups that help rehome pets for people with serious medical conditions. She now has a resource should this scenario come up again. Putting a precise and actionable plan into place helps us achieve our goal.

## Barriers to Moral Action

A majority of small animal veterinarians report facing the ethical dilemma of client financial restrictions compromising desired care at least daily: 49% of these veterinarians reported moderate to substantial burnout, and 77% cited this dilemma as a source of that stress (Kipperman et al. 2017). Despite a majority of practitioners agreeing that it would be helpful in relieving the cause of the distress, only a minority of these practitioners had tried to implement a problem-based strategy, as 31% discussed the cost of care and 23% discussed pet insurance with clients. Lack of time and belief that it would not affect client behavior were the most common reasons cited for why they had not implemented these measures.

These results reveal two significant barriers to problem-based coping: time and moral residue. Morally focused action requires time to analyze and implement. Complicated ethical dilemmas require time to resolve in a satisfactory way, and time is something that is often in short supply in a clinical veterinary setting (Fawcett 2020). This is an area where organizational structure within a clinic could assist in encouraging moral resiliency. Simply, if we are to address veterinary well-being and moral distress, we must be given the time to do so. In addressing practitioner concern that our actions will not affect client behavior we may be seeing evidence of moral residue in the veterinary profession.

Prolonged or recurrent moral distress often results in feelings of helplessness, emotional dysregulation, and a diminished moral responsiveness that prevents objective identification, analysis, and action toward resolution of ethical dilemmas. This is referred to as "moral residue" (Rushton 2016; Carse and Rushton 2017). This creates a vicious cycle where the practitioner feels emotionally overwhelmed by their moral distress and therefore does not act to resolve it, which can result in further distress. This emphasizes the importance of emotional regulation. We must be able to process our previous moral distress in order to take appropriate action to reduce further exposure to ethical conflicts that may cause the distress.

## Cultivating Physical and Emotional Self-Care

Addressing moral residue prepares us to better implement problem-based solutions and has value in moral resiliency (Carse and Rushton 2017). Unfortunately, not all ethical dilemmas can be fully resolved in the moment and therefore a solely problem-based approach has limitations (Morris 2012; Carse and Rushton 2017). A balanced approach that includes problem-based coping as well as emotional-based coping is therefore recommended. Given the relatively high rates of mental health concerns such as anxiety and depression within the veterinary profession (Nett et al. 2015; Volk et al. 2020), a focus on psychological well-being to support these coping mechanisms cannot be overemphasized.

Basic self-care strategies, such as maintaining reasonable work hours, exercise, sleep, and hydration, have benefits to cognition and well-being (Mandolesi et al. 2018; Volk et al. 2020). In many cases, deficiencies in these basic aspects of self-care have been directly linked to measures of burnout, mood disorders, and impaired cognitive abilities in healthcare workers (Shapiro et al. 2019). For example, a study of physicians and nurses revealed that 45% were clinically dehydrated by the end of their shift and those that were dehydrated had significant cognitive impairments (El-Sharkawy et al. 2016).

Instead of simply listing these self-care priorities, an emphasis on planning is important. Veterinarians who reported a self-care plan had lower rates of serious psychological distress and higher well-being than their colleagues who did not have such plans (Volk et al. 2020).

While personal responsibility for self-care is important, we should also consider the cultural and workplace norms that exacerbate deficiencies of self-care among veterinary professionals. Scheduling and safety standards can make access to necessities like food, water, and even bathroom breaks difficult to achieve for many clinicians (Shapiro et al. 2019). In one online survey of 460 veterinarians, 36% reported having no regular lunch break, indicating an organizational barrier to reasonable self-care (Jurney 2019). Furthermore, 41% of veterinarians who had a scheduled lunch break reported missing it more than 50% of the time, which indicates an organizational issue such as overscheduling and/or a cultural one where clinical supervisors place the needs of patients above their own employees. In developing healthy work environments, organizations must create plans conducive to the self-care of their employees. These practices are the cornerstone upon which thoughtful and emotionally regulated actions are built. Simply put, sleep deprivation, dehydration, urine retention, and hunger do not promote one's capacity to address complicated ethical dilemmas, so we must start our planning for emotional regulation here.

Once the basics of physical health are addressed, further attention can be paid to emotional health and regulation. There are various cognitive exercises that have been proven to mitigate the negative consequences of certain personality types. For instance, the practice of self-compassion can mediate consequences of maladaptive perfectionism

(Ferrari et al. 2018), and also has been specifically recommended for the reduction of moral distress (Papazoglou et al. 2020). The "best possible self" exercise, where a person writes about themselves at their best, and the "three good things" exercises, where a person lists three things that they are grateful for daily, have both been shown to have positive effects on well-being in individuals with high neuroticism (Ng 2016). The reader is referred to the Greater Good Science Center at University of California at Berkeley's website (https://greatergood.berkeley.edu) (particularly the section the "Keys to Well-Being"), as well as their podcast series entitled "The Science of Happiness," and the books *The Happiness Advantage* by Anchor and *Emotional Intelligence 2.0* by Bradberry, for further discussion of these techniques.

These positive mental activities can be undertaken as an individual, or some may find it useful to receive guidance from a mental health professional. Mental health care is an underutilized resource in the veterinary profession. Unfortunately, only 52% of veterinarians in serious psychological distress will seek out mental health care (Volk et al. 2020). This has largely been attributed to stigma against treatment, but other obstacles include access to care due to limited availability and affordability (Karaffa and Holk 2019; Volk et al. 2020). Organizations such as Not One More Vet (https://nomv.org), Veterinary Social Work at the University of Tennessee (https://vetsocial work.utk.edu), and The Veterinary Mental Health Initiative (https://www.shanti.org/programs-services/veterinary-mental-health-initiative/) have programs that provide free access to mental health care professionals.

### Fostering Hope, Finding Meaning

Moral distress often causes a feeling of powerlessness and futility in the face of what can seem like senseless suffering or insurmountable obstacles (Rushton 2016; Carse and Rushton 2017; Dürnberger 2020). These frustrations can feel validated by our inability to completely resolve many of the moral dilemmas we face in practice. The complexity of these situations, combined with the intersection of other stakeholder's competing values, and barriers to moral action, can lead to unsatisfying outcomes. By fostering hope and seeking meaning in difficult situations, veterinary professionals can find greater purpose in their actions.

Hope, defined as "one's perceived ability to generate sufficient energy ... in the pursuit of one's goals," has been shown to mediate personal growth (Meyers et al. 2015). Correlations have been found among nurses between resilience and hope (Rushton et al. 2015). In order to act, we must first believe that the action will have positive benefit. Particularly when dealing with moral distress, believing in our own agency to impact the cause of our distress can moderate that distress. In a study of nursing students, one's belief in your own ability to achieve a goal was a key factor in moral resilience (Krautscheid et al. 2020).

The presence of meaning or "the degree to which people ...feel a sense of purpose or mission in their lives," has a positive effect on well-being and has been correlated with professional satisfaction in healthcare workers (Rushton et al. 2015; Li et al. 2020). Based on responses from surveys of work satisfaction in veterinarians, Cake et al. (2015) found that veterinary well-being is best rooted in the Aristotelian concept of *eudaimonia*. Eudaimonia is the happiness that is experienced by "living a life that is fulfilling and deeply satisfying" (Cake et al. 2015). Cake's work underlies the importance of a strong connection to meaning and purpose for veterinary professionals.

The daily experiences of a veterinary professional may be difficult, even traumatic, but by focusing on our broader ideals, we can allow for a perspective shift that is beneficial to resilience. Specific techniques, such as cognitive reappraisal, where one reconsiders the traumatic situation with the intent to form a less maladaptive view, have been suggested for alleviation of moral distress (Papazoglou et al. 2020). This technique allows for an opportunity to explore alternative narratives for a distressing scenario (Case Study 22.3).

---

**Case Study 22.3   Perceived non-beneficial intervention**

Original experience:

Dr. J is an intern at a private equine practice. The horses they treat are high value, and the clients are often wealthy. Dr. J has a patient, Lacey, who is suffering and has a very poor prognosis. Standard therapy has failed. Lacey's owners have refused euthanasia, and have instructed Dr. J to "do everything, money is no object." Dr. J now feels compelled to offer treatments he does not believe will work. He feels helpless. This feeling is compounded by the fact that he is an intern and is not authorized to refuse further care. Dr. J is also bothered by the fact the clients have not visited Lacey in the hospital. This leaves him feeling like these owners don't care for Lacey. He feels like he is being forced to participate in futile, painful procedures that makes him feel stressed.

Cognitive reappraisal:

Dr. J reflects on when his own horse was sick, and how fearful he felt. Perhaps the owners haven't visited because it is too emotional for them. He still wishes they would visit, but he can understand being frightened when your horse is ill. He wonders if the clients are very upset by how sick Lacey is, and because of the depth of their love for her are not ready to let her go. There is other evidence that suggests they care. For instance, they always immediately answer the phone no matter what time he calls. In this reframing, Dr. J concludes his clients are offering the only resource they have to help Lacey, which is money. Even if he can't save Lacey, he is being given the opportunity to give her every possible chance. While her prognosis is poor, there is a small chance she might recover. Dr. J then reflects on one of the reasons he took this internship – so that he would have the opportunity to practice high-level medicine without financial restrictions. This lets him see this case as an opportunity to learn new treatments and techniques that will help him better serve patients in the future.

It's easy to understand Dr. J's frustration in this scenario. He is distressed by Lacey's condition, but his narrative of the client as unfeeling toward their horse and the potential therapies as pointless and cruel is complicating his distress. By considering an alternative narrative, he was able not only to connect with a more compassionate view of the owner's relationship to the horse, but also reconnect to hope for Lacey's recovery, as well as his greater purpose of learning and practicing medicine. In this example, we see how cultivating a narrative that reconnects the clinician to feelings of hope and meaning can mitigate the negative emotional impact of moral distress (Rushton 2016).

---

## Conclusion

Veterinary medicine will never be a stress-free profession. Some experience of moral distress is inevitable, so we must instead work to become resilient to it. Time and focusing on one's personal and professional moral landscape provide the tools to be thoughtful in tough moments. Actionable self-care strategies, practiced regularly, ensure we are in the best possible state to handle complicated scenarios when they arise. Mindful and objective analysis of these distressing situations allows us to find the best possible short- and long-term solutions. Finally, seeking regular connection to hope and meaning grounds us in the very thing that bring us happiness as veterinary professionals. With focus and effort, one can learn to navigate the rocky waters of veterinary medicine. The intangible rewards the profession provides, such as living a life of purpose in service of our patients, make that a truly worthwhile endeavor.

## References

Aldao, A., Nolen-Hoeksema, S., and Schweizer, S. (2010). Emotion-regulation strategies across psychopathology: A meta-analytic review. *Clinical Psychology Review* 30 (2): 217–237.

Bartram, D.J. and Baldwin, D.S. (2010). Veterinary surgeons and suicide: A structured review of possible influences on increased risk. *Veterinary Record* 166: 388–397.

Batchelor, C.E.M. and McKeegan, D.E.F. (2012). Survey of the frequency and perceived stressfulness of ethical dilemmas encountered in UK veterinary practice. *Veterinary Record* 170: 19.

Batchelor, C.E.M., Creed, A., and McKeegan, D.E.F. (2015). A preliminary investigation into the moral reasoning abilities of UK veterinarians. *Veterinary Record* 177: 124.

Cake, M.A., Bell, M.A., Bickley, N. et al. (2015). The life of meaning: A model of the positive contributions to well-being from veterinary work. *Journal of Veterinary Medical Education* 42 (3): 184–193.

Calderón-Amor, J., Luna-Fernández, D., and Tadich, T. (2017). Study of the levels of human–human and human–animal empathy in veterinary medical students from Chile. *Journal of Veterinary Medical Education* 44 (1): 179–186.

Carse, A. and Rushton, C.H. (2017). Harnessing the promise of moral distress: A call for re-orientation. *Journal of Clinical Ethics* 28 (1): 15–29.

Chun, M.S., Joo, S., and Jung, Y. (2019). Veterinary ethical issues and stressfulness of ethical dilemmas of Korean veterinarians. In: *Sustainable Governance and Management of Food Systems: Ethical Perspectives* (Eds. E. Vinnari and M. Vinnari), 193–202. Wageningen, the Netherlands: Wageningen Academic Publishers.

Cooke, G.P., Doust, J.A., and Steele, M.C. (2013). A survey of resilience, burnout, and tolerance of uncertainty in Australian general practice registrars. *BMC Medical Education* 13 (1): 2.

Cornish, A.R., Caspar, G.L., Collins, T. et al. (2016). Career preferences and opinions on animal welfare and ethics: A survey of veterinary students in Australia and New Zealand. *Journal of Veterinary Medical Education* 43 (3): 310–320. https://doi.org/10.3138/jvme.0615-091R2

Crane, M.F., Bayl-Smith, P., and Cartmill, J. (2013). A recommendation for expanding the definition of moral distress experienced in the workplace. *Australian and New Zealand Journal of Organizational Psychology* 6: e1. doi: 10.1017/orp.2013.1

Crane, M.F., Phillips, J.K., and Karin, E. (2015). Trait perfectionism strengthens the negative effects of moral stressors occurring in veterinary practice. *Australian Veterinary Journal* 93 (10): 354–360.

Dürnberger, C. (2020). Am I actually a veterinarian or an economist? Understanding the moral challenges for farm veterinarians in Germany on the basis of a qualitative online survey. *Research in Veterinary Science* 133: 246–250. https://doi.org/10.1016/j.rvsc.2020.09.029

El-Sharkawy, A.M., Bragg, D., Watson, P. et al. (2016). Hydration amongst nurses and doctors on-call (the HANDS on prospective cohort study). *Clinical Nutrition* 35 (4): 935–942.

Enns, M.W., Cox, B.J., and Clara, I.P. (2005). Perfectionism and neuroticism: A longitudinal study of specific vulnerability and diathesis-stress models. *Cognitive Therapy and Research* 29 (4): 463–478.

Fawcett, A. (2020). Moral distress in veterinarians: Why ethical challenges impact wellbeing. Proceedings of VetFest 2020. https://vetfest.ava.com.au (accessed 30 September 2020).

Fawcett, A. and Mullan, S. (2018). Managing moral distress in practice. *In Practice* 40 (1): 34–36.

Fender, K. (2019). Veterinarians more likely to be neurotic than regular folks. DVM 360. www.dvm360.com/view/veterinarians-more-likely-be-neurotic-regular-folks (accessed 30 September 2020).

Ferrari, M., Yap, K., Scott, N. et al. (2018). Self-compassion moderates the perfectionism and depression link in both adolescence and adulthood. *PLoS ONE* 13 (2): e0192022.

Fink-Miller, E.L. and Nestler, L.M. (2018). Suicide in physicians and veterinarians: Risk factors and theories. *Current Opinion in Psychology* 22: 23–26.

Ganster, D.C. and Rosen, C.C. (2013). Work stress and employee health: A multidisciplinary review. *Journal of Management* 39: 1085–1122.

Guillemin, M. and Gillam, L. (2015). Emotions, narratives, and ethical mindfulness. *Academic Medicine* 90 (6): 726–731.

Hamachek, D.E. (1978). Psychodynamics of normal and neurotic perfectionism. *Psychology: A Journal of Human Behavior* 15: 27–33.

Hancock, J., Roberts, M., Monrouxe, L. et al. (2015). Medical student and junior doctors' tolerance of ambiguity: Development of a new scale. *Advances in Health Sciences Education: Theory and Practice* 20 (1): 113–130. http://dx.doi.org/10.1007/s10459-014-9510-z

Hayes, G.M., LaLonde-Paul, D.F., Perret, J.L. et al. (2020). Investigation of burnout syndrome and job-related risk factors in veterinary technicians in specialty teaching hospitals: A multicenter cross-sectional study. *Journal of Veterinary Emergency and Critical Care* 30: 18–27.

Hazel, S.J., Signal, T.D., and Taylor, N. (2011). Can teaching veterinary and animal-science students about animal welfare affect their attitude toward animals and human-related empathy? *Journal of Veterinary Medical Education* 38: 74–83.

Hernandez, E., Fawcett, A., Brouwer, E. et al. (2018). Speaking up: Veterinary ethical responsibilities and animal welfare issues in everyday practice. *Animals* 8 (1): 15.

Holden, C.L. (2020). Characteristics of veterinary students: Perfectionism, personality factors, and resilience. *Journal of Veterinary Medical Education* 47 (4): 488–496.

Howlett, M., Doody, K., Murray, J. et al. (2015). Burnout in emergency department healthcare professionals is associated with coping style: A cross-sectional survey. *Emergency Medicine Journal* 32 (9): 722–727.

Institute for Employment Studies (IES) Report (2019). The 2019 survey of the veterinary profession. A report for the Royal College of Veterinary Surgeons. https://www.rcvs. org.uk/news-and-views/publications/the-2019-survey-of-the-veterinary-profession (accessed 28 October 2020).

Jameton, A. (1984). *Nursing Practice: The Ethical Issues.* Engelwood Cliffs, NJ: Prentice Hall.

Jurney, C. (2019). Diagnosing well-being: A deeper look at veterinary wellness. ACVIM Forum. Phoenix, Arizona, USA (6–8 June).

Karaffa, K.M. and Hancock, T.S. (2019). Mental health stigma and veterinary medical students' attitudes toward seeking professional psychological help. *Journal of Veterinary Medical Education* 46 (4): 459–469.

Killinger, S.L., Flanagan, S., Castine, E. et al. (2017). Stress and depression among veterinary medical students. *Journal of Veterinary Medical Education* 44 (1): 3–8. https://doi.org/10.3138/jvme.0116-018R1

Kipperman, B.S., Kass, P.H., and Rishniw, M. (2017). Factors influencing small animal veterinarians' opinions and actions regarding cost of care and effects of economic limitations on patient care, outcomes and professional career satisfaction and burnout. *Journal of the American Veterinary Medical Association* 250 (7): 785–794.

Kipperman, B., Morris, P., and Rollin, B. (2018). Ethical dilemmas encountered by small animal veterinarians: Characterization, responses, consequences and beliefs regarding euthanasia. *Veterinary Record* 182 (19): 548. doi: 10.1136/vr.104619

Kipperman, B., Rollin, B., and Martin, J. (2020). Veterinary student opinions regarding ethical dilemmas encountered by veterinarians and the benefits of ethics instruction. *Journal of Veterinary Medical Education* 48: 330–342.

Kogan, L.R., Wallace, J.E., Schoenfeld-Tacher, R. et al. (2020). Veterinary technicians and occupational burnout. *Frontiers in Veterinary Science* 7: 328.

Krautscheid, L., Mood, L., McLennon, S.M. et al. (2020). Examining relationships between resilience protective factors and moral distress among nursing students. *Nursing Education Perspectives* 41 (1): 43–45.

Lahey, B.B. (2009). Public health significance of neuroticism. *American Psychologist* 64 (4): 241.

Lazarus, R.S. and Folkman, S. (1984). *Stress Appraisal and Coping.* New York: Springer.

Li, J.B., Dou, K., and Liang, Y. (2020). The relationship between presence of meaning, search for meaning, and subjective well-being: A three-level meta-analysis based on the meaning in life questionnaire. *Journal of Happiness Studies* 22 (1): 467–489.

Liss, D.J., Kerl, M.E., and Tsai, C.L. (2020). Factors associated with job satisfaction and engagement among credentialed small animal veterinary technicians in the United States. *Journal of the American Veterinary Medical Association* 257 (5): 537–545.

Lokhee, S. and Hogg, R.C. (2021). Depression, stress and self-stigma towards seeking psychological help in veterinary students. *Australian Veterinary Journal* https://doi. org/10.1111/avj.13070

Mandolesi, L., Polverino, A., Montuori, S. et al. (2018). Effects of physical exercise on cognitive functioning and wellbeing: Biological and psychological benefits. *Frontiers in Psychology* 9: 509.

Mariti, C., Pirrone, F., Albertinei, M. et al. (2018). Familiarity and interest in working with livestock decreases the odds of having positive attitudes towards non-human animals and their welfare among veterinary students in Italy. *Animals* 8 (9): 150. https://doi.org/10.3390/ani8090150

McArthur, M., Mansfield, C., Matthew, S. et al. (2017). Resilience in veterinary students and the predictive role of mindfulness and self-compassion. *Journal of Veterinary Medical Education* 44 (1): 106–115.

Meyers, M.C., van Woerkom, M., de Reuver, R.S. et al. (2015). Enhancing psychological capital and personal growth initiative: Working on strengths or deficiencies. *Journal of Counseling Psychology* 62 (1): 50.

Morris, P. (2012). *Blue Juice: Euthanasia in Veterinary Medicine*. Philadelphia, PA: Temple University Press.

Moses, L., Malowney, M.J., and Boyd, J.W. (2018). Ethical conflict and moral distress in veterinary practice: A survey of North American veterinarians. *Journal of Veterinary Internal Medicine* 32 (6): 2115–2122.

Nett, R.J., Witte, T.K., Holzbauer, S.M. et al. (2015). Risk factors for suicide, attitudes toward mental illness, and practice-related stressors among US veterinarians. *Journal of the American Veterinary Medical Association* 247 (8): 945–955.

Ng, W. (2016). Use of positive interventions: Does neuroticism moderate the sustainability of their effects on happiness? *The Journal of Positive Psychology* 11 (1): 51–61.

O'Connor, E. (2019). Sources of work stress in veterinary practice in the UK. *Veterinary Record* 184: 19.

Ogden, U., Kinnison, T., and May, S.A. (2012). Attitudes to animal euthanasia do not correlate with acceptance of human euthanasia or suicide. *Veterinary Record* 171: 7.

Oh, Y. and Gastmans, C. (2015). Moral distress experienced by nurses: A quantitative literature review. *Nurse Ethics* 22 (1): 15–31.

Ouedraogo, F.B., Lefebvre, S.L., Hansen, C.R. et al. (2021). Compassion satisfaction, burnout, and secondary traumatic stress among full-time veterinarians in the United States (2016–2018). *Journal of the American Veterinary Medical Association* 258 (11): 1259–1270.

Papazoglou, K., Blumberg, D.M., Kamkar, K. et al. (2020). Addressing moral suffering in police work: Theoretical conceptualization and counselling implications. *Canadian Journal of Counselling & Psychotherapy/Revue Canadienne De Counseling Et De Psychothérapie* 54 (1): 71–87.

Patronek, G. and Crowe, A. (2018). Factors associated with high live release for dogs at a large, open-admission, municipal shelter. *Animals* 8 (4): 45.

Rollin, B.E. (1987). Euthanasia and moral stress. *Loss, Grief & Care* 1 (1–2): 115–126.

Rollin, B.E. (2006). *An Introduction to Veterinary Medical Ethics*, 2e. Ames, IA: Blackwell Publishing.

Rollin, B.E. (2011). Euthanasia, moral stress, and chronic illness in veterinary medicine. *Veterinary Clinics of North America: Small Animal Practice* 41 (3): 651–659.

Rushton, C.H. (2016). Moral resilience: A capacity for navigating moral distress in critical care. *AACN Advanced Critical Care* 27 (1): 111–119.

Rushton, C.H., Batcheller, J., Schroeder, K. et al. (2015). Burnout and resilience among nurses practicing in high-intensity settings. *American Journal of Critical Care* 24 (5): 412–420.

Scotney, R.L., McLaughlin, D., and Keates, H.L. (2015). A systematic review of the effects of euthanasia and occupational stress in personnel working with animals in animal shelters, veterinary clinics, and biomedical research facilities. *Journal of the American Veterinary Medical Association* 247 (10): 1121–1130.

Shapiro, D.E., Duquette, C., Abbott, L.M. et al. (2019). Beyond burnout: A physician wellness hierarchy designed to prioritize interventions at the systems level. *American Journal of Medicine* 132 (5): 556–563.

Shapiro, S.L., Jazaieri, H., and Goldin, P.R. (2012). Mindfulness-based stress reduction effects on moral reasoning and decision making. *Journal of Positive Psychology* 7 (6): 504–515.

Shivley, C.B., Garry, F.B., Kogan, L.R. et al. (2016). Survey of animal welfare, animal behavior, and animal ethics courses in the curricula of AVMA Council on Education-accredited veterinary colleges and schools. *Journal of the American Veterinary Medical Association* 248 (10): 1165–1170.

Smith, M.M., Saklofske, D.H., and Nordstokke, D.W. (2014). The link between neuroticism and perfectionistic concerns: The mediating effect of trait emotional intelligence. *Personality and Individual Differences* 61: 97–100.

Strand, E. (2019). The big five personality: What we know about DVM's and how you can get the most from yours. *VMX Small Animal and Exotics Proceedings*, Orlando, Florida (19–23 January). PM254–256. USA: NAVK

Thomas, M.L., Kaufmann, C.N., Palmer, B.W. et al. (2016). Paradoxical trend for improvement in mental health with aging: A community-based study of 1,546 adults aged 21–100 years. *Journal of Clinical Psychiatry* 77 (8): 8771.

Tomasi, S.E., Fechter-Leggett, E.D., Edwards, N.T. et al. (2019). Suicide among veterinarians in the United States from 1979 through 2015. *Journal of the American Veterinary Medical Association* 254 (1): 104–112. https://doi.org/10.2460/javma.254.1.104

Vaclavik, E.A., Staffileno, B.A., and Carlson, E. (2018). Moral distress: Using mindfulness-based stress reduction interventions to decrease nurse perceptions of distress. *Clinical Journal of Oncology Nursing* 22: 3.

Volk, J.O., Schimmack, U., Strand, E.B. et al. (2018). Executive summary of the Merck Animal Health Veterinary Wellbeing Study. *Journal of the American Veterinary Medical Association* 252 (10): 1231–1238.

Volk, J.O., Schimmack, U., Strand, E.B. et al. (2020). Executive summary of the Merck Animal Health Veterinarian Wellbeing Study II. *Journal of the American Veterinary Medical Association* 256 (11): 1237–1244.

Wallace, J.E. (2017). Burnout, coping and suicidal ideation: An application and extension of the job demand-control-support model. *Journal of Workplace Behavioral Health* 32: 99–118.

Wallace, J.E. and Buchanan, T. (2019). Status differences in interpersonal strain and job resources at work. A mixed methods study of animal health-care providers. *International Journal of Conflict Management* 31 (2): 287–308. https://doi.org/10.1108/IJCMA-08-2019-0135

Weber, E. and Gray, S. (2017). How should integrity preservation and professional growth be balanced during trainees' professionalization? *AMA Journal of Ethics* 19 (6): 544–549.

Witte, T.K., Spitzer, E.G., Edwards, N. et al. (2019). Suicides and deaths of undetermined intent among veterinary professionals from 2003 through 2014. *Journal of the American Veterinary Medical Association* 255 (5): 595–608.

Yang, H.H., Ward, M.P., and Fawcett, A. (2019). DVM students report higher psychological distress than the Australian public, medical students, junior medical officers and practicing veterinarians. *Australian Veterinary Journal* 97 (10): 373–381.

Yeates, J.W. and Main, D. (2011). Veterinary opinions on refusing euthanasia: Justifications and philosophical frameworks. *Veterinary Record* 168: 263.

Zenner, D., Burns, G.A., Ruby, K.L. et al. (2005). Veterinary students as elite performers: Preliminary insights. *Journal of Veterinary Medical Education* 32 (2): 242–248.

23

# The Future of Veterinary Ethics

History, Diagnosis, and Prognosis of an Evolving Research Field

*Svenja Springer and Herwig Grimm*

## The Brief History: Veterinary Ethics in Research and Practice

In recent decades, ethical challenges have been investigated in veterinary ethics, a field which has experienced enormous development. Starting in the 1990s with Tannenbaum (1995) and Rollin (2006 [1999]), veterinary ethics has been institutionalized not only as a research field in academia but as a discipline that aims to provide guidance and support for veterinary professionals. Veterinarians have always faced ethical challenges, but the subject matter as well as the perception and responses to these challenges have changed over time (Woods 2013). Especially at the time when veterinary medicine became a legally recognized profession and veterinarians gained the right to treat animals with corresponding duties (e.g. 1948 Veterinary Surgeons Act in the UK) (Woods 2013; Kimera and Mlangwa 2015), considerable changes in the normative self-understanding of veterinarians have led to an increasing awareness of ethical questions such as "What must I do to be a proper veterinarian?" or "What do I consider as legitimate and what do I refuse to accept as part of my job?" Veterinarians have increasingly considered such concerns (Woods 2013) and have received support from professional ethicists (Tannenbaum 1995; Rollin 2006 [1999]).

The recognition of the varied and sometimes conflicting interests of animals, owners, the public, veterinary professionals, and legal requirements is at the core of debates in veterinary ethics. Expectations from these groups confront veterinarians with challenging situations and force them to rethink their responsibilities as professionals in society (Woods 2013). The fruitful collaboration of veterinarians and ethicists with a background in philosophy and theology as well as sociologists in dealing with challenging questions has been called veterinary ethics.

Although starting off as a problem-oriented discipline, veterinary ethics has evolved as an academic field. In doing so, it strongly borrowed from the debates in medical ethics, animal ethics, research ethics, and animal welfare (Kimera and Mlangwa 2015). However, it quickly became apparent that veterinarians' real-life problems can only be addressed and solved by considering the contextual complexity and requirements of the veterinary profession that result from the relationship between the animal, the client, and the veterinarian. Hence, it is the aim of veterinary ethics to address evolving problems by not only developing solutions but also reflecting on the problems' nature, e.g. in terms of their origin and normative background. To give an example of how the

*Ethics in Veterinary Practice: Balancing Conflicting Interests*, First Edition. Edited by Barry Kipperman and Bernard E. Rollin.
© 2022 John Wiley & Sons, Inc. Published 2022 by John Wiley & Sons, Inc.

profession is oriented along normative goals, the protection and promotion of animal welfare is illustrative, which has often been understood as the paradigm to act in the best interest of the animal (Rollin 2006 [1999]; Grimm et al. 2018; Coghlan 2018; Gray and Fordyce 2020) (see Chapter 7). However, most veterinary oaths acknowledge that veterinarians are faced with additional duties related to other stakeholders such as clients or society that go beyond the best interest of the animal. Accordingly, the question arises if the patient's best interests alone should be the sole normative goal and orientation in a highly diverse profession.

## Diagnosis: Moral Diversity and Context-Specific Responsibilities

Although the interest of animal patients is often proposed as the main responsibility of veterinarians (Coghlan 2018; Kipperman et al. 2018), the veterinary profession is a medical profession with various responsibilities toward different stakeholders. Students are trained as generalists and are equipped with skills and knowledge that are not only suitable to maintain animal health and welfare, but also human or public health. Veterinary students encounter the diversity of their profession on a regular basis in their study programs as is shown in the first of four examples we will use to develop and illustrate our arguments (Case Study 23.1).

---

**Case Study 23.1   Diverse fields of work – Different responsibilities**

Sara is in her final year studying veterinary medicine and meets with two of her study colleagues after she has completed her obligatory experience with a farm animal veterinarian and shares her experiences. One of her classmates mentions that she would like to work in the farm animal sector even though she knows that medical treatments for farm animals are often limited due to economic constraints and its functionality in the production process. The other colleague mutters angrily that she would never work for such a system in which animals only receive proper veterinary treatment if it pays off economically for the farmer and veterinary decisions are not based on the well-being of the animal. She goes on to tell Sara: "That's why you studied veterinary medicine? To support this corrupted system where animals are treated as production units?"

---

In fact, most students start their veterinary training because they want to help animals and put their interests first (Kipperman et al. 2020). However, due to context-specific responsibilities in different fields of work, veterinarians are not always able to pursue animals' best interests but have to take owners' or the public's interests into account as well. Getting a structured overview of the main ends of veterinary medicine and related goals of treatment in order to understand the diversity better, is a first step to any possible strategy of dealing with it.

Table 23.1 demonstrates two important concepts: first, animals are seen differently in different veterinary working contexts; and second, how animals are treated is linked to the goals of the specific contexts. For instance, within the field of companion animal medicine, veterinary interventions are generally directed to the animal as a patient and the overall aim is to promote patients' health and well-being and prevent disease (Rollin 2006 [1999]). This recent development led authors to the normative claim that veterinarians should act in the best interest of the animal and give them first allegiance in their decision-making and actions (Rollin 2006 [1999]; Coghlan 2018). Even though decision-making processes can be strongly influenced by factors related to the client (e.g. financial constraints or strong emotional attachment) and/or the veterinarians themselves (e.g. working background and/or level of specialization) (Springer et al. 2021), consensus can be found in the fact that the animal's best interest constitutes an important basis to justify veterinary interventions. If a particular treatment is in the best interest of the patient and carried out, something good has been done (Grimm et al. 2018). More challenging cases are those where it is questionable whether a treatment option is in the best interest of the animal, such as excessive treatment or undertreatment.

However, it is important to note that not every treatment that is not aligned with the best interest of the animal is immoral. Even though the duty to act in the patient's best interest structures the scope of veterinary actions, veterinary practice, for instance in the farm animal sector, is characterized by medical interventions that are often not (exclusively) aimed at the best interest of the animal. For instance, take the ovarian cyst in dairy cattle. The cow's ovarian cyst receives medical attention as an obstacle to effective reproduction, and hence milk production, that results in financial losses for the farmer (Huth et al. 2019). This illustrates the fact that the health of the animal can become a means for other ends, like efficient production. Consequently, the primary goal of therapy is to restore production efficiency and not to focus primarily on the

**Table 23.1** Status of the animal, goals of veterinary treatment, and ends of veterinary medicine in different fields of the profession.

| Field of work | Status of the animal | Goal of veterinary treatment | End of veterinary medicine |
|---|---|---|---|
| Companion animals | Patient | Patient's health and well-being (in consultation with the client) | Patient's health and well-being |
| Farm animals | Production unit | Functionality and economic prosperities | Animals are means to human ends |
| Zoo animals | Object of conservation, observation, and study | Entertainment, education, and conservation | Animals are means to human ends |
| Public health | Vector or disease carrier | Human public health | Health and well-being of others |
| Laboratory animals | Research instrument | Gain knowledge | Health and well-being of others |

patient's well-being and health. Even though the best interest principle provides a strong normative basis in companion animal medicine, that cannot be easily transferred to other contexts. Farm animal medicine and laboratory animal medicine are indispensable for secure food production, medical knowledge, and public health.

Against this background, an important task of veterinary ethics is to recognize the prevailing diversity within the profession. With respect to the aspiration of veterinary ethics – to provide guidance for veterinary professionals in dealing with ethical challenges – it is crucial to appreciate emerging uncertainties and investigate the profession's diverse moral infrastructures. Although the literature in veterinary ethics often favors bringing the veterinary profession under one single vision and voice (FVE 2019), it raises the question of whether the profession can be aligned along a single normative ideal (e.g. following the best interest principle of the patient) or if a plurality of normative ideals is more appropriate to respond to multidimensional challenges. Hence, veterinarians might not be well advised to prioritize the interests of the animal irrespective of the context they are working in, since they might lose sight of further significant moral ideals. In the small animal clinic, veterinarians are expected to *care and cure* by focusing on the animal's best interest. Whereas in the case of a zoonotic and/or epidemic outbreak, veterinarians are legally bound to *kill and cull* in order to safeguard public health.

Keeping this in mind, the field of veterinary ethics can promote awareness and discussions within the profession as well as in public, and should aim to reflect on the diverse moral infrastructures and context-specific responsibilities that emerge in different fields of work. But what follows from that with a view to the future of veterinary ethics? A recently published executive summary of the Veterinary Future Commission (VFC 2019) indicates intrinsic aspects of the future veterinary professional culture. Among other things, the authors summarize that ethical reasoning, compassion, critical thinking, problem solving, and intra-professional collaborations are decisive competencies in order to meet future challenges of the profession. Why is that? Well, if we know one thing that the future will bring, it is change. Most of the addressed likely changes in the VFC (2019) are articulated in relation to the advancement and digitalization of the veterinary profession, which not only enhance the quality of patient care but additionally lead to new challenges.

In the following section, we aim to focus on ethical challenges that emerge due to the advancement and digitalization of veterinary medicine. Second, we will present the potential and limitations of different tools to support practicing veterinarians in ethically challenging decision-making processes. Finally, we will discuss proposals for teaching within the field of veterinary ethics that can support future veterinarians.

## Prognosis: Responses, Support, and Education for an Evolving Profession

### Responding to Future Challenges

In recent years, the veterinary profession has experienced enormous advancements with respect to patient care. Especially, the implementation of digital technologies for diagnostics (e.g. magnetic resonance imaging [MRI] and computerized tomography

[CT]) and health monitoring (e.g. wearable devices), or the development of innovative methods and sophisticated skills (e.g. minimally invasive surgery) that allow detection of diseases at an earlier stage or enable treatment of animals where this was not possible previously. A driving force of these advancements is digitalization, a global phenomenon finding its way into all spheres of life, and which constitutes an indispensable part of veterinarians' professional lives. For instance, digital tools for herd management (e.g. livestock management software) have been established with the potential not only to improve feeding efficiency, disease, and reproduction management, but also to support clinical decision-making (Fejzic et al. 2019). Further, digital information and communication tools within clinical practices lead to an improvement in patient care and practice management by including electronic health records, billing, and financial analysis (Fejzic et al. 2019). Against this background, the increasing digitalization not only leads to more reliable disease detection, diagnosis, treatment, and continuous real-time monitoring, but also increases the productivity and efficiency of the professional by saving time and human resources (ECCVT 2019; VFC 2019).

However, such developments have their challenges and downsides as well. Case Studies 23.2 to 23.4 highlight challenging aspects that might occur due to the increasing use of advanced diagnostics and treatments in veterinary medicine. The overall aim is not to prescribe what the right or wrong decision or action would be, but rather to stimulate the reader to reflect on possible (future) challenging situations.

---

**Case Study 23.2   Disagreement with respect to patient care between a veterinary specialist and general practitioner**

A general practitioner (GP) refers Prince, a five-year-old male Great Dane for digital x-ray imaging because he is non-weight bearing on the left front limb and physical exam shows a painful swelling of the distal radius. The digital x-rays show a lytic and proliferative lesion compatible with osteosarcoma (bone cancer). Prince has previously had knee surgery performed on both limbs but has no apparent hind limb issues presently. Staging shows a few small nodules in the lungs, potentially compatible with early metastatic disease. The GP knows that the owner has a very close and emotional relationship with Prince and wants to do everything for him. The specialist at the referral clinic suggests amputation and follow-up chemotherapy and the owner agrees with this plan. The GP is of the opinion that the proposed treatment is of questionable benefit for Prince and goes too far.

---

It is a main characteristic of challenging situations that there are several possible ways to deal with them. On the one hand, the GP could advise the client not to follow the proposed treatment plan and inform the client about her doubts. On the other hand, the GP could contact the specialist colleague to discuss her concern regarding suspected overtreatment of the dog. Or the GP might accept the plan despite her concern because she credits the specialist with the expertise and/or because the owner has already agreed to the treatment. Regardless of which option is chosen, important considerations regarding morals, knowledge, and trust arise that are strongly intertwined:

1. *Moral considerations*: Whether or not all available methods for treatment *should* be exhausted by veterinarians and/or clients and whether the treatment is or is not in the best interest of the patient (i.e. over/undertreatment).
2. *Professional assessment*: Different levels of specialization and/or experience may lead to different assessments of the risks and benefits of therapies.
3. *Trusting colleagues' judgment*: Increasing availability of specialists and referring patients requires not only a trustful and respectful relationship between the client and the veterinarian but also between veterinary colleagues.

Nowadays, veterinary medicine, and companion animal medicine in particular, is able to offer options for diagnostics and therapies that are, in some respects, as advanced as in human medicine (Springer et al. 2019a). At the same time, an increasing challenge for veterinary professionals is to reflect on when it is appropriate to advise advanced treatment options and when to advise only palliative or no treatment or euthanasia (Yeates 2010; Grimm et al. 2018). No matter if innovative methods are involved or conventional treatment options are in place, overtreatment is described as a treatment that is not in the patient's best interest and causes more harm than potential benefit for the patient (Yeates 2010; Knesl et al. 2017). Especially in relation to the ever-increasing possibilities in veterinary medicine, the problem of disproportionate use of diagnostics or therapies will be a central topic in the future. Clients' personal preferences and emotional relationships to their animals, financial motivation on the veterinarian's side, as well as the growth of veterinary specialization are contributing factors for this problem (Yeates 2010; Springer et al. 2019a). As a consequence, the concept of the best interest principle will increasingly move to the fore by focusing not on the question of what is medically feasible, but rather whether the medically feasible option is in the best interest of the animal or against it.

There is no doubt that the plethora of medical options goes hand in hand with an increase in veterinary specialization since the use of diagnostic tools (e.g. MRI or CT) and therapies (e.g. radiation or sophisticated surgeries) requires specific knowledge and skills. As in human medicine, clients increasingly expect advanced care and make more use of specialists in veterinary medicine (Springer et al. 2019a). In doing so, GPs see an advantage in referring their patients to university hospitals or referral clinics since they know their limits – both in terms of their expertise and the availability of advanced diagnostic tests and treatments (Tannenbaum 1995; Springer et al. 2019a). However, these aspects of veterinary specialization can cause challenges at the same time. For instance, the specialist might focus only on issues relative to their expertise and therefore might lose sight of the "big picture" or the patient as a whole and tend to initiate more diagnostics and therapies than necessary (Springer et al. 2019a).

Even though the combination of specialization and a specific working background such as at a university hospital may justify enhanced use of technologies and new methods (Springer et al. 2019a), it can also lead to disagreements about the suggested diagnostic and/or treatment plans, as indicated in Case Study 23.2. The availability of advanced tools paired with veterinarian's skills and ambition to make use of them might lead a specialist to go further with therapies compared with GPs. Such disagreements among veterinary colleagues can be stressful (Moses et al. 2018). Therefore, the availability of advanced diagnostics and treatment options paired with the need for specialized knowledge and relevant skills will not only influence veterinarians' and clients' decision-making but will also impact discussions among colleagues with varying working backgrounds and levels of specialization.

Accordingly, besides the recognition of positive aspects in relation to veterinary specialization and the possibility of referring patients, acknowledgment of the value of both *general* veterinary practice and *specialized* fields in future veterinary medicine will be important. As a consequence, increasing attention on developing trustful relationships between the client and the veterinarian as well as among veterinary professionals (Tannenbaum 1995) enabling transparent communication during referring processes (American Veterinary Medical Association [AVMA] 2021) will prepare for the future. Thereby, digital communication tools can facilitate discussions about specific cases and exchange between professionals.

---

**Case Study 23.3  Veterinarians as both healthcare and service providers**

A veterinarian works in a well-equipped referral clinic, where he has, among other things, CT imaging. At the annual "open house" of the clinic, he presents the CT unit to the visitors. During his presentation, a visitor confronts him with the following critical statement: "How can it be possible for animals to be examined and receive a CT without delay, yet my mother, who suffers from chronic pain, had to wait several weeks for her CT appointment?"

---

This scenario reveals the following three aspects that are strongly interwoven:

1. *Clients' expectations*: Clients' demands for high-standard patient care and expectations of immediate and bespoke service.
2. *Privately financed healthcare*: He who pays the piper calls the tune.
3. *Role of veterinary professionals*: Veterinary medicine as a healthcare profession *and* service provider.

Many companion animals enjoy the status of friends or family members. Undoubtedly, the moral status of companion animals (see Chapter 1) and the emotional relationships between owners and their animals impact veterinary services (Timmins 2008; Waters 2017; Pyatt et al. 2020). Even though it can be assumed that the impetus for the development of veterinary medicine lies in the aspiration to improve patient care, the specific status of companion animals and clients' increasing expectations toward veterinary service also represent an important driver (Springer et al. 2019a).

Companion animal medicine can meet these expectations, which are often measured up to the standard of human medicine regarding the provision of medical options. However, even though we can draw parallels between companion animal and human medicine, there remains a specific distinction with respect to the provision of medical services: in comparison to human medicine, veterinary medicine is privately financed and strongly embedded in the service model. Veterinary medicine is provided in the form of a service that is paid for and is consequently structured via economic factors. To put this more straightforwardly: only those clients who are willing and able to pay for diagnostic tests such as a CT scan will get one. And since (in most cases) clients must pay for this service privately, there is an increasing expectation that this service will be performed and delivered immediately (Springer et al. 2019a; Pyatt et al. 2020).

With a view to Case Study 23.3, as long as clients have to pay out of pocket for veterinary services, a comparison between companion animal medicine and human medicine on this level seems to be questionable. Even if the topic of animal health insurance is increasingly coming to the fore (Springer et al. 2022a), veterinary medicine will continue to be dependent on clients' financial backgrounds. Therefore, veterinary medicine will provide services not only with a view to the question of what is medically necessary for the individual patient, but also what is expected and can be financed by clients. It can be assumed that the idea of veterinary medicine as service providers will increase in the future in relation to clients' expectations and the increasing numbers of specialist practices. Thereby, the responsibility of the veterinary profession – as a health and service sector – lies in the provision of the best possible care of the individual patient under the consideration of the client's wishes, needs, and expectations (Springer et al. 2021). As indicated in Case Study 23.3, this can lead to critical debates about existing differences between the mainly established public healthcare system in human medicine and the private healthcare system in veterinary medicine with regard to the availability and immediate access of medical care.

It can be assumed that the gap between companion animal and human medicine regarding possible diagnostic tests and treatment plans will be increasingly narrowed in the near future. Veterinarians should be aware of the advantages of working in a privately financed sector, because they can choose whom they want to serve (AVMA 2019) and are mostly able to offer all available medical services without delay. Hence, the fact that veterinary medicine as a private healthcare sector has advantages as well as disadvantages should be considered when developing and preparing the profession for the future.

---

**Case Study 23.4   Client's use of Internet resources**

A veterinarian has been offering telemedicine in addition to her consultation hours in practice. A new client contacts the veterinarian asking for a telemedicine appointment. During the online consultation, the client informs the veterinarian about Charlie, her five-year-old terrier, who is suffering from severe vomiting, diarrhea, and dehydration. Further, the client reports that she has obtained information from veterinary webpages and requests specific medication. The veterinarian informs the new client that she needs to establish a relationship with the patient including an examination in order to provide medicine appropriately and to go on with possible further diagnostic steps before prescribing any medications. The client tells the veterinarian that she cannot come to the clinic in the next few days and that she only wants the veterinarian to prescribe the proper dose and duration of the medication for Charlie that she has ordered via the Internet.

This scenario reveals two important aspects that might increasingly lead to challenges in veterinary medicine:

1. *Professional authority in the age of "Dr. Google"*: Clients' use of Internet sources prior to consultation with the veterinarian.
2. *Virtual practice*: The option of telemedicine and its potential and limitations in veterinary practice.

Clients have unlimited access to information by using Internet resources (Kogan et al. 2012). In addition, social media platforms and Internet forums provide space for exchanges among animal owners as well as between owners and their veterinarians (Kogan et al. 2012; Widmar et al. 2020; Springer et al. 2022b). However, this can also lead to challenging situations as indicated in Case Study 23.4. Based on Internet sources, clients might consult the veterinarian with a "home-cooked" diagnosis and request medications, etc. without following the standard procedure with clinical examination or diagnostic tests. Further, a common problem that is recognized in relation to clients' use of the Internet is that owners may often consult their veterinarian too late (Springer et al. 2019a). Before they see their veterinarian, they try to treat their animal by themselves in order to save time and/or money. Such situations are especially challenging, since veterinarians know that if the client had come in earlier, the patient's prognosis would have been better. Aside from the fact that the patient's health status can be negatively affected, late consultation can further result in higher cost of care, because the condition of the animal has worsened.

But how should veterinarians deal with such situations? It is likely that professionals might increasingly doubt that their knowledge is understood or appreciated by their clients, which might undermine their professional authority. Since it can be expected that clients' use of Internet sources will increase in the future (Kogan et al. 2017), professionals might be well prepared if they actively address challenges in relation to clients gaining medical information from the Internet.

Here we would like to indicate a few points: first and foremost, having well-informed clients is not a bad thing. In general, clients' use of Internet sources can have a positive impact since it can increase their understanding of suggested diagnostic tests or treatment plans. Further, it can simplify communication if owners know about possible options that are available and the discussions about further procedures can be kept on a higher level if clients are well informed. But what is the added value from the veterinarian's perspective? Typically, professionals are better equipped to judge the quality of information retrieved from the Internet – an expertise that the majority of clients do not have. Further, to process the relevance of the information gained and translate it into a contextualized treatment option is also something one would not expect from clients (Kogan et al. 2012, 2017). Veterinarians are the professionals who are trained and equipped to make use of this medical knowledge to come up with appropriate decisions and actions. Thus, while the professionals' advantage in knowledge may not be as great as it was when owners could not retrieve information from the Internet, the evaluation, application, and contextualization of knowledge remain the expertise of the veterinarian.

It is foreseeable that veterinarians will increasingly have to respond to clients' "home-cooked" recipes from the Internet but can do so without the concern that they have to compete with them or lose their professional authority. Quite the opposite, it will become apparent why and how veterinarians add important expertise in knowing *how*. For instance, since veterinarians cannot prevent clients from carrying out Internet research, they might use it as an opportunity by making clients aware of using the *right* Internet resources, by assessing those and providing a list of approved websites. This in turn can have a positive impact on patient care and, of course, also on the relationship between the client and the veterinarian.

As well as the challenge of clients' use of Internet resources, Case Study 23.4 addresses the increasing demand for telemedicine in veterinary practice. Even though the physical clinical consultation is still the predominant means to provide veterinary service, telemedicine and telehealth are increasingly coming to the fore. In recent years, veterinary associations have responded to this development by discussing its potentials and challenges (AVMA 2017; Royal College of Veterinary Surgeons [RCVS] 2018). The AVMA (2021) distinguishes between both terms and states that "[t]elehealth is the overarching term that encompasses all uses of technology to deliver health information, education or care remotely." Telehealth includes several categories such as teleconsulting between the veterinarian and a specialist or consultant, telecommunication between the veterinarian and the healthcare team, and telemedicine between the veterinarian and the client that "includes the delivery of information specific to a particular patient" (AVMA 2021). An established veterinarian–client–patient relationship (VCPR) still constitutes an important requirement to provide telemedicine in an appropriate manner (AVMA 2017). Provided that a valid VCPR is established, telemedicine is acknowledged as a positive way to expand veterinary services, especially in rural areas that are undersupplied by veterinarians (Watson et al. 2019). It is possible that telemedicine can save time for both the veterinarian and the client and reduce stress for animals because there is no need for transport.

It is quite likely that this form of consultation will be further established and the demand for it will increase. As indicated in Case Study 23.4, an important task for veterinarians will be to advise the client that it cannot replace physical consultations in all cases since this remains an important requirement to offer high-quality telemedicine. For the further successful establishment of telemedicine, it is therefore important not only to support veterinarians in ensuring that technical, legal, and institutional aspects are secured, but clients must also be informed when and in which cases this form of consultation is most beneficial without misusing it (e.g. circumventing the necessity of physical consultation).

Increasing digitalization creates opportunities for the veterinary profession such as improvement and expansion of patient care, practice management, and communication strategies. These changes are also accompanied by concurrent challenges that the profession must meet in the near future. Herewith, we do not make the claim that these addressed challenging aspects are exhaustive or that they cannot be viewed and discussed from other perspectives. Nevertheless, one of the most pressing tasks of veterinary ethics is to recognize and proactively react to these changes that will shape the future profession. Besides the recognition of changes and providing responses to occurring challenges, a further crucial area of responsibility lies in the provision of support for veterinary professionals when dealing with challenges in difficult decision-making processes.

## Preparing Veterinarians for the Future

Veterinarians are trained to assimilate information regarding their patients from a medical perspective. During study and later in daily practice, they learn to integrate this medical information in order to decide on and justify patient care strategies. This always starts with a medical history followed by a physical examination and necessary diagnostic investigations. Based on findings and laboratory results, veterinarians are able to suggest possible treatment options and can provide a prognosis for the patient. This valid structure helps professionals to identify and organize aspects of the clinical case in "order to carry out the reasoning process necessary for diagnosis and therapy" (Jonsen et al. 2015). At the same time, there is the increasing recognition that veterinarians need to be equipped to identify and manage ethically challenging situations and conflicting interests that go beyond clinical aspects (Springer et al. 2021). Jonsen et al. (2015) note that "[j]ust as clinical cases require a method for sorting data, so too ethical cases must have some method to collect, sort, and order the facts and opinions raised by the case." Keeping this in mind, veterinary ethics can help to facilitate challenging decision-making and communication among stakeholders.

### Ethical Tools and Guidelines for Clinical Decision-Making

Various clinical decision-making tools and guidelines have been developed and published to support veterinarians in structuring the prevailing interests and concerns of involved stakeholders (Edney 1989; Grimm et al. 2018; AVMA 2020). These tools often address difficult end-of-life decisions in which veterinary professionals are challenged to assess the quality of life of old and/or sick patients, especially because decisions about interventions for these patients often demand a high level of client willingness and risk (e.g. worsening patient condition or losing the animal through death or euthanasia) as well as time and financial resources to provide adequate and necessary care. As a consequence, the developed tools aim at supporting veterinarians not only to structure but also to justify their decision for further therapies or euthanasia by focusing on relevant aspects that emerge during end-of-life decisions. These guidelines and tools have changed over time.

To illustrate these changes, we use Edney's (1989) seven analytical questions to structure complex decisions, published under the title "Killing with Kindness": Is the animal capable of walking and staying on its feet? Is the animal able to drink and eat independently? Is it able to pass urine and feces regularly and without problems? Can it breathe without difficulty? Is the animal free from painful inoperable tumors? Is it free from pain, suffering or discomfort that cannot be effectively treated? It becomes apparent that these six questions focus exclusively on the animal. Only one question relates to the client by asking whether the owner is physically and mentally able to care for the sick animal in order to meet the veterinary requirements of the therapy plan. He concludes that if the answer to any of these seven questions is negative, then euthanasia is justified. It becomes apparent that Edney's (1989) questions address mainly patient-based factors and do not include further aspects such as the client's capacity to pay that might lead to challenging decision-making processes.

In contrast, the AVMA Guidelines for the Euthanasia of Animals (2020) include varying factors related to the patient, the client, and the veterinarian that need to be considered during decision-making. Hence, besides the recommendation of appropriate methods and preparations for euthanasia, it provides comprehensive support for professional judgment by proposing a decision-making tree and a graphically illustrated structure for evaluating the decision. For instance, general aspects related to the professional's integrity and conscience, transparency of the decision process, consideration of the best possible balance of benefits and harms, as well as questions related to public and legal aspects are considered that should help to evaluate the morality of decisions (AVMA 2020).

Grimm et al. (2018) developed a comprehensive tool that responds to the increasing complexity of clinical decision-making by raising context-specific questions and concerns. Even though veterinary medicine constantly improves the care of patients and is able to treat animals that could not be treated previously, the authors argue that not every possible (life-prolonging) therapy is morally justified. In order to make a sound decision for or against further therapies, they propose a veterinary ethics tool (VET) that compares animal-centered factors (justificatory reasons) with secondary factors (explanatory reasons) (Table 23.2). In relation to the animal-centered reasons, the tool emphasizes the relationship between the veterinarian and the patient by focusing on the professional's clinical responsibility. Questions such as "Do you perceive the proposed treatment to be in the best interests of the patient?" or "Will the proposed treatment improve the patient's health?" are proposed to consider in relation to these animal-centered reasons.

Secondary factors consider the professional responsibility by focusing on the relationship between clinician–profession, client–patient, and client–clinician. A concluding question refers to the important concern of whether secondary factors are more influential compared with animal-centered factors in the clinical decision. The answers to the posed questions indicate whether veterinarians should consider alternative treatment options (X), reconsider the proposed procedure and the clinician's responsibility (–), or the reasons are valid for the proposed clinical procedure (✓). Hence, the tool is not binary coded (yes/no) but rather highlights different options based on the outcome to generate a sound basis for a decision.

Even though such tools and guidelines support veterinarians in structuring difficult decision-making processes, the question arises to what extent they are used in everyday practice and actually provide assistance in challenging situations. Recent studies in this context raise doubts in regard to the practicability and acceptance among professionals (Springer 2013; Kipperman et al. 2018; Quain et al. 2021). Conversely, practical training in dealing with moral challenges, exchanges with colleagues, and access to support services to reduce moral stress from ethical dilemmas are considered as helpful sources (Kipperman et al. 2018; Springer et al. 2019b; Quain et al. 2021). This raises the question of whether criteria in a standardized tool can support professional judgment and minimize uncertainties and what further methods of assistance may be more useful in practice.

**Table 23.2** Veterinary ethics tool (VET) to facilitate decision-making in clinical veterinary medicine (Grimm et al. 2018).

| | Relationship | Questions to facilitate ethical deliberation | No | I don't know | Possibly | Definitely |
|---|---|---|---|---|---|---|
| **Animal-centered factors** (justificatory reasons) | **Clinician–patient** (clinical responsibility) | *A.* Do you perceive the proposed treatment to be in the best interests of the patient? | X | – | ✓ | ✓ |
| | | *A1.* Will the proposed treatment improve the patient's health? | X | – | ✓ | ✓ |
| | | *A2.* Will the proposed treatment improve the patient's quality of life: *(a)* immediately? | X | – | ✓ | ✓ |
| | | *(b)* long term? | X | – | ✓ | ✓ |
| | | *B.* Is the proposed treatment option the one with the least potential to cause harm and suffering while still achieving the intended clinical goal? | – | – | ✓ | ✓ |
| | | *C.* Have measures been taken to minimize the potential for harm and suffering? | – | – | ✓ | ✓ |
| | | *D.* Do the expected benefits outweigh the potential harm and suffering inflicted on the animal or are they at least in balance? | X | – | ✓ | ✓ |
| **Secondary factors** (explanatory reasons) | **Clinician–profession** (professional responsibility) | *E.* Does the primary clinician/team have experience in carrying out the proposed treatment and/or is it a well-documented recognized treatment? | – | – | ✓ | ✓ |
| | | *F.* Is this case an example of good ethical decision-making for students/trainees/colleagues? | – | – | ✓ | ✓ |
| | | *G.* Would you feel comfortable justifying the proposed treatment to professional colleagues? | – | – | ✓ | ✓ |
| | **Client–patient** | *H.* Would proceeding with the proposed treatment have a positive impact on the owner–animal relationship? | – | – | ✓ | ✓ |
| | | *I.* Would proceeding with the proposed treatment have a positive impact on the client's quality of life and/or financial benefits (e.g. the proposed treatment will allow breeding from a valuable animal)? | – | – | ✓ | ✓ |
| | **Clinician–client** | *J.* Is the proposed treatment financially viable for the client? | X | – | ✓ | ✓ |
| | | *K.* Is the client capable of providing a suitable home environment and/or administrating medication during the recovery period? | X | – | ✓ | ✓ |
| **Priority check** | **Professional responsibility** | *L.* Are the secondary factors E–K (explanatory reasons) more influential in your clinical decision than the animal-centered factors A–D (justificatory reasons)? | ✓ | – | X | X |

X  Consider alternative treatment options.

–  Reconsider procedure and the clinician's responsibility.

✓  Valid reasons for clinical procedure.

### Clinical Ethics Support Services

Clinical ethics support services (CESS) are coming to the fore in veterinary practice (Rosoff et al. 2018; Springer et al. 2018), although they are still in their infancy. CESS help to identify and analyze the value conflicts of the involved parties and achieve a resolution. In human medical ethics, such formats were developed from the early 1970s onwards to support responsible persons in the medical field in making ethically reflective decisions (Rosner 1985; Fournier 2015). The methods and models that have been established since then can be used as a starting point for their utilization in the veterinary context.

In general, two main models can be distinguished: first, moral case deliberation (MCD); and second, clinical ethics consultation services (CECs) (Fournier 2015). CECs provide support for clinical cases that require a specific decision for an actual patient (Fournier 2015; Molewijk et al. 2015). Following this approach, the norms, values, and principles relevant to a specific case are identified and weighed in a decision-making process. In comparison, MCD offers the opportunity to discuss principles, norms, and values that play a role within the profession without discussion about a clinical case. In recent years, several groups have been introduced that follow the idea of CESS with the aim to provide discursive formats for veterinary professionals dealing with ethical concerns.

A working group "Ethics in the Equine Hospital" was established at the University of Veterinary Medicine, Vienna, in 2015 (Springer et al. 2018). The group comprises veterinarians and animal caretakers as well as an ethicist, and discusses cases in which veterinarians are confronted with difficult decision-making processes relating to end-of-life decisions. The aim of this working group is to identify and structure responsible decision-making and try to find well-reasoned solutions that all participants can agree on. The authors' experience is that a high degree of flexibility in regard to availability of involved parties is needed in order to convene the group to discuss challenging cases. Beneficially, discussion of previous cases increases efficiency when dealing with new cases since veterinarians refer back to their knowledge previously gained, which helps them to address similar issues (Springer et al. 2018).

A second example was described by Rosoff et al. (2018). They present their model of CESS in the form of a clinical ethics committee established at the North Carolina State University Veterinary Hospital in the United States. The aim of this ethics committee is, on the one hand, to address normative issues in veterinary medicine, such as goals of care in clinical veterinary medicine. On the other hand, the committee serves as an advisory body in critical clinical cases (Rosoff et al. 2018). Consequently, based on Fournier's (2015) differentiation between MCD and CECs, it can be stated that the ethics consultation service established at North Carolina State University combines both models. The authors note that the service facilitated outcomes that were acceptable to all parties in all cases in which it was utilized (Rosoff et al. 2018).

However, the question remains whether such models can prove to be of practical relevance outside of universities. Since the implementation and use of CESS is still young, future investigations should focus on evaluation of the effectiveness of different models and formats. Limitations in the use of such formats in practitioners' daily work lives include the short duration of most hospital stays reduces the likelihood of recognition of an ethical conflict, asking for a consultation, and having it done in the timeframe during which decisions must be made. Consequently, consults may be more apt to be retrospective. Organizational and structural challenges such as maintaining client privacy concerns may also present obstacles. Keeping this in mind, we argue that future empirical studies might be helpful to pave the way for the elaboration of effective and suitable designs of such services – not only at universities, but also for veterinarians working in practice. For instance, a possible future perspective could be to establish and offer such services in the form of teleconsultation services with veterinary ethicists that can be easily integrated in veterinarians' workplaces.

**Teaching Future Veterinarians**

An important pillar of veterinary ethics lies in educational programs for veterinary students, the future veterinarians. Students receiving ethics training value the opportunity to develop necessary competencies for their future professional work life (Verrinder and Phillips 2014; Magalhães-Sant'Ana et al. 2014; Kipperman et al. 2020). However, the establishment and integration of ethics training programs is rather inconsistent (Boo and Knight 2005; Gray 2014; Shivley et al. 2016) and many of today's veterinarians begin their professional life with minimal training or knowledge in relation to recognizing and addressing ethical problems (Kipperman et al. 2018; Richards et al. 2020; Quain et al. 2021). Against this background, one of the major goals of the discipline should lie in the expansion of educational programs at veterinary schools. In doing so, we suggest that the profession might focus on the following three questions: *What* should be taught? *When* should students be taught? *How* should students be taught?

Naturally, a constant effort should lie in the development and reconsideration of content and topics to achieve not only the best possible knowledge outcome for veterinary students but also to meet their future demands and challenges. With regard to the content of established veterinary ethics courses, four main topics can be identified that strongly interrelate with other disciplines such as animal welfare, animal ethics, law, and communication (Magalhães-Sant'Ana et al. 2014; Magalhães-Sant'Ana 2016). First, students should develop an *ethical awareness* to recognize ethical issues in veterinary practice as well as the values and viewpoints of others. Second, *knowledge* of normative aspects should help students to identify veterinary duties and access relevant codes of conduct and legal requirements. Third, *ethical skills* should be developed by students including the development of ethical reasoning, the ability to reflect upon ethical issues, communication skills, and informed decision-making skills. Finally, *individual and professional qualities* should be reinforced during their training with the aim to educate students in their development of a personal and professional identity and to sensitize them to their societal role (Magalhães-Sant'Ana et al. 2014).

There is no doubt that these themes constitute an important basis for educational programs. However, even though there exists a major intersection between animal ethics, animal welfare and protection, law, communication, and veterinary ethics, it is important to address their distinctions and limitations at the same time. For instance, not all ethical theories foster moral duties to care for animal welfare or protection (e.g. contractarian theories) (see Chapter 4). Further, legal requirements may not necessarily align with one's moral views but are still binding (see Chapter 5). The case of culling animals to prevent economic losses might help to illustrate this point where veterinarians' actions are legally permitted or even obligatory but may be perceived to be wrong. Hence, they should be able to reflect on why something can feel morally wrong even though it is legally permissible by thinking about the differences between the moral and legal aspects of their actions.

A further concern of teaching veterinary ethics points to the question of *when* ethical competencies should be taught and developed. Many veterinary ethics courses are scheduled and taught in the first semesters of school (Magalhães-Sant'Ana et al. 2014). At this point, while still quite idealistic, few students may have the capacity to recognize ethical conflicts associated with animal patients. Most ethical dilemmas they may encounter occur during clinical training, which is usually scheduled in the middle or even at the end of their studies. Based on that, efforts should be made to teach students especially in their later semesters to increase the effectiveness and applicability of their gained knowledge in this field.

This comes in line with the question of *how* topics and contents should be taught in the field of veterinary ethics. Studies indicate the need to educate students with practical reference to problems that may emerge in their future work life (Magalhães-Sant'Ana and Hanlon 2016; Knights and Clarke 2018; Springer et al. 2019b; Richards et al. 2020). Keeping this in mind, the use of case vignettes can build a good starting point for further discussions within veterinary ethics courses. This not only increases the context applicability of discussion, but also engages students in their communication of values and beliefs and helps them to make more informed decisions while being confronted with different points of view (Magalhães-Sant'Ana and Hanlon 2016; Hobson-West and Millar 2021).

A very promising format for future teaching programs is the expansion of e-learning courses in veterinary ethics, via distance learning classes (Dürnberger et al. 2018). Such asynchronous Internet courses provide flexibility as they can be accessed on the students' schedule rather than at a predetermined time. Since ethics requires individuals to think, such formats allow them to choose when they are in the right mood to engage in reflecting on normative issues. Acknowledging the limited time resources for ethics courses during studies, the integration of e-learning courses allows educators to train students with necessary theoretical concepts and frameworks remotely and only meet in a few units of in-person sessions for in-depth discussion of cases and experiences during their practical training during study. Against this background, there is great potential in the concept of "blended learning" for teaching future veterinary generations by combining classroom-based and e-learning courses (Hrastinski 2019). Additionally, such e-learning courses can also provide access to veterinary ethics knowledge and skills for students who do not yet have the option of such educational programs at their particular school as well as for veterinarians after graduation. Hence, the establishment of e-learning courses can allow for ethics training with more flexibility regarding time and location and seems to be a promising way of teaching in the future.

## Conclusion

Veterinary ethics is an interdisciplinary and flourishing field in research and practice that takes an active role in shaping the profession and supporting and fostering self-reflection of veterinary professionals. Hence, the future of veterinary ethics as a research discipline is not an "appendix" anymore but has an integral role to play by aiming to investigate and address the ethical challenges that veterinary professionals will encounter in their daily work life. The future of veterinary ethics lies in appreciating the complexities and dynamic diversity in the veterinary profession and addressing them on both a practical and theoretical level. Further, an aspiration should be to recognize and respond to possible risks and opportunities as well as the veterinarian's role and responsibilities that specifically arise due to the increasing digitalization, advancements, and use of information and communication technologies. In doing so, an essential task is not only the provision of ethical tools or support services to help practicing veterinarians, but also to properly educate veterinary students to equip them with relevant knowledge and skills to manage their future challenges. Ideally, teaching teams including ethicists and veterinarians who have knowledge of both ethical theories and principles as well as clinical examples of ethical conflicts would equip students with what they will most likely need when they encounter moral challenges as veterinary professionals in the future. Although – as the comedian Karl Valentin put it some decades ago – forecasts are difficult, particularly if they concern the future, it is not inconceivable that veterinary ethics thus should enable students to navigate through the uncertainties they are likely to encounter as practitioners.

## References

American Veterinary Medical Association (AVMA) (2017). Final report on telemedicine. https://www.avma.org/sites/default/files/resources/Telemedicine-Report-2016.pdf (accessed 29 June 2021).

American Veterinary Medical Association (AVMA) (2019). Principles of veterinary medical ethics of the AVMA. https://www.avma.org/resources-tools/avma-policies/principles-veterinary-medical-ethics-avma (accessed 19 June 2021).

American Veterinary Medical Association (AVMA) (2020). AVMA Guidelines for the Euthanasia of Animals. https://www.avma.org/sites/default/files/2020-01/2020-Euthanasia-Final-1-17-20.pdf (accessed 29 June 2021).

American Veterinary Medical Association (AVMA) (2021). Telehealth: The basics. https://www.avma.org/resources-tools/practice-management/telehealth-telemedicine-veterinary-practice/veterinary-telehealth-basics (accessed 29 June 2021).

Boo, J. and Knight, A. (2005). Concepts in animal welfare: A syllabus in animal welfare science and ethics for veterinary schools. *Journal of Veterinary Medical Education* 32 (4): 451–453.

Coghlan, S. (2018). Strong patient advocacy and the fundamental ethical role of veterinarians. *Journal of Agricultural & Environmental Ethics* 31: 349–367.

Dürnberger, C., Weich, K., Springer, S. et al. (2018). Log-in for VEthics – Applying E-learning in veterinary ethics. In: *Professionals in Food Chains: Ethics, Roles and Responsibilities* (eds. S. Springer and H. Grimm), 317–322. Wageningen, the Netherlands: Wageningen Academic Publishers.

Edney, A.T.B. (1989). Killing with kindness. *Veterinary Record* 124: 320–322.

European Coordinating Committee on Veterinary Training (ECCVT) (2019). Embracing digital technology in veterinary practice. https://fve.org/cms/wp-content/uploads/020-ECCVT-joint-seminar_final.pdf (accessed 29 June 2021).

Federation of Veterinarians of Europe (FVE) (2019). FVE – Federation of Veterinarians of Europe: welcome new members. https://fve.org/cms/wp-content/uploads/WELCOME-TO-FVE-dec2019.pdf. (accessed 21 March 2022).

Fejzic, N., Seric-Haracic, S., and Mehmedbasic, Z. (2019). From white coat and gumboots to virtual reality and digitalisation: Where is veterinary medicine now? *IOP Conference Series: Earth and Environmental Science* 333 (1): 012009.

Fournier, V. (2015). Clinical ethics: Methods. In: *Encyclopedia of Global Bioethics* (ed. H. Ten Have), 553–562. Cham, Switzerland: Springer.

Gray, C. (2014). Similar but not the same: The teaching of veterinary and medical ethics. *Veterinary Record* 175 (23): 590–591.

Gray, C. and Fordyce, P. (2020). Legal and ethical aspects of "best interests" decision-making for medical treatment of companion animals in the UK. *Animals* 10: 1009.

Grimm, H., Bergadano, A., Musk, G.C. et al. (2018). Drawing the line in clinical treatment of companion animals: Recommendations from an ethics working party. *Veterinary Record* 182 (23): 664.

Hobson-West, P. and Millar, K. (2021). Telling their own stories: Encouraging veterinary students to ethically reflect. *Veterinary Record* doi: 10.1002/vetr.17

Hrastinski, S. (2019). What do we mean by blended learning? *Tech Trends* 63: 564–569.

Huth, M., Weich, K., and Grimm, H. (2019). Veterinarians between the frontlines?! The concept of one health and three frames of health in veterinary medicine. *Food Ethics* 3 (1–2): 91–108.

Jonsen, A.R., Siegler, M., and Winslade, W.J. (2015). *Clinical Ethics: A Practical Approach to Ethical Decisions in Clinical Medicine*. New York: McGraw Hill Medical Publishers.

Kimera, S.I. and Mlangwa, J.E.D. (2015). Veterinary ethics. In: *Encyclopedia of Global Bioethics* (ed. H. Ten Have), 1–12. Cham, Switzerland: Springer.

Kipperman, B., Morris, P., and Rollin, B. (2018). Ethical dilemmas encountered by small animal veterinarians: Characterisation, responses, consequences and beliefs regarding euthanasia. *Veterinary Record* 182 (19): 548.

Kipperman, B., Rollin, B., and Martin, J. (2020). Veterinary student opinions regarding ethical dilemmas encountered by veterinarians and the benefits of ethics instruction. *Journal of Veterinary Medical Education* 48: 330–342. doi: 10.3138/jvme.2019-0059

Knesl, O., Hart, B.L., Fine, A.H. et al. (2017). Veterinarians and humane endings: When is it the right time to euthanize a companion animal? *Frontiers in Veterinary Science* 4: 45. doi: 10.3389/fvets.2017.00045

Knights, D. and Clarke, C. (2018). Living on the edge? Professional anxieties at work in academia and veterinary practice. *Cultural Organisation* 24: 134–153.

Kogan, L.R., Schoenfeld-Tacher, R., and Viera, A.R. (2012). The internet and health information: Differences in pet owners based on age, gender, and education. *Journal of the Medical Library Association* 100 (3): 197–204.

Kogan, L.R., Oxley, J.A., Hellyer, P. et al. (2017). United Kingdom veterinarians' perceptions of clients' internet use and the perceived impact on the client–vet relationship. *Frontiers in Veterinary Science* 4: 180. doi: 10.3389/fvets.2017.00180

Magalhães-Sant'Ana, M. (2016). A theoretical framework for human and veterinary medical ethics education. *Advances in Health Sciences Education* 21 (5): 1123–1136.

Magalhães-Sant'Ana, M. and Hanlon, A. (2016). Straight from the horse's mouth: Using vignettes to support student learning in veterinary ethics. *Journal of Veterinary Medical Education* 43 (3): 321–330.

Magalhães-Sant'Ana, M., Lassen, J., Millar, K.M. et al. (2014). Examining why ethics is taught to veterinary students: A qualitative study of veterinary educators' perspectives. *Journal of Veterinary Medical Education* 41 (4): 350–357.

Molewijk, B., Slowther, A., and Aulisio, M. (2015). Clinical ethics: Support. In: *Encyclopedia of Global Bioethics* (ed. H. Ten Have), 562–570. Cham, Switzerland: Springer.

Moses, L., Malowney, M.J., and Boyd, J.W. (2018). Ethical conflict and moral distress in veterinary practice: A survey of North American veterinarians. *Journal of Veterinary Internal Medicine* 32 (6): 2115–2122.

Pyatt, A.Z., Walley, K., Wright, G.H. et al. (2020). Co-produced care in veterinary services: A qualitative study of UK stakeholders' perspectives. *Veterinary Sciences* 7 (4): 149.

Quain, A., Mullan, S., McGreevy, P.D. et al. (2021). Frequency, stressfulness and type of ethically challenging situations encountered by veterinary team members during the COVID-19 pandemic. *Frontiers in Veterinary Science* 8: 647108. doi: 10.3389/fvets.2021.647108

Royal College of Veterinary Surgeons (RCVS) (2018). Review of the use of telemedicine within veterinary practice – Summary analysis. https://www.rcvs.org.uk/document-library/telemedicine-consultation-summary (accessed 29 June 2021).

Richards, L., Coghlan, S., and Delany, C. (2020). "I had no idea that other people in the world thought differently to me": Ethical challenges in small animal veterinary practice and implications for ethics support and education. *Journal of Veterinary Medical Education* 47 (6): 728–736.

Rollin, B. (2006 [1999]). *Veterinary Medical Ethics: Theory and Cases*. Ames, IA: Blackwell Publishing.

Rosner, F. (1985). Hospital medical ethics committees: A review of their development. *Journal of the American Medical Association* 253: 2693–2697.

Rosoff, P.M., Moga, J., Keene, B. et al. (2018). Resolving ethical dilemmas in a tertiary care veterinary specialty hospital: Adaptation of the human clinical consultation committee model. *American Journal of Bioethics* 18 (2): 41–53.

Shivley, C.B., Garry, F.B., and Kogan, L.R. (2016). Survey of animal welfare, animal behavior, and animal ethics courses in the curricula of AVMA Council on Education-accredited veterinary colleges and schools. *Journal of the American Veterinary Medical Association* 248 (10): 1165–1170.

Springer, S. (2013). Praxis Der Euthanasie in Der Kleintiermedizin. Diploma thesis, 70–71. University of Veterinary Medicine.

Springer, S., Auer, U., Jenner, F. et al. (2018). Clinical ethics support services in veterinary practice. In: *Professional in Food Chains: Ethics, Roles and Responsibilities* (eds. S. Springer and H. Grimm), 308–313. Wageningen, the Netherlands: Wageningen Academic Publishers.

Springer, S., Sandøe, P., Lund, T.B. et al. (2019a). "Patients' interests first, but..." – Austrian veterinarians' attitudes to moral challenges in modern small animal practice. *Animals* 9 (5): 241.

Springer, S., Moens, Y., Hartnack, S. et al. (2019b). Soft skills for hard problems: What prepares Austrian veterinarians to effectively manage end-of-life issues? In: *Sustainable Governance and Management of Food Systems* (eds. E. Vinnari and M. Vinnari), 79–85. Wageningen, the Netherlands: Wageningen Academic Publishers.

Springer, S., Sandøe, P., Grimm, H. et al. (2021). Managing conflicting ethical concerns in modern small animal practice – A comparative study of veterinarian's decision ethics in Austria, Denmark and the UK. *PLoS ONE* 16: 6.

Springer, S., Lund, T.B., Grimm, H., et al. (2022a). Comparing veterinarians' attitudes to and the potential influence of pet health insurance in Austria, Denmark and the UK. *Veterinary Record*, e1266.

Springer, S., Lund, T.B., Sandøe, P., et al. (2022b). Digital opportunities to connect and complain – the use of Facebook in small animal practice. *Veterinary Record Open 9*. doi:10.1002/vro2.29.

Tannenbaum, J. (1995). *Veterinary Ethics: Animal Welfare, Client Relations, Competition and Collegiality*. Mosby, St Louis.

Timmins, R.P. (2008). The contribution of animals to human well-being: A veterinary family practice perspective. *Journal of Veterinary Medical Education* 35 (4): 540–544.

Verrinder, J.M. and Phillips, C.J.C. (2014). Identifying veterinary students' capacity for moral behavior concerning animal ethics issues. *Journal of Veterinary Medical Education* 41 (4): 358–370.

Veterinary Futures Commission (VFC) (2019). Executive Summary: The Future of Veterinary Medicine – AVMA – AAVMC Veterinary Futures Commissions. https://www.aavmc.org/assets/Site_18/files/Newsletter_Files/Feb%20VME%20Future%20of%20Vet%20Med.pdf (accessed 29 June 2021).

Waters, A. (2017). What will the future bring? *Veterinary Record* 180 (14): 340–340.

Watson, K., Wells, J., Sharma, M. et al. (2019). A survey of knowledge and use of telehealth among veterinarians. *BMC Veterinary Research* 15 (1): 474.

Widmar, N., Bir, C., Lai, J. et al. (2020). Public perceptions of veterinarians from social and online media listening. *Veterinary Science* 7: 75.

Woods, A. (2013). The history of veterinary ethics in Britain, ca.1870–2000. In: *Veterinary and Animal Ethics: Proceedings of the First International Conference on Veterinary and Animal Ethics* (eds. C.M. Wathes, S.A. Corr, S.A. May, S.P. McCulloch and M.C. Whiting), September 2011. 3–18. Chichester, UK: Wiley-Blackwell.

Yeates, J.W. (2010). When to euthanase. *Veterinary Record* 166 (12): 370.

# Index

Note: page numbers in italics refer to figures; those in bold to tables

*Ethics in Veterinary Practice: Balancing Conflicting Interests,* First Edition. Edited by Barry Kipperman and Bernard E. Rollin.
© 2022 John Wiley & Sons, Inc. Published 2022 by John Wiley & Sons, Inc.